Basics of Blood Management

Basics of Blood Management

Second edition

Petra Seeber MD
Institute for Blood Management
Gotha, Germany

Aryeh Shander MD, FCCM, FCCP
Chief of Anesthesiology, Critical Care Medicine and Hyperbaric Medicine
Englewood Hospital and Medical Center
Englewood, NJ, USA;
Clinical Professor of Anesthesiology, Medicine and Surgery
Mount Sinai School of Medicine
Mount Sinai Hospital
New York, NY, USA

(W)WILEY-BLACKWELL
A John Wiley & Sons, Ltd., Publication

Library of Congress Cataloging-in-Publication Data

Seeber, Petra.

Basics of blood management / Petra Seeber, Aryeh Shander. – 2nd ed.

p. cm.

Includes bibliographical references and index.

ISBN 978-0-470-67070-5 (pbk. : alk. paper)   1. Transfusion-free surgery.   2. Blood–Transfusion.   3. Blood banks.   I. Shander, Aryeh.   II. Title.

RD33.35.S44 2013

362.17'84–dc23

2012014993

A catalogue record for this book is available from the British Library.

Contents

Preface

Much has been done in blood management since the first edition. This is not only true for the many scientific studies that elevate blood management out of the low plains of experience-driven action into the realms of evidence-based medicine. Many of the things that blood managers over the decades have observed have now been proven in randomized clinical trials. Other things in blood management that may have been driven by tradition and belief have come into question. These developments contribute greatly to the maturation of this new specialty of blood management.

It is interesting, though, to note that the definition of blood management is still not accepted by all who claim to practice blood management. Some use the term blood management to efficiently distribute the ever more scarce resource of banked blood to those patients who are deemed to be in the greatest need. Others consider blood management as the outcome-oriented part of transfusion medicine that delivers allogeneic blood products in an evidence-based manner. Still others see blood management as a mix of transfusion medicine and hematology. And another group of medical practitioners consider blood management to be a religiously motivated restriction of modern medicine. However, blood management is none of these. At the core of blood management are two foci: one is the patient's own blood as a precious, live-saving, and potentially finite resource; and the other is the patient's outcome. To manage the patient's resource "blood" skillfully to optimize his or her outcome is the philosophy that drives blood management.

Practically speaking, blood management is a multidisciplinary, multimodality concept that focuses on the patient by improving his/her outcome. Every medical specialty, from neonatology to geriatrics, from anesthesiology to urology, and including all clinical specialties as well as laboratory-based specialties such as diagnostic laboratory medicine, can contribute to a successful blood management program.

As in the first edition, the book introduces the reader to blood management and explains how to improve medical outcomes by avoiding undue blood loss, enhancing the patient's own blood, and improving tolerance of anemia and coagulopathy until any of the underlying conditions are successfully remedied. While the first edition considered transfusion avoidance as a very important outcome improvement, the second edition shifts its focus from this aspect of improving outcomes to the even more important reduction of morbidity and mortality. This does not mean that transfusion avoidance is not a noble goal. But it means that–lacking good (scientific) reasons to transfuse–there is no point in trying to avoid something that has no proven value in itself. It should be self-evident that such non-proven therapies should be let go. Mounting evidence shows that the outcomes of patients treated by current principles of transfusion medicine are not superior to those obtained in transfusion-free environments, and that in some subgroups even the contrary might be the case. Therefore, it seems timely to advance patient care beyond this point and focus attention on interventions that have proven value in improving patient outcome. We therefore again invite you cordially to continue your efforts to improve your patient's outcome by optimal blood management.

Petra Seeber and Aryeh Shander
March 2012

Preface to the First Edition

The benefit-to-risk ratio of blood products needs constant evaluation. Blood products, as therapeutic agents, have had the test of time but still lack the evidence we expect from other medicinals. Blood, an organ, is used as a pharmaceutical agent by the medical profession, due to the achievements in collection, processing, banking, and distribution. The fact that the most common risk of blood transfusion is blood delivery error supports the notion that blood must be handled as a pharmaceutical agent. Over the last few decades, the risk of blood transfusion and associated complications has raised concerns about the safety of blood by both the public and healthcare providers. At the same time, experience with patients refusing blood and data on blood conservation have brought to light the real possibility of other modalities to treat perisurgical anemia and to avoid it with blood conservation methods. In addition to risks and complications, data have become available that demonstrate the behavioral aspect of transfusion practice versus an evidence-based practice. In this book, we address many aspects of modern transfusion medicine, known blood conservation modalities, and new approaches to the treatment of perisurgical anemia, as well as special clinical considerations. This approach, now termed "blood management" by the Society for the Advancement of Blood Management (SABM, www.sabm.org), incorporates appropriate transfusion practice and blood conservation to deliver the lowest risk and highest benefit to the patient. In addition, it brings all these modalities to the patient's bedside and above all is a patient-centered approach. Blood management is a multidisciplinary, multimodality concept that focuses on the patient. Patient outcome is improved, making this one of the most intriguing and rewarding fields in medicine.

Blood management requires an understanding of all elements of blood and transfusions. It includes the philosophy, biology, physiology, and ethical considerations, as well as demonstrating the practical application of various techniques. This publication introduces the reader to blood management and explains how to improve medical outcomes by avoiding undue blood loss, enhancing the patient's own blood, and improving tolerance of anemia and coagulopathy until any of these underlying conditions are successfully remedied.

This introduction to blood management is intended for training and early practicing clinicians. It is meant to be both informative and practical, and spans many of the medical specialties that encounter blood and transfusions as part of their daily practice. It will aid in tailoring individual care plans for different patients. Finally, it addresses the structure and function of a blood management program, a novel approach to blood conservation, and improved patient outcome.

In this book, blood management is considered from an international perspective, so attention is paid to conditions encountered in developing as well as industrial countries. Techniques such as cell salvage are performed differently in economically deprived countries; HIV, hepatitis, and malaria may or may not be a threat to the blood supply, depending on geographical location; oxygen, intravenous fluids, and erythropoiesis-stimulating proteins may be readily available in some countries or inaccessible in others. The book is intended to broaden the readers' horizons, discussing working conditions encountered by blood managers around the world. Many of the clinical scenarios and the exercises that follow are intended to allow the reader to adapt the information to the prevailing circumstances in their location.

This book is unique in the fact that it is the first dedicated in its entirety to the concept of blood management. The authors hope that this book will stimulate its readers to further advance blood management through shared experience and research. It is intended to be informative, practical, enjoyable, and hopefully will stimulate debate and discussion as well as help patients in need.

Petra Seeber and Aryeh Shander
March 2007

1 History and Organization of Blood Management

Blood management has evolved from humble beginnings into a viable, rapidly-developing medical specialty. Its development was initiated by the wish of Jehovah's Witnesses for a transfusion-free treatment and has been shaped by influences coming from transfusion medicine and the military's experiences. Blood management has today been introduced into mainstream medicine. The vivid history of blood management is described in this chapter.

Objectives

1. To identify the historical developments that have led to today's concept of blood management.
2. To demonstrate the benefits of blood management.
3. To identify blood management as "good clinical" practice.
4. To show that blood management and its techniques should be used in all cases who qualify.
5. To help understand how a blood management program works.

Definitions

Bloodless medicine and surgery: Bloodless medicine is a multimodality, multidisciplinary approach to safe and effective patient care *without* the use of allogeneic blood products. Bloodless medicine and surgery utilize pharmacological and technological means as well as medical and surgical techniques to provide the best possible care without the use of donor blood.

Transfusion-free medicine and surgery: Since "bloodless medicine" is something of a misnomer, the term "transfusion-free medicine" was coined and is used instead.

Blood conservation: "Blood conservation is a global concept engulfing all possible strategies aimed at *reducing* patient's exposure to allogeneic blood products" [1]. This concept does not exclude the use of allogeneic blood entirely.

Blood management: Blood management is the philosophy to improve patient outcomes by caring for and managing the patient's own blood as a precious, life-saving resource. It is a patient-centered, multidisciplinary, multimodal, planned approach to patient care. Blood management is not an "alternative" to allogeneic transfusions; it is the standard of care.

Patient blood management: In order to clarify that blood management is not confused with an outcome-oriented transfusion therapy, the term "patient" is added, denoting that it is not the blood in the blood bank that is managed but the patient's own blood that is taken good care of and managed in accord with the philosophy of blood management.

A brief history

Bloodless medicine, transfusion-free medicine, blood conservation, and blood management

The term "bloodless medicine" is often associated with the belief of Jehovah's Witnesses that they should refrain from the use of blood, therefore ruling out the option of

Basics of Blood Management, Second Edition. Petra Seeber and Aryeh Shander.
© 2013 John Wiley & Sons, Ltd. Published 2013 by John Wiley & Sons, Ltd.

blood transfusion. The essence of bloodless medicine, and lately, blood management, however, is not restricted to the beliefs of a religious group. To get a better understanding as to what bloodless medicine and blood management mean, let us go back to the roots of these disciplines.

One is not completely wrong to attribute the origin of the term "bloodless medicine" to the endeavor of Jehovah's Witnesses to receive treatment without resorting to donor blood transfusion. Their attitude toward the sanctity of blood greatly influences their view of blood transfusion. This was described as early as 1927 in their journal *The Watchtower* (December 15, 1927). Although the decision to refuse blood transfusion is a completely religious one, the Witnesses have frequently used scientific information about the side effects of donor blood transfusion to convince their physicians that their decision is a reasonable one and is corroborated by scientific evidence. The booklet entitled *Blood, Medicine and the Law of God* (published in 1961) explained the Witnesses' religious stand, but also addressed issues such as transfusion reactions, transfusion-related syphilis, malaria, and hepatitis.

Refusing blood transfusions on religious grounds was not easy. Repeatedly, patients were physically forced to take donor blood, using such high-handed methods as incapacitation by court order, strapping patients to the bed (even with the help of police officers), and secretly adding sedatives to a patient's infusion. In the early 1960s, representatives of Jehovah's Witnesses started visiting physicians to explain the reasons why transfusions were refused by the Witness population. They often offered literature that dealt with techniques that were acceptable to Witness patients, informing physicians of the availability of so-called transfusion alternatives. In 1979 the governing body of the Jehovah's Witnesses announced the formation of Hospital Liaison Committees (see Chapter 20). These continued to "support Jehovah's Witnesses in *their* determination to prevent their being given blood transfusions, to clear away misunderstandings on the part of doctors and hospitals, to establish a more cooperative spirit between medical institutions and Witness patients (our italics)" and to "alert hospital staff to the fact that there are valid alternatives to the infusion of blood". Occasionally, the Witnesses even went to court to fight for their rights as patients. In a great number of cases, the Witnesses' position was upheld by the courts.

Although many physicians had difficulty with the concept of bloodless medicine, some took up the challenge to provide the best possible medical care without

the use of blood transfusions. These were in fact the earliest blood managers. As their experience in performing "bloodless" surgery increased, more complex procedures, such as open heart surgery, orthopedic surgery, and cancer surgery, could be performed. Even children and newborns could successfully be treated without transfusing blood. Before long, these pioneering physicians published their results with Witness patients, thereby encouraging other doctors to adopt the methods used in performing such surgical interventions.

Among the first to rise to the challenge was the heart surgeon Denton Cooley of Texas. In the early 1960s, his team devised methods to treat Witness patients. He described the techniques in an article, "Open heart surgery in Jehovah's Witnesses," published in 1964 in *The American Journal of Cardiology*. In 1977, Cooley reported his experiences with more than 500 patients [2].

Cooley's example was followed by many other courageous physicians. For instance, in 1970 Dr Pearce performed bloodless open heart surgery in New Orleans. His efforts did not go unnoticed. Newspapers reported on these spectacular cases. Perhaps out of curiosity or out of the earnest desire to learn, many colleagues visited Dr Pearce's team in the operating room to learn how to do "bloodless hearts." Jerome Kay, from Los Angeles, also performed bloodless heart surgery. In 1973 he reported that he was now performing bloodless heart surgery on the majority of his patients. The call for bloodless treatments spread around the whole world. Sharad Pandey, of the KEM Hospital in Mumbai, India, adopted bloodless techniques from Canada and tailored them to Indian conditions. Centers in Europe and the rest of the world started adopting these advances as well.

It is understandable that Witness patients preferred to be treated by physicians who had proven their willingness and ability to treat them without using donor blood. The good reputation of such physicians spread and so patients from far away were transferred to their facilities. This laid the foundation for organized "bloodless programs." One of the hospitals with such a program was the Esperanza Intercommunity Hospital in Yorba Linda, California, where a high percentage of patients were Witnesses. Herk Hutchins, an experienced surgeon and a Witness himself, was known for his development of an iron-containing formula for blood-building. Among his team was the young surgeon Ron Lapin, who was later famed for his pioneering work in the area of bloodless therapies. Critics labeled him a quack. Nevertheless, he continued and was later honored for opening one of the first organized bloodless centers in the world, as well as for publishing the first journal on this topic, and for his efforts to teach his colleagues. During his career, he performed thousands of bloodless surgeries.

The pioneers of blood management had to rise to the challenge of using and refining available techniques, adjusting them to current needs, and individualizing patient care. They adopted new technologies as soon as was reasonable. Much attention was paid to details of patient care, thus improving the quality of the whole therapy. They also fought for patients' rights and upheld those rights. Many involved in the field of blood management confirm the good feeling that comes from being a physician in the truest sense. There is no need to force a particular treatment. Such an attitude is a precious heritage from the pioneers of blood management. Now, at the beginning of the 21st century, this pioneering spirit can still be felt at some meetings dedicated to blood management.

Currently, strenuous efforts are being made to incorporate blood management further and deeper into mainstream medicine. This elicits various responses. Transfusionists, who are actually well suited to spearhead blood management, sometimes insist that their current realm of activity defines blood management. However, transfusion medicine so far is a discipline in itself and defines only certain aspects of blood management, such as cell salvage or the rare provision of specific, purified blood products, e.g., fibrinogen concentrates. Other aspects of blood management include surgical techniques, pharmacological hemostasis, diagnostic procedures, etc. At the core of blood management, however, is the patient's own blood as a precious, life-saving commodity. To emphasize this further, recently the term blood management has been replaced by the term patient blood management by some groups. Although not all parties agree with the definition of blood management, the World Health Organization (WHO) endorsed blood management as a specialty worth developing further. During its 63rd World Health Assembly in 2010, the WHO defined blood management as the previously published three-pillar model (preoperative anemia management, reduction of blood loss, improvement of anemia tolerance). Although this model includes only one aspect of blood management, the WHO's endorsement represents an important historical development.

Military use of blood and blood management

Over the centuries, the armies of different nations have contributed to the development of current blood man-

agement, but not on religious grounds. Instead, the military made many crucial contributions to blood management by taking care of the thousands of wounded operated on before transfusions became feasible, thereby actually performing "bloodless surgery." It was on the battlefield that hemorrhage was recognized as a cause of death. Therefore, it was imperative for military surgeons to stop hemorrhage promptly and effectively, and to avoid further blood loss. To achieve this, many techniques of bloodless medicine and blood management were invented. The experience of the early surgeons serving near the battlefield is applicable in today's blood management schemes. William Steward Halsted, a surgeon on the battlefield, described uncontrolled hemorrhage [3] and later taught his trainees at Johns Hopkins the technique of gentle tissue handling, surgery that respects anatomy, and meticulous hemostasis (Halstedian principles). His excellent work provides the basis of the surgical contribution to a blood management program.

Since war brought a deluge of hemorrhaging victims, there was a need for a therapy. As soon as transfusions became practical, they were adopted by the military, but experience from the First and Second World Wars also showed their drawbacks, such as storage problems and transfusion-transmissible diseases. So, while the world wars propelled the development of transfusion medicine, they simultaneously spurred the development of alternative treatments. Intravenous fluids had been described in the earlier medical literature [4, 5], but the pressing need to replace lost blood and the difficulties involved in transfusions provided a strong impetus for military medicine to change its practice. In this connection, the following comment in the *Providence Sunday Journal* of May 17, 1953 is pertinent: "The Army will henceforth use dextran, a substance made from sugar, instead of blood plasma, for all requirements at home and overseas, it was learned last night. An authoritative Army medical source, who asked not to be quoted by name, said 'a complete switchover' to the plasma substitute has been put into effect, after 'utterly convincing' tests of dextran in continental and combat area hospitals during the last few months. This official said a major factor in the switchover to dextran was that use of plasma entails a 'high risk' of causing a disease known as serum hepatitis—a jaundice-like ailment. Not all plasma carries this hazard, he emphasized, but he added that dextran is entirely free of the hazard. 'We have begun to fill all orders from domestic and overseas theaters with dextran instead of plasma.'"

The military readily adopted other promising products in blood management. For example, the surgeon Gerald

Klebanoff, who served in the Vietnam War, introduced a device for autotransfusion in military hospitals. Another example is "artificial blood." Efforts to develop a "blood substitute" were intensified by the US military in 1985, with major investments supporting research at either contract laboratories or military facilities [6]. The driving force for this was not the search for a plasma expander but the search for an oxygen carrier. A third example is the recombinant clotting factor VIIa. Although officially declared to be a product for use in hemophiliacs, the Israeli army discovered its potential to stop life-threatening hemorrhage and therefore used it in the treatment of injured soldiers.

After the attack on the World Trade Center in New York on September 11, 2001, physicians of the US military approached the Society for the Advancement of Blood Management for advice on blood management. Consequently, specialists in the field of blood management met with representatives of the US military, the result of which was an initiative named STORMACT® (Strategies to Reduce Military and Civilian Transfusion). The consensus of this initiative was a blood management concept to be used to treat victims of war and disaster as well as patients in a preclinical setting.

Recently, the military has spearheaded research in the management of massive bleeding and coagulopathy in polytraumatized patients. This research has addressed the immediate application of a tourniquet to a bleeding extremity and the use of hemostatic combat dressings. Military research is even challenging deeply entrenched mnemonics, changing the ABCDE algorithm for trauma care into cABCDE, highlighting the c for catastrophic bleeding as being even more important than airway management.

Transfusion specialists support blood management

Interestingly, right from the beginning of transfusion medicine, the development of blood transfusion and transfusion alternatives was closely interwoven. "Alternatives" to transfusion are as old as transfusion itself.

The first historically documented transfusions in humans were performed in the 17th century and their aim was to cure mental disorders rather than the substitution of lost blood. However, the first transfusion specialists were in fact also the first to try infusions that were later called transfusion alternatives: it was reported that Christopher Wren was involved in the first transfusion experiments as well as being the first to inject asanguin-

ous fluids, such as wine and beer. After two of Jean Baptiste Denise's (a French transfusionist) transfused patients died, transfusion experiments were prohibited in many countries. Even the Pope condemned those early efforts and transfusions ceased for many years.

At the beginning of the 19th century, the physician James Blundell was looking for a method to prevent the death of women due to profuse hemorrhage related to childbirth. His excellent results with retransfusion of the women's shed blood rekindled the interest of the medical community in transfusion medicine. Due to his work with autotransfusion, he was named in the list of the "fathers of modern transfusion medicine." Other physicians followed his example, giving new impetus to transfusion medicine. However, in 1873 Jennings published a report of 243 transfusions in humans, of which almost half of the cases died [7]. Frustration around this situation led some researchers to look for alternative treatments in the event of hemorrhage. Barnes and Little suggested normal saline as a blood substitute [8] and this was introduced into medical practice. Hamlin tried milk infusions [9]. The use of gelatin was also experimented with. One of the advocates of normal saline, W.T. Bull, wrote in 1884 [10]: "The danger from loss of blood, even to two-thirds of its whole volume, lies in the disturbed relationship between the caliber of the vessels and the quantity of blood contained therein, and not in the diminished number of red blood corpuscles; and this danger concerns the volume of the injected fluids also, it being a matter of indifference whether they be albuminous or containing blood corpuscles or not."

In the early 1900s, Landsteiner's discovery of the blood groups was probably the event that propelled transfusion medicine to where it is today. Some 10–15 years later, when Reuben Ottenberg introduced routine typing of blood into clinical practice, the way was paved for blood transfusions. About that time, technical problems had been solved with new techniques and anticoagulation was in use. Russian physicians (Filatov, Depp, and Yudin) stored cadaver blood. The groundwork for the first blood bank was laid in 1934 in Chicago by Seed and Fantus [11], and as already mentioned, the wars of the first half of the 20th century brought about changes in transfusion medicine. Following the two world wars the medical community had a seemingly endless and safe stream of blood at their disposal. Adams and Lundy suggested that the threshold for transfusion should be a hemoglobin level of 10 mg/dL and a hematocrit of 30% [12]. For nearly four decades thereafter, physicians transfused to their liking, convinced that the benefits of allogeneic transfusions outweighed their potential risks.

Over time reports about the transmission of blood-borne diseases increased. In 1962, when the famous article of J.G. Allen [13] again demonstrated a connection between transfusion and hepatitis, an era of increased awareness about transfusion-transmissible diseases began. However, the risk of hepatitis transmission did not concern the general medical community, and it became an acceptable complication of banked blood. It was not until the early 1980s that the medical community and the public became aware of a transfusion-transmissible acquired immunodeficiency syndrome, and the demand for safer blood and "bloodless medicine" increased. Other problems with allogeneic transfusions, such as immunosuppression, added to the concerns. Lessons learned from the work with the Jehovah's Witnesses community were ready to be applied on a wider scale. In the United States, the National Institutes of Health launched a consensus conference on the proper use of blood. Adams and Lundy's 10/30 rule was revised, and it was agreed that a hemoglobin level of 7 mg/dL would be a better transfusion threshold in otherwise healthy patients.

With time, the incentives for effective blood management changed. The immunomodulatory effects of allogeneic blood came to the fore and offered compelling reasons for carefully handling the patient's own blood. The incremental increase of the costs of blood products is another compelling reason for blood management. Lastly, the experience with tens of thousands of patients treated successfully without allogeneic blood transfusions has led some physicians to see allogeneic transfusions having the same fate as the ancient blood-letting.

Blood management today and tomorrow

Currently, there are more than 100 organized bloodless programs in the United States. Many are transitioning to become blood management programs. This is not unique to the United States, since many more programs have been established worldwide. Most were formed as a result of the initiatives of Jehovah's Witnesses, but a growing number now realize the benefits that all patients can receive from this care. The increasing number of patients asking for treatment without blood demonstrates a growing demand in this field. Concerns about the public health implications of transfusion-related hazards have led government institutions around the globe to encourage and support the establishment of these programs. Private and government initiatives have been taken so far

that in 2011, the first state-wide blood management program was launched in Western Australia.

The growing interest in blood management is reflected by the activities described below. Major medical organizations (see Appendix B) now include blood management issues on the agenda of their regular meetings. Many transfusion textbooks and medical journals have incorporated the subject of blood management. A growing body of literature invites further investigation (see Appendix B). In addition, professional societies dedicated to furthering blood management have been founded throughout the world (see Appendix B). It is their common goal to provide a forum for the exchange of ideas and information among professionals engaged in the advancement and improvement of blood management in clinical practice and by educational and research initiatives. Clearly, from humble beginnings as an "outsider" specialty, blood management has evolved to be in the mainstream of medicine. It improves patient outcome, reduces costs, and brings satisfaction for the physician—a clear win–win situation. Blood management is plainly good medical practice.

What are the future trends in blood management? As long as there is a need for medical treatment, blood management will develop. Many new drugs and techniques are on the horizon. There are already many techniques available to reduce or eliminate the use of donor blood. It is the commitment to blood management that will change the way blood is used. The authors of this book hope that the information provided by its pages will be another piece in the puzzle that will eventually define future blood management by a new generation of physicians.

Blood management as a program

The organized approach to blood management is a program. These programs are named according to the emphasis each places on the different facets of blood management, such as bloodless programs, transfusion-free programs, blood conservation programs, or global blood management programs. Recently, some programs have been renamed "patient blood management programs." No matter what a hospital calls its program, some basic features are common to all good quality programs, as described below. The step-by-step approach to the development of an organized blood management program is described in Chapter 19.

The administration

The basis for establishing a program is not primarily a financial investment but rather a firm commitment on the part of the hospital. Administrators, physicians, nurses, and other personnel need to be involved, as outlined in the recommendations of the Society for the Advancement of Blood Management. Only the sincere cooperation of those involved will make a program successful.

The heart and soul of a program is its coordinator with his/her in-hospital office [14, 15]. Historically, coordinators were often Jehovah's Witnesses. However, as such programs become more widely accepted, there are an increasing number of coordinators from other backgrounds. Usually, coordinators are employed and salaried by the hospital.

During the initial phases of development of the program, the coordinators may be burdened with significant workload. Together with involved physicians, the coordinator has to recruit additional physicians who are willing and able to participate in the program. Since successful blood management is a multidisciplinary endeavor; specialists from a variety of fields need to be involved. The coordinator needs to meet with the heads of the clinical departments and work toward mutual understanding and cooperation. Each participating physician needs to affirm his/her commitment to the program and to enhance his/her knowledge of the basic ethical and medical principles involved. To ensure a lasting and dependable cooperation between physicians and the program, both parties sign a contract. This contract outlines the points that are crucial for blood management: legal, ethical, and medical issues.

The coordinator is also instrumental for the initial and continuous education of participating and incoming staff. He/she may use in-service sessions, invite guest speakers, collect and distribute current literature, obtain information on national and international educational meetings, and help staff interested in hands-on experience in the field of blood management. Ideally, participating staff members take care of their blood management-related education themselves.

From the beginning of the program, there needs to be a set of policies and procedures. Guidelines for cooperation with other staff members need to be drawn up. It is prudent to have the hospital lawyer review all such documents. Each individual hospital must find a way to educate patients and to document their wishes, to ensure that patients are treated according to their wishes and that these are clearly identifiable. Transfer of patients to and from the hospital needs to be organized. A mode of emergency transfer needs to be established. Procedures already in existence, such as storage and release of blood products and rarely used drugs for emergencies, need to be reviewed. Most probably, available medical procedures in the hospital just need to be adapted to the needs of the program. Additional blood management procedures and devices need to be introduced to the hospital staff. The use of hemodilution, cell salvage, platelet sequestration, autologous surgical glue, and other methods needs to be organized. Besides, departments not directly involved in patient care can contribute to the development of policies and procedures. This holds true for the administration offices, blood bank, laboratory and technical departments, pharmacy, and possibly the research department. There is also a variety of issues that need legal and ethical clarification. In keeping with national and international law, issues concerning pediatric and obstetric cases need to be clarified well before the first event arises. Forms need to be developed and a protocol for obtaining legal consent and/or advance directive must be instituted.

To assure continuing support on the part of the administration and the public, some measures of quality control and assurance need to be implemented. Statistical data from the time before the establishment of a certain procedure should be available for comparison with those obtained after its institution and during the course of its implementation. These data are a valuable instrument to demonstrate the effectiveness of procedures and their associated costs. They also serve as an aid in decision-making regarding possible and necessary changes. If records are kept up-to-date, developments and trends can be used as an effective tool for quality assurance and for the identification of strong and weak points in a program. Such records are also helpful for negotiations with sponsors and financial departments, discussions with incoming physicians, and public relations.

The coordinators, and later their staff, need to be well informed about policies and procedures in their hospital and the level of care the facility can provide. There may be times when the burden of cases or the severity of a patient's condition outweigh the faculty's capacity or capability. In such cases, a list of alternative hospitals better suited to perform a certain procedure should be available.

Good communication skills are essential for the daily activities of the coordinator since he/she is the link between patients and physicians. The coordinator is in constant contact with the patient and his/her family and is involved in the development of the care plan for every patient in the program. The coordinator informs the staff involved in the care of the patient about issues pertaining to blood management. In turn, staff members inform the coordinator about the progress of the patient. Planned procedures are discussed and any irregular development is reported. Thus, developing problems can be counteracted at an early stage, thereby avoiding major mishaps.

There is virtually no limit to the ingenuity of a coordinator. He/she is a pioneer, manager, nurse, teacher, host, helper, and friend. No successful program is possible without a coordinator.

The physician

Several studies on transfusion practice in relation to certain procedures demonstrate a striking fact: A great institutional variability exists in transfusion practice, for no medical reason. For example, in a study on coronary bypass surgery the rate of transfusions varied between 27% and 92% [16]. What was the reason? Did those physicians who transfused frequently care for sicker patients? No, the major differing variable was the institution—and with it the physicians. This is in fact good news. If a physician's behavior can be modified to appropriately limit the transfusion rate, then a blood management program can effectively reduce the number of transfusions.

Basic and continuous education is crucial for physicians participating in a blood management program. To start with, physicians should intercommunicate about currently available techniques of blood management that relate to their field of practice and compare their knowledge and skills with those of others. This honest comparison will identify the strong and weak areas in a physician's practice of blood management. Then, new approaches, techniques, and equipment should be added as needed. However, remember that not all techniques suit all physicians and not all physicians suit all techniques. After all, it is not a sophisticated set of equipment that makes for good blood management—it is a group of skilled physicians. That is why it is desirable that all physicians in a blood management program be aware of the experiences and skills of their colleagues, in order to make these available to all patients.

Another group of professionals that is essential for the program to succeed are the nurses. Nurses play a vital role as they contribute much to patient identification, education, and care. Nursing staff must therefore also be included in the process of initial and continuing education.

Commitment, education, cooperation, and communication are key factors for a successful blood management

program. To make each treatment a success, it requires the concerted effort by physicians, coordinators, nurses, administrators, and auxiliary staff on the one hand, and the patient with his/her family on the other.

Key points

• Blood management is a good clinical practice that should be applied to all patients.
• Blood management is best practiced in an organized program.
• Blood management improves outcomes, and is patient centered, multidisciplinary, and multimodal.
• Respect for patients, commitment, education, cooperation, and communication are the cornerstones of blood management.

Questions for review

1. What role did the following play in the development of modern blood management: Jehovah's Witnesses, physicians, the military, and transfusion specialists?
2. What do the following terms mean: bloodless medicine, transfusion-free medicine, blood conservation, blood management, and patient blood management?
3. What are the important facets of a comprehensive blood management program?

Suggestions for further research

1. What medical, ethical, and legal obstacles did early blood managers have to overcome?
2. How did they do this?
3. What can be learned from their experience?

Exercises and practice cases

Read the article by Adams and Lundy [12] that builds the basis for the 10/30 rule.

Homework

Analyze your hospital and answer the following questions:

1. What measures are taken to identify patients for blood management?
2. What is done to comply with legal requirements when documenting a patient's preferences for treatment?
3. What steps are taken to ensure a patient's wishes are heeded?

References

1. Baele P, Van der Linden P. Developing a blood conservation strategy in the surgical setting. *Acta Anaesthesiol Belg* 2002;**53**:129–136.
2. Ott DA, Cooley DA. Cardiovascular surgery in Jehovah's witnesses. Report of 542 operations without blood transfusion. *JAMA* 1977;**238**:1256–1258.
3. Halsted WS. *Surgical Papers by William Steward Halsted*. John Hopkins Press, Baltimore, 1924.
4. Mudd S, Thalhimer W. *Blood Substitutes and Blood Transfusion*, Vol. 1. C.C. Thomas, Springfield, 1942.
5. White C, Weinstein J. *Blood Derivatives and Substitutes. Preparation, Storage, Administration and Clinical Results Including Discussion of Shock. Etiology, Physiology, Pathology and Treatment*, Vol. 1. Williams and Wilkins, Baltimore, 1947.
6. Winslow RM. New transfusion strategies: red cell substitutes. *Annu Rev Med* 1999;**50**:337–353.
7. Jennings C. *Transfusion: It's History, Indications, and Mode of Application*. Leonard & Co, New York, 1883.
8. Diamond L. A history of blood transfusion. In: *Blood, Pure and Eloquent*. McGraw-Hill, New York, 1980.
9. Spence R. Blood substitutes. In: Petz LD, Kleinman S, Swisher SN, Spence RK (eds) *Clinical Practice of Transfusion Medicine*. Churchill Livingstone, New York, 1996, pp. 967–984.
10. Bull W. On the intravenous injection of saline solutions as a substitution for transfusion of blood. *Med Rec* 1884;**25**: 6–8.
11. Fantus B. Therapy of the Cook County Hospital (blood preservation). *JAMA* 1937;**109**:128–132.
12. Adams RC, Lundy JS. Anesthesia in cases of poor surgical risk. Some suggestions for decreasing the risk. *Surg Gynecol Obstet* 1942;**74**:1011–1019.
13. Allen J. Serum hepatitis from transfusion of blood. *JAMA* 1962;**180**:1079–1085.
14. Vernon S, Pfeifer GM. Are you ready for bloodless surgery? *Am J Nurs* 1997;**97**:40–46; quiz 47.
15. deCastro RM. Bloodless surgery: establishment of a program for the special medical needs of the Jehovah's Witness community—the gynecologic surgery experience at a community hospital. *Am J Obstet Gynecol* 1999;**180**:1491–1498.
16. Stover EP, Siegel LC, Body SC, *et al.* Institutional variability in red blood cell conservation practices for coronary artery bypass graft surgery. Institutions of the MultiCenter Study of Perioperative Ischemia Research Group. *J Cardiothorac Vasc Anesth* 2000;**14**:171–176.

2 Physiology of Anemia and Oxygen Transport

Tolerance of anemia while it is being treated is one of the cornerstones of blood management. This chapter explains the physiological and pathophysiological mechanisms underlying the body's oxygen transport and use of oxygen. This furthers understanding of how the body deals with states of reduced oxygen delivery and the efforts to increase delivery. Furthermore, it enables the reader to reflect critically on current and future therapeutic measures to increase oxygen availability to tissue.

Objectives

1. To review factors that influence oxygen delivery.
2. To learn how to calculate oxygen delivery and consumption.
3. To identify the mechanisms the body uses to adapt to acute and chronic anemia.
4. To define the vital role of the microcirculation.
5. To describe tissue oxygenation and tissue oxygen utilization.

Definitions

Anemia: Anemia is a reduction in the total circulating red blood cell mass, usually diagnosed by a decrease in hemoglobin concentration. Thresholds for anemia depend on the age and gender of the patient. Typically, anemia is said to exist in an adult male when hemoglobin is below 13.5 g/dL, and in an adult female when below 13 g/dL.

Normal physiology

A single equation describes the whole concept

Let us jump right into the subject using the well-known equation (Eqn 2.1) where oxygen delivery is simply calculated by multiplying the cardiac output by the arterial oxygen content:

$$DO_2 = Q \times (Hb \times 1.34 \times SaO_2 + 0.003 \times PaO_2) \times 10$$
$$\text{(Eqn. 2.1)}$$

where DO_2 is oxygen delivery; Q is flow in L/min; Hb is hemoglobin in g/dL; 1.34 is Hufner's number; SaO_2 is oxygen saturation of hemoglobin as a %; 0.003 is the oxygen solubility in plasma; and PaO_2 is the partial pressure of oxygen in arterial blood in mmHg.

The equation describes the concept of systemic oxygen transport (macrocirculation), the knowledge of which constitutes a sound basis for understanding therapeutic interventions that enhance oxygen delivery.

One of the crucial factors of oxygen transport is the flow (Q) or cardiac output (CO), which is determined by the stroke volume (SV) and heart rate (HR) (CO = SV × HR). Flow is essential for oxygen delivery since otherwise neither red cells nor any other blood constituent would reach their target.

Another crucial player in oxygen transport is hemoglobin. In healthy individuals, most of the oxygen in blood is bound to hemoglobin. One molecule of hemoglobin can hold a maximum of four oxygen molecules.

Basics of Blood Management, Second Edition. Petra Seeber and Aryeh Shander.
© 2013 John Wiley & Sons, Ltd. Published 2013 by John Wiley & Sons, Ltd.

In vivo, 1 g of hemoglobin has the potential to bind approximately 1.34 mL of oxygen (Hufner's number). In order to know exactly how much oxygen is bound to hemoglobin, another variable must be known. This is the oxygen saturation (SaO_2), the percentage of hemoglobin molecules that actually have oxygen bound to them.

Besides the oxygen bound by hemoglobin, a small amount of oxygen is physically dissolved in plasma. This amount is linearly dependent on the partial pressure of oxygen "above" the plasma, namely the inspiratory oxygen fraction (FiO_2). The higher the FiO_2, the more oxygen is dissolved. The amount of oxygen physically dissolved in plasma also depends on the specific Bunsen solubility coefficient "alpha" of oxygen. A Bunsen solubility coefficient of 0.024 means that there is 0.024 mL of oxygen dissolved in 1 mL of blood at normal body temperature (37 °C) at a pressure of 1 atm. Using the Henry Dalton equation, it can be calculated that 0.003 mL of O_2/mL of blood is physically dissolved in normal arterial blood (PO_2 = 95 mmHg, PCO_2 = 40 mmHg). Thus, the number 0.003 in Eqn 2.1 is the amount of physically dissolved oxygen in the blood under "normal" conditions. Although the amount of physically dissolved oxygen might appear insignificant compared to the amount of oxygen transported by hemoglobin, it should be borne in mind that every single molecule of oxygen bound to hemoglobin has to have been physically dissolved in blood before it entered the red cell. Later it will be shown that the amount of physically dissolved oxygen is crucial for patients with severe anemia.

Does a single equation describes the whole concept?

Imagine a patient with a very low serum calcium level. What treatment should be given? Supplementing the body's calcium stores sounds reasonable, and a doctor could prescribe the patient pebbles to swallow. The body's content of calcium would certainly increase dramatically. Most would object, "But that is complete nonsense," and they would be right, because it is obvious that the calcium contained in the pebbles does not reach the place where it is needed and cannot be used by the body. On the contrary, it may even cause harm to the patient.

The same holds true for patients suffering from a lack of oxygen-carrying red cells. Initially the idea of a "refill" may sound reasonable. However, the main question is easily overlooked if only macrocirculatory oxygen delivery is kept in mind; namely, Do I achieve the goal of delivering oxygen to the tissue? And one step further: Do

I succeed in maintaining aerobic metabolism? Just increasing the hemoglobin level through transfusion may, at times, be similar to feeding a pebble to a patient with a low calcium level. A number is changed, but the condition is not improved. For this reason the second part of oxygen delivery needs to be taken into consideration: the microcirculation.

How do red cells take up oxygen?

How about accompanying red cells on their journey through the human body? The journey starts in the capillary bed of the lungs. Here is where the red cells deliver carbon dioxide and take up oxygen.

Pulmonary gas exchange is governed by Fick's law of diffusion, stating that the flux of diffusing particles (here oxygen and carbon dioxide) is proportional to their concentration gradient. Driven by this gradient, oxygen and carbon dioxide molecules move across membranes in the lung, vessel walls, and red cells, as well as randomly through fluids. Due to the immense surface area of the lung across which oxygen and carbon dioxide gradients develop, the exchange of oxygen and carbon dioxide is rapid. Hemoglobin molecules further support the uptake of oxygen by red cells as hemoglobin molecules diffuse within the cell, also following a gradient. Once hemoglobin is oxygenated by means of oxygen diffusion across the red cell membrane, it diffuses into the center of the red cell, whereas deoxyhemoglobin diffuses toward the cell membrane, ready for oxygen uptake.

The processes of carbon dioxide release and oxygen uptake interact closely. As the partial pressure of carbon dioxide decreases, the affinity of hemoglobin for oxygen increases (Haldane effect). This effect supports the oxygenation of red cells in the lung.

The rate of oxygen uptake by human red cells is approximately 40 times slower than the corresponding rate of oxygen combination with free hemoglobin. The reason for this is that the hemoglobin in red cells is surrounded by several layers: cytoplasm, cell membrane, and a fluid layer adjacent to the red cell membrane. Oxygen therefore has to diffuse over a long distance before it can penetrate the cell. In particular, the unstirred layers around the red cell pose a barrier to oxygen uptake. The impact of the red cell membrane on resisting gas exchange is a subject of controversy and may in fact be negligible [1, 2]. The uptake of oxygen by red cells appears mainly to depend on the thickness of the unstirred fluid layers [1] (and less on pH, 2,3-diphosphoglycerate [2,3-DPG] level, and membrane resistance).

How do red cells reach the microvasculature in the tissue?

Let us follow the red cells even further. As already described, they bring carbon dioxide for exhalation to the lung and take up oxygen. Now the red cells are ready for their next mission. They have to travel to the microcirculation to deliver the oxygen.

The blood is pumped by the heart from large vessels into the narrower areas of the human vasculature. Here the red cells slow down. The reduction in red cell velocity leads to a reduction in hematocrit in a determined segment of vessel relative to the hematocrit of blood entering or leaving the vessel. This dynamic reduction of the intravascular hematocrit is called the Farhaeus effect [3]. The hematocrit in the microcirculation is about 30% of that in the systemic circulation and it remains constant until the systemic hematocrit is lowered to less than 15% [4].

As the red cells travel toward the smallest capillaries, they tend to aggregate and build "rouleaux" formations, which look like stacks of coins [3]. This is due to macromolecular bridging and osmotic water exclusion from the gap between neighboring red cell membranes. Red cells line up in the center of the vessel where they have the maximum velocity. A plasma layer at the vessel wall works like a kind of lubricant to help the cells pass through the capillary. This arrangement of cells and plasma leads to a marked reduction in the viscosity so that blood viscosity in the microcirculation is close to that of plasma [3]. This effect was described by Farhaeus and Lindqvist when they wrote, "Below a critical point at a diameter of about 0.3 mm the viscosity decreases strongly with reduced diameter of the tube" [5].

The smallest capillaries have a diameter of less than 3 μm and red cells a diameter of about 7–8 μm. Red cells are therefore much bigger than the capillaries they have to travel through, but this poses no real problem since red cells are as soft as a sponge and are easily deformable. They literally squeeze through the capillaries. It is obvious then, that red cell deformability is essential for the perfusion of the microcirculation [6].

Now, the red cells have arrived in the microcirculation and are eager to release their oxygen to the tissue. But where exactly? Formerly, the Krogh model was used to explain tissue oxygenation. It described a single capillary with a surrounding cylinder of tissue. Oxygen gradients between the tissue and the vasculature were thought to be the driving forces of tissue oxygenation. Capillaries were the only structures thought to participate in the oxygen exchange with the tissue. Tissue farthest from the capillary received the least oxygen. More recent research, however, has revealed that tissue oxygen distribution is even across all tissue between vessels. The capillary–tissue oxygen gradient is very low, namely only about 5 mmHg. Capillaries are nearly at equilibrium with the tissue and deliver oxygen to pericapillary regions only [7]. Thus, capillaries do not contribute significantly to tissue oxygenation. Most of the oxygen is delivered to the tissues via arterioles. Oxygen gradients were found to be greatest between arterioles and tissue. Significant amounts of oxygen (30%) leave the vessels at the arteriolar level. This is surprising since the tissue surrounding the arterioles does not have a metabolic demand high enough to justify an uptake of large amounts of oxygen. In fact, only 10–15% of the losses can be explained by the oxygen consumption of the tissue surrounding the arterioles. There is no good explanation for where the other 85–90% of the oxygen is consumed, but it probably serves the high metabolic demand of the endothelium [7]. Such demand may be explained by the enormous amount of endothelial synthesis (e.g., nitric oxide, renin, interleukin, prostaglandins, and prostacyclin, etc.), transformation (of bradykinin, angiotensin, etc.), and constant work to adjust vascular tone.

Before continuing with the red cells' journey, let us step back and look at the whole microcirculation. Tissue as a whole depends on a network of capillaries (microvasculature), not only for delivery of oxygen but also for removal of metabolites. According to Fick's law, the size of the area of diffusion is a main component in the exchange of oxygen and metabolites. In the microcirculation, the area of diffusion depends on the number of vessels available for exchange. The term "functional capillary density" (FCD) has been coined to describe the "size" of the microvasculature. This term refers to the number of functional (i.e., perfused) capillaries per unit tissue volume [8]. Decreased FCD lowers tissue oxygenation uniformly (without causing oxygenation inhomogeneity) [7] and is associated with poor outcome.

To maintain tissue survival, adequate FCD is essential. Several factors modify FCD. The diameter of the capillaries depends on the surrounding tissue and internal pressure. This means that capillaries embedded in tissue cannot increase their diameter, but they can collapse if they are not properly perfused. Sufficient arterial pressure and an adequate volume status are therefore needed for capillary perfusion. Another factor that modifies FCD and capillary blood flow is the metabolic requirement of the tissue. Demand increases blood flow and oxygen excess decreases blood flow. This mechanism is partially mediated by nitric oxide. Hemoglobin is able to scavenge nitric oxide and, therefore, constrict vessels. Hence, it seems red cells counteract their own function of delivering oxygen by blocking (constricting) their own path (vessels). This is not the case, however. The explanation for this phenomenon lies in the fact that hemoglobin comes in two different forms: R (relaxed, with high oxygen affinity) and T (tense, with low oxygen affinity). In the R form, hemoglobin not only transports oxygen but can also take up a nitric oxide compound (S-nitrosylation). When hemoglobin arrives at precapillary resistance vessels, it loses some oxygen and starts its transition from the R to T form. This change liberates the nitric oxide and causes dilatation of the arterioles [9]. With this mechanism, oxygen-loaded red cells open their doors to the tissue in order to deliver oxygen.

How do red cells give up oxygen and how is it taken up by tissue?

The quantity of oxygen released by red cells depends greatly on the oxygen affinity of hemoglobin molecules. It is this affinity that translates oxygen flow into available oxygen. A common method to depict the behavior of hemoglobin is the oxygen dissociation curve (Figure 2.1). The oxygen dissociation curve is sigmoid-shaped. This is due to conformational changes in the hemoglobin molecule that occur when it loads or releases oxygen. The uptake of each oxygen molecule alters the hemoglobin conformation and this enhances the uptake of the next oxygen molecule. A change in hemoglobin's oxygen affinity profoundly affects oxygen release to the tissue, whereas the oxygen uptake by hemoglobin is scarcely affected.

There are several factors that can influence the hemoglobin's affinity for oxygen per se (Figure 2.1). Those factors include temperature, carbon dioxide, H$^+$, and 2,3-DPG [10]. Red blood cells deliver oxygen to metabolically active tissues. Such tissues release carbon dioxide that diffuses into the red cells. With carbonic anhydrase, CO_2 and H_2O react to form H$^+$ and HCO_3^-. The resulting HCO_3^- is exchanged with extracellular Cl$^-$, which leads to an intracellular acidification. The resulting decrease in pH facilitates oxygen dissociation from hemoglobin. Also, 2,3-DPG, a glycolytic intermediate, binds to deoxyhemoglobin and stabilizes hemoglobin in the deoxy form, thus reducing hemoglobin's oxygen affinity and supporting oxygen release. In fact, this 2,3-DPG is so important that no oxygen can be unloaded by the red cells if it is completely lacking.

After being released from the hemoglobin molecule, oxygen has to pass through several fluid layers until it reaches the tissue. In contrast to oxygen uptake by red cells, release of oxygen depends mainly on the affinity of hemoglobin in the red cell and not so much on the thickness of the surrounding unstirred fluid layers [1]. Deoxy-

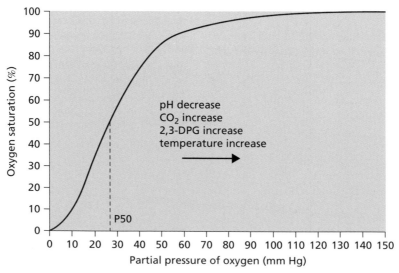

Figure 2.1 Oxygen dissociation curve. 2,3-DPG, 2,3-diphosphoglycerate.

genation therefore depends on pH and 2,3-DPG (lowered pH and increased 2,3-DPG levels facilitate release of oxygen) [1]. Only at very low hemoglobin concentrations do chemical reactions limit release of oxygen from hemoglobin.

After oxygen is released by hemoglobin and has passed all barriers on its way to the tissue, it is accepted by the mitochondria. Oxygen may have traveled via free flow or by means of a "coach" to a myoglobin molecule. The latter is called myoglobin-facilitated oxygen diffusion. "Deoxymyoglobin captures oxygen immediately as it crosses the interface: the newly formed oxymyoglobin diffuses away. The effect is to make the oxygen pressure gradient from capillary lumen to the sarcoplasma more steep, thereby enhancing the oxygen flux" [11]. This effect maintains oxygen flow to the mitochondria under conditions of low extracellular oxygen pressure.

Does the tissue use oxygen?

The human body depends on oxygen for adenosine triphosphate (ATP) generation and maintenance of aerobic metabolism. ATP, the body's main energy source, is generated in the mitochondria using molecular oxygen. Oxygen is only utilized if it can be used by the mitochondria. This means that oxygen utilization is defined by the mitochondria.

Interestingly, there is a genetic component to the function of the mitochondria. Inherited or acquired changes in the enzyme supply determine how effectively oxygen can be used. Drugs such as propofol, which inhibit oxidative phosphorylation, can influence the mitochondria and thus the use of delivered oxygen [12]. Other factors influence tissue (and mitochondrial) use of oxygen as well. The energy demand of the tissue influences how much oxygen is used. In turn, factors that influence the tissue's metabolism also influence the rate of its oxygen use. Nitric oxide inhibits mitochondrial respiration, and thus oxygen consumption. On the other hand, lack of nitric oxide increases metabolism and tissue oxygen consumption [13]. The influence of body temperature on oxygen extraction is well known: higher body temperature increases oxygen demand, extraction [14], and utilization. There are many more factors that alter the body's energy requirement and thus the oxygen demand of the tissue: physical activity, hormones (catecholamines, thyroid hormones), infections, psychological stress, pain and anxiety, digestion and repair of tissues, just to name a few.

All organs and tissues, with the exception of the central nervous system, are able to use the delivered oxygen to the full, i.e., 100%. This is true of the myocardium [15]. In a healthy individual, however, there is a wide safety margin. Oxygen delivery in healthy resting humans exceeds need four-fold. The body as a whole uses only about one in four of hemoglobin's oxygen molecules. The amount of oxygen used is called the oxygen consumption (VO_2). Another way to express the use of oxygen is the oxygen extraction ratio (O_2 ER). It describes the percentage of oxygen extracted from a hemoglobin molecule. The total body's normal resting O_2 ER is about 20–25%, but the organ-specific oxygen extraction varies. Kidneys extract only 5–10% and the heart at rest 55% [4]. It can be seen from such percentages that oxygen delivery is not the only determinant of the body's oxygen balance. Only the concerted efforts of all systems involved in oxygen supply and use make aerobic life possible.

Pathophysiology of anemia

The human body is a marvel of creation. It is equipped with amazing mechanisms to maintain its function and to ensure that its tissue and organ systems tolerate a broad range of conditions. This is true for diminished levels of hemoglobin. Oxygen delivery remains sufficient over a wide range of hemoglobin levels, and even when hemoglobin levels have decreased markedly, the body can survive. All this is due to a variety of compensatory mechanisms, some of which are reviewed below.

The initial adaptation to blood loss is not mainly a reaction to a decrease in oxygen-carrying capacity but rather to hypovolemia. If left untreated, the human body initiates a series of changes: first, to restore blood volume and second, to restore red cell mass. Within minutes, heart rate and stroke volume increase. The adrenergic system and the renin–angiotensin–aldosterone system are stimulated, releasing vasoactive hormones. This leads to the constriction of vascular sphincters in the skin, skeletal muscle, kidneys, and splanchnic viscera. The blood flow is redistributed to high-demand organs, namely the heart and brain [16]. To restore intravascular volume, fluids are first shifted from the interstitial space to the vessels, and later from the intracellular to the extracellular space. Due to adaptations in renal function, water and electrolytes are conserved. The liver is stimulated to produce osmotically active agents (glucose, lactate, urea, phosphate, etc.), which results in a net shift of fluid into the vasculature [16] and thus preload increases. Unless these compensatory mechanisms fail, cardiac output is restored within 1–2 minutes [17].

If the body's compensatory mechanisms do fail, cardiac output and oxygen delivery decrease. At that point, restoration of blood volume (not red cell volume) is mandatory. If fluids are infused, cardiac output can be increased and the untoward effects of hypovolemia averted. Blood flow is restored and the body is able to repair damage and replenish the loss of red cell mass.

In the following paragraphs, the journey of the red blood cell through the human body is repeated—this time under anemic, yet normovolemic, conditions. The assumptions are that the patient is already volume-resuscitated and adaptive mechanisms are mainly due to reduced red cell mass rather than reduced intravascular volume.

Adaptation of the body: Acute is not the same as chronic

It is not uncommon to meet persons with a hemoglobin value of less than 4 g/dL going about their normal daily lives—the only clinically observable effect being reduced exercise tolerance. On the other hand, some patients with the same hemoglobin level are hardly capable of lifting their head. Responses to blood loss and anemia are obviously not uniform. How the body responds to anemia depends on the rapidity of blood loss, the underlying condition of the patient, drugs taken, pre-existing hemoglobin level, etc. [18]. Some adaptive mechanisms are more pronounced in acute anemia while others are more common in chronic anemia.

Adaptive mechanisms to anemia: Macrocirculation

Leonardo da Vinci said: "Movement is the cause of all life." This also holds true for blood loss and anemia. In anemia, increased flow, i.e., cardiac output, compensates for the losses in hemoglobin. In the acute setting, cardiac output increases with increasing levels of volume-resuscitated anemia. This is mainly due to increases in stroke volume. The influence of the heart rate in increasing the cardiac output is a subject of debate. Results conflict depending on the animal species studied and the patients and their conditions (anesthetized versus awake, influence of drugs taken). It seems, however, that an increase in the heart rate is not the main determinant in increasing the cardiac output of acutely anemic, volume-resuscitated individuals [18, 19].

Two major mechanisms are responsible for increased cardiac output. The most important is a reduction in blood viscosity. This results in increased venous flow with increased flow to the right heart. Preload increases, result-ing in an enhanced cardiac output. Afterload is reduced by the decrease in blood viscosity. The other important cause of the increase in cardiac output is stimulation of the sympathetic nervous system. Via this system and catecholamine release, myocardial contractility (and heart rate) increases, and again, the cardiac output increases.

Both in acute and chronic anemia, cardiac output is increased by means of viscosity reduction and sympathetic nerve stimulation. If anemia is becoming chronic, the heart adapts to the increased workload with left ventricular hypertrophy.

In the discussion of macrocirculatory adaptations to anemia, special consideration must be given to the heart. The myocardium requires more oxygen than any other organ and has a high O_2 ER even at rest. When the heart's oxygen demand increases, e.g., by increased cardiac workload, the heart can slightly increase its oxygen extraction. The major increase in oxygen delivery to the heart, however, is due to vasodilatation of the coronary arteries. Normally, there is a great reserve in myocardial blood flow [20]. However, if myocardial blood flow cannot be increased, the heart may not be able to receive the oxygen it needs for its vital work. On the one hand, increased myocardial work is beneficial to compensate for anemia. But then, increased myocardial work increases the heart's oxygen demand. Since an increase in the cardiac output is a crucial factor in compensating for the loss of oxygen-carrying capacity, it is vital for the heart to be able to increase its output on demand. Several factors can impair the heart's ability to increase output. Coronary stenosis, myocardial insufficiency, sepsis, anesthetics, and other drugs may compromise the work of the heart [21]. In such situations, the increase in cardiac output may not be sufficient to compensate for the lost red cell mass. It has been shown that patients with different heart pathologies are more susceptible to ischemia than other patient populations and tolerate anemia less well than the same patients without cardiac pathology.

Closely related to anemia-induced changes in cardiac output is the alteration of vascular tone. Again, the sympathetic nervous system plays an important role in this [18]. Increased activity of aortic chemoreceptors has been postulated to change vasomotor tone, and thus afterload [4]. Part of the reduction in afterload may also be due to hypoxic vasodilatation.

An increase in cardiac output and a reduction in vascular tone leads to increased blood flow. The flow is directed to high-demand organs, with the brain and heart first in line to receive a major portion of the blood

[22]. Even under normal conditions, they extract most of the oxygen offered by the hemoglobin [4] and are therefore supply dependent. Redistribution of the blood flow takes place at the expense of non-critical organs [23], e.g., the skin.

Volume-resuscitated anemic patients have a greater plasma volume than healthy, non-anemic humans. This volume serves to transport physically dissolved oxygen. While the portion of physically dissolved oxygen is almost insignificant in non-anemic patients (see above), it must not be underestimated in severely anemic patients. At times, it may constitute a major portion of the total oxygen delivered by the blood [24].

Another adaptive mechanism of anemia tolerance is increased oxygen extraction. As shown above, given normal conditions, on average only one of the four oxygen molecules carried by a hemoglobin molecule is extracted by the body. Most tissues would be able to extract much more oxygen from the hemoglobin. In fact, in severe states of anemia, most tissues can extract nearly 100% of the oxygen offered. The increase in O_2 ER is thus a valuable tool to compensate for decreased oxygen carriers.

The extent to which the above-mentioned adaptive mechanisms are used by the body differs from patient to patient: The degree of anemia as well as the condition of the patient, his/her comorbidities, and the rapidity of the development of anemia play a role. If anemia becomes a chronic state, systemic vascular resistance returns to normal. Cardiac output is not increased to the same high degree as in acute anemia. Redistribution of blood flow from some organs, with excess flow to other organs, takes place [4]. A combination of adaptive mechanisms enables a chronically anemic body to meet oxygen demand, even at times when hemoglobin levels are extremely low.

As a combined effect of reduction of blood viscosity, increase in cardiac output, etc., delivery of oxygen increases as the hematocrit starts to decrease. Oxygen delivery reaches its maximum at a hematocrit of 25–33% [4]. At hematocrits above 45% and below 25%, oxygen delivery decreases. Adaptation in cardiac output compensates for decreased oxygen-carrying capacity. This results in an almost constant delivery of oxygen to the capillaries, as long as red cell losses do not exceed about 50% in healthy persons [13].

Adaptive mechanisms to anemia: Microcirculation

As shown above, the microcirculation plays a crucial role in oxygen delivery to the tissues. It does not come as a surprise, then, that at the microcirculatory level there are also many mechanisms that compensate for decreased red cell mass. In fact, the microcirculation is where the advantages of hemodilution matter most [19].

How do red cells take up oxygen?

Adaptive mechanisms again begin in the lung, the place where red cells exchange gases. Despite a reduction of the blood's capacity for carrying oxygen and carbon dioxide, even severe anemia is associated with remarkable stability of pulmonary gas exchange [25]. Compensatory mechanisms kick in, ensuring that oxygen transport and carbon dioxide elimination are not impaired [26].

In anemia, lung perfusion is altered. Fewer hemoglobin molecules are available for interaction with nitric oxide, which preserves the vasodilatatory effect of nitric oxide. Resistance to pulmonary blood flow is thus decreased [27]. This leads to an increased flow of blood through the pulmonary vasculature. This flow increases the shear stress in the endothelium, thus further increasing the production of vasodilatating nitric oxide. Those vasodilatatory effects counteract hypoxic pulmonary vasoconstriction [25]. In anemia there is a tendency toward reduced heterogeneity of pulmonary blood flow. Selective constriction of pulmonary vessels diverts blood to better ventilated alveoli [28]. Nitric oxide may also alter airway tone, leading to a redistribution of ventilation. All this results in improved gas exchange in the lung. It has been shown that arterial partial pressure of oxygen in anemic patients may even be greater than in non-anemic patients.

How do red cells reach their target, the microvasculature in the tissues?

There is a clear relationship between hematocrit and viscosity. As the hematocrit decreases, blood viscosity decreases and red cells travel at a higher speed. When traveling at this high speed, they do not have sufficient time to release oxygen on their way to the tissue. Therefore, in anemic conditions red cells arrive in the microcirculation with more oxygen than in non-anemic conditions [4].

Since FCD is important for tissue survival, several mechanisms are employed in anemia to recruit capillaries. The blood flow in the capillaries of anemic patients is more homogenous than in non-anemic ones [19]. Several mechanisms account for this. Hemoglobin has a very high affinity for nitric oxide. This property is a crucial factor for regulating the interaction of red cells and the endothelium. Red cells have the ability to constrict the vascular bed by scavenging the vasodilatator nitric oxide. This effect is concentration dependent; i.e., the lower the hematocrit, the more the vasodilatation and the better the tissue perfusion. A faster flow of blood in anemic states results. "Physical stimuli such as fluid shear stress, pulsatile stretching of the vessel wall, or a low arterial PO_2, also stimulate the release of NO above the basal level" [29]. Furthermore, in anemia, red cells do not aggregate readily and are able to pass through the narrowest capillary. Arterial/venular diffusional shunting is diminished because of the increased blood velocity and the decreased red cell residence time in the vessels [13]. While in the acute anemic setting, the body is only able to recruit available capillaries; in the chronic anemic setting new vessels develop (neoangiogenesis).

Capillary vessels need arterial pressure to remain open. As blood viscosity decreases in anemia, flow increases because less arterial pressure is lost struggling with high blood viscosity. Thus, the lowered blood viscosity improves capillary perfusion. For this reason hemodilution is used therapeutically to improve tissue oxygenation. However, the beneficial effect of reducing the blood viscosity is only apparent as long as the heart can compensate for lost hemoglobin by improving flow. Hemodilution beyond this point reduces viscosity still further, inducing vasoconstriction and thus reducing FCD. At that point, a therapeutic maneuver may be employed to improve tissue perfusion again. Vessels are dependent on shear stress to open. By artificially increasing blood viscosity, shear stress to the vessels can be exerted, eliciting a vasodilatatory response. This may result in recovery of FCD [8, 13, 30].

Summarizing some interesting findings about the relationship of blood viscosity and transfusions, Tsai and Intaglietta stated: "Microcirculatory studies show that the organism compensates for reduced blood viscosity only up to reductions coincident with the conventional transfusion trigger and that reductions beyond this point lower functional capillary density. These studies show that the critical limit for tissue survival at the transfusion trigger is functional capillary density. Functional capillary density is important, primarily, for the extraction of tissue metabolism byproducts and, secondly, for tissue oxygenation. Thus, the transfusion trigger signals a condition where the circulation no longer compensates for significantly lowered viscosity due to hemodilution. Continued hemodilution with high-viscosity plasma expanders beyond the transfusion trigger is shown to maintain functional capillary density and improve tissue perfusion,

suggesting that the conventional transfusion trigger is a viscosity trigger" [31]. After a discussion of the benefits of higher blood viscosity after reaching the "transfusion trigger," the authors concluded: "It is a corollary to these considerations that the level of oxygen carrying capacity required to safely oxygenate the tissue may be much lower than that dictated by medical experience if microvascular function is maintained" [13].

How do red cells release oxygen and how do tissues take up oxygen?

In states of anemia, the oxygen affinity of hemoglobin is lowered, as reflected in a right shift in the oxygen dissociation curve (see Figure 2.1). This facilitates oxygen release to the tissues. The right shift in the oxyhemoglobin dissociation curve is the result of increases of 2,3-DPG in red cells [18]. In contrast to chronic anemia, however, facilitated oxygen dissociation does not play as large a role in acute anemia where 2,3-DPG levels do not change significantly [20]. Theoretically, in anemia also a shift in pH toward greater acidity may enhance oxygen release (Bohr effect). However, this effect is probably not clinically relevant since immense changes in pH are needed to release significant amounts of oxygen from red cells [18].

Oxygen reserves are used in anemia, and this is reflected in an increased O_2 ER. Normally, the tissue extracts only about 20–30% of the total oxygen delivered. In anemia, the tissue may extract much more so that the body's O_2 ER as a whole increases to 50–60%. As a consequence, the mixed venous oxygen partial pressure decreases.

In extreme anemia, oxygen uptake by the tissues seems to be limited. This may be due to the increased flow and the decreased transit time of red cells in the microvasculature. Time available for oxygen diffusion may be insufficient [32]. Also, erythrocyte spacing (increased distance between adjacent red cells during anemia) and the diffusion distance may contribute to this phenomenon [33].

Do the tissues use oxygen?

The last stop on this journey through the anemic body is again the tissues with the mitochondria, the place where a decrease in oxygen delivery should matter most. Intracellular mechanisms sense the decrease of oxygen in the tissues. In response, hypoxia-dependent gene expression is stimulated. A key factor in this process is the hypoxia-inducible factor 1α (HIF 1α). It "induces the expression of genes that influence angiogenesis and vasodilatation, erythropoiesis and increased breathing, as well as glycolytic enzyme genes for anaerobic metabolism" [34]. Interestingly, the basic mechanisms of hypoxia tolerance are shared by different species, including humans. The following model was described for animals.

So, what happens if a cell senses a decrease in oxygen supply? Does the cell die? Not right away. The cell needs oxygen mainly to produce energy (ATP). So it makes sense that in anticipation of reduced oxygen (that is, energy) supply, energy demand is reduced. What does a cell need energy from ATP for? Almost all energy is needed for protein synthesis and degradation, maintenance of ion gradients, and synthesis of glucose and urea. In fact, in an initial defense phase, cells greatly (>90%) and rapidly suppress their protein, glucose, and urea synthesis. Interestingly, ion gradients across membranes remain constant, although the pumping activity of ion pumps is reduced to save energy. The cells use different mechanisms to accomplish this miracle. For instance, liver cells reduce cell membrane permeability, a process called channel arrest. Nerve cells reduce their firing frequency (spike arrest). By employing such measures, many cells can attain an energy balance at a lower level (ATP demand = ATP supply). This may ensure long-term survival in hypoxia. Hypoxia-sensitive cells, however, do not attain a new balance.

After the defense phase, a second "rescue" phase follows. Cells are now aiming at long-term hypoxia survival. To that end, cells reactivate some protein biosynthesis to prepare the cell for survival with extremely low ATP turnover. Hypoxia-dependent expression of key factors (such as HIF 1α) regulates this process. Housekeeping genes consolidate and stabilize the cell, and enzymes for anaerobic ATP production are upregulated [34, 35]. With changes like these, cells can function for a while with a very low oxygen delivery.

Relationship between oxygen delivery and oxygen consumption

As mentioned initially, the aim of anemia therapy is to match the tissues' demand for oxygen with supply. This demand is reflected by tissue oxygen consumption (VO_2). There is a relationship between oxygen delivery and oxygen consumption (Figure 2.2). Oxygen consumption remains constant over a wide range of delivery. At the point where oxygen consumption becomes supply dependent, tissue hypoxia may occur. This point is called "critical oxygen delivery" (DO_{2crit}). This, however, is not a fixed number, leaving room for therapeutic interventions.

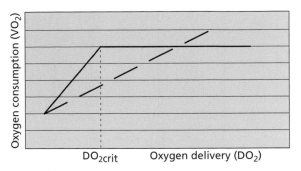

Figure 2.2 Relationship between oxygen delivery and oxygen consumption. Continuous line, healthy individuals; dashed line, pathological as in severe disease (with a wider range of dependence of oxygen consumption [VO_2] on oxygen delivery [DO_2], and a higher critical DO [DO_{2crit}]).

Practical implications

The oxygen delivery equation (see Eqn 2.1) may serve as a mnemonic for available anemia treatments. Every variable in the equation can be considered, based on which therapeutic interventions can be evaluated to optimize oxygen delivery. The cardiac output can be optimized by administering balanced amounts of intravenous fluids and removing negative inotropic influences or increasing positive inotropics as tolerated. The hemoglobin level can be increased, not only by speeding up endogenous hematopoiesis, but also by avoiding undue hemoglobin losses. Arterial oxygen partial pressure and oxygen saturation can be increased, using supplemental oxygen and mechanical ventilation as indicated. In addition, the amount of oxygen dissolved in plasma can be increased further by increasing the atmospheric pressure (hyperbaric oxygen).

A more complete picture of anemia therapy, though, is achieved when not only an increase of oxygen delivery is aimed at, but also a reduction of oxygen demand is contemplated. Oxygen delivery and consumption are related, since $VO_2 = DO_2 \times O_2$ ER. While not many interventions are available to increase oxygen extraction, quite a few things can be done to reduce oxygen consumption. "The four pillars of anemia therapy" (Figure 2.3) summarize how an understanding of physiology and pathophysiology may translate into a care plan. With the appropriate combination of factors that not only increase oxygen delivery but also reduce oxygen consumption, even hemoglobin levels well below the supposed critical level can be tolerated for some time without lasting damage

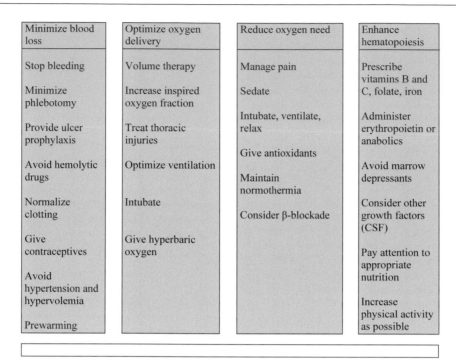

Minimize blood loss	Optimize oxygen delivery	Reduce oxygen need	Enhance hematopoiesis
Stop bleeding	Volume therapy	Manage pain	Prescribe vitamins B and C, folate, iron
Minimize phlebotomy	Increase inspired oxygen fraction	Sedate	
Provide ulcer prophylaxis	Treat thoracic injuries	Intubate, ventilate, relax	Administer erythropoietin or anabolics
Avoid hemolytic drugs	Optimize ventilation	Give antioxidants	Avoid marrow depressants
Normalize clotting	Intubate	Maintain normothermia	Consider other growth factors (CSF)
Give contraceptives	Give hyperbaric oxygen	Consider β-blockade	Pay attention to appropriate nutrition
Avoid hypertension and hypervolemia			Increase physical activity as possible
Prewarming			

Figure 2.3 The four pillars of anemia. CSF, colony stimulating factor.

[36], and even severely anemic patients can be treated successfully.

Key points

• Many mechanisms are used by the body to survive even severe anemia, including:
  ◦ Increased cardiac output
  ◦ Redistribution of blood flow to organs with high oxygen demand
  ◦ Increased oxygen extraction by tissues
  ◦ Improved FCD
  ◦ Decreased oxygen affinity of hemoglobin
  ◦ Metabolic adaptations to tolerate lower oxygen delivery.
• Therapeutic interventions are aimed at finding a new balance between oxygen delivery and oxygen consumption, by either increasing oxygen delivery or reducing oxygen consumption, or both at the same time.

Questions for review

1. What mechanisms support red cell oxygen uptake and oxygen release?
2. Where is oxygen release from the red cells to the tissues regulated?
3. What does the term functional capillary density mean? How can it be influenced?
4. How do red cells respond when decreasing oxygen levels are detected?
5. How is blood flow altered in anemic states?
6. How do adaptation methods for acute and chronic anemia differ?

Suggestions for further research

What different forms of hypoxia are there and how do they differ?

Exercises and practice cases

Read the following published case [37].

> A 37-year-old woman with a long history of Crohn's disease presented for bowel resection and drainage of an abdominal abscess. Her preoperative hematocrit was 30%. She consented to surgery but asked for therapy without the use of donor blood. The patient was taken to the operating room and surgery started. After the abdominal cavity was opened, she started hemorrhaging and in a period of 1 hour she lost 3 L of blood. Her hematocrit during surgery was 17%. After surgery, her hematocrit dropped to 4% (hemoglobin approx 1.3 g/dL). At that point, the patient was intubated and given morphine, muscle relaxants, oxygen ($FiO_2 = 1.0$), crystalloids, and colloids. Her body temperature was 30 °C, blood pressure 130/70 mmHg, heart rate 88, and cardiac output 5.3 L/min.

Using the following questions, try to understand the pathophysiology of her condition.
1. How did the patient adapt to the chronic anemia with a hematocrit of 30%?
2. Which pathophysiological mechanisms were activated in the patient when she had an intraoperative hematocrit of 17%?
3. Calculate how much oxygen was delivered to the patient when she had a hematocrit of 4%? How was the oxygen delivered?

Homework

Read the chapter again, drawing sketches as you read. These sketches will serve as the basis for education material in your future blood management program. Keep the drawings simple and use terms that are understandable to patients.

References

1. Vandegriff KD, Olson JS. Morphological and physiological factors affecting oxygen uptake and release by red blood cells. *J Biol Chem* 1984;**259**:12619–12627.
2. Coin JT, Olson JS. The rate of oxygen uptake by human red blood cells. *J Biol Chem* 1979;**254**:1178–1190.
3. Pries AR, Secomb TW, Gaehtgens P. Biophysical aspects of blood flow in the microvasculature. *Cardiovasc Res* 1996;**32**: 654–667.
4. Tuman KJ. Tissue oxygen delivery: the physiology of anemia. *ACNA* 1990;**8**:451–469.
5. Farhaeus R, Lindqvist T. The viscosity of the blood in narrow capillary tubes. *Am J Physiol* 1931;**96**:562–568.
6. Langenfeld JE, Machiedo GW, Lyons M, Rush BF Jr, Dikdan G, Lysz TW. Correlation between red blood cell deformability and changes in hemodynamic function. *Surgery* 1994;**116**: 859–867.
7. Intaglietta M, Johnson PC, Winslow RM. Microvascular and tissue oxygen distribution. *Cardiovasc Res* 1996;**32**: 632–643.
8. Mazzoni MC, Tsai AG, Intaglietta M. Blood and plasma viscosity and microvascular function in hemodilution. A perspective from La Jolla, California. *Eur Surg Res* 2002;**34**:101–105.
9. Stamler JS, Jia L, Eu JP, *et al*. Blood flow regulation by S-nitrosohemoglobin in the physiological oxygen gradient. *Science* 1997;**276**:2034–2037.
10. Longmuir IS. The effect of hypothermia on the affinity of tissues for oxygen. *Life Sci* 1962;**1**:297–300.
11. Wittenberg BA, Wittenberg JB. Transport of oxygen in muscle. *Annu Rev Physiol* 1989;**51**:857–878.
12. Clay AS, Behnia M, Brown KK. Mitochondrial disease: a pulmonary and critical-care medicine perspective. *Chest* 2001;**120**:634–648.
13. Intaglietta M. Microcirculatory basis for the design of artificial blood. *Microcirculation* 1999;**6**:247–258.
14. Schumacker PT, Rowland J, Saltz S, Nelson DP, Wood LD. Effects of hyperthermia and hypothermia on oxygen extraction by tissues during hypovolemia. *J Appl Physiol* 1987;**63**: 1246–1252.
15. Zander R. Oxygen supply and acid-base status in extreme anemia. *AINS* 1996;**31**:492–494.
16. Stehling L, Zauder HL. How low can we go? Is there a way to know? *Transfusion* 1990;**30**:1–3.
17. Zander R. Pathophysiology of hypovolemic shock. *Anasthesiol Intensivmed Notfallmed Schmerzther* 2001;**36** (Suppl 2):S137–S139.
18. Hebert PC, Szick S. The anemia patient in the ICU: how much does the heart tolerate? *AINS* 2001;**26**:S94–S100.
19. Landrow L. Perioperative hemodilution. *Can J Surg* 1987;**30**: 321–325.
20. Wahr JA. Myocardial ischaemia in anaemic patients. *Br J Anaesth* 1998;**81** (Suppl 1):10–15.
21. Morgan TJ, Endre ZH, Kanowski DM, Worthley LI, Jones RD. Siggaard-Andersen algorithm-derived p50 parameters: perturbation by abnormal hemoglobin-oxygen affinity and acid-base disturbances. *J Lab Clin Med* 1995;**126**: 365–372.
22. Borgstrom L, Johannsson H, Siesjo BK. The influence of acute normovolemic anemia on cerebral blood flow and

oxygen consumption of anesthetized rats. *Acta Physiol Scand* 1975;**93**:505–514.

23. Van der Linden P, Gilbart E, Paques P, Simon C, Vincent JL. Influence of hematocrit on tissue O2 extraction capabilities during acute hemorrhage. *Am J Physiol* 1993;**264**: H1942–H1947.

24. Habler O, Kleen M, Kemming G, Zwissler B. Hyperoxia in extreme hemodilution. *Eur Surg Res* 2002;**34**:181–187.

25. Deem S, Hedges RG, McKinney S, Polissar NL, Alberts MK, Swenson ER. Mechanisms of improvement in pulmonary gas exchange during isovolemic hemodilution. *J Appl Physiol* 1999;**87**:132–141.

26. Deem S, Alberts MK, Bishop MJ, Bidani A, Swenson ER. CO$_2$ transport in normovolemic anemia: complete compensation and stability of blood CO$_2$ tensions. *J Appl Physiol* 1997;**83**:240–246.

27. Agarwal JB, Paltoo R, Palmer WH. Relative viscosity of blood at varying hematocrits in pulmonary circulation. *J Appl Physiol* 1970;**29**:866–871.

28. Lopez-Barneo J. Oxygen-sensing by ion channels and the regulation of cellular functions. *Trends Neurosci* 1996;**19**: 435–440.

29. Motterlini R, Vandegriff KD, Winslow RM. Hemoglobin-nitric oxide interaction and its implications. *Transfus Med Rev* 1996;**10**:77–84.

30. Deem S, Berg JT, Kerr ME, Swenson ER. Effects of the RBC membrane and increased perfusate viscosity on hypoxic pulmonary vasoconstriction. *J Appl Physiol* 2000;**88**: 1520–1528.

31. Tsai AG, Intaglietta M. Hemodilution and increased plasma viscosity for the design of new plasma expanders. *TATM* 2001;**3**:17–23.

32. Gutierrez G, Marini C, Acero AL, Lund N. Skeletal muscle PO$_2$ during hypoxemia and isovolemic anemia. *J Appl Physiol* 1990;**68**:2047–2053.

33. Hogan MC, Bebout DE, Wagner PD. Effect of hemoglobin concentration on maximal O$_2$ uptake in canine gastrocnemius muscle in situ. *J Appl Physiol* 1991;**70**:1105–1112.

34. Csete M. Respiration in anesthesia pathophysiology and clinical update: cellular response to hypoxia. *ACNA* 1998;**16**: 201–210.

35. Hochachka PW, Buck LT, Doll CJ, Land SC. Unifying theory of hypoxia tolerance: molecular/metabolic defense and rescue mechanisms for surviving oxygen lack. *Proc Natl Acad Sci U S A* 1996;**93**:9493–9498.

36. Welte M. Is there a "critical hematocrit?" *Anaesthesist* 2001;**50** (Suppl 1):S2–S8.

37. Lichtenstein A, Eckhart WF, Swanson KJ, Vacanti CA, Zapol WM. Unplanned intraoperative and postoperative hemodilution: oxygen transport and consumption during severe anemia. *Anesthesiology* 1988;**69**:119–122.

3 Anemia Therapy I: Erythropoiesis-Stimulating Agents

Untreated and progressive anemia increases both morbidity and mortality of patients. Anemia, therefore, should be screened for, properly diagnosed, and treated. Under normal circumstances, the patient's own bone marrow should be able to produce the required cell lines, including red blood cells.

This chapter is one of two that address anemia and anemia therapy. Here, we will consider hormone and cytokine therapy of anemia, and in the next chapter we will address the products for blood restoration.

Objectives

1. To review the physiological role of hormones and cytokines in erythropoiesis.
2. To increase knowledge of recombinant human erythropoietin (rHuEPO) as a medication.
3. To define the risk–benefit ratio of rHuEPO in different settings.
4. To compare EPO with its analogs.

Definitions

Erythropoietin: EPO is a naturally occurring hormone that stimulates erythropoiesis, i.e., the synthesis of red blood cells. A recombinant equivalent of human EPO (rHuEPO) and chemically produced stimulants are available for therapeutic use.

Anabolic steroids: These are the hormones derived from androgens. They not only influence metabolism, but also have effects on erythropoiesis.

A brief history

For decades, it has been known that there is a factor that stimulates the production of red blood cells. It was possible to transfer this factor from one individual to another. Transfusing the plasma from an anemic individual into someone else caused acceleration of hematopoiesis [1]. It was not until 1977, however, that Miyake *et al.* [2] isolated the factor from the urine of patients with aplastic anemia. Early experiments used material extracted from urine. The cumbersome process of purification limited the use of this factor for research. Yet, it was possible to identify the gene for EPO. In 1985, Lin *et al.* [1] and Jacobs *et al.* [3] cloned that gene, and EPO became the first hematopoietic growth factor to be cloned [4]. This laid the foundation for the mass production of rHuEPO and accelerated research in this field. In 1987, Sawyer *et al.* described the receptor for EPO [5, 6] and shed further light on the interaction of the hormone and its target.

With record speed, rHuEPO found its way into clinical practice. Kidney failure as the cause of anemia due to a lack of EPO was the first condition that was successfully treated with rHuEPO. More recently, other potential clinical benefits of EPO have been discovered, suggesting an expanded use of rHuEPO in other disease states.

Erythropoietin in normal erythropoiesis

EPO is a naturally occurring hormone. Prior to birth, it is produced in the liver. Within weeks, the main production shifts to the kidneys. After total nephrectomy,

Basics of Blood Management, Second Edition. Petra Seeber and Aryeh Shander.
© 2013 John Wiley & Sons, Ltd. Published 2013 by John Wiley & Sons, Ltd.

residual EPO is detectable as some (in adults <5%) EPO is synthesized in the liver.

Basal EPO secretion has a circadian cycle with levels higher in the evening than in the morning. There are no stores of preformed EPO [4]. EPO is produced on demand. Current thinking is that the main, but not only, stimulus for secretion of EPO is hypoxia. This may be caused by anemia, lung disease, or high-altitude living. The EPO gene has an enhancer where hypoxic-inducing factor (HIF)-1 (a transcription factor that is induced by hypoxia) attaches and induces EPO gene transcription and subsequent EPO synthesis.

Normal EPO levels in non-anemic persons range between 6 and 32 U/L. The levels are similar in men and women. In severe hypoxia or anemia, EPO levels may rise 1000 times above normal. Provided there is enough EPO, basal erythropoiesis may increase six- to eight-fold [7].

The target of this hormone is the EPO receptor. This receptor consists of extracellular, transmembrane, and intracellular domains. EPO binds to its receptor on the cell surface. Afterward, it is ingested into the cell by receptor-mediated endocytosis. Tyrosines on the intracellular domain of the receptor are phosphorylated and an intracellular signaling process is initiated. As a result, gene expression in the nucleus is modulated. This effects the changes EPO mediates.

EPO acts as a "survival factor" in erythropoiesis (Table 3.1). It is not involved in the commitment of the erythroid lineage. EPO mainly promotes survival, proliferation, and differentiation of erythroid progenitors. Therefore, it saves cells from natural cell death (apoptosis). In hematopoiesis, the main EPO targets are progenitor cells: burst-forming unit erythroid (BFU-E) and colony-forming unit erythroid (CFU-E) [8]. BFU-Es possess only a small number of EPO receptors and are relatively resistant to the influence of EPO. The main EPO receptors in the erythroid lineage are CFU-Es. They react even at low concentrations of EPO. Erythro-

Table 3.1 Review: steps in erythropoiesis.

Totipotent stem cell	Undifferentiated hematopoietic cell with a high degree of proliferation capability. Stem cells self-renew or differentiate, depending on the environment and extrinsic factors, e.g., cytokines. Descendants of stem cells develop into specialized cells (= "commitment")
CFU-S ↓	This is one of the two forms that can originate from stem cells. CFU-S is the origin of colony-forming units for leukocytes and platelets. It is also the precursor of the red cell lineage
BFU-E* ↓	BFU-E are stimulated by EPO and other growth factors
CFU-E* ↓	CFU-Es are mainly stimulated by EPO
Proerythroblast ↓	One proerythroblast is the origin of 16 mature red cells
Basophilic erythroblast ↓	
Polychromatophilic erythroblast ↓	
Orthochromatic erythroblast ↓	It has a pyknotic nucleus that is extruded at this stage of development
Reticulocyte ↓	It is released from the bone marrow typically 2–3 days after nucleus extrusion. It contains Golgi apparatus, small amounts of RNA, and mitochondria that are lost 24–48 hours after release from bone marrow
Erythrocyte	Mature red cells

Follow the lines in the table from top to bottom and review how a red cell develops out of a totipotent stem cell.
*The terms BFU-E and CFU-E describe the cell's growth patterns under laboratory conditions.
CFU-S, colony-forming units spleen; BFU-E, burst-forming units erythroid; CFU-E, colony-forming units erythroid.

poietin receptors are also found on proerythroblasts. In the late erythroid precursors, EPO receptors diminish. There are no EPO receptors on reticulocytes and erythrocytes. Besides influencing the survival of erythroid progenitors, EPO accelerates the release of reticulocytes from the bone marrow. Therapy with rHuEPO also increases the amount of fetal hemoglobin by increasing the number of reticulocytes.

Recombinant human erythropoietin as a drug

rHuEPO is a sialylglycoprotein. It has three N-linked oligosaccharide chains. The carbohydrate part of rHuEPO with its sialic acid is used for biological activities in the body. If it were not for sialic acid residues, EPO would be removed from the circulation within minutes.

Under laboratory conditions, it is possible to synthesize rHuEPO through different cell lines. Nowadays, Chinese hamster ovary cells or other cultured cells are used for the pharmacological production of rHuEPO. rHuEPO is biologically active and reacts in a way similar to the natural hormone purified from urine. To date, several forms of rHuEPO are commercially available: EPO alpha, EPO beta, and EPO omega. They have slightly different carbohydrate residues but are equally effective in stimulating erythropoiesis. In addition, so-called "biosimilars" are emerging. These are generic compounds typically produced after the patent rights of the original products have expired. Anticipated reduced costs will hopefully result from the introduction of these chemically produced agents. The biosimilar agents have somewhat different protein structures that may lead to side effects, possibly including antibody formation. However, clinically they should have efficacy similar to the original EPO in enhancing erythropoiesis.

rHuEPO requires parenteral application (either intravenously or subcutaneously) to stimulate erythropoiesis. Intraperitoneal application is also possible. Patients on peritoneal dialysis may prefer this route of administration. The half-life of rHuEPO given intravenously is 3–16 hours, but this declines after multiple doses. If given subcutaneously, the half-life is about 12–28 hours. It takes 5–18 hours until maximum serum concentration is reached. Bioavailability of subcutaneously administered rHuEPO is approximately 30%.

The metabolic "fate" of rHuEPO is poorly understood. When used by erythrocyte precursors, it is removed from the circulation by being taken up into these cells. Less than 5% of the administered rHuEPO is excreted unchanged through the kidneys. Parts of the remaining hormone are desialylated and metabolized by the liver.

Dose and response relationship

The onset of hematocrit recovery in normal postsurgical patients with severe anemia shows a 1-week lag if no rHuEPO is given. This is because endogenous EPO has to be synthesized and iron stores need to be mobilized. In contrast, the erythropoietic effect of rHuEPO starts almost immediately. It takes some time until the results can be detected by laboratory testing. The higher the initial doses of rHuEPO, the faster hematocrit recovery occurs [9]. Reticulocytosis can be detected within 2–3 days. Some laboratories are also able to count the immature reticulocyte fraction (IRF). IRF may be a valuable tool in detecting early response to rHuEPO therapy.

rHuEPO dosage is calculated on an individual basis. Much depends on the patient's underlying medical condition and the response to therapy. Daily administration is warranted in patients with severe anemia and in those in need of rapid increase in red cell mass. Other dosing schedules of rHuEPO, including three times or once a week, may be used for patients for whom there is sufficient time to prepare for elective surgery. It appears that rHuEPO therapy on a weekly schedule for some weeks prior to surgery is as effective as daily perioperative rHuEPO dosing [10]. Refer to Table 3.2 for dosage recommendations to administer rHuEPO in different clinical settings [11–28].

Side effects

rHuEPO is remarkably safe and well tolerated by patients. Only about 10% of patients receiving rHuEPO experience self-limiting flu-like symptoms with bone pain. This is an expression of hemopoiesis activation. Other than in cases of renal disease, significant side effects have only rarely been reported.

A hypertensive response after rHuEPO administration has been observed mainly in patients with chronic renal failure. This hypertension may be the result of the reversal of anemic vasodilatation and the increase in hematocrit. Hemodynamic adaptation to the reversal of anemia may be too slow in uremic patients and so hypertension may develop. Controlled slow increase of hematocrit levels in such patients reduces the risk of severe hypertension. Hypertension may resolve spontaneously by continuing EPO therapy. Regular blood pressure monitoring is advisable for patients receiving rHuEPO. If necessary, antihypertensive therapy can be started.

Table 3.2 Typical rHuEPO dose regimens.

Setting	Dose
Preparation for surgery—elective (days 21, 14, 7 and 0)	150–300 IU/kg s.c. 3×/week
Preparation for surgery—urgent (daily starting 10 days before day 0)	10 000–40 000 IU as soon as possible
Hematological diseases (sickle cell disease, thalassemia, aplastic anemia)	200–400 IU/kg daily or as needed
Anemia in chronic inflammatory processes, such as rheumatoid arthritis, inflammatory bowel disease	40–300 IU/kg 2×/week for 3 months
Critically ill patients (40 000 U once weekly or 10 000 3x/weekly)	300–600 IU/kg daily or every other day
Chronic renal failure	50–100 IU/kg in the correction phase and 25–100 IU/kg in the maintenance phase, each 3×/week; some patients require more; longer-acting erythropoietic agents may be better for chronic phase
Anemia in pregnancy	300 IU/kg 2×/week
Cancer-related anemia	Starting with 40 000 IU and continuing to reach pre-set hemoglobin levels
Premature babies	300 IU/kg 2×/week

Seizures were also observed in dialysis patients receiving rHuEPO, especially during the initial treatment phase when the hematocrit can rise rapidly. Often, there is a combination of hypertension and seizures. The danger of provoking a seizure is reduced if rHuEPO is administered in a way that induces a gradual increase in hematocrit.

Minor allergic reactions after administration of rHuEPO have been reported (such as urticaria). Another type of immune response is the development of antibodies to rHuEPO (and naturally occurring EPO), leading to pure red cell aplasia (PRCA). This was reported mainly in patients on long-term treatment and in those with uremia and myelodysplastic syndromes. While this is very rare, it is a serious side effect. If PRCA occurs, rHuEPO must be stopped immediately. Switching to another brand of rHuEPO does not improve the situation. Actually, rHuEPO is contraindicated if antibodies develop. However, hematide, an EPO-receptor agonist without structural similarity to naturally occurring EPO, may normalize erythropoiesis in PRCA. Another approach to the therapy of PRCA is a short-term regimen of immunosuppressive therapy with corticoids, cyclosporine, cyclophosphamide, immunoglobulins, or plasmapheresis. Spontaneous reversal of the PRCA can occur, but is extremely rare.

While rHuEPO mainly influences the erythroid precursors, it has also some influence on megakaryocytes and on precursors of leukocytes. Increased platelet counts and monocyte counts were observed in patients with renal failure, although levels remained within normal limits. On rare occasions, thrombocytosis, requiring low-dose aspirin therapy, has been reported.

Some of the side effects or rHuEPO are actually beneficial. Mild defects in hemostasis observed in uremic and severely anemic patients were corrected by using rHuEPO [17]. "Tests performed in small numbers of hemodialysis patients at baseline and following normalization of hematocrit with epoetin therapy have demonstrated improved cerebral blood flow, information processing, overall cognitive function, mood state, subjective health and physical activity, and decreased dialysis-related and general treatment-related stress, and fatigue, following correction of anemia." Anemia therapy using rHuEPO was shown to reverse insulin resistance as well as amino acid and lipid abnormalities in dialysis-dependent patients [29]. Reduced fatigue and improved well-being are also observed in patients with cancer-related anemia that is treated with rHuEPO [17].

In addition to the above-mentioned side effects, venous thrombosis and cancer progression have been attributed to rHuEPO therapy [30]. Whether EPO is causative or only related to these disorders is yet to be established. However, some findings provide potential explanations for the development of thrombosis and for cancer progression after rHuEPO therapy (see below).

Effects not directly related to erythropoiesis

In recent years, insight has been gained into the biological role of EPO. As mentioned above, EPO acts as a hormone. In this endocrine function, it originates mainly in the kidneys and is transported by the blood plasma to the target tissues. EPO receptors are distributed throughout the body, including the central nervous system. The heart, retina, vessels, lungs, liver, gastrointestinal tract, ovaries, and uterus also carry EPO receptors. Apart from the kidneys and liver, other tissues are able to produce EPO and EPO-like molecules but do not release EPO into the circulation. The synthesized EPO is used by neighboring cells (paracrine) or by the producing cell itself (autocrine).

In the paracrine and autocrine process, EPO has a wide spectrum of actions, which can be mimicked by exogenously administered rHuEPO. It protects tissues by preventing vascular spasm, cell death (apoptosis), and inflammatory responses. Erythropoietin promotes growth of vessels and improves tissue regeneration. This seems to be beneficial in patients with myocardial infarction, after heart surgery, in chronic heart failure, and for wound and skin graft healing. rHuEPO is able to protect the brain and spinal cord, myocardium, and other tissues from hypoxia [31]. Experimental evidence supports the assumption that EPO plays a role in the regeneration after brain and spinal injury [32–34]. rHuEPO may therefore not only be beneficial in increasing red cell mass, but may also protect tissues until hypoxia is resolved. This effect has been shown to occur even if rHuEPO is given shortly prior to or immediately following the insult [35]. These protective and proliferative effects are probably also exerted on tumor cells, which may at least partially explain the above-mentioned finding that rHuEPO can promote cancer progression. Whether the benefit to be gained from EPO outweighs its potential damage is the subject of current clinical studies.

EPO also has an effect on muscles. Minutes after administration, muscle strength is detectably increased. EPO acts so quickly that it can exert considerable beneficial effects in cardiopulmonary arrest [36]. EPO can even be found in human milk. Epithelial tissue in the mammary gland produces EPO and secretes it with the milk. The suckling baby may benefit from the oral intake of EPO.

Erythropoietin hyporesponsiveness

The term "erythropoietin hyporesponsiveness" (or erythropoietin resistance) refers to situations where—despite sufficiently high doses of rHuEPO—the erythropoietic response is undetectable or minimal. Several conditions cause EPO hyporesponsiveness. Many of them are treatable. However, causes of EPO hyporesponsiveness that are not treatable do not necessarily constitute a contraindication to rHuEPO therapy. Patients who do not respond to the initial dose may respond to higher doses of rHuEPO.

Treating EPO hyporesponsiveness is imperative if the patient is to derive any benefit. Continuation of the rHuEPO therapy in cases of obvious EPO hyporesponsiveness may be of no benefit. Often, the reason for EPO hyporesponsiveness can be elucidated and treated.

Erythropoiesis can be increased above the basal level. This potential increase, however, is limited by iron availability. Healthy humans can provide sufficient iron to triple their basal erythropoiesis. If erythropoiesis is increased more than three-fold, a functional iron deficiency develops. This happens even in the presence of full iron reserves (= relative iron deficiency). Patients who require rHuEPO may also exhibit absolute iron deficiency. Dialysis patients, for instance, lose blood from frequent testing and the process of dialysis itself. Occult gastrointestinal hemorrhage may further increase blood loss and subsequently lead to depletion of iron stores. No matter whether or not a patient has a measurable iron deficiency, patients who receive rHuEPO therapy require iron supplementation.

Also, iron overload may also cause EPO hyporesponsiveness. Even in this case, functional iron deficiency can occur. Treatment with supplemental iron may resolve this problem, but it may also contribute to further iron overload. To circumvent this effect, ascorbic acid infusions (e.g., 200–500 mg i.v., three times a week) were proposed instead of iron infusions [37]. Ascorbic acid is able to mobilize iron from the stores and increases iron utilization in the erythroid progenitor cells. Ascorbic acid infusions in iron overload may not only increase the hematocrit when given with rHuEPO, but may also reduce rHuEPO requirements.

Closely related to iron metabolism is aluminum metabolism. Both metals are bound to transferrin. Aluminum inhibits iron uptake in the gastrointestinal tract, decreases iron utilization, and interferes with heme biosynthesis. Therefore, it can cause EPO hyporesponsiveness. Patients on dialysis are particularly prone to aluminum overload. Monitoring aluminum serum levels is warranted in such patients, and chelation therapy with available chelating medications may be prescribed in case of overload.

Infection and inflammation in chronic diseases can also cause EPO hyporesponsiveness. Cytokines involved in the inflammatory process act on different stages of erythropoiesis. Interferon-γ downregulates the EPO receptor at the surface of erythroid precursors [4]. Tumor necrosis factor suppresses EPO production in the kidneys. Optimizing the treatment of infection and inflammation reduces certain cytokine levels and may recover EPO responsiveness. In some cases, however, it may be necessary to treat inflammation-related anemia with high doses of rHuEPO, since higher doses may overcome the inhibitory effects of cytokines in these cases [38].

Hyperparathyroidism may diminish the body's response to rHuEPO. High serum levels of parathyroid hormone exert toxic effects on EPO synthesis and erythropoiesis. Furthermore, it can cause marrow fibrosis, interfering with red cell production. Surgical or medical (vitamin D analogs) correction of hyperparathyroidism improves the response to rHuEPO [38].

Logically, the lack of substrates for erythropoiesis also causes EPO hyporesponsiveness. Deficiency of any of the hematinics (as discussed in Chapter 4) can be the culprit. This is true not only for iron but also for folate, vitamins B_6 and B_{12}, and L-carnitine. Replenishing deficient vitamins and their derivatives may resolve EPO hyporesponsiveness and may even decrease rHuEPO requirements and costs.

Several other factors can cause EPO hyporesponsiveness. Among these are uremia, severe metabolic acidosis, and oxalosis [39]. Patients with hemoglobinopathies, red cell enzyme deficiencies, and other red cell abnormalities may not respond to the usual doses of rHuEPO [40].

Various medications may interfere with rHuEPO therapy. Theophylline, an adenosine antagonist, lowers plasma levels of EPO in normal humans. The rate of EPO secretion is related to the activity of the renin–angiotensin system [39] and is therefore influenced by some antihypertensive medications, specifically angiotensin-converting enzyme inhibitors.

Flow charts like the one shown in Figure 3.1 are helpful for the efficient work-up of patients with EPO hyporesponsiveness.

Adjuvant therapy

The therapy with rHuEPO can be costly. Adjuvant therapies are available to increase the effectiveness of rHuEPO therapy and hence reduce total costs. While studies on adjuvant therapies usually involve patients on dialysis, the basic principles apply to other patient groups as well. Below we consider some supplements that are valuable as adjuvants to rHuEPO therapy.

Iron

As long as there is no contraindication to iron therapy, it should be given to all patients on rHuEPO. In the majority of cases and when possible, intravenous iron is preferable.

Ascorbic acid

Ascorbic acid can resolve functional iron deficiency even in patients with iron overload. It facilitates the uptake of iron in the gastrointestinal tract and supports hematopoiesis.

Vitamin D

The erythropoiesis in patients with secondary hyperparathyroidism can be improved with vitamin D therapy and its analogs, since the unwanted effects of high parathyroid hormone levels are alleviated. It is still a matter of discussion whether therapy with vitamin D analogs is also beneficial for patients without hyperparathyroidism. Some patients experience an improvement in their anemia by taking calcitriol, even if they do not have hyperparathyroidism. However, the routine use of vitamin D analogs is not recommended for anemia therapy since studies are still in their preliminary phase [39, 41].

Vitamins of the B group

Vitamins of the B group, such as B_{12}, B_6, and folic acid, are needed for erythropoiesis. Since their turnover is increased in accelerated erythropoiesis, patients should receive sufficient amounts of those vitamins [39].

L-Carnitine

L-Carnitine is able to increase the reticulocyte count and hematocrit even if no rHuEPO is given. It may also

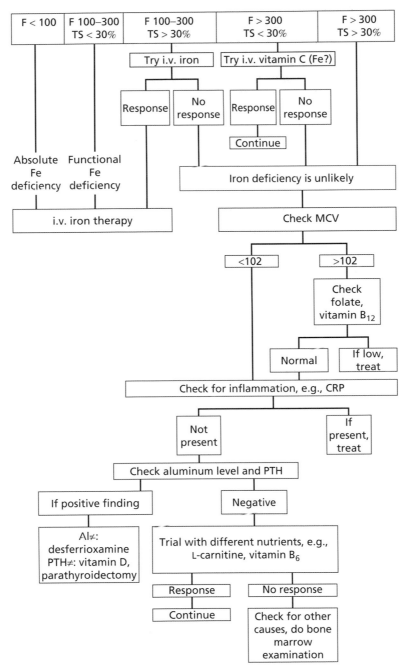

Figure 3.1 Erythropoietin hyporesponsiveness. MCV, mean corpuscular volume; CRP, C-reactive protein; PTH, parathyroid hormone; F, ferritin; TS, transferrin saturation.

increase erythrocyte membrane stability and has a beneficial effect on erythrocyte survival. Several studies demonstrate a reduced requirement for rHuEPO if L-carnitine
is given concomitantly [42]. Because of lack of available
data, recommendations for the routine use of L-carnitine
are not available. A trial of L-carnitine may be indicated
in patients with suspected deficiency [39, 42].

Patient selection

rHuEPO is one of those medications used illicitly by ath-
letes to enhance their athletic performance. This vividly
demonstrates that rHuEPO is a potent medication that
works in healthy people as well. It also helps in accelerating recovery from anemia due to a variety of causes. The
indications of rHuEPO therapy can be classified as stimulation of:
• Normal erythropoiesis with appropriate levels of EPO
to prevent either initiation or progression of anemia
(prophylactic use)
• Normal erythropoiesis with low levels of EPO
• Impaired erythropoiesis with low, normal, or high
levels of EPO.

Prevention is better than cure

Patients who are expected to develop anemia in the
course of their treatment are candidates for preventive
measures. Patients scheduled for chemotherapy and
those who were anemic at the onset of their chemotherapy have been shown to benefit from preventive and
therapeutic rHuEPO therapy, respectively. Patients who
develop anemia during their first therapy cycle also
benefit from rHuEPO administration. rHuEPO helps
such patients to maintain an acceptable hemoglobin level
by boosting their own erythropoiesis. Transfusions are
reduced [43].

rHuEPO also prevents anemia in the surgical setting.
Acute normovolemic hemodilution is facilitated by an
increased preoperative hematocrit. More units can be
drawn before the patient reaches the lowest acceptable
hemoglobin level. The more units that are drawn before
reaching this level, the lower the likelihood of allogeneic
transfusion exposure. Patients who do not donate their
blood before surgery benefit as well [44–46]. The hemoglobin level is a key predictor for the use of perioperative
allogeneic transfusions. Increasing the preoperative
hematocrit to high–normal values increases the tolerable
blood loss [24] and decreases the use of allogeneic transfusions. Perioperative hematocrit values of 45–50% are
usually well tolerated.

Practice tip Prescribing rHuEPO before surgery

Here is an example of a therapeutic regimen for a slightly
anemic adult patient who will undergo hip replacement in
14 days:
rHuEPO 20 000 U s.c. on Monday, Wednesday, and Friday
   for 2 weeks
   Plus daily:
Iron tablets 200 mg—1–1–1
Vitamin B$_{12}$ tablets 500 μg—1–0- 0
Folate tablets 20 mg—1–1–1
Vitamin C tablets 100 mg—1–1–1
   Monitoring:
Finger stick hemoglobin every Friday and blood pressure
   measurement with every dose

Stimulating normal erythropoiesis

There are situations where erythropoiesis is already stimulated by endogenous EPO but, for some reason, a more
rapid recovery of the blood count is needed. Since the
speed of hemoglobin recovery depends on the serum
levels of EPO, giving additional rHuEPO accelerates the
replenishment of the red blood cells. Usually, mid to high
doses of rHuEPO are given to expedite recovery.

Blood loss is a normal feature of childbirth and has
become an accepted feature of some surgical procedures.
If the blood loss is significant or the patient had been sent
to surgery with a low hemoglobin, these patients are likely
to be anemic postoperatively. rHuEPO is used to improve
postoperative and postpartum red cell mass recovery
[47]. Patients reach an acceptable hemoglobin level
earlier and may be able to leave the hospital and resume
normal activity sooner.

rHuEPO also plays a role in pregnancy complicated by
anemia. Anemia during pregnancy and gestation may
endanger mother and child. It increases the risk of miscarriage, infections, and peripartal hemorrhage. If iron
and vitamin therapy alone are not sufficient, rHuEPO can
be added [18].

When erythropoietin is missing

Some forms of anemia are due to low levels of endogenous EPO. The prototype of erythropoietin deficiency
develops in kidney failure. rHuEPO is effective treatment
for the anemia developing under such circumstances.
Also, premature babies have a relative EPO deficiency.
The immature kidneys are unable to produce sufficient
amounts of EPO. This is especially true during the phase

when erythropoietin production is switched from the liver to the kidney. During this time, babies may benefit from rHuEPO therapy [48, 49].

When erythropoiesis is impaired

A great variety of hematological disorders are accompanied by anemia. In such settings, the use of rHuEPO is often very effective. Here are two examples:

• **Sickle cell disease:** Patients with sickle cell disease have been shown to benefit from rHuEPO therapy. In the course of their disease, they suffer hemolysis and painful crises. The underlying defect is the presence of the abnormal sickle hemoglobin. If patients are given rHuEPO, the level of fetal hemoglobin increases and the amount of sickle hemoglobin decreases. This improves the condition of the patients [11].

• **Aplastic anemia:** rHuEPO alone, or in combination with other hematopoietic growth factors, has been successfully used in the treatment of some patients with aplastic anemia [12].

Erythropoiesis is also impaired in patients with chronic inflammatory disease. Inflammatory cytokines hinder EPO's ability to attach to its receptor and to stimulate erythropoiesis. They decrease the sensitivity of erythrogenic progenitor cells to EPO [13]. As a means of compensation, higher levels of endogenous EPO circulate in the plasma. Anemia may exist despite high levels of endogenous EPO. Nevertheless, rHuEPO may be beneficial. Very high doses of rHuEPO partially counteract the effects of inflammatory cytokines and abolish anemia.

Some relatively common chronic disorders were studied in order to evaluate the potential benefits of rHuEPO therapy. The following are examples:

• **Rheumatoid arthritis:** Inflammatory cytokines may affect hematopoiesis. If an optimal anti-inflammatory therapy cannot improve anemia, rHuEPO is available to increase hematocrit levels [50, 51].

• **Inflammatory bowel disease:** Plasma concentration of EPO is raised in patients with inflammatory bowel disease. Despite these raised levels, concentrations are inadequate to reverse anemia. rHuEPO is effective in increasing the hemoglobin level [14].

• **Anemia associated with acquired immunodeficiency syndrome (AIDS):** Anemia is common among patients with AIDS. This is not only due to the presence of the disease but also due to the administered therapies (e.g., zidovudine). rHuEPO can be used to reverse the anemia developing in AIDS patients [52].

• **Malignancy:** rHuEPO is useful when dealing with anemia in cancer patients [53]. Anemia may develop due to an inhibition of erythropoiesis by cytokines, blood loss, and/or hemolysis. In addition, chemotherapy induces anemia due to myelosuppression or nephrotoxicity. rHuEPO either increases the hematocrit levels or prevents it from falling. It also allows for a more intensive therapy regimen [19]. Stem cell and bone marrow harvesting as well as bone marrow transplantation are facilitated by rHuEPO therapy. Mild anemia associated with cancer, which is typically not considered an indication for allogeneic transfusion, has an impact on patients' well-being since patients frequently feel tired. Fatigue caused by anemia is another setting where rHuEPO is used. This dramatically improves the patient's quality of life.

Despite these beneficial effects, concerns have been raised regarding rHuEPO therapy in cancer patients, as outlined above. Therefore, rHuEPO therapy is recommended for use only in accordance with current guidelines, e.g., those published by the National Comprehensive Cancer Network (NCCN), European Organization for the Research and Treatment of Cancer (EORTC), American Society for Clinical Oncology (ASCO) or American Society of Hematology (ASH) [54].

• **Critical illness:** Patients in an intensive care unit are often anemic and approximately 85% of those admitted to the intensive care unit for more than 1 week receive donated red blood cells, typically for chronic rather than acute blood loss. Hospitalized and especially critically ill patients develop anemia over the course of time. This multifactorial process includes a reduced erythropoietic response due to inflammation and iatrogenic blood loss. rHuEPO is able to alleviate the anemia of critical illness [16] and has been shown to improve outcome.

Practice tip Use of erythropoiesis-stimulating agents (ESAs) for patients with cancer undergoing chemotherapy

• Rule out other causes of anemia (iron deficiency, blood loss, hemolysis, etc.)
• Discuss ESA therapy with the patient, informing him/her of the 1.6-fold higher risk of thromboembolic complications
• Set an individual target hemoglobin
• Initiate ESA therapy when hemoglobin level falls below 10 g/dL (consider ESA therapy in patients with an Hb between 10 and 12 g/dL, depending on the risk–benefit evaluation and patient preference)

Continued

- Start with 40 000 IU or 150 IU/kg rHuEPO weekly or 2.25 µg/kg darbepoetin weekly or 500 µg darbepoetin every 3 weeks
- Increase dose according to FDA recommendations if there is no response after 4 weeks
- Modify dosing according to FDA recommendations when there is >1 g/dL increase in Hb in any 2-week period
- Discontinue therapy after 8 weeks if there is no response despite optimal anemia management
- Add iron therapy, e.g., initially 100 mg i.v./week, or depending on continually monitored iron stores

Source: Rizzo *et al.* [54].

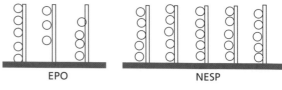

■ Protein backbone
▭ Carbohydrate chain
○ Sialic acid residue

Figure 3.2 Structure of erythropoietin (EPO) and novel erythropoietin-stimulating protein (NESP; engineered to contain five N-linked carbohydrate chains carrying sialic acid residues).

Other erythropoiesis-stimulating agents

In addition to rHuEPO, many other medications have been developed to stimulate hematopoiesis. Among them are the novel erythropoiesis-stimulating protein (darbepoetin), the continuous EPO receptor activator (CERA), and hematide (peginesatide) [55–59].

Novel erythropoiesis-stimulating protein (darbepoetin)

EPO depends on its sialic acid molecules for a prolonged plasma half-life. If these molecules are lost, EPO is rapidly cleared from the blood. In turn, the half-life of EPO is increased when it contains more sialic acid molecules. Based on this fact, it was hypothesized that increasing the amount of sialic acid would increase the serum half-life, and indeed it did. An analog of EPO, a novel erythropoiesis-stimulating protein (NESP; darbepoetin), was engineered by adding two additional oligosaccharide chains with sialic acid residues to the EPO molecule (Figure 3.2). This prolonged the half-life of the new agent considerably. Darbepoetin remains in the blood stream approximately three times longer than does rHuEPO [60].

Darbepoetin is a molecule that is somewhat larger than EPO (38 000 compared to 30 400 Da). It also attaches to the EPO receptor [61], but with a somewhat lower affinity than EPO.

The greatest advantage of darbepoetin is its prolonged half-life. This allows for less frequent administration. A single dose once a week or even once every 2–3 weeks is sufficient to maintain erythropoiesis. Especially patients dependent on long-term EPO substitution benefit from this. Several studies conducted in dialysis patients dem-

onstrated the clinical value of darbepoetin [62]. The same is true for cancer patients [63, 64]. Darbepoetin is useful in the initiation of anemia therapy as well as long-term maintenance therapy.

Continuous EPO receptor activator

Taking the addition of half-life–prolonging molecules to EPO a step further, methoxy-polyethyleneglycol was added to erythropoietin. This resulted in the creation of an erythropoietic agent called continuous EPO receptor activator (CERA) with a half-life of about 130 hours. Therefore, only one or two doses per month are needed. CERA was approved only recently and is used mainly in renal failure. Therapeutic trials are underway to explore the utility of CERA in tumor patients.

Hematide (peginesatide)

Unrelated to the protein structure of the original EPO but still capable of activating the EPO receptor is hematide, a small, peptide-based EPO-mimetic. It is administered parenterally and stimulates erythropoiesis. An advantage is that antibodies to EPO do not cross-react with hematide, so that the latter is an apt candidate for anemia therapy in PRCA. Besides, it has the potential to be useful in anemia due to renal failure. Since it is excreted by the kidneys, it has a prolonged half-life in kidney failure and needs to be given only once per month. It has yet to be approved for clinical use.

Anabolic steroids

The average hematocrit of men is higher than that of women. This is the result of the androgen testosterone stimulating formation of EPO. It increases endogenous EPO production and enhances the sensitivity of erythroid progenitors to available EPO. Persons with bilateral nephrectomy do not benefit much from androgen therapy, since the presence of at least one kidney is needed for a favorable response to androgen therapy in anemia.

Anabolic steroids are derivatives of androgens. Among them are 19-nortestosterone derivatives and 17-alkylated androgens. Examples of androgens used for anemia therapy are nandrolone (e.g., 200 mg/week i.m.) [65–68] and danazol [69–71].

Androgen therapy has been tried for a variety of anemia types, such as in bone marrow failure and myelofibrosis. About half of patients with anemia, particularly cases with bone marrow involvement, respond with an increase in red cell mass. Aplastic anemia may also respond well to androgens. Before the advent of rHuEPO, androgens were also used in the management of anemia in dialysis patients [72]. When used in elderly males (>50 years) on dialysis, it increases hemoglobin levels to a similar degree as equivalent doses of rHuEPO would [65].

The cost of anabolics is considerably lower than that of equivalent doses of rHuEPO. This finding has led to a renaissance of androgen therapy. Androgen therapy alone or in combination with rHuEPO may lower the costs of anemia therapy.

Androgen therapy has significant side effects. A consistent effect of androgens is the retention of water and sodium chloride, resulting in significant edema. This responds to the use of diuretics. Androgens have a virilizing effect (deep voice, hirsutism), which is especially disturbing for women. Only if the prescribed androgens are withdrawn as soon as the first outward effects appear, can a complete recovery be expected. If androgens are given to females for a prolonged time, the virilizing effect remains even after the discontinuation of the agent. Androgens also have a virilizing effect in both male and female children, and cause premature closure of epiphyses. Some androgens have a feminizing effect, which may cause gynecomastia. Anabolic effects increase albumin and body weight, an effect not considered to be disturbing. In addition, triglycerides are increased by the administration of androgens. This is reversible after discontinuation of the therapy. Liver dysfunction and liver cancer were also reported in patients receiving androgens, particularly in those given of 17-alkylated androgens [65]. Therapy with androgens generally is contraindicated in pregnancy since they can pass the placenta, causing fetal virilization. Carcinoma of the prostate and disturbed liver function are contraindications to the use of androgens as well.

Prolactin

Prolactin is a hormone with anabolic properties. It was shown to act on hematopoietic precursors as these have a prolactin receptor. This receptor is similar to the EPO receptor.

Recombinant human prolactin has been used successfully to reduce anemia in animals treated with the myelosuppressive agent azidothymidine [73] and in humans with bone marrow failure [74].

Indirectly increasing endogenous prolactin by means of metoclopramide therapy has proven effective for anemia as well. Patients with Diamond–Blackfan anemia can be treated with metoclopramide for extended periods and may mean they are not transfused [75, 76].

Melatonin

An endogenous hormone for sleep and wake rhythm, melatonin has been postulated to have modulatory effects on hematopoesis. Based on this assumption, some trials have attempted to show a beneficial effect of melatonin in mitigating the ill effects of cyclophosphamide on hematopoiesis. The results of these trials are conflicting [77].

Key points

• rHuEPO is a safe and effective tool in the therapy of anemia. The response to rHuEPO therapy depends on the dose given. To prevent or treat functional iron deficiency, iron therapy, unless contraindicated, should accompany rHuEPO therapy at all times. If EPO hyporesponsiveness is present, adjuvant therapies are warranted. Adjuvant therapy may overcome EPO hyporesponsiveness and may decrease the need for rHuEPO. With or without other techniques of blood management, rHuEPO therapy may reduce the patient's exposure to donor blood.
• Darbepoetin is a synthetic analog of rHuEPO. Its half-life is prolonged. This may allow for less frequent dosing.
• Newer preparations that may be used to enhance erythropoiesis include: CERA, hematide, anabolics, prolactin, and metoclopramide. When used appropriately, these may provide effective hematopoietic therapy for selected patients.

Questions for review

1. How does human erythropoiesis take place?
2. What is the role of EPO in human erythropoiesis?

3. Which erythropoietic agents are available? What are their properties?
4. How is rHuEPO used for blood management?
5. How is EPO hyporesponsiveness overcome?

Suggestions for further research

What are hypoxia-inducible factor (HIF) stabilizers, GATA inhibitors, and hematopoietic cell phosphatase (HCP) inhibitors? What role do they play in the enhancement of erythropoiesis?

Homework

Get a package insert for rHuEPO and NESP, read and file it.

Ask a sales representative to provide you with current articles on EPO/NESP.

Inquire about the cost and availability of the following medications: rHuEPO, NESP, danazol, nandrolone, recombinant human prolactin, and metoclopramide. Use the "Medication detail" as your source. Note the information.

Exercises and practice cases

Read the following published case [37].

A 39-year-old patient with placenta previa who has heavy vaginal hemorrhage is taken to your emergency room. She does not give consent to blood transfusion. Her hematocrit is 37% at admission. You take her to the operating room immediately and her problem is resolved surgically. After surgery, she has a hematocrit of 22%. The next day, her hematocrit is 5.6%. She is no longer hemorrhaging. Your colleague has already given her oxygen and 6% hetastarch. The patient is sedated and has sufficient analgesia [78].

1. What do you prescribe for her today? Please, give exact dosing.
2. How do you follow-up?
3. Do you expect side effects from your treatment? If so, which? How would you treat them?

Read the original case report in the literature [78] to find out how this patient was actually treated. Would you have done something different?

References

1. Tabbara IA. Erythropoietin. Biology and clinical applications. *Arch Intern Med* 1993;**153**:298–304.
2. Miyake T, Kung CK, Goldwasser E. Purification of human erythropoietin. *J Biol Chem* 1977;**252**:5558–5564.
3. Jacobs K, Shoemaker C, Rudersdorf R, *et al.* Isolation and characterization of genomic and cDNA clones of human erythropoietin. *Nature* 1985;**313**:806–810.
4. Lacombe C, Mayeux P. The molecular biology of erythropoietin. *Nephrol Dial Transplant* 1999;**14** (Suppl 2):22–28.
5. Sawyer ST, Krantz SB, Luna J. Identification of the receptor for erythropoietin by cross-linking to Friend virus-infected erythroid cells. *Proc Natl Acad Sci U S A* 1987;**84**: 3690–3694.
6. Fisher JW. Landmark advances in the development of erythropoietin. *Exp Biol Med (Maywood)* 2010;**235**:1398–1411
7. Goodnough LT, Skikne B, Brugnara C. Erythropoietin, iron, and erythropoiesis. *Blood* 2000;**96**:823–833.
8. van Iperen CE, Biesma DH, van de Wiel A, Marx JJ. Erythropoietic response to acute and chronic anaemia: focus on postoperative anaemia. *Br J Anaesth* 1998;**81** (Suppl 1):2–5.
9. Atabek U, Alvarez R, Pello MJ, *et al.* Erythropoietin accelerates hematocrit recovery in post-surgical anemia. *Am Surg* 1995;**61**:74–77.
10. Goldberg MA. Perioperative epoetin alfa increases red blood cell mass and reduces exposure to transfusions: results of randomized clinical trials. *Semin Hematol* 1997;**34** (Suppl 2):41–47.
11. Bourantas K, Makrydimas G, Georgiou J, Tsiara S, Lolis D. Preliminary results with administration of recombinant human erythropoietin in sickle cell/beta-thalassemia patients during pregnancy. *Eur J Haematol* 1996;**56**: 326–328.
12. Bessho M, Hirashima K, Asano S, *et al.* Treatment of the anemia of aplastic anemia patients with recombinant human erythropoietin in combination with granulocyte colony-stimulating factor: a multicenter randomized controlled study. Multicenter Study Group. *Eur J Haematol* 1997;**58**:265–272.
13. Murphy EA, Bell AL, Wojtulewski J, Brzeski M, Madhok R, Capell HA. Study of erythropoietin in treatment of anaemia in patients with rheumatoid arthritis. *BMJ* 1994;**309**: 1337–1338.
14. Schreiber S, Howaldt S, Schnoor M, *et al.* Recombinant erythropoietin for the treatment of anemia in inflammatory bowel disease. *N Engl J Med* 1996;**334**:619–623.

15. Corwin HL, Gettinger A, Rodriguez RM, *et al.* Efficacy of recombinant human erythropoietin in the critically ill patient: a randomized, double-blind, placebo-controlled trial. *Crit Care Med* 1999;**27**:2346–2350.

16. Gabriel A. High-dose recombinant human erythropoietin stimulates reticulocyte production in patients with multiple organ dysfunction syndrome. *J Trauma* 1998;**44**: 361–367.

17. Faulds D, Sorkin EM. Epoetin (recombinant human erythropoietin). A review of its pharmacodynamic and pharmacokinetic properties and therapeutic potential in anaemia and the stimulation of erythropoiesis. *Drugs* 1989;**38**: 863–899.

18. Breymann C, Major A, Richter C, Huch R, Huch A. Recombinant human erythropoietin and parenteral iron in the treatment of pregnancy anemia: a pilot study. *J Perinat Med* 1995;**23**:89–98.

19. Estrin JT, Ford PA, Henry DH, Stradden AP, Mason BA. Erythropoietin permits high-dose chemotherapy with peripheral blood stem-cell transplant for a Jehovah's Witness. *Am J Hematol* 1997;**55**:51–52.

20. Pronzato P, Cortesi E, van der Rijt CC, *et al.* Epoetin alfa improves anemia and anemia-related, patient-reported outcomes in patients with breast cancer receiving myelotoxic chemotherapy: results of a European, multicenter, randomized, controlled trial. *Oncologist* 2010;**15**:935–943.

21. Braga J, Marques R, Branco A, *et al.* Maternal and perinatal implications of the use of human recombinant erythropoietin. *Acta Obstet Gynecol Scand* 1996;**75**:449–453.

22. Niemeyer CM, Baumgarten E, Holldack J, *et al.* Treatment trial with recombinant human erythropoietin in children with congenital hypoplastic anemia. *Contrib Nephrol* 1991;**88**:276–280; discussion 281.

23. Braga M, Gianotti L, Gentilini O, Vignali A, Di Carlo V. Erythropoietic response induced by recombinant human erythropoietin in anemic cancer patients candidate to major abdominal surgery. *Hepatogastroenterology* 1997;**44**: 685–690.

24. Sowade O, Warnke H, Scigalla P, *et al.* Avoidance of allogeneic blood transfusions by treatment with epoetin beta (recombinant human erythropoietin) in patients undergoing open-heart surgery. *Blood* 1997;**89**:411–418.

25. Yazicioglu L, Eryilmaz S, Sirlak M, *et al.* Recombinant human erythropoietin administration in cardiac surgery. *J Thorac Cardiovasc Surg* 2001;**122**:741–745.

26. Shimpo H, Mizumoto T, Onoda K, Yuasa H, Yada I. Erythropoietin in pediatric cardiac surgery: clinical efficacy and effective dose. *Chest* 1997;**111**:1565–1570.

27. Messmer K. Consensus statement: using epoetin alfa to decrease the risk of allogeneic blood transfusion in the surgical setting. Roundtable of Experts in Surgery Blood Management. *Semin Hematol* 1996;**33** (Suppl 2):78–80.

28. Chun TY, Martin S, Lepor H. Preoperative recombinant human erythropoietin injection versus preoperative autologous blood donation in patients undergoing radical retropubic prostatectomy. *Urology* 1997;**50**:727–732.

29. Mak RH. Effect of recombinant human erythropoietin on insulin, amino acid, and lipid metabolism in uremia. *J Pediatr* 1996;**129**:97–104.

30. Lippi G, Franchini M, Favaloro EJ. Thrombotic complications of erythropoiesis-stimulating agents. *Semin Thromb Hemost* 2010;**36**:537–549.

31. Lewis LD. Preclinical and clinical studies: a preview of potential future applications of erythropoietic agents. *Semin Hematol* 2004;**41** (Suppl 7):17–25.

32. Erbayraktar S, Grasso G, Sfacteria A, *et al.* Asialoerythropoietin is a nonerythropoietic cytokine with broad neuroprotective activity in vivo. *Proc Natl Acad Sci U S A* 2003;**100**: 6741–6746.

33. Ehrenreich H, Hasselblatt M, Dembowski C, *et al.* Erythropoietin therapy for acute stroke is both safe and beneficial. *Mol Med* 2002;**8**:495–505.

34. Calvillo L, Latini R, Kajstura J, *et al.* Recombinant human erythropoietin protects the myocardium from ischemia-reperfusion injury and promotes beneficial remodeling. *Proc Natl Acad Sci U S A* 2003;**100**: 4802–4806.

35. Taniguchi N, Nakamura T, Sawada T, *et al.* Erythropoietin prevention trial of coronary restenosis and cardiac remodeling after ST-elevated acute myocardial infarction (EPOC-AMI): a pilot, randomized, placebo-controlled study. *Circ J* 2010;**74**:2365–2371.

36. Morley PT. Drugs during cardiopulmonary resuscitation. *Curr Opin Crit Care* 2011;**17**:214–218.

37. Tarng DC, Huang TP. A parallel, comparative study of intravenous iron versus intravenous ascorbic acid for erythropoietin-hyporesponsive anaemia in haemodialysis patients with iron overload. *Nephrol Dial Transplant* 1998;**13**:2867–2872.

38. Danielson B. R-HuEPO hyporesponsiveness—who and why? *Nephrol Dial Transplant* 1995;**10** (Suppl 2):69–73.

39. Horl WH. Is there a role for adjuvant therapy in patients being treated with epoetin? *Nephrol Dial Transplant* 1999;**14** (Suppl 2):50–60.

40. Kuhn K, Nonnast-Daniel B, Grützmacher P, *et al.* Analysis of initial resistance of erythropoiesis to treatment with recombinant human erythropoietin. Results of a multicenter trial in patients with end-stage renal disease. *Contrib Nephrol* 1988;**66**:94–103.

41. Fusaro M, D'Angelo A, Naso A, *et al.* Treatment with calcimimetic (cinacalcet) alters epoetin dosage requirements in dialysis patients: preliminary report. *Ren Fail* 2011;**33**: 732–735.

42. Bommer J. Saving erythropoietin by administering l-carnitine? *Nephrol Dial Transplant* 1999;**14**:2819–2821.

43. Wolchok JD, Klimek VM, Williams L, Chapman PB. Prophylactic recombinant epoetin alfa markedly reduces the need for blood transfusion in patients with metastatic melanoma

treated with biochemotherapy. *Cytokines Cell Mol Ther* 1999;**5**:205–206.

44. Colomina MJ, Bagó J, Pellisé F, Godet C, Villanueva C. Preoperative erythropoietin in spine surgery. *Eur Spine J* 2004;**13** (Suppl 1):S40–S49.

45. Christodoulakis M, Tsiftsis DD. Preoperative epoetin alfa in colorectal surgery: a randomized, controlled study. *Ann Surg Oncol* 2005;**12**:718–725.

46. Weber EW, Slappendel R, Hémon Y, *et al*. Effects of epoetin alfa on blood transfusions and postoperative recovery in orthopaedic surgery: the European Epoetin Alfa Surgery Trial (EEST). *Eur J Anaesthesiol* 2005;**22**:249–257.

47. Breymann C, Zimmermann R, Huch R, Huch A. Erythropoietin zur Behandlung der postpartalen Anä mie. Hä matologie, *München Sympomed* 1993;**2**:49–55.

48. Kumar P, Shankaran S, Krishnan RG. Recombinant human erythropoietin therapy for treatment of anemia of prematurity in very low birth weight infants: a randomized, double-blind, placebo-controlled trial. *J Perinatol* 1998;**18**:173–177.

49. Ohls RK. Erythropoietin to prevent and treat the anemia of prematurity. *Curr Opin Pediatr* 1999;**11**:108–114.

50. Goodnough LT, Marcus RE. The erythropoietic response to erythropoietin in patients with rheumatoid arthritis. *J Lab Clin Med* 1997;**130**:381–386.

51. Wilson A, Yu HT, Goodnough LT, Nissenson AR. Prevalence and outcomes of anemia in rheumatoid arthritis: a systematic review of the literature. *Am J Med* 2004;**116** (Suppl 7A):50S–57S.

52. Fischl M, Galpin JE, Levine JD, *et al*. Recombinant human erythropoietin for patients with AIDS treated with zidovudine. *N Engl J Med* 1990;**322**:1488–1493.

53. Stasi R, Amadori S, Littlewood TJ, Terzoli E, Newland AC, Provan D. Management of cancer-related anemia with erythropoietic agents: doubts, certainties, and concerns. *Oncologist* 2005;**10**:539–554.

54. Rizzo JD, Brouwers M, Hurley P, *et al*. American Society of Hematology/American Society of Clinical Oncology clinical practice guideline update on the use of epoetin and darbepoetin in adult patients with cancer. *Blood* 2010;**116**: 4045–4059.

55. Del Vecchio L, Cavalli A, Tucci B, Locatelli F. Chronic kidney disease-associated anemia: new remedies. *Curr Opin Invest Drugs* 2010;**11**:1030–1038.

56. Macdougall IC, Rossert J, Casadevall N, *et al*. A peptide-based erythropoietin-receptor agonist for pure red-cell aplasia. *N Engl J Med* 2009;**361**:1848–1855.

57. Minutolo R, Zamboli P, Chiodini P, *et al*. Conversion of darbepoetin to low doses of CERA maintains hemoglobin levels in non-dialysis chronic kidney disease patients. *Blood Purif* 2010;**30**:186–194.

58. Auerbach M, Silberstein PT, Webb RT, *et al*. Darbepoetin alfa 300 or 500 mcg once every 3 weeks with or without intravenous iron in patients with chemotherapy-induced anemia. *Am J Hematol* 2010;**85**:655–663.

59. Cano F, Alarcon C, Azocar M, *et al*. Continuous EPO receptor activator therapy of anemia in children under peritoneal dialysis. *Pediatr Nephrol* 2011;**26**:1303–1310.

60. Glaspy J. Phase III clinical trials with darbepoetin: implications for clinicians. *Best Pract Res Clin Haematol* 2005;**18**: 407–416.

61. Macdougall IC. Novel erythropoiesis stimulating agents: A new era in anemia management. *Clin J Am Soc Nephrol* 2008;**3**:200–207.

62. Brunkhorst R, Bommer J, Braun J, *et al*. Darbepoetin alfa effectively maintains haemoglobin concentrations at extended dose intervals relative to intravenous or subcutaneous recombinant human erythropoietin in dialysis patients. *Nephrol Dial Transplant* 2004;**19**:1224–1230.

63. Schwartzberg LS, Yee LK, Senecal FM, *et al*. A randomized comparison of every-2-week darbepoetin alfa and weekly epoetin alfa for the treatment of chemotherapy-induced anemia in patients with breast, lung, or gynecologic cancer. *Oncologist* 2004;**9**:696–707.

64. Cvetkovic RS, Goa KL. Darbepoetin alfa: in patients with chemotherapy-related anaemia. *Drugs* 2003;**63**:1067–1074; discussion 1075–1077.

65. Teruel JL, Aguilera A, Marcen R, Navarro Antolin J, Garcia Otero G, Ortuño J. Androgen versus erythropoietin for the treatment of anemia in hemodialyzed patients: a prospective study. *J Am Soc Nephrol* 1996;**7**:140–144.

66. Gascon A, Belvis JJ, Berisa F, Iglesias E, Estopiñán V, Teruel JL. Nandrolone decanoate is a good alternative for the treatment of anemia in elderly male patients on hemodialysis. *Geriatr Nephrol Urol* 1999;**9**:67–72.

67. Teruel JL, Aguilera A, Marcen R, Navarro Antolin J, Garcia Otero G, Ortuño J. Androgen therapy for anaemia of chronic renal failure. Indications in the erythropoietin era. *Scand J Urol Nephrol* 1996;**30**:403–408.

68. Teruel JL, Marcén R, Navarro JF, *et al*. Evolution of serum erythropoietin after androgen administration to hemodialysis patients: a prospective study. *Nephron* 1995;**70**:282–286.

69. Cervantes F, Alvarez-Larrán A, Domingo A, Arellano-Rodrigo E, Montserrat E. Efficacy and tolerability of danazol as a treatment for the anaemia of myelofibrosis with myeloid metaplasia: long-term results in 30 patients. *Br J Haematol* 2005;**129**:771–775.

70. Cervantes F, Hernández-Boluda JC, Alvarez A, Nadal E, Montserrat E. Danazol treatment of idiopathic myelofibrosis with severe anemia. *Haematologica* 2000;**85**:595–599.

71. Harrington WJ, Sr, Kolodny L, Horstman LL, Jy W, Ahn Y. Danazol for paroxysmal nocturnal hemoglobinuria. *Am J Hematol* 1997;**54**:149–154.

72. Hardman J. *Goodman and Gilman's The Pharmacological Basis of Therapeutics*. McGraw-Hill, New York, 1995, p. 1441ff.

73. Woody MA, Welniak LA, Sun R, *et al*. Prolactin exerts hematopoietic growth-promoting effects in vivo and partially counteracts myelosuppression by azidothymidine. *Exp Hematol* 1999;**27**:811–816.

74. Jepson JH, McGarry EE. Effect of the anabolic protein hormone prolactin on human erythropoiesis. *J Clin Pharmacol* 1974;May–June:296–300.

75. Akiyama M, Yanagisawa T, Yuza Y, *et al.* Successful treatment of Diamond-Blackfan anemia with metoclopramide. *Am J Hematol* 2005;**78**:295–298.

76. Abkowitz JL, Schaison G, Boulad F, *et al.* Response of Diamond-Blackfan anemia to metoclopramide: evidence for a role for prolactin in erythropoiesis. *Blood* 2002;**100**: 2687–2691.

77. Pacini N, Borziani F. Action of melatonin on bone marrow depression induced by cyclophosphamide in acute toxicity phase. *Neuroendocrinol Lett* 2009;**30**:582–591

78. Koenig HM, Levine EA, Resnick DJ, Meyer WJ. Use of recombinant human erythropoietin in a Jehovah's Witness. *J Clin Anesth* 1993;**5**:244–247.

4 Anemia Therapy II: Hematinics

Erythropoiesis depends on three prerequisites to function properly: a site for erythropoiesis, i.e., the bone marrow; a regulatory system, i.e., cytokines acting as erythropoietins; and substrates for erythropoiesis, among them hematinics. This second chapter on anemia therapy will introduce the latter, their role in erythropoiesis, and their therapeutic value.

Objectives

1. To review the physiological basis for the use of hematinics.
2. To relate the indications for the therapeutic use of hematinics.
3. To define the role of hematinics in blood management.

Definitions

Hematinics: Hematinics are vitamins and minerals essential for normal erythropoiesis. Among them are iron, copper, cobalt, and vitamins A, B_6, B_{12}, C, E, folate, riboflavin, and nicotinic acid.

Iron: Iron is a trace element that is vital for oxidative processes in the human body. Its ability to switch easily from the ferrous form to the ferric state makes it an important player in oxygen binding and release.

Physiology of erythropoiesis and hemoglobin synthesis

Hematinics are the fuel for erythropoiesis. When treating a patient with anemia, it is frequently necessary to administer hematinics in order to support the patient's own erythropoiesis in restoring a normal red blood cell mass. A review of erythropoiesis and hemoglobin synthesis will provide the necessary background information to prescribe hematinics effectively.

Erythropoiesis starts with the division and differentiation of stem cells in the bone marrow. In the course of erythropoiesis, deoxyribonucleic acid (DNA) needs to be synthesized, new nuclei need to be formed, and cells need to divide. For all these processes, hematinics are needed. Folates and vitamin B_{12} are important cofactors in the synthesis of the DNA. They are necessary for purine and pyrimidine synthesis. Folates provide the methyl groups for thymidylate, a precursor of DNA synthesis.

Erythropoiesis continues while the newly made red cell precursors synthesize hemoglobin. This synthesis consists of two distinct, yet interwoven, processes: the synthesis of heme and the synthesis of globins. The synthesis of heme, a ring-like porphyrin with a central iron atom, starts with the production of δ-aminolevulinic acid (ALA) in the mitochondria (Table 4.1). ALA then travels to the cytoplasm. There, coproporphyrinogen III is synthesized from several ALA molecules. This then travels back to the mitochondria where it converts to protoporphyrin IX. With the help of the enzyme ferrochelatase, iron is introduced into the ring structure and the resulting molecule is heme.

Parallel to the synthesis of heme, the synthesis of globin chains takes place. Physiologically, this matches the needs of erythropoiesis. After the globins are synthesized, the pathways of globin synthesis and heme synthesis merge. This final pathway, the assembly of the hemoglobin molecule, occurs in the cytoplasm of the red cell precursor. In the process of folding the primary amino acid sequence, each globin molecule binds a heme molecule. After this process, dimers of an alpha-chain

Basics of Blood Management, Second Edition. Petra Seeber and Aryeh Shander.
© 2013 John Wiley & Sons, Ltd. Published 2013 by John Wiley & Sons, Ltd.

Table 4.1 Hemoglobin synthesis.

Step	Enzyme	Place	Cofactor
Succinyl CoA + glycine forms ALA	ALA synthase, pyridoxal phosphatase	Mitochondria	Pyridoxal phosphate
2 × ALA form porphobilinogen	ALA dehydratase	Cytoplasm	
4 × porphobilinogen form uroporphyrinogen III	Two-step process: hydroxymethylbilane synthase (= porphobilinogen deaminase); uroporphyrinogen III cosynthase	Cytoplasm	
Uroporphyrinogen converted to coproporphyrinogen III	Uroporphyrinogen decarboxylase, converting four acetates to methyl residues	Cytoplasm	
Coproporphyrinogen III converted to protoporphyrin IX	Two-step process: coproporphyrinogen III oxidase for decarboxylation of propionate to vinyl residues; protoporphyrin oxidase for oxidation of the methylene bridges between pyrrole groups	Mitochondria	
Insertion of iron in protoporphyrin IX	Ferrochelatase	Mitochondria	

ALA, delta-aminolevulinic acid; CoA, coenzyme A.

Table 4.2 Human hemoglobin types.

Type of hemoglobin	Globin chains
Embryonic hemoglobins	Gower 1: zeta × 2 plus epsilon × 2 Gower 2: alpha × 2 plus epsilon × 2 Portland: zeta × 2 plus gamma × 2
Fetal hemoglobin	HbF: alpha × 2 plus gamma × 2
Adult hemoglobin	HbA: alpha × 2 plus beta × 2 HbA2: alpha × 2 plus delta × 2

and a non–alpha-chain form. Later, the dimers are assembled into the functional hemoglobin molecule.

During life, the human body synthesizes different kinds of hemoglobins. The differences between those hemoglobins are the result of the type of globin chains produced (Table 4.2). Apart from a short period in embryogenesis, healthy humans always have hemoglobins that consist of two alpha-chains and two non–alpha-chains. During fetal life and 7–8 months thereafter, considerable amounts of hemoglobin F are present. After this period, hemoglobin A is the major hemoglobin present, with trace amounts (<3%) of hemoglobin A2. Alpha-chains are encoded for on chromosome 16, whereas the non–alpha-chains are encoded for on chromosome 11. A set sequence of non–alpha-globins is found on chromosome 11, in the sequence from the 5′ to the 3′ end of the DNA epsilon, gamma, delta, and beta. The genes are activated in this sequence during human development. Based on the molecular pattern encoded by the globin genes, RNA and globin chains are synthesized.

Iron therapy in blood management

Physiology of iron

Iron plays a key role in the production and function of hemoglobin. It is able to accept and donate electrons, thereby easily converting from the ferrous (Fe^{2+}) to the ferric form (Fe^{3+}) and vice versa. This property makes iron a valuable commodity for oxygen-binding molecules. On the other hand, iron molecules may be toxic if not bound to transport proteins. Excess iron stored in the body can inhibit erythropoiesis. In addition, iron can damage tissues by promoting the formation of free radicals. If the storage capacity of ferritin is superseded (in conditions when body iron stores are in excess of 5–10 times normal), iron may cause organ damage. The same happens if iron is rapidly released from macrophages. Another interesting feature of iron is that its metabolism is tightly interwoven with immune functions. Since iron promotes the growth of bacteria *in vitro* and possibly promotes cancer growth, iron metabolism is modified when patients have infections or cancer. In these conditions, the body employs several mechanisms to reduce the availability of iron.

The body iron stores of normal humans contain about 40–50 mg/kg body weight of iron in the adult male and somewhat less in the adult female. More than two-thirds of this iron is found in the red cell pool. Most of the remaining iron is stored in the liver and the reticuloendothelial macrophages. Storage occurs as iron bound to ferritin, and mobilization of iron from ferritin occurs by a reducing process using riboflavin-dependent enzymes.

Iron is recycled by the body, i.e. it is not normally excreted, but stored and reused as required. Old red cells are taken up by macrophages that process the iron contained in them and load it to transferrin for reuse. This recycling process provides more than 90% of the iron needed for erythropoiesis. Only a small amount of new iron (1–2 mg) enters the body each day. There are no mechanisms to actively excrete iron. Iron is lost by shedding endothelial cells containing iron and by blood loss (1–2 mg/day).

Since the maintenance of adequate iron stores is of vital importance, many mechanisms help in the regulation of iron uptake and recycling. Dietary iron is taken up by enterocytes in the duodenum. These enterocytes are programmed, during their development, to "know" the iron requirements of the body. The low gastric pH in conjunction with a brush border enzyme called ferrireductase helps to convert the iron from its ferrous form (Fe^{2+}) to ferric iron (Fe^{3+}). A divalent metal transporter 1 (DMT1) is located close to the ferrireductase in the membrane of the enterocytes. This transports iron through the apical membrane of the enterocyte after it has been reduced by the ferrireductase. The absorption of iron in the gut is regulated by several mechanisms. After a meal rich in iron, enterocytes stop taking up iron for a few hours ("mucosal block"), probably "believing" that there is sufficient iron in the body (although this may not be the case). Iron deficiency can cause a two- to threefold increase in iron uptake by the enterocytes. Furthermore, erythropoietic activity is able to increase iron absorption, a process that is independent of the iron stores in the body. Acute hypoxia is also able to stimulate iron absorption [1].

The absorbed iron is either stored in the enterocyte, bound to ferritin (up to about 4500 iron atoms per ferritin molecule), or transported through the basolateral membrane into the plasma. The transporter in the basolateral membrane is known to need hephaestin (which is similar to the copper transporter ceruloplasmin) to carry the iron into the plasma. After being transported into plasma, iron is converted back to the Fe^{3+} form. Probably, hephaestin aids in this conversion [2]. Transferrin in the plasma accepts a maximum of two incoming Fe^{3+} ions.

Iron-loaded transferrin attaches to transferrin receptors on the cell surface of various cells, among them red cell precursors. The receptors are located near clarithrin-coated pits. The clarithrin-coated pits hold the transferrin receptor and the transferrin–iron complex together. In addition, a DMT1, which is close to the membrane that contains the clarithrin-coated pit, is incorporated. As a result, the pits are ingested by the cell by endocytosis and form endosomes. A proton pump in the membrane of the endosomes lowers the pH in the endosome. This leads to changes in the protein structure of the transferrin and triggers the release of free iron into the endosome. The DMT1 pumps the free iron out of the endosome and the endosome membrane fuses with the cell membrane, again releasing the transferrin receptor and the unloaded transferrin for further use. In erythroid cells, the free iron in the cytoplasm is absorbed by mitochondria. This process is facilitated by a copper-dependent cytochrome oxidase. The iron in the mitochondria is used to transform protoporphyrin into heme. In non-erythroid cells, iron is stored as ferritin and hemosiderin [1].

An interesting mechanism for the regulation of iron metabolism was more recently identified. This suggests that the liver not only stores iron but also acts as the command center for iron metabolism. While searching for antimicrobial principles in body fluids, Park *et al.* [2] found a new peptide in the urine that had antimicrobial properties. The same peptide was found in plasma. Due to the peptide's synthesis in the liver (hep-) and its antimicrobial properties (-cidin), the peptide was called hepcidin. Hepcidin seems to regulate the transmembrane iron transport. It binds to its receptor ferroportin. Ferroportin is a channel through which iron is transported. When hepcidin binds to ferroportin, ferroportin is degraded and iron is locked inside the cell [3]. By this mechanism, hepcidin locks iron in cells and blocks the availability of iron in the blood. Conversely, when hepcidin levels are reduced, more iron is available.

Table 4.3 Regulation of hepcidin.

Hepcidin decreases	Hepcidin increases
In anemia and hypoxia	In inflammation
By non–transferrin-bound iron (as in thalassemias, some hemolytic anemias, hereditary hemochromatosis, hypo-/a-transferrinemia)	In iron ingestion and parenteral iron application After transfusion
A lack of hepcidin causes:	Superfluous hepcidin causes:
• Iron accumulation • Hyperabsorption of iron • Increased release of storage iron • Release of iron from macrophages with resulting decrease of iron in the spleen	• Decreased iron stores • Microcytic hypochromic anemia • Reduced iron uptake in the small intestine • Inhibition of release of iron from macrophages • Inhibition of iron transport through the placenta to the fetus

A closer look at hepcidin revealed its unique properties in the regulation of iron metabolism. In the initial studies, one urine donor developed an infection and hepcidin levels in the urine increased by about 100 times. This finding led to more research, the results of which are summarized in Table 4.3 [4, 5].

It is evident from Table 4.3 that anemia causes a decrease in hepcidin, making iron available for erythropoiesis. In contrast, inflammation and infection increase hepcidin levels and reduce the availability of iron. This may be protective when bacteria or tumor tissue is present, since the growth of both of these may rely on iron. However, under such circumstances, increased hepcidin may also induce anemia due to iron deficiency. Overproduction of hepcidin during inflammation may thus be responsible for anemia during inflammation [6].

The concept of hepcidin as a key regulator of iron metabolism offers potential for diagnostic and therapeutic use. Patients with hemochromatosis, who are deficient in hepcidin, could be treated with hepcidin or similar peptides, once they become available. In chronic anemia due to inflammation, detection of hepcidin pro-

vides a new diagnostic and possibly therapeutic tool for anemia.

Therapeutic use of iron

Iron deficiency anemia is the most common form of treatable anemia. Absolute iron deficiency develops if the iron intake is inadequate or if iron is lost through blood loss. Iron uptake is impaired if the diet is insufficient in iron, if the pH of the gastric fluids is too high (antacids), and if other divalent metals compete with the iron on the DMT1 protein. After bowel resection, the surface area available for iron absorption is reduced, also limiting the iron uptake. This can also occur in gastritis (due to *Helicobacter pylori* infection), bowel inflammation, and other diseases causing malabsorption. Iron loss is increased in all forms of blood loss, such as gastrointestinal hemorrhage, parasitosis, menorrhagia, pulmonary siderosis, trauma, phlebotomy, etc.

Relative or functional iron deficiency develops as a result of inflammation and malignancy. The term "functional iron deficiency" refers to iron need despite sufficient or even supranormal iron levels in the body stores. Iron is trapped in the macrophages, but it is not recycled and cannot be mobilized easily for erythropoiesis. Anemia develops despite these normal or supranormal iron stores. Under certain circumstances, iron therapy may be warranted in these cases. This may be true for patients with anemia due to infection or chronic inflammation who are being treated with recombinant human erythropoietin (rHuEPO).

Iron therapy is indicated in states of absolute or functional iron deficiency. If patients are eligible for oral iron therapy, this is the treatment of choice. There are many oral iron preparations available. Ferrous salts (ferrous sulfate, gluconate, fumarate) are equally tolerable. Controlled release of iron causes less nausea and epigastric pain than conventional ferrous sulfate. Most cases of absolute iron deficiency, especially the chronic ones, can be managed by oral iron administration. Iron absorption is best when the medication is taken between meals. Occasional abdominal upset after taking the iron can be reduced if iron is taken with meals. For iron stores to be replenished, the treatment with iron supplements must be continued over several months.

Several additional factors increase or interfere with the iron absorption from the intestine. Ascorbic acid (vitamin C) prevents the formation of less-soluble ferric iron and increases iron uptake. Meat, fish, poultry, and alcohol enhance iron uptake as well, while phytates (inositol phosphates, soya), calcium (in calcium salts, milk, cheese), polyphenols (tea, coffee, red wine [with tannin]), and eggs inhibit iron absorption [7].

Unlike patients with mild-to-moderate iron-deficiency anemia, some groups of patients do not respond or tolerate oral iron medication. Non-responders are usually those with an infection, a malignant disease, or another inflammatory state. A stress response, such as to surgery, will result in the production of hepcidin that leads to prevention of iron uptake. Other patients require a rapid replenishment of their iron reserves. For some patients, oral iron may be contraindicated if it will add to the damage already caused by chronic inflammatory bowel diseases. In all these cases, parenteral iron therapy is more likely to be beneficial than oral iron therapy. The conventional intravenous iron preparation used to be a high-molecular-weight iron dextran. Although generally well-tolerated, some major side effects raised concerns, including flushing, dizziness, backache, anxiety, hypotension, and occasionally respiratory failure and even cardiac arrest. Similar symptoms have been observed with the newer, low-molecular-weight iron dextrans. However, although many of the symptoms are consistant with anaphylactic reactions, some may only be a self-limiting phenomenon called the Fishbane reaction. True anaphylaxis is most likely due to the dextran in the product. Also, a specific effect of free iron contributes to the symptoms. Since high-molecular-weight dextran is partly responsible for the adverse effects of iron dextran, it was proposed that iron preparations with low-molecular-weight dextran or without dextran might be safer. Sodium ferric gluconate, a high-molecular-weight complex, contains iron hydroxide, as does iron dextran. However, it is stabilized in sucrose and gluconate but not in dextran. The dextran-free products cause similar side effects, such as nausea and vomiting, malaise, heat, back and epigastric pain, and hypotension but, in contrast to high-molecular-weight iron dextran, these reactions are short-lived and milder. It is recommended that, due to their better safety profile, dextran-free products should be favored when they are available [8]. Even patients who have had allergic reactions to iron dextran can safely be managed with any of the other products. Low-molecular-weight dextran products may be equally safe, unless the patient is allergic to them.

When intravenous iron therapy is warranted, the amount of iron to be given can be infused in a single dose (total iron dose) or in divided doses, depending on the clinical need and the iron preparation chosen. It is recommended that iron be diluted in normal saline (not in dextrose, since administration with sugar is more painful).

The amount of iron can be calculated using the following equations:

$$\text{Dose in mg of Fe} = 0.0442 \times (13.5 - \text{hemoglobin current}) \times \text{lean body weight} \times 50 + (0.26 \times \text{lean body weight}) \times 50$$

Or

$$\text{Dose in mg of Fe} = (3.4 \times \text{hemoglobin deficit} \times \text{body weight in kg} \times \text{blood volume in mL/kg body weight})/100$$

A male has a blood volume of 66 mL/kg and a female about 60 mL/kg.

1000 mg should be added to the amount of iron calculated by this formula to replenish iron stores.

For example, a 70-kg female has a hemoglobin level of 8 g/dL and is scheduled for parenteral iron therapy. How much iron does she need?

If we consider a hemoglobin level of 13 g/dL to be normal for this woman, she has a deficit of 5 g/dL. Therefore, calculate:

$$(3.4 \times 5 \text{ g/dL} \times 70 \text{ kg} \times 60 \text{ mL/kg} = 71\,400)/100$$
$$= 714 \text{ mg}$$

This means the woman has an iron deficit of about 714 mg and a further 1000 mg is also needed to replenish the iron stores.

Practice tip

A simpler way to estimate the iron needs of an adult is to multiply the hemoglobin deficit by 200 mg. An additional 500 mg should be given to replenish iron stores.

The above-mentioned patient would receive approximately 1500 mg of iron ([5 × 200] + 500) using this calculation method.

There are different iron products available for parenteral use. Table 4.4 gives important information [9] for their practical use.

Markers of iron deficiency

It is usually simple to recognize and diagnose iron-deficiency anemia. Microcytic and hypochromic anemia

Table 4.4 Commonly used parenteral iron formulas.

Iron preparation	Iron dextran, high molecular weight	Iron dextran, low molecular weight	Iron sucrose	Iron gluconate	Ferric (iron) carboxymaltose
Allergic reactions	Relatively common	Rare	Rare	?	rare
Anaphylactoid reactions, e.g., due to free iron	Rare	Rare	Rare	Occasionally (iron complex instable)	rare
Availability of iron	Takes 4–7 days until iron available		Immediately	Immediately	
Stability	Very stable	Stable	Moderate	Unstable	stable
Recommended dose given in one session (shortest time of session)	Do not exceed 20 mg/kg body weight (4–6 h); it has been reported that up to 3–4 g have been given over several hours	Total dose iron (whole deficit), max. 20 mg/kg body weight (4–6 h)	500 mg, do not exceed 7 mg/kg body weight (3.5 h)	62.5–125 mg (slowly i.v. or over 20–60 min)	1.000 mg in 15 min possible (max. 15 mg/kg), maximum 1 × / week
Test dose required	Yes	Yes	No	No	no
Remarks	There are different types of iron dextran with slightly different properties	More than 1.5 g given over 6–8 h possible		Contains preservatives that may be dangerous for newborns	

Other available parenteral iron preparations include chondroitin sulfate iron colloid, ferumoxytol, and iron sorbitol.

together with a low ferritin level are the classical findings. However, there is an increasing number of patients whose iron needs are not easily monitored by the classical iron markers. Among them are patients with functional iron deficiency. Since iron status and immunity are closely related, most biochemical markers of the iron status are affected by inflammation and/or infection. Table 4.5 describes commonly used and newer markers of the iron reserves [10–13].

Most hospitals do not offer all the tests listed in Table 4.5 to monitor iron status. Nevertheless, a reasonably reliable differential diagnosis (Table 4.6) is possible using combinations of commonly available tests. For instance, in addition to the red cell count and the red cell indices (MCV, MCHC), ferritin, transferrin saturation, and percentage of hypochromic red cells is a good combination. Another, recently introduced combination of tests consists of the soluble transferrin receptor, ferritin, and reticulocyte hemoglobin. The results of the tests are used to calculate the ferritin index, which is then plotted against the reticulocyte hemoglobin (the so-called

Thomas plot) [14]. The plot tells not only which kind of iron deficiency is likely, but also gives recommendations regarding therapy.

Copper therapy in blood management

Copper deficiency can cause anemia. This is interesting, since hemoglobin does not contain copper. The reason for this is that a lack of copper influences hematopoiesis by interfering with iron metabolism due to impaired iron absorption, iron transfer from the reticuloendothelial cells to the plasma, and inadequate ceruloplasmin activity mobilizing iron from the reticuloendothelial system to the plasma. Additionally, copper is a component of cytochrome-c oxidase, an enzyme that is required for iron uptake by mitochondria to form heme. Defective mitochondrial iron uptake due to copper deficiency may lead to iron accumulation within the cytoplasm, forming sideroblasts. Copper deficiency may also shorten red cell survival [15].

Table 4.5 Available essays for the determination of iron deficiency.

Assay	Reference values	Description	Use and limitations
Bone marrow aspirate	Normal: stainable iron present	"Gold standard;" if stainable iron is missing, iron deficiency is present	Too invasive for routine use in the diagnosis of iron deficiency
Classic biochemical markers			
Serum iron	50–170 µg/dL or female: 10–26 µmol/L; male: 14–28 µmol/L (µmol/L × 5.58 = µg/dL)	Iron bound to transferrin	Diurnal variations (higher concentrations late in the day); diet-dependent; infection and inflammation lower serum iron
Transferrin	2.0–4.0 g/L in adults; higher in children	Iron-binding transport protein in plasma and extracellular fluid	Increased by oral contraceptives; decreased in infection or inflammation
Total iron-binding capacity (TIBC)	Normal: 240–450 µg/dL	Measures indirectly the transferrin level (TIBC in µmol/L = transferrin in g/L × 22.5)	High in iron deficiency anemia, late pregnancy, polycythemia vera; low in cirrhosis, sickle cell anemia, hypoproteinemia, hemolytic, and pernicious anemia
Transferrin saturation (TS)	20–50%	Ratio of the serum iron to the TIBC	Oral contraceptives cause inappropriately low TS
Ferritin (F)	<100 µg/L in healthy individuals predicts functional Fe deficiency; <12–20 µg/L is highly specific for iron deficiency	Storage protein of iron; currently accepted laboratory test for iron deficiency; however, disagreement on the lower reference value that indicates iron deficiency	Acute-phase protein; increased in infection/ inflammation, hyperthyroidism, liver disease, malignancy, alcohol use, oral contraceptives; does not reflect iron stores in anemia of chronic disease
Newer biochemical markers			
Serum transferrin receptor (sTfR)	Male: 2.16–4.54 mg/dL; female: 1.79–4.63 mg/dL (extremely dependent on method)	Truncated form of the tissue transferrin receptor; reflects total body mass of cellular transferrin; concentration of circulating sTfR is determined by erythroid marrow activity: estimate of red cell precursor mass which is inversely related to erythropoietin concentrations	Not an acute-phase reactant; higher in patients with iron deficiency than in non-iron deficiency, but not sufficient to discriminate between both; decreased in hypoplastic anemia, increased in hyperplastic anemia and iron deficiency
R/F ratio	>1.5–4.0: absolute iron deficiency; <0.8–1.0 for iron deficiency in inflammation	= sTfR/F, most sensitive method to distinguish between anemia of iron deficiency and anemia of chronic disease	Estimates body iron stores; value limited in liver disease and inflammation/infection (C-reactive protein [CRP] screening recommended to identify patients with infection)
Erythrocyte zinc protoporphyrin (ZPP)	ZPP <40 mmol/mol Hb may exclude iron deficiency	In case of iron deficiency, zinc instead of iron is incorporated into protoporphyrin, and ZPP accumulates in the red cells	ZPP reflects intracellular iron deficiency/supply of iron to red cells; ZPP is also increased in hemolyticanemia, anemia of chronic disease, lead intoxication

Table 4.5 (*Continued*)

Assay	Reference values	Description	Use and limitations
Red cell and reticulocyte indices			
% of hypochromic red cells (%HYPO)	Pathological: >2.5–6.0%; highly pathological: >10%	Cells with a mean corpuscular Hb concentration <280 g/L	It takes prolonged iron deficiency to develop pathological %HYPO; also increased with reticulocytosis
Reticulocyte count	0.5–2.0%	Seen as response to red cell synthesis: it takes 18–36 h for reticulocytes to be seen in the circulation	Estimate of response to anemia therapy, e.g., with rHuEPO; increases in reticulocyte count after iron therapy indicates iron deficiency
Hemoglobin content of reticulocytes (CHr; in pg/ cell)	Pathological if <29 pg in some patients, e.g., children; generally pathological if <20–24 pg		Not useful in thalassemias since reticulocytes already have a low CHr; not useful in chemotherapy since megaloblastic/macrocytic erythropoiesis causes increased CHr
Immature reticulocyte fraction		Reticulocytes with medium-to-high fluorescence based on fluorescence intensity (of RNA residues)	

Serum transferrin receptor/ferritin; RNA, ribonucleic acid; Hb, hemoglobin.

Table 4.6 Differential diagnosis of absolute and functional iron deficiency.

	Absolute iron deficiency	Functional iron deficiency
Serum iron	Low	Low (or normal)
Transferrin	High	Low (or normal)
Transferrin saturation	low	Low (or normal)
Ferritin	low	(Normal or) high
TfR in serum	Increased	Normal
Serum iron-binding capacity		Low
R/F ratio	High	Low

TfR, transferrin receptor; R/F, serum transferrin receptor/ ferritin.

The average daily Western diet contains 0.6–1.6 mg of copper. Meats, nuts, and shellfish are the richest sources of dietary copper. Because of the ubiquitous distribution of copper and the low daily requirement, acquired copper deficiency is rare. However, it has been reported in pre- mature and severely malnourished infants, in patients with malabsorption, in patients receiving parenteral nutrition without copper supplementation, and with ingestion of massive quantities of zinc or ascorbic acid. Copper and zinc are absorbed primarily in the proximal small intestine. Zinc interferes directly with intestinal copper absorption.

When copper deficiency anemia is present, the patient presents with macrocytic or microcytic anemia, occa- sionally accompanied by neutropenia or thrombocytope- nia [16–19]. Erythroblasts in the bone marrow are vacuolized. The serum copper level is lower than the normal level of 70–155 μg/dL. The ceruloplasmin level may also be lower than normal. Treatment of copper deficiency is with copper sulfate solution (80 mg/kg/day) per os or an intravenous bolus dose of copper chloride [20].

Vitamin therapy in blood management

Vitamins play an important role in blood management. They not only influence hematopoiesis, but also have an impact on other aspects of blood such as the prevention of hemorrhage. The following paragraphs shed light on the background to and use of vitamins.

Vitamin B$_{12}$

The term vitamin B$_{12}$ stands for a group of chemical compounds called cobalamins. In common they have a corrin ring with a central cobalt ion but differ with regard to the chemical groups added to this atom.

Cobalamins are found in food. The highest levels are found in animal products such as meat. The ingested vitamin is freed from the food by acid in the stomach and by enzymatic activity. Most of the vitamin B$_{12}$ is bound to the so-called R protein and transported to the duodenum where the protein is degraded by pancreatic proteases. The free vitamin now binds to the intrinsic factor, a protein produced by parietal cells of the gastric mucosa. The complex of the intrinsic factor and the vitamin is resistant to further enzymatic degradation and continues its journey down to the ileum where it binds to receptors for the intrinsic factor. These facilitate the uptake of vitamin B$_{12}$. A small amount of the ingested vitamin B$_{12}$ (about 1%) is taken up without the use of intrinsic factor. Vitamin B$_{12}$ is transported by a plasma protein called transcobalamin II and is absorbed by the liver where it is stored, bound to transcobalamin I.

The normal requirement of vitamin B$_{12}$ is 1–2 μg/day. The human body stores the vitamin, and it may take 2–4 years for the stores to be depleted. Only after that length of time do the typical clinical symptoms of vitamin B$_{12}$ deficiency appear. A lack of vitamin B$_{12}$ occurs if the dietary intake is too low, if intrinsic factor is lacking (after gastrectomy or due to autoimmune processes), in pancreatic insufficiency (with a lack of proteases for the degradation of R protein), or if malabsorption is present (in cases of colonization of the small intestine with bacteria, Crohn's disease, celiac disease).

A lack of vitamin B$_{12}$ stops the function of folate coenzymes, which is necessary for DNA synthesis. Since vitamin B$_{12}$ is a cofactor for enzymes that aid in the conversion of folate, its lack causes "folate trapping," a condition of functional deficiency of folate. Folate is available but cannot be changed into the form the body typically uses, namely tetrahydrofolate (THF) (see below). DNA synthesis is impaired. Cell division and formation of the nucleus in red cell precursors are hindered. Therefore, megaloblasts accumulate in the bone marrow and immature red cells are found in the blood. The lack of vitamin B$_{12}$ affects the blood count. If a vitamin B$_{12}$ deficiency is manifest, megaloblastic anemia results. In addition, neurological sequelae develop. Some-times, bleeding diathesis with thrombocytopenia may be present.

When clinical signs and basic laboratory results suggest a deficiency in vitamin B$_{12}$, specific tests are warranted. The measurement of serum vitamin B$_{12}$ (normal level is about 160–960 ng/L) is a step in the right direction. Homocysteine and methylmalonic acid levels are raised early in vitamin B$_{12}$ deficiency. These are more sensitive markers for vitamin B$_{12}$ deficiency than serum B$_{12}$ levels, but they are less specific.

Vitamin B$_{12}$ for pharmaceutical use contains cyano, methyl, or hydroxyl groups (cyanocobalamin, methylcobalamin, and hydroxycobalamin). These different forms of vitamin B$_{12}$ differ in their retention rate, i.e., the amount of vitamin found in the body 28 days after parenteral administration. While about 30% of hydroxycobalamin is retained after 28 days, only 10% of cyanocobalamin is retained. Calculation of the amount of vitamin needed should take these differences into account.

Traditionally, vitamin B$_{12}$ is given as an intramuscular or subcutaneous dose to circumvent gastroenteral passage and the need for intrinsic factor, etc., for uptake. However, since about 1% of the ingested vitamin is taken up passively, daily high-dose vitamin B$_{12}$ (500–1000 μg) given sublingually or orally meets the needs of patients with a lack of vitamin B$_{12}$, even if the intrinsic factor is lacking [21]. If vitamin B$_{12}$ needs to be administered to patients who cannot take it orally, injections are recommended. Doses of 500–1200 μg are commonly given. Alternatively, nasal spray containing hydroxycobalamin is available. If vitamin B$_{12}$ is given as an adjunct to a blood-building regimen, adults typically receive 1–2 mg/week parenterally and children 0.21 μg/kg body weight/week.

Absolute vitamin B$_{12}$ deficiency is clearly an indication for vitamin B$_{12}$ therapy. In patients undergoing rHuEPO therapy or in those recovering from other kinds of anemia, B$_{12}$ supplementation is recommended to meet the increased vitamin needs of erythropoiesis and to prevent neurological sequelae resulting from vitamin B$_{12}$ deficiency. Patients with sickle cell disease should be monitored closely for vitamin B$_{12}$ deficiency, since the hyperhomocysteinemia associated with this condition may worsen sickle cell disease [22]. (Hyperhomocysteinemia is a risk factor for endothelial damage contributing to sickle cell vaso-occlusive disease.)

Folates

Folates, e.g., dihydrofolates (DHFs) or tetrahydrofolates (THFs), are derived from folic acid. They are used by the body to accomplish the transfer of carbon groups. The synthesis of purines, pyrimidines, and thymidylates for DNA synthesis depends on such carbon group transfers.

Folates in food (i.e., polyglutamates from plants) are hydrolyzed in the bowel to monoglutamates and are absorbed in the small intestine. In the mucosa, they are transformed to methyltetrahydrofolate and enter the plasma and cells as such.

Hematological changes based on a lack of folate include a megaloblastic blood smear, and later, anemia. In addition, thrombocytopenia and a bleeding diathesis can develop. The clinical differentiation between anemia due to vitamin B_{12} or folate deficiency cannot be made without vitamin assays. It is possible to monitor folate levels in serum or in red cells. While the serum folate is immediately affected by folate ingestion or acute loss in hospitalized patients, red cell folate may be a better indicator of the long-term folate level of a patient. However, a low vitamin B_{12} level also causes low red cell folate even when there is no actual lack of folate.

Folates are readily available in fresh vegetables, but are destroyed by cooking. Patients with a poor diet are at risk for folate deficiency. Also, patients with disorders of the gastrointestinal tract that lead to malabsorption may suffer from folate deficiency (such as celiac disease). Alcohol and some drugs (sulfasalazine, cholestyramine) impair the absorption of folates as well. A lack of folate can occur in states of increased requirement, such as pregnancy and lactation, and conditions of rapid cell turnover. In general, folate may be required by all patients with a rapid cell turnover. The increased need for folate in hematological disorders such as hemolytic anemia and myelofibrosis is of special interest. Folates may also be lacking in patients with erythropoietin hyporesponsiveness. Even if folate serum levels are within the normal range, the mean corpuscular volume increases during rHuEPO therapy, suggesting an increased folate demand in patients undergoing rHuEPO therapy [23]. If folate is given as part of a blood-building program, e.g., in conjunction with erythropoietin and iron, adults receive a daily dose of 5 mg p.o. and children 0.1 mg/kg body weight/day p.o. Folate serum levels may also be within the normal or near-normal range in critically ill patients who suddenly develop a syndrome consisting of hemorrhage, severe thrombocytopenia, and a megaloblastic bone marrow. When this occurs, even if no megaloblastic anemia may be present, folate therapy may be considered, since it has been shown to rapidly reverse this condition. Folates are even recommended as a prophylactic treatment for critically ill patients as the folate deficiency is common among this group [24].

Riboflavin

Riboflavin was isolated from milk in 1879. Its biologically active forms are flavin adenine dinucleotide (FAD) and flavin mononucleotide (FMN). Small amounts of free riboflavin are present in food, but FAD and FMN are the most common forms. In order to be absorbed by the small intestine, FAD and FMN are hydrolyzed to riboflavin. Absorption is facilitated by a saturable active transporter. In the enterocytes, riboflavin undergoes changes and enters the plasma either as riboflavin or as FMN. Riboflavin is also found in the colon, most probably as the result of the biological activity of the bacterial flora in the colon. This microbial source may be more important than previously thought. In the blood, riboflavin is bound to albumin and immunoglobulins.

Riboflavin deficiency is endemic in many regions of the world, especially in populations whose diets do not include milk and meat, and those who do not have a balanced vegetable diet. In industrial nations, riboflavin is often added to various products. Elderly persons are prone to a lack of riboflavin. Since riboflavin is sensitive to light, hyperbilirubinemic newborns treated with phototherapy may also have riboflavin deficiency.

Anemia may be the result of riboflavin deficiency. Patients with this pathology develop erythroid hypoplasia and reticulocytopenia (pure red cell aplasia). Also, a lack of riboflavin impairs iron utilization [25]. Since riboflavin is required for the activation of red cell glutathione reductase, the activity of this enzyme is reduced in riboflavin deficiency.

Therapeutic doses of riboflavin were shown to cause a rise in hemoglobin when given to young adults [26].

Vitamin C

Ascorbic acid is derived from glucose, using L-gulonolactone oxidase. Humans do not have this enzyme and therefore cannot perform this metabolic step. Therefore, the intake of ascorbic acid is essential for humans.

Vitamin C is required for folic acid reductase, the enzyme synthesizing the active form of folate (THF). Ascorbic acid is also used in the uptake of iron and its mobilization from its stores.

A lack of vitamin C is rare in patients with a reasonable nutrition. If it occurs, scurvy results—a condition that leads to hemorrhage due to impaired vessel integrity and hemostasis. About 80% of patients with scurvy are also anemic.

Intravenous vitamin C was shown to increase hemoglobin in iron-overloaded patients. The vitamin facilitates iron release from iron stores and increases the iron utilization [27]. Furthermore, it enhances iron uptake from oral iron preparations. Ascorbic acid was also shown to reverse the adverse effects of certain psychopharmaceuticals on coagulation, such as serotonin reuptake inhibitors.

Typical doses of oral vitamin C in blood management range from 100 to 500 mg/day p.o. in the adult patient.

L-Carnitine

L-Carnitine is a derivative of butyrate. It is ingested with food and synthesized in the body itself. States of L-carnitine deficiency may develop when its biosynthesis is impaired, such as in cirrhosis and renal failure, or it is lost during hemodialysis. Other conditions may also decrease carnitine levels, such as catabolism in critically ill patients, prematurity, or drugs such as valproate and zidovudine.

Typically, L-carnitine is needed for the oxidation of fatty acids in the mitochondria. L-Carnitine also exerts pharmacological effects. It seems to reduce apoptosis in erythroid precursors. Besides this, it stabilizes the membrane of the red cells and increases their osmotic resistance [28].

L-Carnitine therapy may be indicated in patients with anemia due to renal failure. It may alleviate erythropoietin hyporesponsiveness and may increase the blood count by other unknown mechanisms. L-Carnitine is also beneficial in patients with thalassemia major as it increases the hemoglobin level and reduces the number of allogeneic transfusions [29]. The recommended dose for thalassemia patients is 50 mg/kg body weight/day, given for at least 6 months.

Vitamin B_6

Vitamin B_6 comes in different forms: pyridoxine, pyridoxal, pyridoxamine, and their phosphates. The different forms seem to have equal vitamin activity since they are interconvertible in the body. The active form of vitamin B_6 is pyridoxal phosphate, which is also the major form transported in the plasma.

Pyridoxine is essential for heme synthesis. The first step of heme synthesis depends on pyridoxal phosphate as a cofactor. A lack of vitamin B_6 leads to sideroblastic anemia. Sideroblastic anemia is characterized by ring sideroblasts in the bone marrow, impaired heme synthesis, and storage of iron in the mitochondria. Sideroblastic anemia is a heterogenous group of disorders. Genetic disorders, toxins (ethanol), and drugs (isoniacid, chlo-

ramphenicol) can trigger sideroblastic anemia. Vitamin B_6 effectively treats various kinds of sideroblastic anemia. Presumably, high doses of pyridoxine counteract the resulting defect in the heme synthesis.

A trial of pyridoxine should be given to patients with sideroblastic anemia. Beginning with 100 mg/day orally, and thereafter a maintenance dose of 50 mg/day, seems to be a reasonable regimen [30]. Short-term intravenous regimens are also applicable, e.g., 180–500 mg/day of pyridoxal phosphate [31].

Other vitamins

Several other vitamins also seem to influence hematopoiesis and are suitable for certain blood-related disorders.

Vitamin A

There is a strong relationship between serum vitamin A levels and the hemoglobin concentration. Vitamin A deficiency results in anemia that is similar to that due to iron deficiency. Serum iron levels are low but the iron stores in the liver and bone marrow are increased. Iron therapy in such cases does not correct the anemia. When vitamin A is given, iron is mobilized from stores and this increases red cell production. An increase in erythropoietin levels was demonstrated after administration of vitamin A. On the other hand, erythropoietin level may be reduced in anemic patients given vitamin A despite their increased red cell mass after vitamin A therapy [32].

Vitamin B complex

Pantothenic acid deficiency is not associated with anemia. In contrast, niacin deficiency (pellagra) is associated with anemia. Niacin promotes iron uptake from food. A thiamine-responsive megaloblastic anemia, a bone marrow disorder presenting with ringed sideroblasts and megaloblasts, has also been described. The anemia typically improves after therapy with thiamine.

Vitamin E

Low-birthweight babies are born with low vitamin E levels and they may develop hemolytic anemia if a diet rich in polyunsaturated fatty acids and iron is given. In such babies, vitamin E therapy corrects the anemia quickly. Patients with cystic fibrosis may develop severe anemia due to a lack of vitamin E. In this case, water-soluble vitamin E preparations are recommended.

Vitamin K

Vitamin K is not considered a hematinic vitamin since it does not contribute directly or indirectly to red cell production. It is used in the therapy of coagulation disorders.

Interactions of hematinics

The list of interactions of hematinics is very long. For example, niacin deficiency is increased by iron deficiency [33]; superfluous zinc intake reduces copper and iron availability, leading to anemia; and riboflavin deficiency interferes with the metabolism of other B vitamins by enzymatic activity. A thorough knowledge of the interactions of hematinics is vital in improving response to therapy and to treat anemia effectively, as well as to avoid side effects of hematinic therapy. You are encouraged to dig a little deeper into this matter. The references at the end of the chapter will help you find more information.

Implications for blood management

Hematinics are vital for blood management. The following is a list of settings where hematinics can be used [34].

Primary prevention of anemia

The primary prevention of anemia includes providing patients, and prospective patients, with all the hematinics they will need under the special circumstances they will find themselves in. In fact, anemia caused by nutritional deficiencies is rarely due to the lack of a single nutrient. Rather, multiple components of hematopoiesis are usually missing in nutritional anemia. In different regions of the world, different hematinics are typically lacking in the population. Certain patient groups also have specific needs. In order to be effective, primary prophylaxis of anemia has to consider these differences.

Among the nutritional anemias, iron deficiency is the leading cause worldwide. In addition, deficiency of vitamins A, B_{12}, C, E, folic acid, riboflavin, and zinc is also attributed to anemia. Many different nutritional supplements are now available for the primary prevention of the anemias prevalent in different regions of the world.

Certain groups of patients are prone to develop nutritional anemia, and primary prevention means supplying them with what they are likely to need. Multiple hematinic deficiency anemia is common in pregnant women. Twenty percent of pregnant women in industrialized countries and up to 75% of pregnant women in developing countries are anemic [35]. In areas with chronic food shortages, as well as frequent pregnancies and prolonged lactation, pregnant women may be deprived of vital hematinics, leaving them anemic [35]. Efforts to prevent anemia in populations with a high prevalence of hematinic deficiency include using micronutrient-fortified foods or medical preparations.

Patients with anemia due to a lack of hematinics are prone to receive blood transfusions. Primary prevention of anemia by the consumption of hematinics may lower the risk of receiving allogeneic transfusions. This is especially true for malnourished women of childbearing age who receive hematinics when they become pregnant and give birth. Elderly, malnourished individuals also receive fewer transfusions when they receive hematinics to boost their blood cell mass prior to possible blood loss. The same may be true for children and patients with certain medical conditions, such as renal failure, Crohn's disease, and cystic fibrosis.

Prevention and therapy of iatrogenically-induced hematinic deficiency

Medical interventions can cause a need for hematinics.

• **Erythropoietin (EPO) therapy:** When EPO encourages the body to build new blood, an increased requirement for hematinics arises. If this is not met, either hematinic deficiency ensues (with resulting sequelae such as neurological damage due to vitamin B_{12} deficiency) or EPO does not work properly (EPO hyporesponsiveness). This should be prevented by concurrent use of EPO and hematinics. In a typical patient on EPO, iron, vitamin B_{12}, folate, and vitamin C should be given and sufficient nutritional intake should be encouraged.

• **Antibiotic therapy:** Some patients on antibiotics have an increased need for hematinics. Many antibiotics when given for prolonged periods destroy the intestinal flora and thereby may cause hematinic deficiency. Other antibiotics directly lead to anemia, such as is the case with isoniacid, the effect of which can be alleviated by concurrent use of vitamin B_6.

• **Blood loss caused by medical/surgical interventions:** Substantial blood loss caused by surgery or phlebotomy may overwhelm the body's reserves to compensate for the loss of iron and other hematinics. They should be replenished. As an example, patients receiving surgery after hip fracture are often elderly and, typically, have or develop iron-deficiency anemia during hospitalization. Parenteral iron application may speed up recovery after surgery. It reduces patients' exposure to allogeneic blood products and seems to reduce the length of hospital stay and mortality [36].

> **Practice tip**
>
> To treat anemia of elderly patients with hip fracture, the following regimen may be used:
>   100 mg of iron sucrose i.v. upon admission and just before surgery, and another 100 mg dose between admission and surgery if the hemoglobin level is below 12 g/dL (= 200–300 mg preoperatively) [36].

Therapy of anemia due to hematinic deficiency

Anemia developing as a result of a lack of hematinics is easily treated with the deficient hematinic.

- **Iron deficiency:** Iron deficiency is the most common hematinic deficiency.
- **Vitamin B complex:** Other commonly encountered deficiencies are those of B_{12}, folate, and riboflavin. As an example, most patients with hemolytic disorders need to have a regular supply of folate to meet their increased requirements.
- **Combined vitamin deficiency:** Patients with chronic blood disorders often present with a deficiency of many hematinics. As an example, patients with sickle cell disease have a greater requirement for vitamins. Regular treatment with an appropriate combination of hematinics in combination with a comprehensive prophylactic and treatment schedule reduces their exposure to transfusions. An impressive example is reduction in transfusion rate from 90% to 2% and of mortality from 20.7% to 0.6% by a Nigerian Sickle Cell Clinic and Club using, among other agents, therapy with hematinics [37].

> **Practice tip**
>
> Patients with sickle cell anemia should receive a combination of hematinics. Here is an example of what can be prescribed for them:
>   5 mg folate once daily; vitamin B compound 3x daily; 100–200 mg vitamin C 3x daily; vitamins A and E 1–3x daily, according to individual need.

Treatment of anemia not related to an absolute deficiency of hematinics

Hematinics can also be used to treat anemia if an absolute deficiency of the hematinic was not the cause of the anemia. In such cases, hematinics are used pharmacologi-
cally, not nutritionally. Vitamin B_6, for example, is recommended in patients with certain kinds of sideroblastic anemia. High-dose vitamin E may compensate for genetic defects (glutathione synthetase, glucose-6-phosphate dehydrogenase deficiency), which limit the red cells' defense against oxidative injury, and it often increases the life span of erythrocytes. Vitamin E also reduces the number of irreversibly sickled erythrocytes in sickle cell disease [20]. While still controversial, certain kinds of myelodysplastic syndromes and leukemia benefit from vitamin substitution, and transfusion reduction or elimination has been reported [38].

Patients with thalassemia and other forms of anemia not due to vitamin deficiency often lack substantial amounts of vitamins, especially of those associated with oxidative stress. When vitamins are lacking, some enzyme system functions are drastically reduced in red cells (catalase, glutathione peroxidase, and reductase), while others are increased (superoxide dismutase). In addition, the red cell membrane is changed. These patients seem to benefit from substituting the deficient vitamins to achieve supranormal levels [39–42].

Hematinics as an adjunct to other medical therapies in blood management

Some hematinics are not used to directly influence erythropoiesis. Vitamin C, for instance, is primarily given to enhance iron uptake in the gastrointestinal tract. The increased availability of iron is the factor that influences erythropoiesis. Riboflavin, vitamin A, and copper act similarly—by also increasing the availability of iron.

Hematinics as therapy for other blood management-related issues

Sometimes, minerals and vitamins are given to treat a condition that leads to increased blood loss rather than to increased erythropoiesis. Vitamin C is a good example. Certain psychotherapeutic drugs impair coagulation. Vitamin C seems to antidote this effect. Another example is vitamin K, which contributes to the coagulation process as well, and sometimes prevents the use of allogeneic blood products.

Key points

- Hematinics fuel hematopoiesis. Without hematinics, hematopoiesis is not possible.
- Anemia due to hematinic deficiency warrants supplementation of the deficient nutrient.

Questions for review

1. What happens when hepcidin increases and how does this take place?
2. Which vitamins play a role in erythropoiesis and how do they do so?
3. Do hematinics influence use of allogeneic transfusions? Do they reduce morbidity and mortality?

Suggestions for further research

What is the relationship between transferrin and lactoferrin? How do they interact with iron, and what role does this play in the defense against bacteria?

Exercises and practice cases

How much iron is needed by a previously healthy male who has lost so much blood during a car accident that his hemoglobin level has dropped to 6 mg/dL?

Homework

Go to your hospital laboratory and find out what parameters can be used to detect (a) a lack of iron and (b) a lack of vitamins.

Ask your hospital pharmacy which oral and parenteral iron preparations are available and what vitamins are stocked. Note the dose per tablet, vial, etc., and the price.

Ask about the availability of all other hematinics mentioned in this chapter and note their prices and dosages also. Note the manufacturers of all the hematinics.

Find out where hematinics are routinely used in your hospital. Check, for instance, with obstetricians, general practitioners, hematologists and oncologists, pediatricians, and surgeons. Note the current standards that are applicable in your hospital with regard to hematinic use.

References

1. Andrews NC. Disorders of iron metabolism. *N Engl J Med* 1999;**341**:1986–1995.
2. Park CH, Valore EV, Waring AJ, Ganz T. Hepcidin, a urinary antimicrobial peptide synthesized in the liver. *J Biol Chem* 2001;**276**:7806–7810.
3. Vyoral D, Petrak J. Hepcidin: a direct link between iron metabolism and immunity. *Int J Biochem Cell Biol* 2005;**37**:1768–1773.
4. Chepelev NL *et al.* Regulation of iron pathways in response to hypoxia. *Free Radical Biol Med* 2011;**50**:645–666.
5. Kearney SL, Nemeth E, Neufield EJ, *et al.* Urinary hepcidin in congenital chronic anemias. *Pediatr Blood Cancer* 2007;**48**:57–63.
6. Roy CN, Andrews NC. Anemia of inflammation: the hepcidin link. *Curr Opin Hematol* 2005;**12**:107–111.
7. Hallberg L, Hulthen L. Prediction of dietary iron absorption: an algorithm for calculating absorption and bioavailability of dietary iron. *Am J Clin Nutr* 2000;**71**:1147–1160.
8. Fishbane S, Kowalski EA. The comparative safety of intravenous iron dextran, iron saccharate, and sodium ferric gluconate. *Semin Dial* 2000;**13**:381–384.
9. Danielson BG. Structure, chemistry, and pharmacokinetics of intravenous iron agents. *J Am Soc Nephrol* 2004;**15**:S93–S98.
10. Brugnara C. Iron deficiency and erythropoiesis: new diagnostic approaches. *Clin Chem* 2003;**49**:1573–1578.
11. van Tellingen A, Kuenen JC, de Kieviet W, van Tinteren H, Kooi ML, Vasmel WL. Iron deficiency anaemia in hospitalised patients: value of various laboratory parameters. Differentiation between IDA and ACD. *Neth J Med* 2001;**59**:270–279.
12. Joosten E, Van Loon R, Billen J, Blanckaert N, Fabri R, Pelemans W. Serum transferrin receptor in the evaluation of the iron status in elderly hospitalized patients with anemia. *Am J Hematol* 2002;**69**:1–6.
13. Brittenham GM, Weiss G, Brissot P, *et al.* Clinical consequences of new insights in the pathophysiology of disorders of iron and heme metabolism. *Hematology (Am Soc Hematol Educ Program)* 2000:39–50.
14. Steinmetz HT, Tsamaloukas A, Schmitz S, *et al.* A new concept for the differential diagnosis and therapy of anaemia in cancer patients. *Support Care Cancer* 2010;**19**:261–269.
15. Hassan HA, Netchvolodoff C, Raufman JP. Zinc-induced copper deficiency in a coin swallower. *Am J Gastroenterol* 2000;**95**:2975–2977.
16. Gregg XT, Reddy V, Prchal JT. Copper deficiency masquerading as myelodysplastic syndrome. *Blood* 2002;**100**:1493–1495.
17. Fuhrman MP, Herrmann V, Masidonski P, Eby C. Pancytopenia after removal of copper from total parenteral nutrition. *JPEN J Parenter Enteral Nutr* 2000;**24**:361–366.
18. Manser JI, Crawford CS, Tyrala EE, Brodsky NL, Grover WD. Serum copper concentrations in sick and well preterm infants. *J Pediatr* 1980;**97**:795–799.
19. Masugi J, Amano M, Fukuda T. Letter: copper deficiency anemia and prolonged enteral feeding. *Ann Intern Med* 1994;**121**:386.
20. Beutler E, *et al. Williams Hematology*, 6th edn. McGraw-Hill, New York, 2001, p. 417ff.

21. Nyholm E, Turpin P, Swain D, *et al*. Oral vitamin B$_{12}$ can change our practice. *Postgrad Med J* 2003;**79**:218–220.

22. Dhar M, Bellevue R, Carmel R. Pernicious anemia with neuropsychiatric dysfunction in a patient with sickle cell anemia treated with folate supplementation. *N Engl J Med* 2003;**348**:2204–2208.

23. Pronai W, Riegler-Keil M, Silberbauer K, Stokenhuber F. Folic acid supplementation improves erythropoietin response. *Nephron* 1995;**71**:395–400.

24. Mant MJ, Connolly T, Gordon PA, King EG. Severe thrombocytopenia probably due to acute folic acid deficiency. *Crit Care Med* 1979;**7**:297–300.

25. Riboflavin. Monograph. *Alternative Med Rev* 2008;**13**(4).

26. Ajayi OA, Okike OC, Yusuf Y. Haematological response to supplements of riboflavin and ascorbic acid in Nigerian young adults. *Eur J Haematol* 1990;**44**:209–212.

27. Handelman GJ. New insight on vitamin C in patients with chronic kidney disease. *J Ren Nutr* 2011;**21**:110–112.

28. Evangeliou A, Vlassopoulos D. Carnitine metabolism and deficit—when supplementation is necessary? *Curr Pharm Biotechnol* 2003;**4**:211–219.

29. El-Beshlawy A, Seoud H, Ibrahim A, *et al*. Apoptosis in thalassemia major reduced by a butyrate derivative. *Acta Haematol* 2005;**114**:155–159.

30. Alcindor T, Bridges KR. Sideroblastic anaemias. *Br J Haematol* 2002;**116**:733–743.

31. Murakami R, Takumi T, Gouji J, Nakamura H, Kondou M. Sideroblastic anemia showing unique response to pyridoxine. *Am J Pediatr Hematol Oncol* 1991;**13**:345–350.

32. Cusick SE, Tielsch JM, Ramsam M, *et al*. Short-term effects of vitamin A and antimalarial treatment on erythropoiesis in severely anemic Zanzibari preschool children. *Am J Clin Nutr* 2005;**82**:406–412.

33. Oduho GW, Han Y, Baker DH. Iron deficiency reduces the efficacy of tryptophan as a niacin precursor. *J Nutr* 1994;**124**:444–450.

34. Hallak M, Sharon AS, Diukman R, Auslender R, Abramovici H. Supplementing iron intravenously in pregnancy. A way to avoid blood transfusions. *J Reprod Med* 1997;**42**:99–103.

35. Makola D, Ash DM, Tatala SR, Latham MC, Ndossi G, Mehansho H. A micronutrient-fortified beverage prevents iron deficiency, reduces anemia and improves the hemoglobin concentration of pregnant Tanzanian women. *J Nutr* 2003;**133**:1339–1346.

36. Cuenca J, García-Erce JA, Martínez AA, Solano VM, Molina J, Muñoz M. Role of parenteral iron in the management of anaemia in the elderly patient undergoing displaced subcapital hip fracture repair: preliminary data. *Arch Orthop Trauma Surg* 2005;**125**:342–347.

37. Akinyanju OO, Otaigbe AI, Ibidapo MO. Outcome of holistic care in Nigerian patients with sickle cell anaemia. *Clin Lab Haematol* 2005;**27**:195–199.

38. Giagounidis AA, Haase S, Germing U, *et al*. Treatment of myelodysplastic syndrome with isolated del (5q) including bands q31–q33 with a combination of all-trans-retinoic acid and tocopherol-alpha: a phase II study. *Ann Hematol* 2005;**84**:389–394.

39. Dhawan V, Kumar KhR, Marwaha RK, Ganguly NK. Antioxidant status in children with homozygous thalassemia. *Indian Pediatr* 2005;**42**:1141–1145.

40. Das N, Das Chowdhury T, Chattopadhyay A, Datta AG. Attenuation of oxidative stress-induced changes in thalassemic erythrocytes by vitamin E. *Pol J Pharmacol* 2004;**56**:85–96.

41. Rachmilewitz EA, Shifter A, Kahane I. Vitamin E deficiency in beta-thalassemia major: changes in hematological and biochemical parameters after a therapeutic trial with alpha-tocopherol. *Am J Clin Nutr* 1979;**32**:1850–1858.

42. Rachmilewitz EA, Kornberg A, Acker M. Vitamin E deficiency due to increased consumption in beta-thalassemia and in Gaucher's disease. *Ann N Y Acad Sci* 1982;**393**:336–347.

5 Growth Factors

Human hematopoiesis is regulated by an intricate system of factors that regulate growth, maturation, and death of hematopoietic cells. In health, this enables the hematopoietic system to adapt to the needs of the organism. The idea of modulating such systems in disease is intriguing. In fact, it has been possible to modulate certain conditions with the use of growth factors. This chapter gives a brief description of the current quest for agents to modify hematopoiesis. It identifies the efforts that have led to success and where further work is needed.

Objectives

1. To summarize what is known about the role of growth factors in hematopoiesis.
2. To become familiar with a variety of hematological growth factors in current use.
3. To understand the role of available growth factors and their current and potential use in blood management.

Definitions

Hormones: Substances that have a specific regulatory effect on the organs. Classically, they are secreted by endocrine glands and are transported by the blood to their target tissues.

Cytokines: Proteins that are secreted by leukocytes and some non-leukocytic cells, which act as intercellular mediators. In contrast to hormones, they are produced by a certain cell type rather than by specialized glands, and act locally in a paracrine or autocrine fashion.

Interleukins: Factors that stimulate the growth of hematopoietic and other cells, and regulate their function.

Colony stimulating factors (in hematology): Glycoproteins that regulate proliferation, differentiation, maturation, and function at different levels of hematopoiesis.

Hematopoietic cell growth factors: Comprise a family of hematopoietic regulators with biological specificities defined by their ability to support proliferation and differentiation of different blood cell lines.

Hematopoiesis and the role of growth factors

Hematopoiesis is the sequential development of the final blood cells, or corpuscles, from a pluripotent stem cell. Different cell lines develop from the stem cell. The result is the production of red cells (see Chapter 3), platelets, or white cells. The cell's division, maturation, and function are regulated by the activities of a variety of cytokines (growth factors). Some cytokines develop multiple cell lines; others are specific for one cell line. Some cytokines contribute only in the initial phase of hematopoiesis, while others act later in the development of blood corpuscles. Refer to Figure 5.1 for an impression of the maturation process of platelets and white cells.

Megakaryopoiesis
Megakaryocytes develop from their stem cells. These undergo endomitosis (i.e., several mitoses without division of their cytoplasm), thereby growing to become the largest cells in the bone marrow. Megakaryocytes carry

Basics of Blood Management, Second Edition. Petra Seeber and Aryeh Shander.
© 2013 John Wiley & Sons, Ltd. Published 2013 by John Wiley & Sons, Ltd.

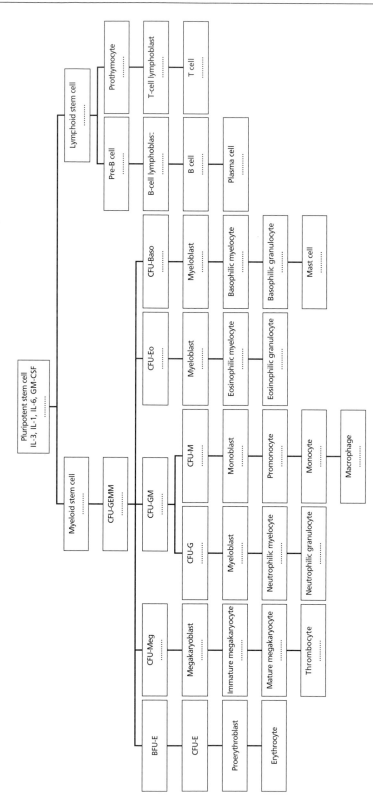

Figure 5.1 Human hematopoiesis, Baso, basophil; BFU, burst-forming units, CFU, colony-forming units; E, erythrocyte; Eo, eosinophil; G, granulocyte; GEMM, granulocyte erythrocyte megakaryocyte; GM, granulocyte–macrophage; M, monocyte/macrophage; MM, monocyte macrophage; Meg, megakaryocyte; MM, monocyte macrophage.

receptors for growth factors, permitting these factors to influence their development. The most prominent of these factors is thrombopoietin (TPO), which acts on its receptor (c-Mpl). About 90% of all thrombopoiesis depends on TPO. If TPO is completely lacking, 10% of the normal platelet level is still reached, suggesting that growth factors other than TPO also contribute to thrombopoiesis [1]. After reaching a certain growth and maturation level, megakaryocytes shed platelets. This happens when megakaryocytes develop proplatelets, long branching processes with bud-like ends that typically reach into the sinusoids of the bone marrow. One hundred to 3000 platelets of 2–3 μm in size are produced from a single megakaryocyte of 50–80 μm in size and this depends on a large pool of so-called demarcation membranes found within the megakaryocyte. These membranes shift to the bud-like ends of the megakaryocyte and form platelets. It takes about 5 days for the stem cell to mature and finally shed platelets. Where the final platelet maturation takes place is currently a matter of debate. Some research points to the bone marrow itself; other research hints at the lung as the place of final platelet maturation [2, 3].

The final platelet has three distinct zones. The outer zone consists of the glycocalyx and the plasma membrane with the platelet receptors. These receptors facilitate the adherence of platelets to collagen and support the aggregation and activation of platelets. They also bind growth factors. The middle platelet zone is the sol-gel zone with tubular systems, microfilaments, and thrombosthenin. The central zone of the platelet is the metabolic (organelle) zone with organelles and granules. The granules contain a variety of substances needed for the function of the platelets. There are dense granules (containing ATP, ADP, calcium, magnesium, serotonin, epinephrine), alpha granules (containing platelet-derived growth factor, platelet factor 4, plasminogen activator inhibitor 1, albumin, and fibrinogen), and lysosomes (containing hydrolytic enzymes).

Leukopoiesis

Leukopoiesis starts with the stem cell. Early during development, two distinct lines of white cells divide: the lymphoid line (lymphopoiesis) and the myeloid line (myelopoiesis). Lymphopoiesis results in the synthesis of T cells and B cells. Leukopoiesis is rarely the target of therapeutic intervention with growth factors. Myelopoiesis, which results in the development of monocytes and granulocytes, is more often the target.

The body stores a reserve of granulocytes for about 11 days. The bone marrow releases granulocytes, and so

there is a constant level in the circulation. However, when infection is present, their level may increase dramatically. This is regulated by granulocyte–colony stimulating factor (G-CSF). Its receptor is found on immature neutrophils. In severe infection, G-CSF levels can increase over 10 000 times. This increase in G-CSF is a result of G-CSF secretion by the bone marrow stroma (which produces G-CSF in a healthy individual) and other white cells (which accelerate G-CSF production in infection). G-CSF binds to its receptors (found on progenitors of the neutrophil line) and regulates their proliferation, maturation, and survival. It also moves neutrophils from the bone marrow into the blood circulation. This shift makes a rapid response to the growth factor possible. Granulocyte–macrophage colony stimulating factor (GM-CSF) contributes to the development of granulocytes and macrophages.

One of the most important functions of the granulocytes and macrophages is the phagocytosis of foreign agents such as bacteria. The function of phagocytes can be divided into phases: chemotaxis (directed motility after recognition), diapedesis (phagocytes pass the endothelium to leave the circulation), endocytosis (of the harmful agent with formation of a phagosome), degranulation (content of the granules digests ingested particles), and killing of the invader.

In addition, mature neutrophils carry receptors for growth factors (e.g., G-CSF). These receptors transduce signals from outside the cell and protect the cell from apoptosis. The granulocyte functions are also regulated by growth factors.

Growth factors for platelets

It has long been known that there must be an agent that specifically controls and accelerates platelet synthesis—a so-called TPO (megapoietin). This cytokine attaches to a platelet receptor called c-Mpl. It was not until the late 1980s that an agent was detected which acted as a cytokine in megakaryosynthesis. This agent was named c-Mpl ligand. In 1994, the native c-Mpl ligand was purified. This proved to be the TPO that had been looked for [4]. It is one of the most potent stimulators of megakaryocyte production, size, and expression of platelet membrane glycoprotein. It acts almost exclusively on the megakaryocyte line. In addition, it has a limited effect on red cell production by enhancing proliferation and survival of erythroid progenitors, and on other primitive hematopoietic stem cells.

The native TPO precursor protein is synthesized primarily in the liver (and possibly also in stroma cells in the bone marrow). It consists of two domains: one for attaching to its receptor and the other to maintain its stability. The liver seems to produce a constant amount of TPO. When autologous platelets are present, TPO attaches to the c-Mpl receptor of platelets, and possibly also to their precursors, and is incorporated into them. The TPO plasma level diminishes. The same is true when allogeneic platelets are transfused [4]. In contrast, when thrombocytopenia exists, TPO is not taken up by the platelets to the same degree and TPO plasma levels are increased. This leads to a stimulation of megakaryocyte synthesis.

As predicted, TPO is a potent megakaryocyte colony stimulating factor and increases the size and number of megakaryocytes. TPO acts synergistically with other growth factors, including many interleukins, to increase myeloid and erythroid precursors. TPO (as well as some other growth factors) increases aggregation of platelets only in non-physiological doses.

Animal experiments suggest that there must be other stimulants for thrombopoiesis, since animals without TPO do not bleed to death, although they are thrombocytopenic with reduced numbers of white and red cell precursors.

Recombinant or synthetic analogs of TPO and other c-Mpl agonists can be used to stimulate natural pathways that result in increased platelet production or enhanced platelet function.

First-generation thrombopoietic growth factors

The initial attempts to find clinically useful agonists for the TPO receptor resulted in the development of three distinct drugs: recombinant human TPO (rHuTPO), pegylated recombinant human megakaryocyte growth and development factor (PEG-rHuMGDF), and the fusion protein promegapoietin (TPO/IL-3 fusion protein) [5].

Recombinant human thrombopoietin

Understanding the role of TPO in megakaryosynthesis helped in the engineering of recombinant agents that were able to attach to the c-Mpl receptor. Among them is rHuTPO. This is the full-length recombinant form of native TPO. It is produced in mammalian cells. It mimics the action of native TPO in increasing the number of megakaryocyte progenitors and hastening the synthesis of platelets. Its effect on the red cell and white cell lines is not consistent and clinically is often negligible.

rHuTPO has been used successfully to mobilize peripheral blood progenitor cells for autologous reinfusion. It has been used in doses of 0.6–5.0 μg/kg i.v. rHuTPO was also given to accelerate platelet recovery after chemotherapy. When rHuTPO was given together with GM-CSF, platelet and granulocyte recovery after chemotherapy was accelerated, and red cell and platelet transfusions were reduced [6]. However, rHuTPO's delayed action has prevented most physicians from using it in acute thrombocytopenia.

Therapy with rHuTPO is usually well tolerated. If given intravenously, it does not seem to cause neutralizing antibody production.

Pegylated recombinant human megakaryocyte growth and development factor

Another recombinant c-Mpl agonist is PEG-rHuMGDF. In contrast to rHuTPO, the recombinant PEG-rHuMGDF is shorter and holds only one domain of the native TPO, namely, its functional part that binds to its receptor [7]. This domain is bound to polyethylene glycol. PEG-rHuMGDF is produced by *Escherichia coli*. As in its native counterpart, TPO, PEG-rHuMGDF enhances the production of platelets, but also of other hematopoietic progenitors. Its effects are enhanced by the coadministration of G-CSF.

PEG-rHuMGDF has been used extensively in humans. It brings about a dose-related increase in platelet counts in healthy volunteers and in patients prior to chemotherapy. It increases the life span of platelets in healthy volunteers and in *in vitro* experiments, it was shown to increase platelet aggregability [8]. In animal experiments, the increase in aggregability did not lead to increased thrombosis formation. PEG-rHuMGDF has been used for the treatment of thrombocytopenia in aplastic anemia, myelosuppression of a variety of origins (chemotherapy), and in other disease-related or iatrogenic states of thrombocytopenia. The sooner PEG-rHuMGDF is administered after myelosuppression, the better the results seem to be as residual hematopoietic progenitors will still be present [9]. PEG-rHuMGDF has also proven safe for patients on long-term treatment.

After initial promising results, the development of PEG-rHuMGDF came to a halt in the United States in 1998. Some patients developed neutralizing antibodies against it. Immunoglobulin G antibodies to PEG-rHuMGDF, which cross-reacted with endogenous TPO and neutralized its biological activity, were responsible

[10]. In some cases, this led to severe thrombocytopenia and research on PEG-rHuMGDF was stopped. The clinical development of rHuTPO has been discontinued for the same reason.

Second-generation thrombopoietic growth factors

The second-generation thrombopoietic growth factors were intended to be TPO receptor agonists (TPO-R, also called TPO mimetics) that did not lead to the development of neutralizing antibodies against native TPO. Avoiding a structural similarity with native TPO, three different groups of second-generation thrombopoietic growth factors were developed: peptide TPO-R, non-peptide TPO-R, and TPO-R agonist antibodies [5].

Peptide TPO receptor agonists

Among the peptide TPO-R agonists are Fab 59, Peg-TPOmp, and Romiplostim (AMG 531). While the first two compounds are not in clinical use, AMG 531 has reached the market and is approved for use in thrombocytopenia.

Romiplostim

Romiplostim consists of parts of the immunoglobulin chains and Fc fragments designed to bind to the human TPO receptor. It competes with human TPO. In a dose-dependent fashion, it enhances megakaryopoiesis, but does not appear to have any adverse effects on red and white cell production. Romiplostim sensitizes platelets to their agonists, such as epinephrine. An increase in platelet count can be appreciated after about 1 week. Romiplostim is administered weekly by the subcutaneous route. It is shipped in vials of 250 and 500 μg. A typical initial dose is 3 μg/kg and up to 10 μg/kg can be given [11, 12].

Side effects are rare and mild. Rebound thrombocytopenia after stopping romiplostim and development of antibodies against romiplostim, but not against endogenous TPO, have been reported. There have also been early reports of the development of a potentially reversible increase in reticulin in the bone marrow without obvious cytopenias. Whether or not this may lead to adverse effects in long-term therapy with romiplostim remains to be seen [13].

Romiplostim is approved for use in primary immune thrombocytopenia (ITP). It has also been tested successfully for the therapy of thrombocytopenia secondary to chemotherapy and radiation, as well as for myelodysplastic syndromes (MDS) [14, 15].

Non-peptide TPO receptor agonists

Among the non-peptide TPO receptor agonists are AKR-501 (formerly YM477) and elthrombopag (SB497115) [5]. Although AKR-501 seemed to be slightly more effective than elthrombopag, the latter received market approval.

Elthrombopag

Elthrombopag is a small organic compound that activates the TPO receptor when given orally. Thus, megakaryopoiesis is stimulated in a dose-dependent fashion, with the first clinically relevant effects seen after 8 days and a peak platelet level after 16 days. Platelet activation is not changed. Elthrombopag does not compete with TPO at the receptor. The beneficial effects of elthrombopag are species specific.

Elthrombopag is readily available after oral administration, providing it is taken on an empty stomach and not together with polyvalent cations such as iron or zinc. It is highly protein bound in the blood stream. After it is metabolized, it is excreted in feces and urine. Blood levels increase as liver function decreases [11, 12].

Commercially, 25 and 50 mg tablets are available. A dose of 25 mg is recommended in severe liver disease and in patients with an East Asian ethnicity; all other patients receive a starting dose of 50 mg. Like romiplostim, elthrombopag is licensed for use in ITP [16]. Besides, it appears to be effective in the treatment of thrombocytopenia in conditions like hepatitis C, myelodysplasia, and after chemotherapy.

TPO agonist antibodies

TPO agonist antibodies are monoclonal antibodies designed to activate the TPO receptor. Two examples under investigation, but far from clinical use, are TPO minibodies [VB22B sc(Fv)2] and domain subclass-converted TPO agonist antibodies (MA01G4G344) [5].

Interleukins to enhance thrombopoiesis

Interleukin 11

Interleukin (IL)-11 is a multifunctional cytokine that has a profound effect on the synthesis of megakaryocytes. IL-11 enhances the growth and maturation of megakaryocyte progenitors, but their proliferation remains almost unaffected. IL-11 works synergistically with other early promoters of hematopoiesis, such as IL-3 and stem cell factor. It also accelerates red cell and neutrophil production. However, as seems to be the case with TPO, IL-11 is not essential for hematopoiesis. It also has immunological effects, stimulates growth of enterocytes, modifies autoimmune phenomena, and maintains female fertility [10].

Recombinant human interleukin-11 (rHuIL-11, oprelvekin) is available for therapy. rHuIL-11 increases platelet counts in a dose-related fashion. The increase starts 5–9 days after the start of therapy and peaks 14–19 days thereafter. rHuIL-11 does not seem to influence platelet function, but it increases fibrinogen and von Willebrand factor levels.

Practice tip

rHuIL-11 is administered subcutaneously. Adults are administered a once-daily dose of 50 μg/kg and children 75–100 μg/kg, due to their accelerated clearance.

---

rHuIL-11 (oprelvekin) is licensed for the prophylaxis of chemotherapy-induced thrombocytopenia in non-myeloid malignancies [17]. It is given as a prophylactic agent, starting 6–24 hours after chemotherapy, before thrombocytopenia develops. rHuIL-11 has also been used as treatment for thrombocytopenia in patients with myelosuppression, undergoing chemotherapy or radiation therapy, stem cell infusion, and autologous bone marrow transplant. rHuIL-11 has successfully been used to treat thrombocytopenia in hypersplenic thrombocytopenia due to hepatic cirrhosis [18].

rHuIL-11 is generally well tolerated. However, it stimulates renal sodium absorption and therefore increases plasma volume by approximately 20%. This results in edema (which can be treated with diuretics), dyspnea, and cardiac arrhythmia in susceptible individuals. Since native IL-11 is a pluripotent agent, acting on many organ systems, it is no surprise that it may cause side effects in many organ systems. These include hyperbilirubinemia, anemia, flu-like symptoms, and hypotension.

Other growth factors

Many more cytokines have been used therapeutically to enhance megakaryopoiesis. However, none of them is used routinely in clinical practice. Table 5.1 summarizes the important features of these drugs [19–26].

Combinations

Mimicking nature, scientists have tried to use a combination of cytokines, either given together or sequentially, to speed up platelet recovery. Combinations of GM-CSF and IL-3, IL-3, and IL-6, as well as IL-3 and IL-11 were tried in animal experiments. Also, the combination of TPO and stem cell factor is intriguing and an attempt has been made to coexpress them in one chimeric protein in *E. coli* [27].

Growth factors for leukocytes

Granulocyte colony stimulating factor

G-CSF is a naturally occurring glycoprotein that supports neutrophil maturation and function. It is synthesized by monocytes, macrophages, fibroblasts, bone marrow stroma, and the endothelium in response to other cytokines. Its levels are increased during infection. It enhances not only the proliferation but also the function of mature granulocytes. G-CSF stimulates progenitors of granulocytes, monocytes, megakaryocytes, and lymphocytes. It has by far the greatest effect on granulocytes. Its effects on cell lines other than the neutrophils seem to be clinically negligible.

There are several recombinant forms of G-CSF available for clinical use. They differ from the native form in their protein sequence or glycosylation. Glycosylation adds to the stability of the agent under different temperatures and pHs, and slows its degradation in the blood.

Practice tip

Therapeutic doses of rHuG-CSF usually range between 5 and 32 μg/kg body weight/day.

The following recombinant G-CSFs are commonly used in clinical practice:
- **Filgrastim (r-metHuG-CSF):** A recombinant non-glycosylated protein expressed in *E. coli*. Its half-life is about 3.5 hours. It can be given intravenously or subcutaneously.
- **Pegfilgrastim (= sustained delivery filgrastim SD/01, PEG-r-methuG-CSF):** Produced by adding a polyethylene glycol residue to the filgrastim molecule (pegylation). This pegylation prolongs the half-life to 15–80 hours and so less frequent doses, as compared to filgrastim, are required. In equivalent doses, it is as effective as filgrastim.
- **Lenograstim:** Glycosylated recombinant form of human colony stimulating factor that is synthesized in Chinese hamster ovary cells [28]. Lenograstim seems to be as effective as filgrastim in stimulating leukocyte

Table 5.1 Miscellaneous growth factors for megakaryopoiesis.

Name	Description	Biological activity	Use	Side effects
Interleukin 3 (IL-3) and analogs (multi-CSF or multipoietin, daniplestim, synthokine [SC-55494], rHuIL-3)	Multilineal cell growth factor; it is secreted by lymphocytes, epithelial cells, and astrocytes	Stimulates clonal proliferation and differentiation of various hematological cell lines; enhances function of mature blood cells	Reactivates megakaryosynthesis after chemotherapeutic myelosuppression; used with mixed results in chemotherapy-induced thrombocytopenia, myelodysplastic syndrome, and aplastic anemia; promising in congenital megakaryocytic thrombocytopenia to reduce bleeding and transfusions	Low-dose regimen: mildflu-like effects (controlled with propranolol); high therapeutic doses: severe side effects limiting the use
Interleukin 1 (IL-1)	Soluble factor produced by monocytes and macrophages	Supports proliferation and differentiation of megakaryocyte progenitors; stimulates platelet production in two phases (peaking on day 8 and 17 after application); reduces neutropenia; enhances the effect of other hematological growth factors; stimulates secretion of cytokines from other cells	Used inpatients to reduce thrombocytopenia in chemotherapy patients	Severeside effects (high fever, severe flu–like syndromes, pain syndromes, and hypotension) limit use
Interleukin 6 (IL-6) (= interferon -β2, B-cell stimulatory factor 2, plasmocytoma, hybridoma growth factor, hepatocyte-stimulating factor, cytotoxic T-cell differentiation factor)		Induces primitive progenitor cells; suppresses erythropoiesis; stimulates megakaryocyte progenitor growth and maturation (together with IL-3); does not affect the megakaryocyte progenitor number; causes smaller platelets to develop	Accelerates platelet production in chemotherapy patients; results mixed	Causes anemia and, due to its many physiological actions, a variety of severe side effects
Granulocyte–macrophage colony stimulating factor (GM-CSF)		Stimulates megakaryocyte colonies	Used to increase platelet count and speed up platelet recovery after autologous transplantation in Hodgkin's disease, myelodysplastic syndrome, and aplastic anemia; results mixed; promising when used in combination with other hematopoietic growth factors	Mild

production during chemotherapy and peripheral blood stem cell transplantation [29].

• **Nartograstim:** A further recombinant form of G-CSF. In comparison to native G-CSF, its N-terminal amino acid sequence is altered. It therefore has a three-fold higher affinity for the G-CSF receptor.

The side effects of recombinant G-CSF are mild to moderate. Immediately after G-CSF is injected, the neutrophil count decreases, with a subsequent marked increase in granulocytes. Other side effects are similar to those of GM-CSF (see below). Overall, both G-CSF and GM-CSF are well tolerated. Up to 30% of patients experience flu-like symptoms with fever, musculoskeletal pain, diarrhea, and headaches. Occasionally, splenomegalia develops. Rashes may occur, but overt allergic reactions are rare [30].

Granulocyte–macrophage colony stimulating factor

The endogenous GM-CSF is not as restricted to the neutrophil white cell line as is G-CSF. GM-CSF was shown to enhance growth and differentiation of neutrophils, eosinophils, monocytes, megakaryocytes, and erythrocytes. It also stimulates the phagocytosis and enzymatic function of mature granulocytes. GM-CSF is naturally synthesized in lymphocytes, monocytes, fibroblasts, bone marrow stroma, and endothelium.

GM-CSF has been produced in a recombinant form and is available for therapy. Commonly used recombinant forms of GM-CSF include the following:

• **Sargramostim:** Differs from the native GM-CSF in its amino acid sequence and its glycosylation. Its half-life is about 2.7 hours when given subcutaneously.

• **Molgramostim:** Non-glycosylated variant of endogenous GM-CSF.

• **Regramostim:** Fully glycosylated variant of endogenous GM-CSF.

Recombinant GM-CSF can be administered subcutaneously or intravenously. When given intravenously, its half-life is 1–3 hours. This is prolonged to about 10 hours when it is given subcutaneously [31].

Apart from the above-mentioned side effects, higher doses of GM-CSF may lead to a capillary leakage syndrome with the development of edema as well as pleural and pericardial effusions. Thrombosis has also been reported. However, these side effects are rare.

Clinical use of G-CSF and GM-CSF

For the majority of patients with neutropenia, G-CSF is the standard therapy. The following conditions associated with neutropenia can also be treated with G-CSF or GM-CSF.

G-CSF is effective in preventing and treating chemotherapy-induced neutropenia [32].

> **Practice tip Recommended prophylactic use of G-CSF in combination with chemotherapy to reduce febrile neutropenia (FN) (EORTC guidelines 2010 [33])**
>
> • If a chemotherapy cycle has a high risk for FN (>20%), G-CSF should be given prophylactically (for comparison of the risk with the common chemotherapy regimen see [33]).
> • If a chemotherapy cycle has an intermediate risk for FN (10–20 %), individual risk factors as assessed before each cycle (65 years or older; low neutrophil count; female; liver, renal or cardiovascular disease; advanced disease; poor performance or nutrition status; anemia) should be taken into consideration.
> • If a patient developed a FN in a previous chemotherapy cycle, they should receive G-CSF in subsequent cycles.
> • When dose-dense or dose-intense chemotherapy regimen (for a list of the regimens see [33]) has the potential to improve survival.
> When a reduced dose or increased interval between chemotherapy cycles may lead to a poor prognosis, G-CSF may be used to continue chemotherapy as scheduled.
> Filgrastim (daily injection), lenograstim (daily injection), and pegfilgrastim (once per cycle injection) seem to be equally effective.

Also, patients undergoing stem cell transplantation have benefited from G-CSF [34, 35]. G-CSF mobilizes stem cells into the blood and speeds up the hematological recovery of patients after transplantation.

Patients with MDS and neutropenia have also benefited from G-CSF. However, due to the concern about the development of overt leukemia, patients with MDS should receive G-CSF only in severe neutropenia associated with infection, a high risk of infection due to other than neutropenic risk factors (e.g., old age), and in conjunction with erythropoietin (EPO) to support red cell recovery. Under such circumstances, G-CSF is given only intermittently.

G-CSF is also indicated in selected cases of leukemia therapy to enhance neutrophil recovery. However, this does not seem to improve the survival rate.

Patients with acquired aplastic anemia may benefit from G-CSF (or GM-CSF) [36]. It was a theoretical concern that growth factors could accelerate the rate of transformation of aplastic anemia to MDS or to acute myeloid leukemia. A large database review did not confirm this worry. However, the continuous use of G-CSF is currently not recommended and it should be restricted to intermittent episodes of infection [37].

Patients with other forms of bone marrow failure or with diseases that cause neutropenia may also benefit from G-CSF or GM-CSF. Among these are Fanconi anemia, dyskeratosis congenital [38], severe chronic neutropenia (as infantile agranulocytosis), cyclic neutropenia, idiopathic neutropenia, Shwachman–Diamond syndrome, Felty syndrome, Chediak–Higashi syndrome, autoimmune neutropenia, and glycogen storage disease 1b. In such conditions, the response rate to G-CSF or GM-CSF is very high, and it has been shown that the continuous use of these agents over years is possible and beneficial.

Neutropenia induced by intoxication (e.g., autumn crocus) [39] and adverse reaction to drug therapy [40] can be successfully managed with G-CSF or GM-CSF.

Neutropenia in human immunodeficiency virus (HIV) infection and HIV antiviral therapy is also ameliorated by G-CSF or GM-CSF [41].

G-CSF and GM-CSF in combination with other hematological growth factors are used to treat accidental or therapeutic radiation injury. It speeds up bone marrow recovery. The sooner it is given after the irradiation, the better the hematological response [31].

Monocyte colony stimulating factor

Monocyte colony stimulating factor (M-CSF) regulates the proliferation and differentiation of monocyte and macrophage progenitors. Native M-CSF is produced in fibroblasts, endothelium, osteoblasts, keratinocytes, and monocytes themselves.

A recombinant form of human M-CSF (rHuM-CSF) is available. It is a glycoprotein produced in *E. coli*. rHuM-CSF is not widely used. It may, theoretically, be beneficial in increasing the monocyte count and with it the cells that produce other growth factors. The therapy of fungal infections may be enhanced by the administration of rHuM-CSF. However, since rHuM-CSF may cause thrombocytopenia, its use is limited.

Pluripotent, multilineal growth factors

To a certain degree, all known hematopoietic growth factors seem to be multilineal agents and are pluripotent.

However, the degree to which they influence organ systems other than a single line of hematopoiesis varies. This may be due to the fact that not much is known about their widespread biological effects, or each agent's activity may indeed be restricted to a few hematopoietic actions. Table 5.2 lists the growth factors that are known to have a pluripotent effect on hematopoiesis [31, 42–45].

General concerns about growth factor use

Although growth factors enhance a natural pathway, concerns have been raised about their use [46]. The most pronounced concern is that growth factors might induce or enhance cancer growth. Growth factors, acting mainly on the white cell lines, raised a special concern about the induction of leukemia or myelodysplasia (MDS). It was indeed shown that patients with long-term use of white cell growth factors developed leukemia. This may be due to the underlying disease itself, as a certain percentage of patients develop leukemia with or without growth factor therapy. The development of leukemia is now a recognized complication of MDS, congenital neutropenia, and aplastic anemia. In patients receiving chemotherapy with G-CSF support, the rate of developing secondary leukemia or MDS seems to be low, but a recent meta-analysis has shown that this risk is doubled when G-CSF is used during chemotherapy. However, the net effect of growth factor use favors overall survival [47].

Another concern was raised regarding the antigenicity of growth factors. As was shown with EPO (see Chapter 4), antibody formation is a realistic concern. Growth factors of the white cell lines and of the megakaryocyte line rarely induce antibody formation and very rarely seem to cross-react with the respective endogenous growth factors.

A third concern is the lineage steal. Worries were voiced that the accelerated proliferation of one cell line with a growth factor does not leave enough progenitor cells for the other cell lines. While neutropenia, anemia, and thrombocytopenia have been observed during therapy with EPO, IL-6, and G-CSF, large-scale studies did not confirm that a lineage steal is a common clinical problem.

Further concerns were raised regarding side effects of supranormal concentrations of growth factors. Many of the factors are proinflammatory. They increase the phagocytosis and chemotaxis of white cells. While this may be beneficial in some instances, it may theoretically

Table 5.2 Growth factors with known pluripotent effects on hematopoiesis.

Name	Description	Biological function	Use	Side effects
Stem cell factor (SCF, steel factor, c-kit ligand, ancestim, r-metHuSCF)	Produced in stroma of bone marrow; ligand for c-kit, a growth factor receptor	Supports survival of hematopoietic cells; stimulates early proliferation and growth of hematopoietic progenitors	Used in experimental settings in patients to induce hematopoiesis; to mobilize peripheral stem cells for future autologous transplantation	Frequent; also due to mast cell activation, therefore antiallergy prophylaxis desirable
Leridistim	Myelopoietin, chimeric growth factor consisting of IL-3 and G-CSF receptor agonists, produced by *E. coli*		Enhances white cell and platelet recovery in radiated monkeys and reduces their use of red cell transfusions; not widely used in humans	Not known
SC-68420	Myelopoietin, consisting of IL-3 and G-CSF, but different to leridistim		Used in animal experiments to recover neutrophil counts	Not known
PIXY 321	Genetic product of an artificial fusion of the genes for GM-CSF and IL-3	Attaches to neither the GM-CSF nor the IL-3 receptor, but to a receptor that attracts both GM-CSF and IL-3	In chemotherapy patients and bone marrow failure induces a slight increase in platelets, white cells, and red cells	Rash, fever, and erythema at the injection site. The effects were reported to be tolerable
Promegapoietin (PMP)	Family of chimeric products, consisting of a thrombopoietin receptor ligand and an IL-3 receptor ligand		Used in animal studies to increase neutrophil and platelet counts	Highly immunogenic, its development has been halted
Flt3 ligand	Fetal liver tyrosine kinase 3 (Flt 3) (receptor found in hematopoietic progenitors, mature blood cells and the heart, lungs, spleen, and muscle) ligand produced in bone marrow stroma	Proliferation, survival of primitive stem cells; supports development of lymphocytes and macrophages; synergistic with G-CSF and GM-CSF, erythropoietin, IL-3 and -11, and many other interleukins	Enhances white cell counts; much more potent when given together with G-CSF	Not known
Progenipoietin	Synthetic combination of Flt3 and G-CSF receptor agonists	Induces proliferation of multiple hematological cell lines	Not available for human use	Not known

G-CSF, granulocyte colony stimulating factor; GM-CSF, granulocyte–macrophage colony stimulating factor; IL-3, interleukin 3.

damage the lung and intestines. Other growth factors downregulate inflammatory responses. Skin reactions, vasculitis, and splenomegalia with atraumatic rupture have been observed after the use of some growth factors. Such reactions seem to be rare.

Growth factors in blood management

Management of thrombocytopenia

A variety of diseases cause thrombocytopenia and thrombocytopenia-related bleeding. Appropriate blood management therefore seeks to avoid thrombocytopenia and its associated bleeding, and enhance endogenous platelet production and function. General supportive measures in the treatment of thrombocytopenic patients seem to improve the clinical outcome (Table 5.3) [48]. To a certain degree, growth factors contribute to this as well. As shown above, several hematopoietic growth factors with thrombopoietic activity have been discovered over

Table 5.3 Supportive care for the thrombocytopenic patient.

All severely thrombocytopenic (<30 000 platelets) patients receive:
Vitamin K

Antifibrinolytic agents, (e.g., aminocaproic acid 1 g every 4 h i.v. or p.o.)

No anticoagulation, acetyl salicylic acid

Proton pump inhibitors

Stool softeners

Early removal of vascular catheters

Also consider: electrical over wet shaving preferred, use of a soft tooth brush or just an antiseptic mouth rinse

If thrombocytopenic patients start to bleed:
Increase antifibrinolytic agent (e.g., aminocaproic acid 4 g every 4 h i.v. or p.o.)

DDAVP

Nasal vasoconstrictors

Hormonal agents in females to prevent excessive blood loss via menses

the last decades. Currently, the second-generation thrombopoietic agents romiplostim and elthrombopag are available for clinical use, as well as IL-11, GM-CSF, and stem cell factor. It was shown that some of these are effective in preventing and treating thrombocytopenia and bleeding.

Patients suffering from thrombocytopenia caused by different diseases have benefited from therapy with thrombopoietic agents. In case reports, patients with thrombocytopenia due to aplastic anemia have benefited from long-term therapy with PEG-rHuMGDF by increasing platelet and erythrocyte levels and reducing bleeding episodes [49]. Other anecdotal evidence reports benefit from a combination of G-CSF with stem cell factor (ancestim) in improving thrombocytopenia in aplastic anemia [50].

Patients with various forms of chronic ITP may also benefit from thrombopoietic agents. Standard of care may consist of glucocorticoids, splenectomy, anti-D-immunoglobulins, rituximab, or other immunomodulatory agents. Results are favorable in up to 70% of patients. In addition to the standard of care, therapy with PEG-rHuMGDF, rHuTPO, and rHuTPO in combination with rHuIL-11 has been attempted [51–53]. Platelet production increased and bleeding episodes decreased. After the cessation of clinical use of the first-generation thrombopoietic agents, extensive studies were started to test the second-generation agents for use in ITP. Thus, elthrombopag and romiplostim found their way into the clinic. They were shown to significantly increase platelet levels and reduce overall bleeding episodes as effectively as standard of care, while having fewer side effects than the latter. So far, the influence of the second-generation agents on overall survival has not been determined [6, 54, 55].

Radiation- and chemotherapy-related thrombocytopenia are other areas where platelet growth factors have been employed. PEG-rHuMGDF, rHuTPO, and rHuIL-11 have proven successful in reducing thrombocytopenia in some patients undergoing myelosuppressive or ablative therapeutic regimens [6, 56–58]. Some general statements can be made about the chances of a thrombopoietic agent being effective. When thrombopoietic agents are administered before chemotherapy, a dose-related increase in platelet count can usually be observed [59]. However, when the agents are administered after the start of chemotherapy, and especially after the onset of thrombocytopenia, an accelerated hematological recovery is not consistently observed. Patients undergoing myeloablative chemotherapy, stem cell transplantation [60–63], and leukemia chemotherapy [64] often do not respond well to first-generation thrombopoietic agents. Second-generation thrombopoietic agents are currently under investigation regarding their ability to increase platelet counts in thrombocytopenic patients undergoing chemotherapy, but results have not been published yet [11].

Some (as yet not well-defined) patients with MDS have benefited from first-generation thrombopoietic agents [65]. The patients responded to such therapy with increased platelet counts, and some of them demonstrated a multilineal response [66]. Second-generation agents are under investigation in the therapy of MDS and preliminary data are promising, showing increased platelet levels and fewer bleeding episodes [67].

HIV infection and its treatment can cause thrombocytopenia, and PEG-rHuMGDF is able to reverse this effect. Whether the second-generation thrombopoietic agents are able to do so is not known, but is likely.

Thrombocytopenia secondary to severe liver disease may be amenable to therapy with thrombopoietic agents. Thrombocytopenia may not only be due to the reduced production of native TPO in severe liver disease, but also to hypersplenism. Studies are underway to test elthrombopag's ability to raise platelet counts in patients with pending invasive procedures [11].

Hepatitis C infection is an example of a chronic liver disease that may also present with thrombocytopenia. This is not only due to reduced TPO levels, but also to autoimmune mechanisms, virus-induced bone marrow suppression, and as a side effect of therapy with interferon and ribavirin. Elthrombopag was successfully used to increase platelet counts and to maintain effective therapy of hepatitis C with interferon and ribavirin [11, 68].

Thrombopoietic agents have also been suggested as treatment for neonatal thrombocytopenia [69, 70]. Taking into consideration that neonatal thrombocytopenia is usually short-lived, clinical benefit may only be seen in patients with an expected longer phase of thrombocytopenia, such as is found in liver disease and viral infection.

Some animal experiments suggest the use of thrombopoietic agents for yet other thrombocytopenic conditions. For instance, preoperative treatment with PEG-rHuMGDF has proven effective in animal models of surgical extracorporeal circulation to reduce bleeding and thrombocytopenia [71]. Also, platelet counts were increased in animals with Kasabach–Merritt syndrome,

and PEG-rHuMGDF has been recommended for use in this setting [72].

Some of the growth factors mentioned have been grouped together under the heading "platelet transfusion and alternatives to transfusion" [73]. Indeed, some of the growth factors are effective in increasing platelet counts and reducing thrombocytopenia-related bleeding. However, as they do not acutely increase platelet counts, they do not seem to be the perfect agents. Foresight, prevention, and earliest possible therapy with those agents are therefore mandatory in preventing platelet counts from falling too low. Whether it is beneficial for patients to receive thrombopoietic agents in an acute thrombocytopenic condition, by simply assuming that the function of the residual platelets is enhanced, cannot be said.

Management of neutropenia

A low neutrophil count is associated with infections. When falling below 1000/μL, the risk for infection is increased, and it is especially high if the count is below 100/μL. The longer the time a patient is exposed to neutropenia, the higher is the risk of acquiring infections. In addition to antibiotics, granulocyte transfusions were sometimes favored. However, they have severe side effects and their efficacy in improving patient outcome is far from proven. Actually, granulocyte transfusions are no more than experimental. Nevertheless, severe neutropenia is life-threatening and calls for intervention. A variety of synthetic growth factors are available for this. rHuG-CSF and rHuGM-CSF are the agents with a relatively long and reassuring efficacy and safety record.

Patients who might be given a leukocyte transfusion are apt candidates for therapy with rHuG-CSF or rHuGM-CSF. Patients who relapse after stem cell transplantation are typically given leukocyte transfusions. rHuG-CSF seems to be a better therapeutic option with fewer side effects [74]. Patients with aplastic anemia or congenital chronic neutropenia, who are considered candidates for white cell transfusion, can be successfully managed with white cell growth factors [30]. rHuG-CSF alone or in combination with rHuGM-CSF or EPO was shown to improve stem cell mobilization into the peripheral blood and accelerate hematological recovery after stem cell transplantation. This translates into fewer transfusions [34, 75, 76].

rHuG-CSF and rHuGM-CSF reduce the duration of neutropenia, shorten hospitalization, and reduce antibiotic therapy in patients undergoing chemotherapy.

Management of multilineal hematological failure

Many forms of hematological failure are multilineal failures. This is true for diseases such as MDS and aplastic anemia. Multilineal failure is also common as a result of chemotherapy and radiation therapy. Prevention or treatment is essential. Some approaches resort to treating every line failure separately, while others try to address the multilineal failure collectively, using early acting growth factors or their interactions.

The approaches that treat the lines individually typically use recombinant EPO (rHuEPO) for red cell line failure, G-CSF or GM-CSF for white cell line failure, and possibly rHuIL-11 or rHuTPO to enhance megakaryosynthesis. However, since this approach, as straightforward as it may sound, may not invariably result in the desired effects, other approaches have been tried. Some early or multifunctional agents were proposed for the treatment of multilineal bone marrow failure. These include IL-3 and stem cell factor, which showed some success. For instance, recombinant human IL-3 (rHuIL-3) has shown a clear effect in improving chemotherapy-induced bone marrow failure, but with a variable response [77].

Another approach to multilineal failure is to use a combination of hematopoietic agents to achieve a synergistic action on hematopoiesis. In nature there is clearly a synergistic action of a variety of factors. Certain factors act only in certain phases of hematopoiesis or on certain lines, while other factors seem to act on more or all hematopoietic lines and almost throughout the whole hematopoietic process. Mimicking the interaction of so many factors is difficult. It is therefore understandable that progress in research has not (yet) yielded the desired universal agent(s) to successfully treat multilineal failures.

A combination of hematopoietic agents can be applied by either administering several single agents to the same patient, or synthesizing chimeric agents. Some combinations indeed achieve a better effect than single factors alone, e.g., rHuEPO and rHuGM-CSF combined for MDS to stimulate erythropoietic response. Most proposed combinations have not lived up to their promise, e.g., rHuEPO in combination with rHuIL-3 [78]. In trials using a variety of growth factors or early acting factors, it was seen that some patients reacted with a limited or even substantial improvement of their condition. Overall, though, there has been no consistent success.

Key points

- Hematopoietic growth factors have tremendously improved selected patient's hematological status.
- G-CSF and its analogs not only reduce neutropenia, but also improve survival in selected patient populations.
- First-generation thrombopoietic growth factors have been withdrawn from the market, while second-generation agents are now licensed for use in ITP, with promising preliminary results in the treatment of thrombocytopenia due to other causes.

Questions for review

1. Which growth factors act primarily on white cell production and which on platelet production? Which ones act on both lines?
2. Which growth factors are already available for therapy and which ones are still in the experimental stage?
3. What is the role of hematopoietic growth factors in blood management? Are thrombopoietic and leukopoietic agents able to increase platelet and white cell count and to reduce bleeding and febrile episodes, respectively? Do they improve outcome?
4. What conditions have benefited from therapy with thrombopoietic and leukopoietic agents?

Suggestions for further research

Complete Figure 5.1 by inserting the growth factors in the boxes of the cell types on which they act (this has already been done for pluripotent stem cell as an example). If necessary, refer to the literature to perform this task.

Exercises and practice cases

Perform a literature search. What growth factors may be relevant for the therapy of patients with the following diseases: sepsis with *Aspergillus*, Diamond–Blackfan anemia, and cyclic ITP?

Homework

Find out which hematopoietic growth factors are available in your hospital and in your country. Are any growth factors licensed or are they used in experimental settings only? Note who produces and markets them.

References

1. Zheng C, Yang R, Han Z, Zhou B, Liang L, Lu Ml. TPO-independent megakaryocytopoiesis. *Crit Rev Oncol Hematol* 2008;**65**:212–222.
2. Geddis AE. Megakaryopoiesis. *Semin Hematol* 2010;**47**:212–219.
3. Thon JN, Italiano JE. Platelet formation. *Semin Hematol* 2010;**47**:220–226.
4. Kuter DJ, Begley CG. Recombinant human thrombopoietin: basic biology and evaluation of clinical studies. *Blood* 2002;**100**:3457–3469.
5. Kuter DJ. New thrombopoietic growth factors. *Blood* 2007;**109**:4607–4616.
6. Somlo G, Sniecinski I, ter Veer A, *et al*. Recombinant human thrombopoietin in combination with granulocyte colony-stimulating factor enhances mobilization of peripheral blood progenitor cells, increases peripheral blood platelet concentration, and accelerates hematopoietic recovery following high-dose chemotherapy. *Blood* 1999;**93**:2798–2806.
7. Neumann TA, Foote M. Megakaryocyte growth and development factor (MGDF): an Mpl ligand and cytokine that regulates thrombopoiesis. *Cytokines Cell Mol Ther* 2000;**6**:47–56.
8. Harker LA, Roskos LK, Marzec UM, *et al*. Effects of megakaryocyte growth and development factor on platelet production, platelet life span, and platelet function in healthy human volunteers. *Blood* 2000;**95**:2514–2522.
9. Miyazaki H, Kato T. Thrombopoietin: biology and clinical potentials. *Int J Hematol* 1999;**70**:216–225.
10. Fetscher S, Mertelsmann R. Supportive care in hematological malignancies: hematopoietic growth factors, infections, transfusion therapy. *Curr Opin Hematol* 1999;**6**:262–273.
11. Stasi R, Bosworth J, Rhodes E, Shannon MS, Willis F, Gordon-Smith EC. Thrombopoietic agents. *Blood Rev* 2010;**24**:179–190.
12. Kuter DJ. Biology and chemistry of thrombopoietic agents. *Semin Hematol* 2010;**47**:243–248.
13. Cuker A. Toxicities of the thrombopoietic growth factors. *Semin Hematol* 2010;**47**:289–298.
14. Sekeres MA, Kantarjian H, Fenaux P, *et al*. Subcutaneous or intravenous administration of romiplostim in thrombocytopenic patients with lower risk myelodysplastic syndromes. *Cancer* 2011;**117**:992–1000.
15. Shirasugi Y, Ando K, Miyazaki K, *et al*. Romiplostim for the treatment of chronic immune thrombocytopenia in adult Japanese patients: a double-blind, randomized Phase III clinical trial. *Int J Hematol* 2011;**94**:71–80.
16. Nieto M, Borregaard J, Ersbøll J, *et al*. The European Medicines Agency review of eltrombopag (Revolade) for the treatment of adult chronic immune (idiopathic) thrombocytopenic purpura: summary of the scientific assessment of the Committee for Medicinal Products for Human Use. *Haematologica* 2011;**96**:e33–40.
17. Reynolds CH. Clinical efficacy of rhIL-11. *Oncology (Williston Park)* 2000;**14** (9 Suppl 8):32–40.
18. Ustun C, Dainer PM, Faguet GB. Interleukin-11 administration normalizes the platelet count in a hypersplenic cirrhotic patient. *Ann Hematol* 2002;**81**:609–610.
19. Guinan EC, Lee YS, Lopez KD, *et al*. Effects of interleukin-3 and granulocyte-macrophage colony-stimulating factor on thrombopoiesis in congenital amegakaryocytic thrombocytopenia. *Blood* 1993;**81**:1691–1698.
20. Smith JW 2nd, Longo DL, Alvord WG, *et al*. The effects of treatment with interleukin-1 alpha on platelet recovery after high-dose carboplatin. *N Engl J Med* 1993;**328**:756–761.
21. Vadhan-Raj S, Kudelka AP, Garrison L, *et al*. Effects of interleukin-1 alpha on carboplatin-induced thrombocytopenia in patients with recurrent ovarian cancer. *J Clin Oncol* 1994;**12**:707–714.
22. Kaushansky K. The thrombocytopenia of cancer. Prospects for effective cytokine therapy. *Hematol Oncol Clin North Am* 1996;**10**:431–455.
23. D'Hondt V, Humblet Y, Guillaume T, *et al*. Thrombopoietic effects and toxicity of interleukin-6 in patients with ovarian cancer before and after chemotherapy: a multicentric placebo-controlled, randomized phase Ib study. *Blood* 1995;**85**:2347–2353.
24. Sakai R, Nakamura T, Nishino T, *et al*. Xanthocillins as thrombopoietin mimetic small molecules. *Bioorg Med Chem* 2005;**13**:6388–6393.
25. Safonov IG, Heerding DA, Keenan RM, *et al*. New benzimidazoles as thrombopoietin receptor agonists. *Bioorg Med Chem Lett* 2006;**16**:1212–1216.
26. Cwirla SE, Balasubramanian P, Duffin DJ, *et al*. Peptide agonist of the thrombopoietin receptor as potent as the natural cytokine. *Science* 1997;**276**:1696–1699.
27. Zang Y, Zhang X, Jiang X, *et al*. Expression, purification, and characterization of a novel recombinant fusion protein, rhTPO/SCF, in Escherichia coli. *Appl Microbiol Biotechnol* 2007;**74**:836–842.
28. Dunn CJ, Goa KL. Lenograstim: an update of its pharmacological properties and use in chemotherapy-induced neutropenia and related clinical settings. *Drugs* 2000;**59**:681–717.
29. Huttmann A, Schirsafi K, Seeber S, Bojko P. Comparison of lenograstim and filgrastim: effects on blood cell recovery after high-dose chemotherapy and autologous peripheral blood stem cell transplantation. *J Cancer Res Clin Oncol* 2005;**131**:152–156.
30. Balint B. Renewed granulocyte support practice and its alternatives. *Vojnosanit Pregl* 2004;**61**:537–545.

31. Thierry D, Gourmelon P, Parmentier C, Nénot JC. Haemat-opoietic growth factors in the treatment of therapeutic and accidental irradiation-induced bone marrow aplasia. *Int J Radiat Biol* 1995;**67**:103–117.

32. Johnston EM, Crawford J. Hematopoietic growth factors in the reduction of chemotherapeutic toxicity. *Semin Oncol* 1998;**25**:552–561.

33. Aapro MS, Bohlius J, Cameron DA, *et al.* 2010 update of EORTC guidelines for the use of granulocyte-colony stimu-lating factor to reduce the incidence of chemotherapy-induced febrile neutropenia in adult patients with lymphoproliferative disorders and solid tumours. *Eur J Cancer* 2011;**47**:8–32.

34. Olivieri A, Scortechini I, Capelli D, *et al.* Combined admin-istration of alpha-erythropoietin and filgrastim can improve the outcome and cost balance of autologous stem cell trans-plantation in patients with lymphoproliferative disorders. *Bone Marrow Transplant* 2004;**34**:693–702.

35. Bishop MR, Tarantolo SR, Geller RB, *et al.* A randomized, double-blind trial of filgrastim (granulocyte colony-stimulating factor) versus placebo following allogeneic blood stem cell transplantation. *Blood* 2000;**96**:80–85.

36. Jeng MR, Naidu PE, Rieman MD, *et al.* Granulocyte-macrophage colony stimulating factor and immunosup-pression in the treatment of pediatric acquired severe aplastic anemia. *Pediatr Blood Cancer* 2005;**45**:170–175.

37. Heuser M, Ganser A. Colony-stimulating factors in the management of neutropenia and its complications. *Ann Hematol* 2005;**84**:697–708.

38. Erduran E, Hacisalihoglu S, Ozoran Y. Treatment of dysk-eratosis congenita with granulocyte-macrophage colony-stimulating factor and erythropoietin. *J Pediatr Hematol Oncol* 2003;**25**:333–335.

39. Gabrscek L, Lesnicar G, Krivec B, *et al.* Accidental poisoning with autumn crocus. *J Toxicol Clin Toxicol* 2004;**42**:85–88.

40. Kotanagi H, Ito M, Koyama K, Chiba M. Pancytopenia asso-ciated with 5-aminosalicylic acid use in a patient with Crohn's disease. *J Gastroenterol* 1998;**33**:571–574.

41. Scadden DT. Cytokine use in the management of HIV disease. *J Acquir Immune Defic Syndr Hum Retroviro* 1997;**16** (Suppl 1):S23–29.

42. Blaise D, Faucher C, Vey N, Caraux J, Maraninchi D, Chabannon C. Rescue of haemopoiesis by a combination of growth factors including stem-cell factor. *Lancet* 2000;**356**:1325–1326.

43. Farese AM, *et al.* Leridistim, a chimeric dual G-CSF and IL-3 receptor agonist, enhances multilineage hematopoietic recovery in a nonhuman primate model of radiation-induced myelosuppression: effect of schedule, dose, and route of administration. *Stem Cells* 2001;**19**:522–533.

44. Farese AM, Casey DB, Smith WG, Vigneulle RM, McKearn JP, MacVittie TJ. Promegapoietin-1a, an engineered chi-meric IL-3 and Mpl-L receptor agonist, stimulates hemat-opoietic recovery in conventional and abbreviated schedules

following radiation-induced myelosuppression in nonhu-man primates. *Stem Cells* 2001;**19**:329–338.

45. Drexler HG, Quentmeier H. FLT3: receptor and ligand. *Growth Factors* 2004;**22**:71–73.

46. Carr R, Modi N. Haemopoietic growth factors for neonates: assessing risks and benefits. *Acta Paediatr* 2004;**93** (Suppl):15–19.

47. Lyman GH, Dale DC, Wolff DA, *et al.* Acute myeloid leuke-mia or myelodysplastic syndrome in randomized controlled clinical trials of cancer chemotherapy with granulocyte colony-stimulating factor: a systematic review. *J Clin Oncol* 2010;**28**:2914–2924.

48. Ford P. *Stem cell transplantation without the use of blood products.* First European Congress on Blood Conservation, Vienna, Austria, 2005.

49. Yonemura Y, Miyake H, Asou N, Mitsuya H. Long-term efficacy of pegylated recombinant human megakaryocyte growth and development factor in therapy of aplastic anemia. *Int J Hematol* 2005;**82**:307–309.

50. Usuki K, Iki S, Arai S, Iijima K, Takaku F, Urabe A. Stable response after administration of stem cell factor combined with granulocyte colony-stimulating factor in aplastic anemia. *Int J Hematol* 2006;**83**:404–407.

51. Nomura S, Dan K, Hotta T, Fujimura K, Ikeda Y. Effects of pegylated recombinant human megakaryocyte growth and development factor in patients with idiopathic thrombocy-topenic purpura. *Blood* 2002;**100**:728–730.

52. Zhao YQ, Wang QY, Zhai M, *et al.* [A multi-center clinical trial of recombinant human thrombopoietin in chronic refractory idiopathic thrombocytopenic purpura.] *Zhong-hua Nei Ke Za Zhi* 2004;**43**:608–610.

53. Liao X, Tang X, Deng C, Niu T, Meng W. [The effects of thrombopoietin and interleukin-11 on bone marrow meg-akaryocytic progenitors in patients with chronic idiopathic thrombocytopenic purpura in vitro.] *Hua Xi Yi Ke Da Xue Xue Bao* 2001;**32**:572–575.

54. Zeng Y, *et al.* TPO receptor agonist for chronic idiopathic thrombocytopenic purpura. *Cochrane Database Syst Rev* 2011;(7):CD008235.

55. Cheng G. Eltrombopag for the treatment of immune throm-bocytopenia. *Expert Rev Hematol* 2011;**4**:261–269.

56. Basser RL, Underhill C, Davis I, Enhancement of platelet recovery after myelosuppressive chemotherapy by recom-binant human megakaryocyte growth and development factor in patients with advanced cancer. *J Clin Oncol* 2000;**18**:2852–2861.

57. Tepler I, Elias L, Smith JR 2nd, *et al.* A randomized placebo-controlled trial of recombinant human interleukin-11 in cancer patients with severe thrombocytopenia due to chem-otherapy. *Blood* 1996;**87**:3607–3614.

58. Turner KJ, Neben S, Weich N, Schaub RG, Goldman SJ. The role of recombinant interleukin 11 in megakaryocytopoie-sis. *Stem Cells* 1996;**14** (Suppl 1):53–61.

59. Gordon MS, McCaskill-Stevens WJ, Battiato LA, *et al.* A phase I trial of recombinant human interleukin-11

(neumega rhIL-11 growth factor) in women with breast cancer receiving chemotherapy. *Blood* 1996;**87**:3615–3624.

60. Schuster MW, Beveridge R, Frei-Lahr D, *et al*. The effects of pegylated recombinant human megakaryocyte growth and development factor (PEG-rHuMGDF) on platelet recovery in breast cancer patients undergoing autologous bone marrow transplantation. *Exp Hematol* 2002;**30**:1044–1050.

61. Fields KK, Crump M, Bence-Bruckler I, *et al*. Use of PEG-rHuMGDF in platelet engraftment after autologous stem cell transplantation. *Bone Marrow Transplant* 2000;**26**: 1083–1088.

62. Bolwell B, Vredenburgh J, Overmoyer B, *et al*. Phase 1 study of pegylated recombinant human megakaryocyte growth and development factor (PEG-rHuMGDF) in breast cancer patients after autologous peripheral blood progenitor cell (PBPC) transplantation. *Bone Marrow Transplant* 2000;**26**: 141–145.

63. Vredenburgh JJ, Hussein A, Fisher D, *et al*. A randomized trial of recombinant human interleukin-11 following autologous bone marrow transplantation with peripheral blood progenitor cell support in patients with breast cancer. *Biol Blood Marrow Transplant* 1998;**4**:134–141.

64. Archimbaud E, Ottmann OG, Yin JA, *et al*. A randomized, double-blind, placebo-controlled study with pegylated recombinant human megakaryocyte growth and development factor (PEG-rHuMGDF) as an adjunct to chemotherapy for adults with de novo acute myeloid leukemia. *Blood* 1999;**94**:3694–3701.

65. Geissler RG, Schulte P, Ganser A. Treatment with growth factors in myelodysplastic syndromes. *Pathol Biol (Paris)* 1997;**45**:656–667.

66. Kizaki M, Miyakawa Y, Ikeda Y. Long-term administration of pegylated recombinant human megakaryocyte growth and development factor dramatically improved cytopenias in a patient with myelodysplastic syndrome. *Br J Haematol* 2003;**122**:764–767.

67. Bryan J, Jabbour E, Prescott H, Kantarjian H. Thrombocytopenia in patients with myelodysplastic syndromes. *Semin Hematol* 2011;**47**:274–280.

68. Tillmann HL, McHutchison JG. Use of thrombopoietic agents for the thrombocytopenia of liver disease. *Semin Hematol* 2010;**47**:266–273.

69. Ferrer-Marin F, Liu ZJ, Gutti R, Sola-Visner M. Neonatal thrombocytopenia and megakaryocytopoiesis. *Semin Hematol* 2010;**47**:281–288.

70. Murray NA. Evaluation and treatment of thrombocytopenia in the neonatal intensive care unit. *Acta Paediatr* 2002;**91** (Suppl):74–81.

71. Nakamura M, Toombs CF, Duarte IG, *et al*. Recombinant human megakaryocyte growth and development factor attenuates postbypass thrombocytopenia. *Ann Thorac Surg* 1998;**66**:1216–1223.

72. Verheul HM, Panigrahy D, Flynn E, Pinedo HM, D'Amato RJ. Treatment of the Kasabach-Merritt syndrome with pegylated recombinant human megakaryocyte growth and development factor in mice: elevated platelet counts, prolonged survival, and tumor growth inhibition. *Pediatr Res* 1999;**46**:562–565.

73. Vaickus L, Breitmeyer JB, Schlossman RL, Anderson KC. Platelet transfusion and alternatives to transfusion in patients with malignancy. *Stem Cells* 1995;**13**:588–596.

74. Bishop MR, Tarantolo SR, Pavletic ZS, *et al*. Filgrastim as an alternative to donor leukocyte infusion for relapse after allogeneic stem-cell transplantation. *J Clin Oncol* 2000;**18**: 2269–2272.

75. Nademanee A, Sniecinski I, Schmidt GM, *et al*. High-dose therapy followed by autologous peripheral-blood stem-cell transplantation for patients with Hodgkin's disease and non-Hodgkin's lymphoma using unprimed and granulocyte colony-stimulating factor-mobilized peripheral-blood stem cells. *J Clin Oncol* 1994;**12**:2176–2186.

76. Schmitz N, Linch DC, Dreger P, *et al*. Randomised trial of filgrastim-mobilised peripheral blood progenitor cell transplantation versus autologous bone-marrow transplantation in lymphoma patients. *Lancet* 1996;**347**:353–357.

77. Rinehart J, Margolin KA, Triozzi P, *et al*. Phase I trial of recombinant interleukin 3 before and after carboplatin/etoposide chemotherapy in patients with solid tumors: a southwest oncology group study. *Clin Cancer Res* 1995;**1**: 1139–1144.

78. Miller AM, Noyes WE, Taetle R, List AF. Limited erythropoietic response to combined treatment with recombinant human interleukin 3 and erythropoietin in myelodysplastic syndrome. *Leuk Res* 1999;**23**:77–83.

6 Fluid Management

Circulating intravascular volume is essential for survival. Therefore, fluid therapy is one of the first measures taken to resuscitate a patient. In the context of blood management, fluids serve several purposes as they expand the plasma volume. They not only guarantee cardiac output by means of the Frank–Starling mechanism, but also carry red cells, oxygen, nutrients, metabolic byproducts, and drugs. Besides, they cause changes in the microvasculature, coagulation profile, and rheology. All intravascular fluids have a profound impact on the water and electrolyte balance of the body. Effects may be beneficial or detrimental. An in-depth understanding of fluids is needed to convey the maximum benefit to the patient from fluid management.

Objectives

1. To explain the importance of fluid therapy in blood management.
2. To learn about the role of blood products in volume therapy.
3. To explain different models of the human fluid balance and their implications for fluid management.
4. To describe how the choice and timing of fluid therapy influences coagulation parameters and blood loss.

Definitions

Plasma substitutes: Any liquids that are used to replace blood plasma. Sometimes, the term *plasma substitute* refers only to colloid solutions.

Crystalloids: Solutions that contain electrolytes or other small solutes. Their molecular weight does not exceed 30 kDa. By definition, crystalloids have zero colloid osmotic pressure.

Colloids: Solutions that contain substances with a molecular weight exceeding 30 kDa. The dispersed particles are between 1 and 10 nm in diameter and cannot be separated by filtration or gravity. Colloids exert a colloid-osmotic pressure.

Volume therapy: The replacement or expansion of plasma volume to achieve an optimal intravascular fluid level, to restore osmotic pressure, to influence rheology, and to ensure microvascular perfusion.

A brief history

The history of intravenously administered fluids dates back to Christopher Wren in the middle of the 17th century when he described the first vascular access by quill and bladder. He and his colleagues at the Royal Society, England, experimented with different fluids as "blood substitutes," including wine, beer, and milk.

A more scientific approach to fluid management was taken about 200 years later. O'Shaughnessy and Brooke observed pathophysiological changes in cholera patients. They wrote: "The blood drawn in the worst of cases of the cholera has lost a large proportion of its water. It has lost also a great proportion of its neutral saline ingredients" [1]. Based on this observation, Thomas Latta administered saline solution intravenously. One source wrote: "The great desideratum of restoring the natural current in the veins and arteries, of improving the color of the blood, and recovering the functions of the lungs, in Cholera Asphyxia, may be accomplished by injecting a weak saline solution into the veins of the patient. To Dr

Basics of Blood Management, Second Edition. Petra Seeber and Aryeh Shander.
© 2013 John Wiley & Sons, Ltd. Published 2013 by John Wiley & Sons, Ltd.

Thomas Latta . . . is due the merit of first having recourse to this practice. . . . To produce the effect referred to, a large quantity must be injected, from *five to ten pounds in an adult*" [2].

Some years later, in 1860, normal saline was used by Barnes and Little to treat hemorrhage. Bull and colleagues recommended the use of saline as a transfusion substitute for blood [3].

In 1880, Sydney Ringer, who experimented with frog hearts, used normal saline as well. Not being content with the results, he added other electrolytes to normal saline, developing a more physiological electrolyte solution. Consequently, he became the father of Ringer's solution. In the 1930s, Alexis Hartmann added a lactate buffer to an electrolyte solution to treat metabolic acidosis. This addition produced what we now call Hartmann's solution.

Finally, as the results of Penfield's work, the first successful use of hypertonic saline solutions for medical purposes was reported in 1919. But it was not until 1980 that DeFelippe and colleagues undertook systematic investigations on the clinical use of hypertonic sodium chloride solutions. Today's sophisticated solutions are the result of innumerable refinements in the type and amount of ions added to resuscitation fluids.

The history of the colloids began in 1861 when Thomas Graham experimented with different solutions. He passed them through a membrane. Some fluids were unable to pass through the membrane. Graham called these fluids colloids, coming from the Latin word "*collo*," meaning glue.

The medical use of colloids began in the early part of the 20th century. During the First World War, Arabian gum solutions were advocated for the treatment of severe hemorrhage. However, their toxicity led them to fall into disrepute by the late 1930s. A more successful approach to volume substitution with a colloid was the use of gelatin. It has been in clinical use since 1915 [4]. In the beginning, gelatin was produced by boiling the connective tissues of animals, which developed a jelly-like fluid. These solutions had the advantage of having a significant oncotic effect. Unfortunately, they tended to gel on cooling—which makes infusion difficult. To overcome this unwanted effect, modified gelatin solutions were introduced. These became known as new-generation gelatins.

During the Second World War, polyvinylpyrrolidone (PVP), a synthetic polymer of vinyl pyrrolidone, was used as a colloid. PVP was soon abandoned as it was found to be stored permanently in the reticuloendothelial system. Attention moved to other colloids. Dextran solutions appeared to be an alternative. Sponsored by the sugar industry, Swedish chemists performed research on sugar beets and identified dextran. In order to detect even small amounts of this sugar, they tried to produce antibodies by injecting dextran into rabbits. However, no matter how hard they tried, the rabbits did not develop antibodies. At the same time and in the same place, other researchers tried to dry blood plasma and ship it to regions where the First World War was raging. From conversations among both groups of researchers, the idea was born to use dextran as a plasma expander, since it seemed to be non-antigenic. The urgent need for such a product accelerated the research and, very soon, the first clinical investigations started [5]. Raw dextran solutions were first used in 1943 in animals. The dextran in these solutions had a very high molecular weight and was highly antigenic. Reducing the size of the dextran molecule by hydrolysis made it fit for human use. In 1947, "Macrodex," a dextran with an average molecular weight of about 75 000 Da, was introduced into clinical practice.

Finally, starch solutions were modified and proved to be a usable colloid. Hydroxyethyl starch (HES) was introduced as plasma replacement in 1957 by Wiedersheim. Its career in clinical use began in the late 1960s and continues to this day.

Why do we need fluid therapy?

Judicious fluid management is thought to correlate with a favorable outcome [6]. Restoration of blood volume, blood pressure, and cardiac output is what classically is aimed at and indicates macrovascular resuscitation. It is hoped that macrovascular resuscitation translates into optimal tissue perfusion, tissue oxygenation, and removal of toxic metabolic byproducts. The ultimate goal of volume therapy, though, is to prevent patients from undue morbidity and mortality.

When considering fluid management, it is prudent to distinguish between the settings that call for fluid therapy. Absolute (physiological) fluid losses, whether in normal or increased quantity, include fluid losses via urine and perspiration. These losses are not accompanied by losses of oncotically active substances. Relative fluid losses, where fluids are not lost to the body, but have left their compartment by fluid shifts across membranes, may occur with or without oncotically active substances, the latter occurring especially when membranes leak. The second form of absolute fluid losses is pathological fluid losses, the most common form being blood loss. Thereby, oncotically active substances are also lost [7].

When clinically relevant, all the above mentioned fluid losses may call for fluid therapy. In the realm of blood management, fluid therapy is needed to replace lost blood. Besides, when fluids are given for reasons other than blood loss, prudent choice of the best possible fluid management may prevent coagulopathy and kidney failure, both of which may counteract optimal blood management.

At first glance, treating like with like, namely treating blood loss and anemia with blood transfusions, seems reasonable. But if increasing the cardiac output is the goal, transfusing red cells and whole blood is not the treatment of choice. Cellular fluids increase the viscosity of blood. Whole blood and erythrocyte transfusions sometimes even reduce blood flow and increase oxygen deficiency in tissue.

Basics of volume balance and intravenous fluids

The human body has an intricate system of volume control. To elucidate the mechanisms controlling the human fluid balance, physiology research has proposed a simplified model of this. It tries to explain what may happen when a particular fluid is infused. The model estimates that the total body water makes up 50–60% of the fat-free body mass. The total body water is divided in compartments or spaces. About 15% of the total body water is found in connective tissue and bones. Water exchange with this compartment takes a long time and in an acute situation, this compartment can be neglected in calculations. There are three further compartments or spaces relevant for clinical considerations regarding fluid management:
• Intracellular fluids (ICF)—55% of total body fluid
• Interstitial fluids (ISF)—20% of total body fluid
• Intravascular fluids (IVF)—about 7.5% of total body fluid.

Based on these estimates, it is assumed that the following volume ratios are true:
ICF/ECF about 2:1
ISF/IVF about 3:1 (approx 75% of the extracellular fluid is in the interstitium and 25% is in the vessels).

It was thought that the fluids in the respective compartments are kept relatively constant. Starling's law, taking the osmotic and hydrostatic pressures on both sides of a membrane into consideration, was thought to govern fluid movements across membranes. These assumptions were used to explain the behavior of the various intravenous fluids after being infused. However, the issue is not as simplistic. Many regulatory mechanisms alter the amount of fluids found in the body's compartments. When changing from the lying to the sitting position, plasma volume is shifted from the intravascular to the interstitial space. Inflammatory reactions (e.g., due to infection, surgical manipulation or trauma) increase vascular permeability, resulting in a shift of fluids from the intravascular to the interstitial space. Atrial natriuretic peptide, which is excreted in conditions of hypervolemia, also increases vascular permeability, causing similar fluid shifts. Such hypervolemia may be caused by an actual increase in intravascular fluids, e.g., by intravenous fluid therapy, or by vasoconstrictory influences. All these findings may be important in guiding effective fluid therapy [8].

Before starting the review of the various fluids, check Table A.6. It contains some definitions of terms that are used in the following paragraphs.

Intravenous fluids

There are two basic groups of intravenous fluids available: crystalloids and colloids. Crystalloids are solutions that contain electrolytes or other small solutes, their molecular weight not exceeding 30 kDa. By definition, crystalloids have zero colloid osmotic pressure. In contrast, colloids contain substances with a molecular weight exceeding 30 kDa. The dispersed particles are between 1 and 1000 nm in diameter and cannot be separated by filtration or gravity. Colloids exert a colloid-osmotic pressure.

Crystalloid solutions
Attempts have been made to classify crystalloids. They can be classified by their clinical use as replacement fluids, maintenance fluids, and fluids for special purposes.

Another way to classify crystalloids is to differentiate between balanced and unbalanced solutions. Balanced solutions are those with electrolyte concentrations similar to normal human plasma. Logically, balanced fluids are recommended for plasma (volume) replacement. Balanced solutions may have fewer side effects than unbalanced solutions.

Sodium chloride 0.9% (normal saline)

Normal saline is the prototype of all crystalloid solutions. It contains 154 mmol sodium and 154 mmol chloride. Although normal saline is referred to as "physiological" sodium chloride solution, its electrolyte levels are not physiological. The sodium level is a little higher than in normal plasma and the chloride level is much higher. Thus, normal saline is an example of an unbalanced crystalloid.

What happens to 1 L of normal saline after rapid intravenous infusion? As already mentioned, the sodium content of normal saline is similar to that found in the extracellular fluid compartment. This limits its distribution to the extracellular space. In theory, the infused solution disperses according to the distribution of the extracellular fluid—namely, 25% remains intravascularly and 75% is shifted interstitially. Theoretically, 25% of the infused liter remains in the vascular system and expands it by about 250 mL. This is the reason behind the historical recommendation to substitute 1 L of blood loss with 3–4 L of normal saline. This recommendation was drawn from the test results of laboratory physiology, but seems to contradict clinical findings [9]. Clinically, when measured in postoperative patients, the plasma volume expansion from infusion of 1 L normal saline amounted to 180 mL only. As will be outlined later, the plasma volume expansion with intravenous fluids in context-sensitive.

Ringer's, Hartmann's, etc.

Besides sodium and chloride, other ions may be added to a crystalloid solution—constituting a distinct solution or brand, e.g., Ringer's solution, Hartmann's solution, E153, and Plasmalyte. Among those added ions are potassium, calcium, and magnesium. Sometimes bicarbonate is added to these solutions. Lactate (or its racemate), gluconate, or acetate may be added as well. They are bicarbonate precursors that are metabolized to bicarbonate in the liver.

The distribution of all pure electrolyte solutions with a near-physiological sodium content in the body's fluid compartment follows the same principles as those that govern the distribution of normal saline, as outlined above.

Glucose solutions

Glucose is a small organic molecule. If dissolved in water, it also constitutes a crystalloid solution. Isotonic glucose solutions (about 5% glucose in water) are used to treat dehydration by providing free water. Hypertonic glucose solutions (>10%) are used to provide metabolic substrate or to treat hyperkalemia (together with insulin).

Glucose solutions are not suitable for volume substitution. Why? According to the fluid compartment model, 1 L of 5% glucose solution given intravenously is rapidly metabolized, leaving free water behind. This free water distributes throughout the whole body water space. Each space receives its share in proportion to its contribution to total body water. We know that only 7.5% of the total body water constitutes the intravascular volume. Consequently, only 7.5% of the liter of glucose solution remains in the blood stream, i.e., only 75 mL. This is less than ideal when it comes to plasma volume expansion. Therefore, glucose solutions are not a good choice for volume substitution.

Other points argue against the use of glucose as mere volume replacement as well. Severely sick patients may not be able to metabolize glucose properly. It is thus metabolized to lactate, which is thought to be toxic. Accumulation of glucose itself exerts osmotic pressure and leads to cell dehydration. If excess glucose is excreted by the kidney, it takes with it water and thereby promotes dehydration. Additionally, carbon dioxide production during metabolism may be problematic to patients on ventilation.

Hypertonic fluids

Hypertonic fluids contain an unphysiologically high percentage of electrolytes and come in varying osmolarities (500–2400 mOsm/kg). Among the most commonly used is hypertonic saline, e.g., with a 1.8% or 7.5% saline content. Rapid volume expansion is expected after infusion of small amounts of such hypertonic fluids (e.g., 250 mL). When iso-osmotic solutions are used, this effect, however, is only transient. The addition of colloids such as dextran or HES to increase the colloid osmotic pressure of the solution is thought to prolong their duration of action in keeping fluid in the intravascular system.

Hypertonic solutions are relatively cheap. It is even possible to prepare hypertonic solutions on the spot.

> ## Practice tip Preparing a hypertonic solution
>
> You can prepare a 1.8% NaCl solution by adding 150 mEq NaCl to 1 L of normal saline (NaCl 0.9%).

The way hypertonic fluids work is very simple. The sodium content of the solution limits its distribution to the extracellular space, since sodium cannot cross cell membranes easily. Water, in contrast, crosses cell membranes with ease and follows the osmotic gradient. The intravenous injection of hypertonic sodium chloride results in an increase of plasma sodium concentration and creates an osmotic gradient across the cell membrane. Like a sponge in a bucket of water, hypertonic sodium chloride draws water out of the tissue into the vessels. Endogenous intracellular fluids are mobilized and the intravascular volume increases. This is a kind of autotransfusion, tapping on the total body water, which is a huge reservoir amounting to more than 30 L in the adult.

Volume expansion is not the only effect hypertonic solutions exert. Due to the resulting volume expansion, cardiac output increases. Possible vasodilatatory effects in combination with venoconstriction lead to a drop in the afterload and overall changes in vascular tone. Taken together, oxygen delivery may improve. Additionally, myocardial performance improves since an increased serum osmolarity acts as an inotrope. Other reported beneficial effects are an enhanced renal perfusion, induction of diuresis, improvement of blood fluidity, re-establishment of spontaneous arteriolar vasomotion, and activation of the sympathetic nervous system. Beneficial effects of hypertonic saline and even more so of hypertonic saline with dextran have also been reported for the microcirculation. Since hypertonic saline draws water out of cells into vessels, swelling of the endothelial cell lining in the vasculature is reduced. Small vessels that have been blocked by this swelling may become patent again. This potentially improves tissue perfusion. Adhesion and activation of neutrophils is reduced by hypertonic solutions as well. Fewer substances that damage the endothelium are released by neutrophils. However, this positive effect was observed only if hypertonic solutions were given early after a physiological insult, such as a trauma, before the activation of neutrophils.

Unfortunately, hypertonic fluids also cause some unwanted effects. Infusion leads to electrolyte imbalance, resulting in hypernatremia, hyperchloremia, hyperosmolarity, and hypokalemia. Rapid infusion is to be avoided due to the danger of causing cardiac arrhythmias and cardiac failure. Severe hypernatremia and other electrolyte imbalances have the potential to cause neurological sequelae.

Hypertonic fluids occasionally irritate the vessel wall, resulting in pain at the injection site and thrombophlebitis. Coagulation disorders due to added dextran are

possible, but unlikely because the solution is given only in increments of 250 mL. There is also the potential for excessive blood loss when the hypertonic solution is given before active hemorrhage is stopped. Increased intravascular volume increases vascular wall tension and interferes with clotting.

Hypertonic solutions are used for so-called small-volume resuscitation. When compared with isotonic crystalloids, a smaller infusion volume is required to provide equal volume expansion. Less edema formation was observed. The volume-sparing effect of hypertonic solutions is especially desirable in cardiac patients and in patients undergoing extensive procedures, which normally require large amounts of fluids.

Despite more than 20 years of research yielding encouraging results, small-volume resuscitation has not changed clinical practice. Over the last few years, trials have been conducted in prehospital trauma patients, after cardiac bypass surgery, burns, endotoxic shock, brain edema, and other conditions. A recent trial with hypertonic saline in the trauma setting yielded discouraging results and the trial was stopped prematurely [10].

Colloid solutions

Plasma proteins such as albumin are the major colloids of human plasma. As such, they are important since they exert osmotic forces across the vessel wall. Due to their size, usually only small amounts of colloids leave the intact vessel. If the vessel wall is damaged, capillary leakage may result, and relatively large molecules may leave the blood vessel and travel to the interstitial space. By mimicking natural plasma colloids, synthetic colloids, called "plasma substitutes," may augment or replace plasma volume and act as a substitute for the osmotic effects of lost endogenous colloids.

The origin of therapeutically used colloids varies. There are naturally occurring colloids, such as albumin, and synthetically produced colloids, such as gelatin, dextran, and starch.

There is a particular terminology that is used in conjunction with colloid solutions:
• **Dispersion** divides colloids in monodisperse and polydisperse solutions. Albumin is a molecule that has a relatively constant molecular weight, being a monodisperse solution. In contrast, the molecular weight of synthetic colloid molecules varies, since their size follows the Gaussian distribution. These solutions are called polydisperse.

• The **molecular weight** indicates the weight of one molecule of the colloid. The actual molecular weight of colloid molecules in the solution follows the Gaussian distribution. The molecular weight indicated on the bottle of such solutions denotes the average weight of all molecules in that bottle. What is clinically important, though, is the so-called intravascular molecular weight. *In vivo*, the average molecular weight may change. This may be due to changes from enzymatic breakdown of the colloid molecule, e.g., starch. Besides, small molecules of a polydisperse colloid, especially if they are below the renal threshold of 50–60 kDa, are rapidly excreted. Other molecules may easily be broken down by blood enzymes. Such molecules do not contribute to the volume effect. What counts are the molecules that actually remain in the circulation for a given time. It is the number of molecules present, and not their size, that is responsible for the osmotic, water-binding effect.

Hydroxyethyl starch solutions

HES is a synthetic colloid made from corn or potato starch. This starch is the basis for the production of amylopectin, a glucose chain. For the production process, corn starch is preferred over potato starch because it already consists of more than 95% amylopectin, whereas potato starch consists of only 80% amylopectin. Hydroxyethyl groups are added to amylopectin (a process called hydroxylation) to synthesize the final product. Hydroxylation protects the HES molecules from degradation by serum amylases.

The pharmacology of HES varies greatly from one solution to another, depending on its properties. To distinguish different forms of HES, certain characteristics are described, namely, the molecular weight, degree, and pattern of substitution and concentration (Table 6.1). Labels on bottles of HES solutions state the characteristics of the fluids, e.g. HES 6% (130/0.4). The percentage gives the concentration of the starch solution. A 6% solution is considered iso-oncotic, a 10% solution hyperoncotic. The first number in the parentheses denotes the average molecular weight of the colloid, and the second number is the substitution degree or molar substitution (MS) of the starch. It describes how many glucose units on average are substituted, i.e., hydroxylated. A substitution degree of 0.4 means that on average there are four hydroxyethyl groups per 10 glucose molecules. Varying substitution degrees produce different starch formulations, such as hetastarch (MS = 0.7), hexastarch (MS = 0.6), pentastarch (MS = 0.5), and tetrastarch (MS = 0.4).

Table 6.1 Classification of hydroxyethyl starches.

Characteristic	Classification	Definition
Molecular weight	High	450–480 kDa (or >400 kDa)
	Medium	130–200 kDa (or 200–400 kDa)
	Low	40–70 (<100) kDa (or <200 kDa)
Concentration	High	10%
	Low	3–6%
Degree of substitution	High	0.6–0.7
	Low	0.4–0.5
Pattern of substitution	High	>8
(C2/C6 ratio)	Low	<8

Another characteristic of HES solutions is the pattern of substitution. This is determined by the position of the glucose groups on the entire HES molecule. It is sometimes expressed as the C2/C6 ratio. A high ratio means that there are many glucose molecules on the second carbon atom in the HES molecules. The more glucose substitution on a C2 molecule in an HES molecule, the longer the starch remains in the circulation. The reason for this is that glucose in the C2 position hinders the breakdown of the HES molecule by amylases. The less hydroxylation, the shorter is the stay in the circulation.

A further characteristic of a starch solution is the carrier solution. Initially, the starches were dissolved in normal saline. More recently, a balanced electrolyte solution has been used.

HES is excreted by the kidney. If this is hindered by the size and substitution pattern of the molecule, accumulation of HES in the reticuloendothelial system occurs. Accumulation is responsible for many of the side effects of HES: renal and immunological impairment, pruritus (notably in long-term administration), changes in the coagulation system, and an increase in blood viscosity. Pruritus is especially troubling for patients. It commences several weeks after HES administration and the effects can last as long as 2 years, with no therapy being effective [11].

HES solutions exert effects on the microvasculature. Some experimental evidence exists for the beneficial effect of HES. It was claimed for some HES that the extravascular leakage of colloids caused by microvascular hyperpermeability may be reduced, but this effect is not universally demonstrated [12]. Postulated underlying mechanisms may include the HES' sealing effect on the capillaries or the inhibition of endothelial activation and damage. HES may also modify severe inflammatory responses and reduce endothelial dysfunction. It may therefore be organ protective in sepsis and surgeries that elicit severe systemic inflammatory responses.

Dextran solutions

Dextran is a glucose polymer. It is synthesized by enzymes of *Leuconostoc mesenteroides*. This bacterium produces dextran of very high molecular weight. Hydrolytic breakdown and fractionation finally lead to different dextran preparations. Dextran solutions are available as dextran 40 (average molecular weight of 40 kDa) and dextran 70 (average molecular weight of 70 kDa). They are available in concentrations of 3–10% [13].

Initially, dextran has an excellent volume-increasing effect but the effect is only short-lived. Because of the small molecule size, dextran is excreted rapidly. Dextran 40 increases plasma volume more and acts for shorter duration than dextran 70.

Although initial experiments with dextran failed to demonstrate the antigenicity of dextran, antibodies are developed occasionally. To prevent anaphylactic reactions, a monovalent hapten, dextran 1, is usually given prior to the infusion of dextran 40 or 70 to block possible antibody development.

Nowadays, the use of dextran is limited and it has largely been replaced with HES. Dextran still has some use in combination with hypertonic saline.

Gelatin solutions

The gelatins available today are the so-called new-generation gelatins. They are modified polypeptides from bovine collagen. Three different modifications are used: cross-linked gelatin (e.g., Gelifundol), urea-linked gelatin (e.g., Polygelin), and succinylated gelatin (e.g., Gelofusine). Gelatin solutions differ with regard to their electrolyte concentrations. This is of clinical importance. Urea-linked gelatin has a high calcium and potassium concentration, while the succinylated preparations are low in calcium and potassium. Gelatin is available in solutions of concentrations of 4%, 6%, and 10%, and is dissolved in sodium chloride solution [13, 14].

The average molecular weight of gelatin is 30–35 kDa. This is far below the renal threshold of approximately 60 kDa. Gelatin is therefore rapidly excreted. The plasma half-life is only short, namely about 2 hours. Repeated doses are needed to maintain an appropriate intravascular volume.

High-viscosity fluids: Alginate solutions

Alginate solutions are not new. Studies with these agents were launched in the 1950s [15]. However, alginate solutions were not widely used clinically. It was only a few years ago that the interest in alginate was rekindled when searching for an agent to increase the viscosity of blood. In animal experiments, high-viscosity alginates are currently under investigation for use as a plasma expander [16].

Last but not least: The albumin story

Albumin is a naturally occurring colloid with an average molecular weight of about 66 kDa. It account for about 55% of the total blood protein pool of healthy persons. It is responsible for approximately 75% of the blood's colloid-osmotic pressure. Albumin solutions for clinical use are prepared from pooled human plasma. Commercially available solutions are either iso-oncotic (4/5%) or hyperoncotic (20/25%) [17].

Some think of albumin as the gold standard of colloid therapy. Others are absolutely against its use. Why? The proponents of albumin therapy cite albumin's ability to maintain the colloid osmotic pressure, its anti-inflammatory and antioxidant properties, its protective effects on the endothelium, and its buffering properties. The opponents not only cite its high costs, but also its pro-oxidant effects, the potential for pathogen transmission, and its lack of additional benefit or even survival over other fluid resuscitation regimens.

One rationale for the use of albumin may be to correct hypoalbuminemia. It is true that the serum albumin level of critically ill patients correlates with their outcome. A low albumin level predicts an unfavorable outcome. Nevertheless, the artificial correction of the albumin level by albumin supplementation does not improve the outcome and may even be associated with a worse outcome [18]. Hypoalbuminemia is best corrected with sufficient nutrition and treatment of the underlying condition.

Another reason that has been given for using albumin is to treat edema since albumin is a colloid that binds water. However, this is not the case. The reason for this is easy to understand when we consider that albumin is also present in the interstitial space. Also, when intravenously administered, albumin disperses freely in the interstitium, an effect that is even more pronounced in critically ill patients with capillary leakage. That is why albumin may even cause edema.

A third reason given for the use albumin is to administer the "ideal" resuscitation fluid. As the protein designed to maintain the colloid osmotic pressure of blood, it is thought to naturally have the lowest rate of side effects, even when solutions produced from donated blood are used. Nevertheless, when albumin solutions were tested in clinical routine for fluid resuscitation, they had little proven advantages over HES or saline [19]. In some groups of patients, albumin seems to be outrightly detrimental, such as in patients with traumatic brain injury. In some other groups of patients, albumin demonstrated some benefit [20]. Based on such contradictory findings, some authors claim that albumin reduces morbidity and mortality, while others refute this claim. To date, it has not been clarified which patients, if any, may benefit and which patients may be harmed by albumin resuscitation.

Side effects of intravenous fluids

Despite decades of research on fluid therapy, the choice of resuscitation fluid is often nothing more than a creed. Taking into consideration what side effects the fluids may elicit may make it easier to decide on the therapy for an individual patient.

Coagulation

Every intravenous fluid has the potential to impair hemostasis. They may dilute clotting factors, flush away newly made clots, and have specific effects on coagulation factors or platelets. Nevertheless, crystalloids may also enhance hemostasis. They were shown to cause a mild hypercoagulopathy, lasting several hours. The clinical impact of intravenous fluids on coagulation is not only fluid-specific but also depends on the amount and manner of fluid administration.

Albumin was thought of as the gold standard of fluid therapy, since it was postulated that it does not cause coagulopathy. Nevertheless, it was shown that albumin exerts an intrinsic anticoagulatory effect and may impair coagulation, especially in higher grades of hemodilution [21]. The same is true of gelatins. They were also thought not to influence coagulation, even in higher doses. However, specialized clotting tests (e.g., ristocetin time) were able to show some influence of gelatin on coagulation [22]. Even so, the influence of albumins and gelatins

on the body's ability to clot is not as pronounced as with dextran or some HES solutions [23].

Dextran is known for its inhibition of thrombocyte aggregation by coating platelets (inhibition of factor VIII) and its ability to increase fibrinolysis. Further, it reduces blood viscosity. Such properties may not be favorable in patients who are hemorrhaging, but they can be used to prevent thrombosis and to improve the blood's rheology.

The effect of HES on coagulation varies with the HES formulation. Some HES formulations cause an acquired von Willebrand syndrome. These may also alter the platelet's ability to participate effectively in the clotting process, either by coating the platelet or by interfering with its receptors. Some HES solutiomns decrease the expression of platelet receptors, while others increase it. DDAVP (1-deamino-8-D-arginine vasopressin) can offset some of the side effects of HES on coagulation [24]. There is a historical restriction of the amount of HES given. In an attempt to prevent coagulopathy, HES infusions were restricted to 20 mL/kg body weight/day. This recommendation was given in the early days of HES therapy, when only HES with a high molecular weight and a high substitution ratio was available. Although not universally agreed upon, medium molecular weight HES with a low substitution ratio and HES with a low molecular weight seem to alter coagulation much less than high molecular weight HES [23, 25]. Thus, it has been said that their maximum daily dose can be increased to 50 mL/kg body weight/day. The magnitude of their effects on the clotting process is comparable with those of gelatin solution [26].

Apart from the colloid itself, its carrier solution may influence the colloid's effects on the coagulation profile. A lack of calcium in the unbalanced solution was proposed to impair clotting. Colloids in calcium-containing carrier solutions may impair clotting less than the same colloid formulated in normal saline [27].

Kidney function

Virtually every colloid may impair kidney function and is associated with a higher rate of renal replacement therapy. For most colloids, this effect is dose dependent. The effect of albumin on kidney function is ambiguous, with some studies demonstrating a renoprotective, others a neutral, and others a detrimental effect. Gelatins are also thought to impair kidney function minimally. HES, and probably especially the high molecular weight formulations, are nephrotoxic and seem to cause higher rates of acute kidney failure and the need for dialysis.

In patients with renal insufficiency, HES should only be given in low concentration and with sufficient co-administration of crystalloids to prevent kidney damage [25].

Allergic reactions

According to a study by Laxenaire *et al.* [28], the following incidences of anaphylactoid reactions after colloid infusion occurred: 0.345% for gelatin, 0.273% for dextran, 0.099% for albumin, and 0.058% for HES. In 20% of the cases, these reactions were serious. Patients with a history of drug allergies were especially at risk of developing an anaphylactoid reaction. Gelatins and dextrans therefore should be avoided in patients with a known history of drug allergies.

Hyperchloremic metabolic acidosis

Hyperchloremic metabolic acidosis is a non-respiratory acidosis with an increase of chloride in plasma. The most common avoidable cause of this acidosis is an intravenous fluid with a high chloride content, as is found in unbalanced fluids and especially in normal saline. Balanced fluids do not cause this derangement. Hyperchloremic metabolic acidosis was reported to have many effects on red cells, coagulation, the gastrointestinal tract, and renal function. Although the clinical relevance of those effects is controversial, it was stated that balanced solutions could be superior to unbalanced solutions in preventing the development of this acidosis.

Fluids at work

When should fluid be given?

Does the timing of fluid resuscitation play a role? In general, the earlier the patient has an adequate fluid status, the better. In surgical and trauma patients, early fluid optimization is more efficacious than delayed resuscitation in maintaining or restoring normal tissue perfusion and oxygenation. The shorter the time a patient is in shock, the lower their risk of developing postinjury coagulopathy. However, early fluid resuscitation to achieve normovolemia and to restore a normal blood pressure in the actively bleeding patient seems to be detrimental. It favors bleeding or rebleeding when administered before definitive surgical hemostasis is achieved. The human body usually initiates clot formation within 10 minutes when the mean arterial blood pressure drops to 60 mmHg. In actively bleeding patients, such low blood pressures may be reached some minutes after the

trauma, depending on the velocity of blood loss [29]. When fluids are administered during this time, i.e., the time the body needs to produce stable clots, intrinsic hemostasis is impaired and only weak clots are produced [30]. Fluid resuscitation increases the blood pressure and fluid volume may wash away the developing clots. Early fluid administration during the initiation of hemostasis may prolong the time to achieve hemostasis, and with it blood loss increases. Fluid administration after the formation of the initial clot triggers rebleeding. Total blood loss increases as well [31. The remaining clotting factors are diluted. Hypothermic coagulopathy may be worsened if the resuscitation fluids are not warmed adequately. Thus, artificially, the patient is rendered coagulopathic and hypothermic. To avoid this, alternative resuscitation strategies for the hypovolemic patient with active or threatened rebleeding have been proposed. These strategies include hypotensive resuscitation and delayed resuscitation.

The goal of hypotensive resuscitation is to maintain a low blood pressure by volume resuscitation. It is only after definite surgical hemostasis that hypotensive resuscitation switches to normotensive resuscitation. In humans, the goal of hypotensive resuscitation is mean arterial pressure of about 40–60 mmHg or mean systolic blood pressure of 80–90 mmHg. When blood pressure measurement is not available, infusions at a fixed rate (one that empirically does not raise the systolic blood pressure above 90 mmHg) are administered. This constitutes so-called controlled resuscitation.

Hypotensive resuscitation was shown in animal models and in some human studies to improve survival of hemorrhagic shock [32]. However, the benefits of hypotensive resuscitation are time-dependent. Evidence suggests that the benefit of low blood pressure is offset by the detriments of this resuscitation strategy after about 1–8 hours (depending on the study) have elapsed.

Another form or resuscitation is delayed resuscitation. In comparison with traditional resuscitation, it reduces blood loss and mortality while maintaining tissue oxygenation. However, mortality increases when resuscitation is delayed for hours. Current evidence suggests delayed resuscitation may be beneficial only when the patient is awake and has a palpable radial pulse, and hemostasis is achievable within about 15 minutes. For all other cases, hypotensive resuscitation may be more appropriate [32].

The timing of fluid therapy may also be important when it comes to surgical procedures. When fluid infusion is delayed until after the phase with potential or actual blood loss, overall surgical blood loss may be reduced without detriment to the patient [33].

What fluid should be given?

There is an ongoing debate about the ideal agent for fluid management. The heated discussions among the proponents and opponents of the different fluids can be followed in the current medical literature. Since no one resuscitation fluid has clear-cut survival benefits over another [11, 34], there is no point in becoming dogmatic about the choice of fluids. Nevertheless, some differences of the available fluids can be kept in mind when the decision about a fluid regimen is to be made for an individual patient.

Benefits may be conveyed when the fluid's effects on the coagulation system, immune system, kidney, and overall fluid volume are taken into account. Also, cost considerations may play a role.

How should fluid be given?

Nowadays, fluids are usually administered intravenously. Questions remain regarding the velocity of infusion. Some fluid management strategies recommend bolus infusions, others continuous infusions. In a recent trial multicenter trial (FEAST) [35], bolus infusions for patients in hypotensive septic shock increased mortality compared with patients treated with continuous fluid resuscitation, and the trial was halted prematurely. The authors of the study speculated that the vasoconstriction in shock may be a protective measure that should not be disturbed by bolus infusion. Besides, reperfusion injury and subclinical effects on the lung, heart, and brain may play a role in the detrimental effect of bolus fluid infusion.

Bolus infusions may also be detrimental in hemorrhagic patients. They may increase bleeding and disturb endogenous clotting, as outlined above [29, 31].

Besides, the infusion rate affects the amount of fluid that is kept in the vasculature. When fluid is administered slowly, more will remain in the vascular bed compared with bolus administration. For instance, more than 90% of a medium molecular weight starch may remain intravascularly when given slowly, while only 60% of the same fluid will remain there when given as a bolus. This may be due to the sudden increase in blood pressure that is elicited by the rapid infusion. Other factors may play a role as well. The rate of intravascular fluid retention depends also on the condition of the patient at commencement of fluid infusion. If the patient is hypovolemic, more fluid remains intravascularly than if the patient is already normovolemic. With the limited evidence we have on this subject, bolus infusions should be discouraged.

When intravenous access is not available or feasible, there are other routes of fluid administration: intraosseous, subcutaneous, oral, rectal, and intraperitoneal. There is not much scientific evidence regarding efficacy, benefits, and risks of the alternative routes of fluid administration. However, when intravenous access is not achievable or in austere environments, administering fluids via alternative routes may be effective in reversing hemorrhagic or hypovolemic shock [36, 37].

How much fluid should be given?

Hypovolemia is detrimental since it precipitates tissue hypoxia. Hypervolemia may be just as detrimental. Hypervolemia finally leads to tissue edema and tissue hypoxia results as well. Besides, hypervolemia may lead to pulmonary edema and paralytic ileus. That is why it is beneficial to know the optimum fluid level of any individual.

Monitoring the volume status of individual patients is an art. There is no number or symptom which tells whether a patient is normovolemic or will benefit from further volume. At the level of the macrocirculation, hypovolemia is usually assumed when there is orthostatic hypotension (which may indicate an estimated volume loss of at least 20%) or when there is supine hypotension (which may indicate an estimated volume loss of at least 30%). Other clinical signs, such as the heart rate, skin temperature, urine output or a dry oral mucosa, may or may not be associated with hypovolemia. Whether or not clinical signs indicative of hypovolemia are present, one cannot tell whether there already is a volume need at the level of the microcirculation in general or in one organ system in particular.

A variety of measurable goals have been defined as surrogate markers for tissue perfusion. Traditionally, volume therapy was targeted at static intravascular pressures, such as the arterial blood pressure, central venous pressure, and pulmonary capillary wedge pressure. Low pressures may indicate hypovolemia, but may also be caused by other factors. Normal pressure, however, does not rule out hypovolemia and tissue hypoxia. Intravascular pressures may be useful if their trends are considered, but a single pressure reading does not indicate how to proceed with the volume therapy. Measures of the global blood flow, such as cardiac output, stroke volume, stroke volume variation or its delta-down component, oxygen delivery, and oxygen consumption, have been assumed to indicate hypovolemia. Volume therapy to achieve goals (goal-directed therapy), such as an appropriate cardiac output, has been shown to improve survival in some patient groups. However, neither intravascular pressures nor variables of the global blood flow answer the important question: Do I optimize tissue perfusion and oxygenation with my current fluid resuscitation strategy? Since tissue oxygenation and perfusion is currently considered the major goal in volume therapy, monitoring of them seems promising. Direct measurements of tissue oxygenation are not available. Some surrogate markers gained by gastric tonometry (an indirect estimate of mucosa perfusion) and near infrared spectroscopy may help estimate tissue oxygenation in selected patients. For the great majority of patients, however, good clinical judgment combined with some clinical and paraclinical parameters should be used to guide fluid therapy.

Influence of fluid therapy on blood management

The last question in this chapter is: Does the choice of fluid affect blood management-related outcome variables, such as blood loss, anemia, coagulation and mortality? Well, it does in so far that blood is not a volume replacement. For volume resuscitation, crystalloids or colloids, but not transfusions, is indicated. In the great majority of settings, acellular fluids are actually superior to blood as far as their ability to optimize cardiac output is concerned.

Avoiding or reducing pharmacologically-induced coagulopathy

Resuscitation fluids themselves may lead to coagulopathy. The right choice of resuscitation fluid does prevent this, at least partially. When a patient undergoes surgery with high anticipated blood loss, when even minor bleeding may be detrimental, or when the patient is coagulopathic to begin with, avoidance of fluid-induced coagulopathy is essential.

Impairment of coagulation by resuscitation fluids has been tested in vitro (e.g., by thromboelastography, factor levels, platelet function assays). The results, however, often do not correlate with clinical endpoints such as blood loss and postoperative anemia [38]. Therefore, it is difficult to extrapolate information gained from in vitro testing to clinical medicine. It is not known which laboratory parameter of coagulation correlates with blood loss and postoperative anemia.

Few high-quality data are available that guide the choice of fluids regarding prevention of coagulopathy. The little information that can be gleaned from the medical literature is summarized below.

In general, crystalloids exert the least influence on coagulation and blood loss. When it comes to colloids, all of them seem to impair one or another in vitro marker of coagulation disturbance. Some studies report that this translates into increased blood loss and transfusions [39]. Physiologically balanced fluids or colloids (HES) dissolved in them seem to lessen blood loss and trigger fewer transfusions than unbalanced fluids. Low molecular weight HES in saline impairs coagulation less than high molecular weight HES in a balanced solution [40]. Gelatin, albumin, and low-to-medium molecular weight HES, preferably in a balanced salt solution, seem to cause the least coagulopathy and increase in blood loss of all colloids [11, 41]. However, few trials comparing different HES solutions head-to-head regarding their effect on blood loss have been published so far [25].

Avoiding or reducing postinjury coagulopathy

Resuscitation fluids are not the only culprit for developing coagulopathy. Trauma patients may develop a special kind of coagulopathy, the so-called postinjury coagulopathy, a condition without an agreed definition. Its pathophysiology is complex. Factors such as tissue injury itself, hemorrhage with concomitant circulatory impairment and immunomodulation, hypothermia, hypocalcemia, clotting factor dilution, acidosis, and pre-existing conditions may all contribute to its development. In addition, resuscitation injury may contribute to the development of postinjury coagulopathy.

Presumably, the development of postinjury coagulopathy can be modified by fluid management. Logically, fluids known for their marked coagulopathic effect should be avoided. All fluids given should be warmed to body temperature in order to avoid hypothermia. Rapid and full volume resuscitation may initially prevent or treat shock effectively, and thus reduce the ischemic and reperfusion component of postinjury coagulopathy. On the other hand, normotensive resuscitation may encourage further bleeding with its concomitant loss of clotting factors, reduced clot strength, and disturbance of intrinsic hemostatic measures [30]. Hypotensive resuscitation of trauma patients reduces this risk. Coagulopathy and coagulopathic bleeding with its resulting mortality is reduced when hypotensive resuscitation is employed [42].

Reducing blood loss

Overall blood loss can be reduced with judicious fluid resuscitation. Hypotensive resuscitation to a goal of a mean arterial pressure of 50 mmHg in trauma patients with hemorrhagic shock reduces transfusions and postoperative mortality [42]. Giving only restricted amounts of fluid during major surgery and postponing full fluid replacement to the end of surgery is reported to reduce intraoperative blood loss and red cell transfusions [33, 43].

Preservation of microcirculation in severe hemodilution/anemia

Another important factor for blood management is the resuscitation fluid's ability to impair or to preserve microcirculation during bleeding and in anemic states. In states of shock, microcirculatory impairment with a reduced functional capillary density results [44]. Similarly, patients resuscitated with large volumes of low-viscosity fluids, such as crystalloids, show signs of impaired microcirculation. Reduced blood viscosity, and not anemia, is the limiting factor in such settings. Fluid management, thus, should aim at restoring or preserving microvascular perfusion.

Among other factors, resuscitation fluid viscosity influences the microcirculation. Viscosity increases the shear stress on the microvasculature and nitric oxide is produced. Vessels dilate and the functional capillary density increases. Once microcirculatory blood flow is restored, signs typically associated with severe anemia may disappear. It is believed that using viscous fluids in severe hemodilution or in hemorrhagic shock may reduce transfusions and improve survival.

Knowing this, preclinical data point to advantages of increasing the viscosity of the resuscitation fluid once a critically low value of blood viscosity has been reached. Different viscosity modifiers have been proposed: sodium alginate, high molecular weight starches, dextrans, PVP, keratin and polyethylene glycol-conjugated albumin [45]. It has been postulated that polyethylene glycol-conjugated albumin yields the best results [46]. Such new viscogenic colloids are in preclinical trials and may provide future resuscitation fluids.

Key points

• Restoring blood volume in hypovolemic patients is more important than correcting anemia. Crystalloids and colloids are equally effective in optimizing the cardiac output, if the correct dose is given at the right time and in the right manner.
• The choice of fluid therapy may influence the total blood loss. Though not tested in large trials, some fluids may be more effective in preventing coagulopathy and other blood loss than others. The timing and manner of fluid resuscitation may be equally important to reduce coagulopathy and bleeding.
• High-viscosity fluids may improve the microcirculation. Normalizing blood viscosity in states of severe hemodilution maintains tissue perfusion and oxygenation.

Questions for review

1. What is the difference between crystalloids and colloids?
2. What crystalloids are there and how do they differ from each other?
3. What colloids are there?
4. What do the following terms mean: polydisperse, substitution degree, hypertonic, and replacement fluid?
5. What four terms are typically used to describe HES?
6. How do timing and manner of fluid resuscitation influence blood management-related outcomes?

Exercises and practice cases

A boxer weighing 100 kg experiences severe epistaxis. He loses 1.5 L of blood.

How much of the following solutions are needed to restore his blood volume?—normal saline, lactated Ringer's, HES 6% (450/0.7); 10% dextran 40, gelatin 3%, and NaCl 7.5%. Explain your answers.

Suggestions for further research

1. What solutions are suitable plasma substitutes for therapeutic plasma exchange, e.g., in myasthenic crisis?
2. What specific considerations are needed for fluid therapy in babies?
3. What fluids are acceptable to strict vegetarians?

Homework

List all available fluids in your hospital, classify them as crystalloid or colloid, and make a table containing all fluids and their content of electrolytes, molecular weights, substitution degree, etc.

Find out where you can get the best available colloids and crystalloids. Record the contact details for the sources (e.g., a pharmacy or a pharmaceutical company).

References

1. O'Shaughnessy D, Brooke W. Experiments on the blood in cholera [letter]. *Lancet* 1831;**1**:490.
2. Lewins R, Latta T. Injection of saline solutions in extraordinary quantities into the veins in cases of malignant cholera. *Lancet* 1831;**32**:243–244.
3. Bull WT. On the intra-venous injection of saline solutions as a substitute for transfusion of blood. *Med Rec* 1884:6–8.
4. Gruber UF. Blutersatz. *Fortschr Med* 1969;**87**:631–634.
5. Gronwall A, Ingelman B. The introduction of dextran as a plasma substitute. *Vox Sang* 1984;**47**:96–99.
6. Myburgh JA. Fluid resuscitation in acute illness—time to reappraise the basics. *N Engl J Med* 2011;**364**:2543–2544.
7. Chappell D, Jacob M, Hofmann-Kiefer K, Conzen P, Rehm M. A rational approach to perioperative fluid management. *Anesthesiology* 2008;**109**:723–740.
8. Iijima T. Complexity of blood volume control system and its implications in perioperative fluid management. *J Anesth* 2009;**23**:534–542.
9. Hartok CS, et al. A systematic review of third-generation hydroxyethyl starch (HES 130/0.4) in resuscitation: Safety not adequately addressed. *Anesth Analg* 2011;**112**:635–645.
10. Bulger EM, May S, Kerby JD, et al. Out-of-hospital hypertonic resuscitation after traumatic hypovolemic shock. A randomized, placebo controlled trial. *Ann Surg* 2011;**253**:431–441.
11. Murphy GS, Greenberg SB. The new generation hydroxyethyl starch solutions: The holy grail of fluid therapy of just another starch? *J Cardiothorac Vasc Anesth* 2010;**24**:389–393.
12. Ando Y, Terao Y, Fukusaki M, et al. Influence of low molecular weight hydroxyethyl starch on microvascular permeability in patients undergoing abdominal surgery: comparison with crystalloids. *J Anesth* 2008;**22**:391–396.
13. Niemi TT, Miyashita R, Yamakage M. Colloid solutions: a clinical update. *J Anesth* 2010;**24**:913–925.
14. Mitra S, Khandelwal P. Are all colloids same? How to select the right colloid? *Indian J Anaesthes* 2009;**53**:592–607.
15. Tomoda M, Inokuchi K. Sodium alginate of lowered polymerization (alginon). A new plasma expander. *J Int Coll Surg* 1959;**32**:621–635.
16. Cabrales P, Tsai AG, Intaglietta M. Alginate plasma expander maintains perfusion and plasma viscosity during extreme hemodilution. *Am J Physiol Heart Circ Physiol* 2005;**288**:H1708–H1716.
17. Rena NM, Wibawa ID. Albumin infusion in liver cirrhotic patients. *Acta Med Indones* 2010;**42**:162–168.
18. Myburgh JA, Finfer S. Albumin is a blood product too—Is it safe for all patients? *Crit Care Resusc* 2009;**11**:67–70.
19. Liberati A, Moja L, Moschetti I, Gensini GF, Gusinu R. Human albumin solution for the resuscitation and volume expansion in critically ill patients. *Intern Emerg Med* 2006;**1**:243–245.
20. SAFE Study Investigators. Impact of albumin compared to saline on organ function and mortality of patients with severe sepsis. *Intensive Care Med* 2011;**37**:86–96.
21. Roche AM, James MF, Bennett-Guerrero E, Mythen MG. A head-to-head comparison of the in vitro coagulation effects of saline-based and balanced electrolyte crystalloid and colloid intravenous fluids. *Anesth Analg* 2006;**102**:1274–1279.
22. Thaler U, Deusch E, Kozek-Langenecker SA. In vitro effects of gelatin solutions on platelet function: a comparison with hydroxyethyl starch solutions. *Anaesthesia* 2005;**60**:554–559.
23. Van der Linden P, Ickx BE. The effects of colloid solutions on hemostasis. *Can J Anaesth* 2006;**53** (Suppl 6):S30–39.
24. Conroy JM, Fishman RL, Reeves ST, Pinosky ML, Lazarchick J. The effects of desmopressin and 6% hydroxyethyl starch on factor VIII:C. *Anesth Analg* 1996;**83**:804–807.
25. Groeneveld AB, Navickis RJ, Wilkes MM. Update on the comparative safety of colloids: A Systematic review of clinical studies. *Ann Surg* 2011;**253**:470–483.
26. Vanhoonacker J, Ongenae M, Vanoverschelde H, Donadoni R. Hydroxyethyl starch 130/0.4 versus modified fluid gelatin for cardiopulmonary bypass priming: The effects on postoperative bleeding and volume expansion needs after elective CABG. *Acta Anesth Belg* 2009;**60**:91–97.
27. Boldt J, Mengistu A. A new plasma-adapted hydroxyethyl starch preparation: In vitro coagulation studies. *J Cardiothorac Vasc Anesth* 2010;**24**:394–398.
28. Laxenaire MC, Charpentier C, Feldman L. Anaphylactoid reactions to colloid plasma substitutes: incidence, risk factors, mechanisms. A French multicenter prospective study. *Ann Fr Anesth Reanim* 1994;**13**:301–310.
29. Fouche Y, Sikorski R, Dutton RP. Changing paradigms in surgical resuscitation. *Crit Care Med* 2010;**38** (Suppl):S411–420.
30. Rezende-Neto JB, Rizoli SB, Andrade MV, et al. Permissive hypotension and desmopressin enhance clot formation. *J Trauma* 2010;**68**:42–50; discussion 50–51.
31. Hirshberg A, Hoyt DB, Mattox KL. Timing of fluid resuscitation shapes the hemodynamic response to uncontrolled hemorrhage: analysis using dynamic modeling. *J Trauma* 2006;**60**:1221–1227.

32. Santry HP, Alam HB. Fluid resuscitation: Past, present and the future. *Shock* 2010;**33**:229–241.

33. Fujita Y, Takeuchi A, Sugiura T. Before-after study of a restricted fluid infusion strategy for management of donor hepatectomy for living-donor liver transplantation. *J Anesth* 2009;**23**:67–74.

34. Bunn F, *et al*. Colloid solutions for fluid resuscitation. *Cochrane Database Syst Rev* 2011;(3):CD001319.

35. Maitland K, Kiguli S, Opoka RO, *et al*; FEAST Trial Group. Mortality of fluid bolus in children with severe infection. *N Engl J Med* 2011;**364**:2483–2495.

36. Grocott MPW. Resuscitation from hemorrhagic shock using rectally administered fluids in a wilderness environment. *Wilderness Environ Med* 2005;**16**:209–211.

37. Cancio LC, Kramer GC, Hoskins SL. Gastrointestinal fluid resuscitation of thermally injured patients. *J Burn Care Res* 2006;**27**:561–569.

38. Schramko A, Suojaranta-Ylinen R, Kuitunen A, Raivio P, Kukkonen S, Niemi T. Hydroxyethylstarch and gelatin solutions impair blood coagulation after cardiac surgery: a prospective randomized trial. *Br J Anaesth* 2010;**104**:691–697.

39. Hecht-Dolnik M, Barkan H, Taharka A, Loftus J. Hetastarch increases the risk of bleeding complications in patients after off-pump coronary bypass surgery: A randomized clinical trial. *J Thorac Cardiovasc Surg* 2009;**138**:703–711.

40. Choi SJ, Ahn HJ, Chung SS, *et al*. Hemostatic and electrolyte effects of hydroxyethyl starches in patients undergoing posterior lumbar interbody fusion using pedicle screws and cages. *Spine (Phila Pa 1976)* 2010;**35**:829–834.

41. Choi YS, Shim JK, Hong SW, Kim JC, Kwak YL. Comparing the effects of 5% albumin and 6% hydroxyethyl starch 130/0.4 on coagulation and inflammatory response when used as priming solutions for cardiopulmonary bypass. *Minerva Anesthesiol* 2010;**76**:584–591.

42. Morrison CA, Carrick MM, Norman MA, *et al*. Hypotensive resuscitation strategy reduces transfusion requirements and severe postoperative coagulopathy in trauma patients with hemorrhagic shock: preliminary results of a randomized controlled trial. *J Trauma* 2011;**70**:652–663.

43. Vretzakis G, Kleitsaki A, Stamoulis K, *et al*. The impact of fluid restriction policy in reducing the use of red blood cells in cardiac surgery. *Acta Anaesth Belg* 2009;**60**:221–228.

44. Komori M, Takada K, Tomizawa Y, Uezono S, Nishiyama K, Ozaki M. Effects of colloid resuscitation on peripheral microcirculation, hemodynamics, and colloidal osmotic pressure during acute severe hemorrhage in rabbits. *Shock* 2005;**23**:377–382.

45. Zhao L, You G, Liao F, *et al*. Sodium alginate as viscosity modifier may induce aggregation of red blood cells. *Artif Cells Blood Substit Immobil Biotechnol* 2010;**38**:267–276.

46. Villela N, Salazar Vázquez BY, Intaglietta M. Microcirculatory effects of intravenous fluids in critical illness: plasma expansion beyond crystalloids and colloids. *Curr Opin Anaesthesiol* 2009;**22**:163–167.

7 Chemistry of Hemostasis

All bleeding eventually stops, but it is a matter of timing whether the patient experiences this phenomenon dead or alive. The faster, the more complete, and the more proficient the hemostasis, the better is the patient's chance of recovery. Mere chemistry may help to achieve such timely hemostasis. Systemically administrable drugs are available to enhance endogenous coagulation factor production, function, and release. Some drugs are able to modify fibrinolysis and enhance platelet function. There are also drugs that promote local hemostasis. Systemically- as well as locally-acting hemostatic drugs have been shown to reduce bleeding and to improve the patient's outcome.

Objectives

1. To describe ways in which blood loss can be reduced by systemically administering drugs.
2. To explain the mode of action and use of agents that promote local hemostasis.
3. To define the use of hemostatically acting drugs in blood management and their impact on outcome.

Definitions

Antifibrinolytics: Agents that prevent fibrinolysis or lysis of a thrombus by prohibiting the conversion of plasminogen to plasmin and the action of plasmin itself. These drugs are used to prevent and control hemorrhage and to enhance hemostasis.

Vitamin K group (antihemorrhagic factors): This group comprises compounds with a naphthoquinone ring and different side chains. Vitamins of the K group are important for the post-translational γ-carboxylation of blood clotting factors, crucial in their ability to enhance clotting.

Conjugated estrogens: Mixtures of compounds containing water-soluble female hormones derived from urine of pregnant mares or synthetically from estrone and equilin with other concomitant conjugates, including 17-α-dihydroequilin, 17-α-estradiol, and 17-β-dihydroequilin.

Tissue adhesive or sealant (formerly called tissue glue): Any substance that polymerizes to an extent that glues tissues together and prevents leakage of body fluids including blood [1].

Hemostatics: Agents that arrest bleeding either by forming an artificial clot or by providing the matrix for physiological clot formation.

A brief history

The oldest methods used to stop a hemorrhage were probably applied directly onto the site of bleeding. A wide variety of agents were used to achieve hemostasis. Among them were agents that initiated clotting using a variety of mechanisms, such as providing a matrix for endogenous platelets to aggregate (flour, cotton ash), reducing the blood flow to the site of bleeding (ice, water, cocaine), adding exogenous clotting factors (freshly slaughtered chicken meat, snake venoms), changing the coagulation milieu in the wound (lemon juice), or acting as caustic

Basics of Blood Management, Second Edition. Petra Seeber and Aryeh Shander.
© 2013 John Wiley & Sons, Ltd. Published 2013 by John Wiley & Sons, Ltd.

agents (hot oil, animal and plant products). Some of these agents proved very effective in locally reducing hemorrhage.

Systemically administered drugs to promote hemostasis were later added to the armamentarium of the physician attempting to stop a hemorrhage. In 1772, William Hewson noted that blood collected under stress clotted rapidly. This finding triggered a series of animal experiments that clarified the role of the stress hormone responsible for this phenomenon: epinephrine (adrenalin). Almost 200 years later it was found that release of coagulation factor VIII (FVIII) followed the injection of epinephrine—with no change in any other known clotting factors. The concept of treating a coagulation disorder simply by releasing the patient's own FVIII was tantalizing, but the means to do so were lacking. Furthermore, epinephrine injections were followed by too many side effects. Subsequent research found that vasopressin and insulin also induced FVIII release. However, these substances also had too many side effects to be used therapeutically in the setting of coagulation disorders. In 1974, desmopressin, the synthetic analog of vasopressin, was shown to release FVIII and von Willebrand factor (vWF). Since the side effects of desmopressin are mild, it proved to be the long-looked-for drug to be used in certain clotting factor deficiencies, and use in humans soon followed [2]. Desmopressin was first shown to be useful in von Willebrand disease (vWD) and hemophilia in 1977 in Italy [2, 3]. Following further studies in other countries, the World Health Organization (WHO) included desmopressin in its list of essential drugs. Since 1986, desmopressin has also been evaluated as a drug that reduces patient exposure to donor blood [2].

Vitamin K was discovered by Henrik Dam in 1935. He was experimenting with cholesterol synthesis and observed that chicken fed with a cholesterol-deficient diet developed a coagulation disorder. The discovery of a vitamin that was obviously involved in coagulation followed. The vitamin was called vitamin K since it has a very close relation to the process of "koagulation", the Danish word for coagulation.

In the 1930s, Kraut et al. and Kunitz et al. worked on aprotinin, which was shown to be an inhibitor of trypsin and kallikrein. This drug was shown to reduce fibrinolysis as well. Other antifibrinolytic drugs were discovered soon after, among them carbazochrome (1954), hemocoagulase (1966), amniocaproic acid (1962), and tranexamic acid (1965). The development of hemostatic drugs came to a halt in the late 1960s and a trend toward the development of antithrombotic and fibrinolytic drugs developed, probably spurred on by the increase in thromboembolic cardiovascular events. The blood-sparing effect of hemostatic drugs received renewed attention in the 1980s when there was a need to reduce the use of transfusions.

Systemic hemostatic drugs

Antifibrinolytics

Physiology of fibrinolysis

Ideally, the coagulation process and fibrinolysis are balanced, and so neither a bleeding diathesis nor an exaggerated intravascular thrombosis occurs. Since blood clots are not meant to be durable structures, they need to be dissolved as soon as the damaged tissues are sufficiently repaired. Fibrin in the clot is the prime target of plasmin, a serine protease that is able to cleave the fibrin molecules. Plasminogen, the plasmin precursor, diffuses through water channels into the fibrin clot. There it is responsible for the fibrinolysis. Tissue plasminogen activator (t-PA), which is released from the vascular endothelium, converts plasminogen to plasmin. Plasminogen binds to the lysine residues of fibrin, where it is converted to plasmin by t-PA, which simultaneously binds to fibrin.

Plasmin, mainly, is active when bound to fibrin. When it is free in plasma, it is rapidly inactivated by α2-antiplasmin. Plasmin seems to be the central antagonist of coagulation. Apart from cleaving fibrin, it also impairs other processes in hemostasis (degradation of cofactors Va and VIIIa, proteolysis of platelet receptors, consumption of α2-antiplasmin, and degradation of fibrinogen).

Role of fibrinolysis in blood management

A variety of procedures and conditions are associated with an increased fibrinolysis or the presence of plasminogen activators. The use of a tourniquet for surgery leads to the local activation of fibrinolysis, which may increase postoperative blood loss. During liver transplantation, there is a time period (anhepatic phase) during which the body does not have a functioning liver synthesis and clearance of metabolites. Fibrinolysis is increased during to this time. Hyperfibrinolysis has also been observed in a considerable number of polytraumatized patients. Patients undergoing a cardiac procedure with cardiopulmonary bypass show signs of increased coagulation and fibrinolysis, which are stimulated not only by the surgery itself, but also by the use of the bypass machine. This activation leads to the consumption of clotting factors, which may lead to excessive postoperative bleeding.

Many body compartments contain naturally occurring plasminogen activators. Among them are the urine and mucosa in the urinary tract, cervical tissue, iris and choroid, as well as the gastrointestinal, tract, including the mouth and saliva. Placental abruption activates the fibrinolytic system as well as the deficiency of C1-esterase inhibitor, as is the case in hereditary angioneurotic edema.

Aprotinin

Aprotinin is a naturally occurring serine protease inhibitor. It occurs in bovine lungs. The mechanisms of action of aprotinin have not been completely identified. It is known, however, that it reversibly forms enzyme–drug complexes with enzymes carrying a serine site. Many enzymes that play roles in the process of coagulation, fibrinolysis, and inflammation carry such serine sites, e.g., trypsin, plasmin, and kallikrein. Therefore, aprotinin prevents plasmin-mediated fibrinolysis. It inhibits the contact activation of blood components (especially important in areas where blood is in contact with foreign material for a prolonged time). Aprotinin preserves the adhesive glycoproteins in the platelet membrane (glycoprotein [GP] Ib). This makes the platelets resistant to damage from increased plasmin levels and mechanical injury. Additionally, aprotinin attenuates the heparin-induced platelet dysfunction. The net effect is that fibrinolysis and the turnover of coagulation factors are decreased. Aprotinin also has anti-inflammatory and antioxidant properties, as well as a weak anticoagulant effect.

Aprotinin given orally is quickly degraded. Therefore, a parenteral route has to be used, typically the intravenous one. After injection, aprotinin distributes rapidly into the extracellular space. After distribution, it has a plasma half-life of 150 minutes. Aprotinin is cleared by the kidneys and reabsorbed in the proximal tubuli. Lysosomal enzymes slowly degrade aprotinin. Aprotinin has a low toxicity and even large doses are well tolerated. Hypersensitivity occurs in 0.1–0.6% of patients treated with aprotinin and seems to be more frequent in patients with repeated exposure to the drug (especially when administration of the drug is repeated within a 6-month period) [4].

In comparison with other antifibrinolytics on the market, aprotinin seems to be the most potent. Up until 2005, there was no concern about possibly increased thrombosis after administration of aprotinin was not confirmed in studies: none of myocardial infarction rate, incidence of deep vein thrombosis, graft occlusion, or mortality after cardiac surgery was shown to increase after aprotinin administration [5]. However, in 2006, Mangano et al. conducted a study that strongly suggested that aprotinin use is associated with renal failure, myocardial infarction, heart failure, stroke, and encephalopathy in patients who underwent cardiac surgery [6]. A high-quality randomized, multicenter trial, the so-called BART study in 2008, confirmed the findings of Mangano et al., showing a higher mortality in cardiac surgical patients using aprotinin compared to other antifibrinolytics [7]. This led to the withdrawal of aprotinin from the world market. The medical literature abounds with emotional controversy about these studies, subjecting their results to different statistical re-analysis. Some authors believe in the net benefit of aprotinin, while others do not [8–12]. The influence of aprotinin on outcome has not been clarified to an extent that it satisfies all authors.

Tranexamic acid

Tranexamic acid is another antifibrinolytic currently on the market and that was also trialed in the BART study [13]. It is a synthetic derivative of the amino acid lysine. It is similar to ε-aminocaproic acid (see below), but binds 6–10 times more potently to plasminogen. Tranexamic acid reversibly blocks lysine-binding sites on plasminogen. The saturation of this site with tranexamic acid prevents the binding of plasminogen to the surface of fibrin. This delays fibrinolysis.

After intake, tranexamic acid diffuses into the mother's milk and into joints. It can also cross the blood–brain and placental barriers. Tranexamic acid is generally well tolerated. Rarely, patients complain of nausea and vomiting or orthostatic reactions. The theoretical concern about increased thrombotic events was not confirmed in studies. Seizures have been reported, especially after high-dose regimen [14]. A rare reaction to the drug is disturbance of color vision. In this event, the drug must be discontinued. To prevent drug-induced hypotension, intravenous application should be slow, not exceeding 100 mg/min. Both, adult and pediatric patients can be treated with tranexamic acid.

Tranexamic acid is available as injectable solution, as tablets, and as syrup. An example of possible dosages in various indications is provided in Table 7.1 [15–17]. Since tranexamic acid is excreted primarily by the kidneys, its dosage needs to be reduced in patients with impaired kidney function. Tranexamic acid can also be combined

Table 7.1 Dose recommendations for tranexamic acid.

Indication	Dosage
Local fibrinolysis	500 mg–1 g i.v. 3x/day or 1.0–1.5 g p.o. 2–3x/day
General fibrinolysis	Single dose of 1 g or 10 mg/kg i.v.
Patients undergoing cardiopulmonary bypass	10 mg/kg before bypass and infusion of 1 mg/kg body weight/h afterward or 10 g i.v. over 20 min as a single injection before sternotomy 30 mg/kg after induction of anesthesia and same dose added to the prime solution of cardiopulmonary bypass 15 mg/kg after systemic heparinization followed by an infusion of 1 mg/kg body weight/h until the end of the surgery
Upper gastrointestinal bleeding	1.5 g 3x/day to 1 g 6x/day for 5–7 days; first i.v., then p.o.
Patients with hemophilia for oral surgery	1–1.5 g 3x/day
Patients under oral anticoagulants for oral surgery	4.8–5.0% mouthwash used for 2 min 4x/day for 7 days
Transurethral prostatectomy	6–12 g p.o. daily for 4 days
Liver transplantation	40 mg/kg body weight/h as i.v. infusion
Menorrhagia	1–1.5 g p.o. 3–4x/day for 3–4 days
(Poly)traumatized patients	1 g immediately i.v., followed by 1 g over 8 h
Acute promyeloic leukemia	4–8 g p.o. in 3–4 doses/day
Postpartum hemorrhage	4 g over 1 h i.v., followed 1 g i.v. every 6 h

with desmopressin, e.g., in patients with vWD or in other conditions that warrant maximal enhancement of hemostasis. Tranexamic acid is said to be contraindicated in hemorrhages of the upper urinary tract because of the risk of clotting in the urinary system. However, antifibrinolytics have been used in this condition with success.

Tranexamic acid has a positive impact on many outcome variables. It reduces perioperative bleeding in patients undergoing a variety of surgeries. Tranexamic acid was shown to reduce postoperative blood loss in cardiac surgery [15, 18], after total knee [19] and hip [20] arthroplasty, spinal surgery [21, 22], oral surgery [23, 24], transurethral prostatectomy, and liver transplantation [25]. Also, in gynecological patients with cervix conization or those suffering from blood loss due to menorrhagia or placental abruption, tranexamic acid has proved beneficial by reducing blood loss. Tranexamic acid can also reduce the rebleeding rate in a variety of conditions, such as intracranial bleeding [26], ocular trauma, and upper gastrointestinal hemorrhage [27]. It is also effective in reducing the number and severity of attacks in patients

with hereditary angioedema. A remarkable recent study, the CRASH-2 trial, included 20 211 adult trauma patients in 40 different countries [28]. It demonstrated a clear survival benefit for patients who receive tranexamic acid immediately after trauma with risk of severe hemorrhage. Overall, tranexamic acid improves the outcome in a variety of settings associated with bleeding, reducing blood loss and increasing survival rates.

Practice tip: Preoperative tranexamic acid

Two tablets of tranexamic acid (1 g) can be easily given orally before surgery with anticipated major blood loss. This is a simple measure to reduce blood loss in a variety of settings and illustrates that blood management can indeed be simple.

ε-Aminocaproic acid

ε-Aminocaproic acid (EACA) is another lysine analog used as an antifibrinolytic agent. It mainly inhibits plasminogen activators and has a slight antiplasmin activity. The mechanism by which EACA treats bleeding in thrombocytopenic patients is not known.

When there is a fibrinolytic component to the bleeding of a patient, EACA can be used successfully. This has been demonstrated in cardiac surgery with or without cardiopulmonary bypass, abruptio placentae, liver cirrhosis, surgery in the urinary tract (prostatectomy, nephrectomy), and hematuria due to severe trauma, shock, or anoxia. EACA was also used successfully in bleeding patients with thrombocytopenia due to immune and non-immune processes. It has been used in bleeding thrombocytopenic patients with hemophilia, aplastic anemia, or acute leukemia, as well as in patients with Kasabach–Merritt syndrome [29].

EACA can be given orally or intravenously. It is taken up rapidly from the gastrointestinal tract. It distributes in the extravascular and intravascular compartments and diffuses into red cells and tissues. The drug is excreted in the urine. The intravenous standard dose is 0.1 g/kg administered over 30–60 minutes (or a loading dose of 5 g), followed by 8–24 g/day or 1 g every 4 hours. When the bleeding ceases, 1 g is usually given every 6 hours. The same dose regimen is used when the patient is able to take the drug per os.

Side effects of EACA are rare. Nasal stuffiness, abdominal complaints with nausea and diarrhea, headaches, allergic reactions, dizziness, and arrhythmias are among them. If given rapidly intravenously, hypotension and bradycardia can occur. A syndrome characterized by myopathy and necrosis of muscle fibers has been described in some patients. If it occurs, the drug has to be stopped for the symptoms to resolve. However, on re-exposure, the same usually happens again.

EACA is able to improve the outcome of patients. It was shown to reduce the blood loss after cardiac and orthopedic surgery [30, 31]. EACA may also be beneficial in stopping intractable upper hematuria, thereby preventing the need for rescue-nephrectomy.

p-Aminomethylbenzoic acid

A third lysine derivative is p-aminomethylbenzoic acid (PAMBA). Saturation of the lysine-binding sites of plasminogen with this inhibitor displaces plasminogen from the fibrin surface. Thereby, PAMBA inhibits fibrinolysis. On a molar basis, tranexamic acid is twice as potent as PAMBA [32–34].

There is not much literature that deals with the role of PAMBA in the transfusion arena. The scarce information that can be gathered suggests that PAMBA may be effective in reducing rebleeding after subarachnoid hemorrhage and in traumatic hyphema [35–37]. It has also been used for perioperative and peripartum bleeding [38, 39]. No valid claim can be made about PAMBA's ability to reduce mortality.

Desmopressin

Desmopressin (also called 1-deamino-8-D-arginine vasopressin or DDAVP) is a synthetic analog of the natural antidiuretic hormone L-arginine vasopressin, which has been altered so that the plasma half-life is prolonged. DDAVP binds to vasopressin receptors of the V2 type, located in the renal tubule and endothelium. It releases the content of endogenous storage sites for the clotting factors (e.g., the Weibel–Palade bodies, which are the secretory granules of the endothelium, and the sinusoid liver endothelial cells). Consequently, the blood levels of vWF, FVIII, and t-PA increase. This effect is observed in factor-deficient patients as well as in healthy individuals. For some coagulation factor deficiencies—vWD and hemophilia A—DDAVP could be likened to an autologous replacement therapy. The expected release of vWF and FVIII depends on the baseline level of the patient and his/her individual response to the drug. The factor levels usually increase three to five times baseline (range: 1.5–20.0 times) [2]. Platelet reactivity and adhesiveness, presumably due to the release of vWF, GPIb/IX, and other, yet unknown mechanisms, increase as well [40]. DDAVP also has a fibrinolytic effect (through the release of t-PA) and is therefore sometimes administered in association with an antifibrinolytic drug, such as EACA [41] or tranexamic acid. Whether this is necessary or not is controversial, since the released t-PA is rapidly complexed and supposedly does not produce fibrinolysis in blood [2]. Occasionally, DDAVP is also given for thromboprophylaxis [42].

DDAVP is a safe and affordable therapy for patients with congenital or acquired vWD [43–45]. This disease is characterized by the lack or malfunctioning of vWF. Three main types of vWD have been identified. Type 1 is the most common (80% of all cases). Most patients with type 1 vWD respond favorably to DDAVP. In contrast, type 2 patients have a functional abnormality of vWF, which is not correctable by DDAVP. However, there are reports of patients with the subtype, type 2A, vWD responding to DDAVP with a shortened bleeding time. In type 2B vWD, DDAVP is considered to be contraindicated, because release of the abnormal vWF can cause platelet aggregation and thrombocytopenia. This, however, is not unanimously agreed upon, since some patients with type 2B vWD respond favorably to the drug [2]. Patients with vWD type 3 do not have any vWF and, therefore, do not respond to DDAVP with a release of vWF.

DDAVP also releases FVIII into the bloodstream. Therefore, hemophiliacs with hemophilia A also benefit from the use of DDAVP. Mild-to-moderate cases can be successfully treated with this drug rather than with blood-derived or recombinant clotting factors.

The response to DDAVP in hemophilia A and vWD differs from patient to patient, but is consistent over time. This finding can be used when a test dose is given to patients who potentially benefit from DDAVP. The magnitude of the increase in the factor under investigation (vWF, FVIII) can also be observed in subsequent administrations, especially when time has elapsed between the test dose and the therapeutic dose [46].

Patients with a variety of platelet disorders respond favorably to DDAVP, namely with an increase in platelet adhesiveness. Congenital defects of the platelets (e.g., in Bernard–Soulier syndrome, but not Glanzmann thrombasthenia) can be treated with DDAVP. Patients with acquired platelet defects can be treated with DDAVP instead of platelet transfusions [47]. DDAVP has been used in bleeding due to drug-induced platelet dysfunctions such as those caused by aspirin, dextran [42], ticlopidin, or heparin [46]. Patients with platelet dysfunction due to uremia or liver cirrhosis (with usually normal-to-high levels of FVIII or vWF) [48] are also good candidates for DDAVP treatment.

Thrombocytopenic bleeding also responds to DDAVP [49]. The mechanism of action of DDAVP in this setting is not clear, but a contributing factor is probably an increase in platelet adhesiveness in the remaining platelets. DDAVP also shortens bleeding time in patients with isolated and unexplained prolongation of their bleeding time [2].

It has been claimed that DDAVP also reduces blood loss and the use of transfusions in patients without congenital platelet abnormalities. However, most of the available studies were unable to demonstrate a significant reduction of blood loss or transfusions in patients with uncomplicated cardiac surgery and in patients without congenital or acquired platelet defects [46]. Cardiac surgery patients benefited from DDAVP only if they had such platelet defects, either due to drugs or prolonged cardiopulmonary bypass [50].

DDAVP is available in an injectable form for intravenous or subcutaneous administration, as well as a spray or liquid formulation for intranasal use. For home treatment, e.g., in women with menorrhagia due to vWD, the intranasal route is the most convenient. Two intranasal "standard puffs" of a total of 300 µg of DDAVP is all that is needed to reduce blood loss due to menorrhagia. If needed, the spray can be used repeatedly, typically after an 8–12-hour interval. Even a low dose of 10–20 µg of DDAVP spray seems to be effective, as shown in uremic children [51]. In the perioperative phase, intravenous administration is recommended. The intravenous route provides slightly better results than the intranasal route. An intravenous or subcutaneous dose of 0.3 µg/kg achieves optimal results in the majority of patients. Perioperatively, DDAVP should be given at least twice, the second dose administered 6–8 hours after the first one.

A reported effect of DDAVP is tachyphylaxis, i.e., a reduced response to treatment when repeated in short succession. However, Lethagen [46] claims: "In the clinical use of desmopressin, tachyphylaxis is rarely a problem, even if prolonged treatment is given." When DDAVP is given three to four times per 24 hours, the FVIII response is reduced by about 30% [2].

DDAVP is a safe drug. Serious side effects are rare. Facial flushing and mild lightheadedness are commonly observed [41]. DDAVP does not exert the vasopressive action of its mother substance vasopressin, but has an antidiuretic effect that continues for about 24 hours after the last administered dose. Patients should be advised to reduce their water intake, especially when repeated doses are needed. Although there are reports of arterial thrombosis in patients treated with DDAVP, studies and a meta-analysis did not show an increased risk of arterial thrombosis after administration of the drug [52].

Vitamins of the K group

Vitamin K is the collective term for different compounds with a common naphthoquinone ring structure and different side chains (Table 7.2).

Vitamins K_1, K_2, and K_3 are the only ones used for human therapy. Upon administration, vitamin K_1 is converted to vitamin K_2. Vitamin K_1 has the quickest onset of action, the most prolonged duration, and is the most potent of all the vitamin K forms.

The natural forms of vitamin K are lipid-soluble and they are stored in the liver. Healthy adults need at least 65–80 µg of vitamin K/day. Children need about one-third of the adult requirements. Approximately half of the vitamin K requirement of humans is produced by intestinal bacteria. The other half is taken up in a healthy diet. The excretion of absorbed vitamin K occurs mainly in the feces, but some is also excreted in the urine.

Table 7.2 Vitamin K complex.

Vitamin K	Description
K₁: Phylloquinone (phytonadione, phytonactone)	Naturally occurring form, found in green plants, part of healthy diet
K₂: Menaquinone (group of menaquinones)	Natural occurring form, synthesized by intestinal bacteria
K₃: Menadione (menodoine/ menaphthone)	Synthetically derived, used as dietary supplements, especially for babies, lipid-soluble
K₄: Menadiol (acetomenaphthone and others)	Synthetically derived, water-soluble dietary supplements for farm animals, food preservatives
K₅₋₉, K-S, MK, etc.	Synthetically derived, dietary supplements for farm animals, food preservatives

Proteins involved in the coagulation process undergo post-translational changes. Certain glutamate molecules are γ-carboxylated and so the factors finally carry γ-carboxyglutamate residues. The post-translational γ-carboxylation of the coagulation factors II (prothrombin), VII (proconvertin), IX (Christmas factor), and X (Stuart–Prower factor), and the anticoagulant proteins C, S, and Z depends on the presence of vitamin K. If the γ-carboxyglutamate is missing, coagulation factors are synthesized, but these lack the carboxy groups that are essential for the interaction between coagulation factors and calcium. Such deficient factors are called des-γ-carboxy molecules or PIVKA (proteins induced by vitamin K absence). By a yet unknown mechanism, vitamin K also influences platelet aggregation. In vitamin K deficiency, the prothrombin time and activated partial thromboplastin time are prolonged.

Vitamin K is the prophylactic of choice to prevent hemorrhagic disease of the newborn. Coagulation factors do not cross the placenta and have to be synthesized by the baby. During normal gestation, the level of vitamin K-dependent coagulation factors is about half that of the adult level, while the other factors reach adult level at birth. After birth, vitamin K provided by the mother's milk is just about sufficient. In case of increased need, e.g., prematurity or if the mother took drugs that inter-

fere with vitamin K metabolism (antibiotics, anticonvulsants, tuberculostatics, vitamin K antagonists), the level of vitamin K-dependent factors may be insufficient for the baby. This may result in gross hemorrhage, a condition easily preventable by peripartal vitamin K therapy. Vitamin K can be given either to the baby or to the expectant mother [53]. The baby is usually administered 1.0 mg of the lipid-soluble form orally or intramuscularly. This dose may even be excessive, since 1–5 μg has been shown to be sufficient [54].

Several other conditions may cause a lack of vitamin K and its dependent factors. Among the common ones are treatment with vitamin K antagonists, such as warfarin, and the absolute lack of vitamin K due to gastrointestinal disturbances, inadequate diet, impaired lipid absorption, malabsorption, and excess intake of fat-soluble vitamins and salicylates. In their effort to rid the body of foreign bacteria, antibiotics may also destroy the normal intestinal flora needed for vitamin K synthesis, causing a deficiency of the vitamin.

Therapeutic doses of vitamin K rapidly normalize the hemostatic disorder, given the liver can provide the necessary factors. The response is so rapid that even some emergency surgery can be performed when patients present with a coagulation disturbance due to a lack vitamin K. Traditionally, fresh frozen plasma or prothrombin complex concentrate was used to provide the necessary factors. However, in many cases vitamin K serves the same purpose. Even if fresh frozen plasma or prothrombin complex concentrate is deemed necessary, vitamin K has to be given to correct the underlying problem.

Given a normal or residual liver function, vitamin K-dependent coagulation factors can be synthesized, once the vitamin is given. For adults, the vitamin K dose for bleeding due to a lack of vitamin K-dependent factors is 2.5–10 mg. If a more rapid response is needed, 10–20 mg (up to 50 mg) may be administered. The response to the vitamin K is fairly rapid and clinical bleeding may subside quickly. However, a measurable improvement in the prothrombin time takes at least 2 hours.

Vitamin K can be given intravenously, intramuscularly, subcutaneously, or orally. In case of an emergency, the intravenous route is preferred [55]. In other cases, oral administration may be sufficient and may even be superior to the subcutaneous route [56].

Side effects of vitamin K depend on the preparation given. Natural vitamins K₁ and K₂ seem to cause much fewer side effects than the synthetic vitamin K₃. A severe hemolytic anemia is occasionally observed in newborns, but not in adults. This reaction may be due to overdosing, as occurred in babies who were given up to 80 mg/kg, whereas the effective prophylactic dose is less than 1.0 mg/kg. The water-soluble vitamin K_3 seems to have a greater ability to induce hemolysis than the natural, lipid-soluble vitamin K_1. In addition, liver damage, deafness, and severe neurological problems, including retardation in infants, have been reported following vitamin K_3 therapy. Care must be taken with intravenous injections of vitamin K, since they can cause facial flushing, excessive perspiration, chest tightness, cyanosis, and shock.

Conjugated estrogens and other hormones

It is well known that estrogens ("the pill") increase the risk of thrombotic events. It was also observed that some women with vWD showed a marked improvement in their bleeding diathesis when pregnant or when taking contraceptives. Bleeding resumed once the baby was born or contraception was discontinued. Obviously, estrogens have an impact on the coagulation system.

Conjugated estrogens increase the level of prothrombin and factors VII, VIII, IX, and X, and decrease fibrinolysis and the level of antithrombin III. Additionally, they increase the norepinephrine-induced platelet aggregability. Estrogens also have a weak anabolic effect.

Conjugated estrogens can be given intravenously, intramuscularly, or orally. They are rapidly absorbed from the gastrointestinal tract. Estrogens are widely distributed in the body and moderately bound to plasma proteins. They are metabolized and inactivated primarily in the liver and eliminated in the urine. Some estrogens are excreted into the bile; however, they are reabsorbed by the intestine and returned to the liver.

Side effects of a short-term course of conjugated estrogens are uncommon. When the drug is given only for about 5–7 days, hormonal activity is negligible. When given for a prolonged time, gallbladder disease, thromboembolic events, hepatic adenoma, elevated blood pressure, glucose intolerance, hypercalcemia, and other symptoms typically occurring in hormonal therapy (increased water retention, changed skin pigmentation, changes in sexual function, depression, etc.) develop.

Abnormal uterine bleeding due to hormonal imbalance in the absence of organic pathology is the typical indication for conjugated estrogens in blood management. One 25-mg injection, intravenously or intramuscularly, may be sufficient. The intravenous route is preferred when a rapid response is needed. Repeated doses every 6–12 hours can be administered, if necessary.

Case reports have shown that patients with vWD benefit from oral contraception or another form of estrogen therapy [57], i.e., control of postmenopausal symptoms. Such patients also benefit from a short course of estrogens given perioperatively, reducing the use of allogeneic blood products. Another potential area for estrogen therapy is in patients with end-stage liver disease with coagulation abnormalities.

Conjugated estrogens shorten prolonged bleeding time and reduce bleeding in patients with uremia. The mechanism of action is unknown. In uremic patients, single daily infusions of 0.6 mg/kg for 4–5 days shorten the bleeding time for at least 2 weeks. Given orally, 50 mg of conjugated estrogens shorten the bleeding time after about 7 days [58]. The effect of the conjugated estrogens lasts 10–15 days [2] and therefore makes the drug ideal when long-term hemostasis needs to be achieved [59]. In uremia, conjugated estrogens are a long-acting alternative to DDAVP.

Topical estrogen has been reported to reduce epistaxis in patients with recurrent bleeding due to hereditary hemorrhagic teleangiectasia, hemophilia or vWD. It has been postulated that this effect is not due to a systemic optimization of coagulation but due to strengthening and thickening of the nasal epithelium.

Other hormones have been used in blood management. As multiple case reports demonstrate, patients with bleeding due to gastrointestinal vascular abnormalities, Osler–Rendu–Weber disease, and angiodysplasia benefit from a certain combination of estrogens and progesterone. Ethynylestradiol (30 mg) and norethisterone (1.0–1.5 mg/day) reduced or eliminated blood transfusions in a subset population of patients [60–62].

Other hemostatic drugs

The above-mentioned drugs are commonly used (Table 7.3) [15, 17, 18, 21, 23–25, 29, 42, 46, 48, 49, 54, 63–77]. In addition to them, a great variety of other hemostatic drugs have been advocated over the years [78]. Quite a few of them are still in clinical use. Extensive efficacy and safety studies are lacking for most of them. The following points outline some of the distinct features of such drugs.

• **Tissue extracts** have a thromboplastin-like action. After intravenous administration, they may accelerate coagulation. Extracts from animal brain, for instance, have been used for this purpose.

• **Oxalic and malonic acid** were once proposed as hemostatic agents, but they were never extensively clinically tested.

Table 7.3 Common uses of hemostatic drugs in clinical practice.

Drug	Examples of successful uses in blood management
Tranexamic acid	Trauma Cardiac surgery, knee or hip arthroplasty, spinal surgery, liver transplantation, oral surgery, also in patients on oral anticoagulants or with hemophilia Hyperfibrinolytic disseminated intravascular coagulation, transurethral prostatectomy, upper gastrointestinal bleeding, menorrhagia, bleeding after placental abruptio and cervix conization, postpartum hemorrhage, ocular hemorrhage after traumatic hyphema, hereditary angioedema, rebleeding after subarachnoidal hemorrhage, acute promyeloic leukemia, bleeding patients with factor XI deficiency (in conjunction with rHuFVIIa)
EACA	Cardiac surgery Hemophilia, aplastic anemia, acute leukemia with thrombocytopenia, Kasabach–Merritt syndrome, spinal fusion, hip arthroplasty, hyperfibrinolysis in liver cirrhosis, hematuria
DDAVP	Cardiac surgery in patients on preoperative aspirin or other non-steroidal antirheumatic drugs; patients for cardiac surgery with expected major blood loss and confirmed platelet abnormality Patients with congenital platelet disorders, e.g., platelet TxA2 receptor abnormality and vWD; drug-induced platelet disorders causing bleeding (aspirin, ticlopidin, heparin, dextran, clopidogrel); thrombocytopenic bleeding due to immune and non-immune causes; bleeding due to liver cirrhosis
Vitamins of the K group	Patients with a lack of vitamin K Hemorrhagic disease of the newborn; patients lacking vitamin K-dependent factors due to liver disease
Conjugated estrogens	Liver transplantation Uremic coagulopathy; dysfunctional uterine bleeding

EACA, ε-aminocaproic acid; DDAVP, 1-deamino-8-D-arginine vasopressin; rHuFVIIa, recombinant human factor VIIa; vWD, von Willebrand disease.

• **Tetragalacturonic acid ester** is obtained from apple pectin. It was recommended for topical and oral use as a hemostatic agent. This substance may inhibit fibrinolysis, but clinical trials have not been performed.

• **Naphthionine** is related to Congo red. It was claimed to be useful in normal and thrombocytopenic patients. It is considered to act by shifting the isoelectric point of fibrinogen, thereby favoring the gel state.

• **Ethamsylate** is also a derivative of Congo red. Although its mode of action is still only vaguely defined, it seems to increase platelet adhesiveness and capillary resistance. It may also have an antihyaluronidase activity and may inhibit prostacyclin. Clinical trials propose its use in menorrhagia as well as in bleeding after dental extraction, adenotonsillectomy, and transurethral prostatectomy.

• **Naftazone** was shown to reduce the use of transfusions in patients undergoing prostatectomy. However, there are only a limited number of clinical trials to support its use.

• **Adrenochrome, carbazochrome:** Adrenochrome is a derivative of epinephrine. When complexed with a salicylate, its stability is increased (carbazochrome). It was claimed to reduce blood loss, but the evidence is sparse.

Local hemostatic agents

Local hemostasis depends on a variety of factors and processes which, under physiological conditions, provide a stepwise approach to tissue repair. Vasoconstriction is an early mechanism to stop bleeding. Activated platelets contribute to this vasoconstriction by releasing vasoactive compounds at the site of injury. Thereupon, vessels constrict and blood flow is reduced. Platelets activated at the site of tissue injury contribute many more hemostyptic effects. They adhere to injured vessels where they begin to form a physical barrier to blood flow; change their outer membrane in a way to facilitate the formation of a blood clot; release compounds that activate plasma clotting, including calcium ions; and generate thrombin, which cleaves fibrinogen to fibrin fibers, the latter of which are stabilized by FXIII. The interaction of platelets, tissue components, red cells, and plasma components of the clotting process finally forms a stable clot and promotes tissue healing. Tissue healing is accompanied by changes in vessel structures. Larger ones are often recanalized by proteolyzing the blood clot. Smaller ones obliterate and growth factors promote revascularization in the repaired tissue.

Chemical local hemostatic agents are valuable adjuncts to the physical means of hemostasis. The use of physical means sometimes depends on visualization of distinct bleeding vessels in order to ligate them. Other physical means for hemostasis use heat to cauterize vessels. This heat may spread sideways and be detrimental to delicate tissues such as neural structures. While chemical agents to stop bleeding are rarely effective in brisk bleeding from large vessels, they are effective in stopping bleeding from small venous and capillary vessels and from the surface of parenchymatous structures where suturing is difficult. Chemical hemostatic agents may also be effective when

a coagulopathic patient lacks the necessary factors for hemostasis. Chemical hemostatic agents can be used in addition to physical means, hence being useful even when brisk bleeding occurs. As for all medical treatments, the success of hemostasis and the avoidance of side effects of hemostatic agents depend on the expertise of the clinicians and their in-depth knowledge of the abilities and potential complications of the agents used.

All of the below-mentioned agents have been used with the intent to reduce bleeding. Empirically, they indeed do so. However, randomized controlled trials are lacking for the majority of the discussed agents. While many of the agents have been shown to have a hemostatic effect, only a minority has been shown to reduce patient exposure to blood transfusions [79–90] (Table 7.4).

Tissue adhesives and other agents accelerating clot formation locally

Tissue adhesives, also referred to as tissue glues, are a heterogenous group of compounds that all have the ability to stick to tissues and to seal them, either by their own action or by promoting physiological processes. In doing so, they can also promote wound healing, seal

Table 7.4 Effects of tissue adhesives on blood loss.

Field of use	Tissue adhesives	Effect on blood loss and use of transfusions
Cardiothoracic surgery	Fibrin sealant	Reduces postoperative blood loss
Aortic dissection	Fibrin sealant	Blood loss reduced
Cardiac surgery	Fibrin spray	Reduces bleeding
Femoral artery cardiac catheterizations	Fibrin sealant given per sheath at the end of procedure (animal study)	Reduces bleeding
Cardiac surgery in pediatrics	Fibrin sealant	Reduces bleeding and transfusions
Hepatic surgery	Microcrystalline collagen powder, fibrin glue	Reduces bleeding
Bleeding gastroduodenal ulcers	Fibrin sealant vs polidocanol	Reduces bleeding
Bone bleeding	Gelatin foam paste, gelatin sponge with thrombin, microfibrillar collagen	Reduces bleeding
Knee replacement	Fibrin spray applied	Reduces blood loss and transfusions
Spinal instrumentation	Fibrin glue	Reduces blood loss, no patients who received fibrin glue were transfused
Burns	Fibrin sealant	Eliminated need for transfusions

tissues to prevent leakage of tissue fluids or air, support sutures, and deliver drugs (e.g., chemotherapeutics, antibiotics) to the target tissues. Above all, they can promote hemostasis.

Fibrin sealants

Probably the most commonly used tissue adhesives are fibrin sealants. They mimic the natural process of clotting by providing the required physiological material for clot formation. This makes fibrin sealants biodegradable, i.e., they are broken down by fibrinolysis. The two main components of fibrin glues are thrombin and fibrinogen. Thrombin may be derived from human plasma or bovine blood, or recombinant thrombin may be used, as is the case in newer products. Fibrinogen is typically taken from human blood. In addition to these two main components, FXIII (for added clot strength), calcium (for the clotting process itself), and antifibrinolytics (for prevention of early clot lysis) may be added. The more fibrinogen is found in glue, the higher is the tensile strength. The more thrombin is found, the more rapid is the clot formation.

Fibrin-based tissue adhesives have a very low complication rate. They are biocompatible and do not cause local irritation, inflammation, or foreign body reactions. Occasionally, allergic reactions to one of their ingredients have been described. Bovine thrombin rarely causes immunological complications. While most of these complications are of allergic origin, they may also result in coagulopathy due to the formation of neutralizing antibodies to human factor V. Those antibodies are reported much less frequently when recombinant ingredients are used for glue preparation. Another side effect of fibrin glues is the transmission of infectious agents. Since commercial fibrin sealants are made from allogeneic blood, they have the potential to transmit diseases. To date, however, only the transmission of parvovirus B19 has been reported. Since the plasma used for fibrin adhesive production is treated by several virus inactivation steps, the risk of infection with HIV and hepatitis viruses is almost non-existent.

Fibrin and thrombin when used together effectively and rapidly promote hemostasis. However, this also brings a challenge since as soon as both agents mix, they clot. Delivery systems are needed that mix those agents only where the adhesive is expected to form the clot. Double-barrel syringes are typically used when commercial preparations are applied. It is also possible to attach a spray mechanism to this syringe. When large surfaces are to be sprayed, fibrinogen may be sprayed

first, followed by thrombin. When no double-barrel syringe is available, the two components of the fibrin sealant can also be attached to one of the ports of a double-lumen central line, and the tip of the line placed into the wound.

Commercially available fibrin sealants made from donor blood are rather consistent in their action. They have predictable, often supranormal, levels of ingredients. In contrast, when the glue is self-made, e.g., from cryoprecipitate or from autologous blood prior to surgery, the clotting factor levels are variable and not as highly concentrated. Nevertheless, autologous glue may be an attractive alternative to avoid disease transmission and immunological reactions. Besides, it may be the only sealant available in countries where commercial sealants are not approved or available. In the future, recombinant fibrinogen and thrombin may eliminate the use of allogeneic blood products altogether.

Indications for the use of fibrin sealants are diverse, including bleeding in cardiac surgery, parenchymatous organs (liver and spleen surgery), bleeding gastroduodenal ulcers, burns, and many other situations. Fibrin glue is also useful in coagulopathic patients with hemophilia A or B, or vWD, or on anticoagulant therapy, etc., since it provides the missing clotting factors [91]. While there are not many high-quality studies of fibrin sealants, they have been shown to improve at least some patient outcome variables [92]. Fibrin sealants may reduce blood loss. It was also suggested that hemophiliac patients are not exposed to as many clotting factor concentrates when fibrin glue is used. When fibrin glue is used in conjunction with laparoscopy during an attempt to stop parenchymatous bleeding, it may save the patient the pain of laparotomy. Besides, higher survival rates in bleeding patients have been shown.

Albumin-based compounds

Another group of tissue adhesives is made of albumin and a glue-like substance. There are a handful of variants: gelatin–resorcinol–formaldehyde glue, gelatin–resorcinol–formaldehyde–glutaraldehyde glue, and glutaraldehyde glue. Albumin-based tissue sealants are biodegradable. Compared with fibrin sealants, their hemostatic activity is weaker. However, these enhance fibroblastic proliferation and thus produce greater tensile strength than fibrin sealants. Therefore, these are mainly used where tissues need strength, as in aortic dissection surgery. So far, cardiovascular procedures are the main realm for the use of albumin-based compounds. In this setting, some have been shown to reduce blood loss.

Side effects of the albumin-based compounds are tissue toxicity and vessel stenosis if used around sutured vessels. The development of inhibitors to human clotting factor V has also been reported.

Bone wax

The traditional bone wax is a mix of beeswax and vaseline. It melts slightly when it comes into contact with the warm hand of the surgeon. Bone wax can be applied to bleeding bones, and there it stops blood flow by providing a mechanical barrier. Traditional bone wax is an inert substance and is not absorbed. It therefore hinders the healing of bones and should not be used when two bone parts are expected to fuse. Traditional bone wax can also cause foreign body reactions and is associated with impaired wound healing and wound infection. It should be used only for the time needed to achieve hemostasis and excess wax must be removed. It must not be used for infected wounds.

To circumvent the ill effects of the inert traditional bone wax, some surgeons have resorted to vancomycin cream as an off-label use to stop bleeding from open bone surfaces, thereby trying to prevent infection. However, newer, biodegradable bone waxes are on the horizon, such as ostene, which is reported to be removed from the bone surface within 2 days and does not substantially impair wound healing.

Cyanoacrylates

Cyanoacrylates are a group of compounds that have strong tissue adhesive properties. However, they are not biodegradable and their use is akin to the implantation of a foreign body. They can provoke immunological and inflammatory responses, including tissue necrosis. They may even be cancinogenic. These adhesives are almost exclusively used to approximate skin. Since they are bacteriostatic, they can also be used in dental procedures. However, they should not be used internally.

Hydrogels

Hydrogels are based mainly on polyethylene glycol polymers. These agents are water soluble and biodegradable. Some of the brands need to be activated by light and so they are not useful for urgent hemostasis.

Gelatin

Gelatin is an animal product that is made from animal skin. The product is boiled and supplied as a paste or sponge. It can be whipped into a foam and dried into a spongy substance. It is also available as powder. When applied alone, it works as a matrix for coagulation. When combined with agents such as thrombin, it actively promotes clot formation.

Gelatin sticks readily to tissues. It can easily be applied with wet pads. However, it is also easily dislodged when soaked in blood. When hemostasis is achieved, residual material should be removed. Since gelatin is resorbable, it is a good alternative to bone wax at sites where fusion is needed.

Gelatin foam has some reported side effects when applied to neuronal tissues, such as inflammatory reactions, paresthesias, pain, and neurological deficiencies. It was reported to induce toxic shock syndrome when used in the nose. Gelatin must not remain in a closed space since it can swell and cause pressure injury to adjacent tissues. Gelatin also accelerates bacteria growth and therefore must not be used in infected areas.

Collagen

Hemostatic collagen is obtained from the collagen of bovine corium. It is available in various forms, e.g., microfibrillar collagen (MFC) and microcrystalline collagen powder. Collagen serves as the matrix that promotes platelet aggregation. It seems to be effective in heparinized patients, but less so in thrombocytopenia. It readily adheres to the tissues and provides rapid hemostasis. MFC is very sticky and it sticks more readily to latex gloves than tissue. Therefore, it must be applied with instruments, and not with gloved hands. It does not swell extensively. Since collagen can increase infection and interferes with the healing process, it should be removed from the surgical site before closure.

Hemostatic collagen can be combined with a variety of other hemostatics to enhance its performance. A mix of collagen and thrombin is available. A composite of MFC and polyethylene glycol has been marketed to treat bone bleeding. It is biodegradable and does not interfere with bone healing.

Oxidized cellulose and oxidized regenerated cellulose

Cellulose is made from wood pulp. During preparation it is formed into a fibrillar material that can be knit into meshes. Cellulose promotes clot formation and hemostasis by mechanical means. It can swell or form a gel. Oxidized cellulose also promotes activation of corpuscular and humoral components of the clotting system. However, it is less effective if the patient is coagulopathic. Cellulose for hemostasis has a low pH and acts as a caustic. The low pH may be the reason why it works as an antiseptic. This makes oxidized cellulose appropriate for use in infected areas.

Oxidized regenerated cellulose (ORC) should be used dry for maximum hemostasis. It should not be combined with thrombin. Since it swells, it must not be packed in closed spaces. Bipolar vessel sealing can be undertaken even through ORC layers. After hemostasis is achieved, ORC can be removed from the wound.

Microporous polysaccharide hemosphere

Microporous polysaccharide hemosphere comes as a powder, which is applied in wounds. It soaks water out of the bleeding wound and concentrates endogenous clotting factors. The powder seems to work only in deep wounds where blood is pooling. When it is applied to heavily bleeding superficial wounds, the blood flow washes the powder away.

Mineral zeolite

As is the case with microporous polysaccharide hemosphere, mineral zeolite powder absorbs liquids in the wound and concentrates clotting factors in the wound, and seems to be effective only in wounds where blood is pooling. The original mineral zeolite containing mainly calcium acts in an exothermic reaction, which increases the temperature in the wound rapidly to 40–42 °C. Burns have been reported after its use. In order to reduce this side effect, in the second-generation zeolite some calcium ions are exchanged for silver ions, which reduces the heat produced.

Zeolite produced as a powder can be poured into a wound. It if comes with a trauma dressing, this should be pressed down onto the bleeding surface for about 60 seconds. There it exerts its hemostatic effects. These depend partially on an intact clotting system. In animal models, zeolite dressings have been shown to reduce blood loss and to improve survival. Whether this is true also for human use will be seen.

Chitosan

Chitosan is commercially produced by deacetylation of chitin. Chitin and chitosan are derivatives from algae products or are made from other marine animals. As a dressing, it is used as a hemostatic (and antibacterial) agent, but its mode of action is still the subject of debate. It may activate platelets and may make red cells stick more readily to the wound. Also, it may have a vasoconstrictive effect and mobilize clotting factors in the wound. It may also be active in coagulopathic patients.

Physics meets chemistry

A smart way to achieve hemostasis is to combine physical and chemical measures. Applying pressure with hemostatic-coated packs adds the physical component of tamponade to the chemical component of clot formation. The packs may either be removed after application and clot formation or remain *in situ*, given they are absorbable. Such combinations make for a robust hemostatic. They can be applied to major bleeding vessels without impairing blood flow beyond the hemostatic. They can also be applied to bleeding parenchymatous organs. Such hemostatic packs are especially valuable in the preclinical setting [93–96].

A hemostatic pack that has been available for decades is a bandage coated with extremely high concentrations of dry fibrinogen and thrombin. When applied to the wound, it accelerates clot formation. In animal studies, it has proven successful in reducing blood loss and has shown promise clinically. However, it is very expensive. Besides, it has to be handled with care since it breaks easily. That is why it cannot be applied to deep wounds in the prehospital setting.

Another, less expensive hemostatic pack employs chitin or its deacetylated form, chitosan. There is some evidence that a pack with chitin or the more efficacious chitosan may reduce blood loss following trauma [97].

A further dressing uniting chemical and physical means to achieve hemostasis is a dressing with a microporous polyacrylamide core. This core has the potential to absorb 1400 times its weight in fluids. In doing so, it expands and becomes heavy. When applied to a wound, it creates local pressure to stop the bleeding, and by its absorption of fluids it may accelerate coagulation.

Practical recommendations for the use of tissue adhesives

Choice of tissue adhesive

Apart from the intrinsic properties of available agents, two major considerations should be taken into account when choosing a suitable tissue adhesive. The first is whether the adhesive is needed urgently or not. If it is urgent, preparations that are supplied in frozen form are not suitable since they take time to thaw. Autologous glues, which require the patient to be phlebotomized, are also not suitable in an emergency situation. In case of emergency, ready-to-use preparations are indicated. The second is the patient's intrinsic ability to form a clot. In coagulopathic patients, tissue adhesives that merely concentrate and accelerate physiological clotting effects are not suitable. In this case, adhesives that exhibit their own clotting ability should be used.

Method of application

Hemostatic agents come in many different forms, i.e., spray, powder, gel, mesh, or wool. Sprays and powders are more suitable if larger areas are to be treated. Gels can be precisely targeted and seem not to dislodge easily in wet areas. Meshes and wools are positioned strategically, and the swelling effect can be used to apply pressure to a bleeding spot. Some hemostatic agents need a dry field for application. Since this is sometimes difficult to achieve, prophylactic use is recommended to prevent anticipated bleeding. Prophylactic use of some tissue sealants may allow for complete polymerization of the agent and maximum clot strength before it is challenged by blood flow. For instance, the sealant can be applied to vascular anastomoses before the clamps are released. When the sealant is finally polymerized, the clamps are opened and blood flow can start.

Vasoconstrictors

Mimicking the first physiological step in hemostasis, namely vasoconstriction, is a simple and effective means to reduce blood loss. As the gold standard, epinephrine is the agent of choice for hemostatic vasoconstriction. Depending on the mode of application, it is typically used in dilutions of 1:10 000–1:2 000 000. Other than epinephrine, vasopressin, terlipressin, norepinephrine, and phenylephrine may also achieve hemostatic vasoconstriction. The agents are either injected locally or are applied directly to the wound, mucosa, or peritoneum. Sprays, sponges, tamponade material, or glues have served as vectors for the application of the vasoconstrictors. Epinephrine can also be nebulized to treat hemorrhage in the oropharynx [98].

Vasoconstrictors have been very successful in reducing bleeding in burn [99, 100] and breast surgery [101–103]. In addition, many other minor and major surgeries have used the hemorrhage reduction induced by vasoconstrictors. They have been proven useful in such diverse interventions as pilonidal sinus surgery [104], bone graft harvest [105], bleeding peptic ulcers [106], head and neck surgery [107, 108], gynecological procedures [109], and postpartum hemorrhage [110].

Usually, local vasoconstrictors are simple and safe to use. However, systemic absorption of the drugs may cause cardiovascular, neurological, and immunological side effects (changes in heart rate and blood pressure, cardiac arrhythmias, myocardial infarction, seizures, allergic reactions, etc.).

Miscellaneous topical agents used to stop bleeding

A heterogenous group of agents have been used to stop bleeding locally. Among them are the above-mentioned fibrinolytics. Aprotinin, EACA, and tranexamic acid have successfully been used to irrigate bleeding areas, resulting in reduction in bleeding. Such therapy has been shown to be successful in heart surgery [111, 112], spinal surgery, as an enema in bleeding colitis, epistaxis, before tonsillectomy, as irrigation for bladder hemorrhage, and after transurethral resection of the prostate. Antifibrinolytics have also been instilled into the pleural cavity to treat hemoptysis. Tranexamic acid as a 5% solution can be used as a mouthwash [113] to reduce bleeding after surgery in patients on oral anticoagulants. Hot water has also been proposed to stop bleeding, e.g., in epistaxis [114].

Apart from antifibrinolytics, a variety of other substances have been shown to reduce bleeding. Among them are barium preparations given as an enema for diverticula bleeding [115] and aluminum salts for bladder hemorrhage [116]. Also, calcium alginate, silver nitrate, trichloroacetic acid [117], and Monsel's solution (20% ferric subsulfate) [118] have been used to stop local bleeding. Some of them are caustic; they leave a layer of damaged tissue that stops bleeding.

An increasingly recommended hemostatic agent is formalin. Instillation of the 4% solution is an effective treatment for patients bleeding from hemorrhagic cystitis or proctitis. It has a caustic effect and therefore, all non-bleeding tissues should be protected from the solution. The perineum can be protected by jelly and formalin-soaked sponge sticks can be used to apply the solution directly to the bleeding bowel, preventing spread of the solution more proximally [119, 120]. The procedure is not without complications but may be helpful in selected cases.

Key points

• Antifibrinolytics are indicated in patients bleeding from exaggerated fibrinolysis. Some are also effective in thrombocytopenic bleeding.
• Desmopressin is helpful in bleeding due to many congenital and acquired platelet disorders, as well as in thrombocytopenia.

• Vitamin K, not fresh frozen plasma, is the therapeutic of choice in patients with vitamin K deficiency, providing there is sufficient time for the vitamin to be effective and a liver that is able to synthesize the necessary factors.

• There are a wide variety of local hemostatic agents. They act as topical sealants, matrices for endogenous clotting, vasoconstrictors, caustics, or by other mechanisms. All of them can reduce bleeding and some have been shown to reduce the use of transfusions. Maximum benefit results when the healthcare practitioner is familiar with their use.

Questions for review

1. What is the role of fibrinolysis in blood management?
2. What are the essential and the adjunct ingredients of fibrin sealants?
3. What different kinds of tissue sealants are available and what are the indications for their use?
4. What agents are available for local hemostasis?

Suggestions for further research

Collect different recipes on how to prepare autologous fibrin sealants. Apart from a patient's blood, what other ingredients are required for the preparation? Which methods are used to prepare fibrin concentrates? How long does it take to prepare autologous sealants?

Exercises and practice cases

Give recommendations for the pharmacological treatment of the following patients. Prescribe one or more drugs you deem beneficial to reduce bleeding. Give the exact dosing, timing, and route of administration.
1. A 54-year-old patient has been on chronic hemodialysis for the past 3.5 years. He is scheduled for emergency laparotomy for peritonitis due to a suspected ruptured appendix.
2. A 98-year-old healthy patient fell when he was on a hiking tour and broke his arm. He is scheduled for open reduction and internal fixation of his humerus.
3. A 14-year-old girl is admitted to hospital for open correction of her scoliosis.

4. You see a 33-year-old female with menorrhagia. She does not have any apparent anatomical lesions in her genitalia.
5. A 55-year-old patient presents in the emergency room because he has severe chest pain. During cardiac catheterization he shows severe stenosis of his coronary arteries. The patient agrees to have coronary artery bypass surgery. He has not taken any drugs until now.
6. A known 61-year-old woman presents for coronary artery bypass graft and aortic valve replacement. She was on aspirin until 3 days ago.
7. A 76-year-old woman fell in her bathroom and broke her hip. She is scheduled for hip replacement tomorrow. She currently takes Coumadin® for a pre-existing atrial fibrillation. Her current INR is 2.9.
8. A 40-year-old obese female with vWD presents for cholecystectomy.
9. A 24-year-old patient with hemophilia A needs to have his wisdom teeth removed. His factor A level is 2.5%.
10. A patient with recurrent epistaxis is known to have liver cirrhosis.

Homework

Visit the different surgical departments of your hospital and inquire about the use of tissue sealants, vasoconstrictors, and other locally acting hemostatic agents. Note the current indications for the agents used.

Go to the pharmacy and note all available means to improve hemostasis. Note the package size and the price, and ask for a package insert from the available products. When you have a complete list of the available products, compare them with the products mentioned in this chapter. Note all missing products and try to find out whether there is a way to purchase them in your country. Record all your findings.

If there is somebody in your hospital who prepares autologous fibrin sealants, ask to join him/her when he/she is preparing it next time.

Check the different delivery devices for tissue adhesives and try to master their assembly procedure and use.

References

1. Reece TB, Maxey TS, Kron IL. A prospectus on tissue adhesives. *Am J Surg* 2001;**182** (2 Suppl):40S–44S.
2. Mannucci PM. Desmopressin (DDAVP) in the treatment of bleeding disorders: the first 20 years. *Blood* 1997;**90**: 2515–2521.

3. Cattaneo M. Review of clinical experience of desmopressin in patients with congenital and acquired bleeding disorders. *Eur J Anaesthesiol* 1997;**14** (Suppl):10–14; discussion 14–18.

4. Peters DC, Noble S. Aprotinin: an update of its pharmacology and therapeutic use in open heart surgery and coronary artery bypass surgery. *Drugs* 1999;**57**:233–260.

5. Rich JB. The efficacy and safety of aprotinin use in cardiac surgery. *Ann Thorac Surg* 1998;**66** (5 Suppl):S6–S11; discussion S25–S28.

6. Mangano DT, Tudor IC, Dietzel C. The risk associated with aprotinin in cardiac surgery. *N Engl J Med* 2006;**354**: 353–365.

7. Fergusson DA, Hébert PC, Mazer CD, *et al*, for the BART Investigators: A comparison of aprotinin and lysine analogues in highrisk cardiac surgery. *N Engl J Med* 2008;**358**: 2319–2331.

8. Henry D, Carless P, Fergusson D, Laupacis A. The safety of aprotinin and lysine-derived antifibrinolytic drugs in cardiac surgery: a meta-analysis. *CMAJ* 2009;**180**: 183–193.

9. Takagi H, Manabe H, Kawai N, Goto SN, Umemoto T. Aprotinin increases mortality as compared with tranexamic acid in cardiac surgery: a meta-analysis of randomized head-to-head trials. *Interact CardioVasc Thorac Surg* 2009;**9**:98–101.

10. Ide M. Lessons from the aprotinin saga: current perspective on antifibrinolytic therapy in cardiac surgery. *J Anesth* 2010;**24**:96–106.

11. Beattie WS, Karkouti K. The Post-BART Anti-Fibrinolytic Dilemma? *Journal of Cardiothorac Vascr Anesth* 2011;**25**: 3–5.

12. Westaby S. Aprotinin: Twenty-five years of claim and counterclaim. *J Thorac Cardiovasc Surg* 2008;**135**:487–491.

13. Raghunathan K, Connelly NR, Kanter GJ. Epsilon-Aminocaproic acid and clinical value in cardiac anesthesia. *J Cardiothoracic Vasc Anesth* 2011;**25**:16–19.

14. Martin K, Knorr J, Breuer T, *et al*. Seizures after open heart surgery: Comparison of epsilon-aminocaproic acid and tranexamic acid. *J Cardiothorac Vasc Anesth* 2011;**25**: 20–25.

15. Dunn CJ, Goa KL. Tranexamic acid: a review of its use in surgery and other indications. *Drugs* 1999;**57**:1005–1032.

16. Armellin G, Vinciguerra A, Bonato R, Pittarello D, Giron GP. Tranexamic acid in primary CABG surgery: high vs low dose. *Minerva Anestesiol* 2004;**70**:97–107.

17. Seto AH, Dunlap DS. Tranexamic acid in oncology. *Ann Pharmacother* 1996;**30**:868–870.

18. Adler SC, *et al*. Tranexamic acid is associated with less blood transfusion in off-pump coronary artery bypass graft surgery: A systematic review and meta-analysis. *J Cardiothorac Vasc Anesth* 2011;**25**:26–35.

19. Cid J, Lozano M. Tranexamic acid reduces allogeneic red cell transfusions in patients undergoing total knee arthro-plasty: results of a meta-analysis of randomized controlled trials. *Transfusion* 2005;**45**:1302–1307.

20. Sukeik M, Alshryda S, Haddad FS, Mason JM. Systematic review and meta-analysis of the use of tranexamic acid in total hip replacement. *J Bone Joint Surg Br* 2011;**93**: 39–46.

21. Gill JB, Chin Y, Levin A, Feng D. The use of antifibrinolytic agents in spine surgery. A meta-analysis. *J Bone Joint Surg Am* 2008;**90**:2399–2407.

22. Sethna NF, Zurakowski D, Brustowicz RM, Bacsik J, Sullivan LJ, Shapiro F. Tranexamic acid reduces intraoperative blood loss in pediatric patients undergoing scoliosis surgery. *Anesthesiology* 2005;**102**:727–732.

23. Zellin G, Rasmusson L, Pålsson J, Kahnberg KE. Evaluation of hemorrhage depressors on blood loss during orthognathic surgery: a retrospective study. *J Oral Maxillofac Surg* 2004;**62**:662–666.

24. Morimoto Y, Yoshioka A, Sugimoto M, Imai Y, Kirita T. Haemostatic management of intraoral bleeding in patients with von Willebrand disease. *Oral Dis* 2005;**11**:243–248.

25. Boylan JF, Klinck JR, Sandler AN, *et al*. Tranexamic acid reduces blood loss, transfusion requirements, and coagulation factor use in primary orthotopic liver transplantation. *Anesthesiology* 1996;**85**:1043–1048; discussion 30A–31A.

26. Sorimachi T, Fujii Y, Morita K, Tanaka R. Rapid administration of antifibrinolytics and strict blood pressure control for intracerebral hemorrhage. *Neurosurgery* 2005;**57**:837–844.

27. Gluud LL, Klingenberg SL, Langholz SE. Systematic review: tranexamic acid for upper gastrointestinal bleeding. *Aliment Pharmacol Ther* 2008;**27**:752–758.

28. CRASH-2 Trial Collaborators, Shakur H, *et al*. Effects of tranexamic acid on death, vascular occlusive events, and blood transfusion in trauma patients with significant haemorrhage (CRASH-2): a randomized, placebo-controlled trial. *Lancet* 2010;**376**:23–32.

29. Bartholomew JR, Salgia R, Bell WR. Control of bleeding in patients with immune and nonimmune thrombocytopenia with aminocaproic acid. *Arch Intern Med* 1989;**149**: 1959–1961.

30. Benfatti RA, Carli AF, Silva GV, Dias AE, Goldiano JA, Pontes JC. Epsilon-Aminocaproic acid influence in bleeding and hemotransfusion postoperative in mitral valve surgery. *Rev Bras Cir Cardiovasc* 2010;**25**:510–515.

31. Eubanks JD. Antifibrinolytics in major orthopaedic surgery. *J Am Acad Orthop Surg* 2010;**18**:132–138.

32. Hellinger J. Fibrinolytic hemorrhage in surgery and its treatment with *p*-aminomethylbenzoic acid. *Folia Haematol Int Mag Klin Morphol Blutforsch* 1967;**87**:32–40.

33. Hellinger J, Vogel G. On the clinical features and therapy of fibrinolytic hemorrhages in surgery with special consideration of the new antifibrinolytic agent *p*-aminomethylbenzoic acid (PAMBA). *Bruns Beitr Klin Chir* 1966;**213**:478–487.

34. Westlund LE, Lunden R, Wallen P. Effect of EACA, PAMBA, AMCA and AMBOCA on fibrinolysis induced by streptokinase, urokinase and tissue activator. *Haemostasis* 1982;**11**:235–241.

35. Kassell NF, Haley EC, Torner JC. Antifibrinolytic therapy in the treatment of aneurysmal subarachnoid hemorrhage. *Clin Neurosurg* 1986;**33**:137–145.

36. Gharabeh A, *et al.* Medical interventions for traumatic hyphema. *Cochrane Database Syst Rev* 2011;(1):CD005431.

37. Heidrich R, Markwardt F, Endler S, Hindersin P. Antifibrinolytic therapy of subarachnoid hemorrhage by intrathecal administration of *p*-aminomethylbenzoic acid. *J Neurol* 1978;**219**:83–85.

38. Shukla KK, Ambastha SS, Dube RK, Dube B. Use of antifibrinolytic therapy in prostate surgery. *Int Surg* 1979;**64**:79–81.

39. Yang H, Zheng S, Shi C. Clinical study on the efficacy of tranexamic acid in reducing postpartum blood lose: a randomized, comparative, multicenter trial. *Zhonghua Fu Chan Ke Za Zhi* 2001;**36**:590–592.

40. Gordz S, Mrowietz C, Pindur G, Park JW, Jung F. Effect of desmopressin (DDAVP) on platelet membrane glycoprotein expression in patients with von Willebrand's disease. *Clin Hemorheol Microcirc* 2005;**32**:83–87.

41. Kobrinsky NL, Israels ED, Gerrard JM, *et al.* Shortening of bleeding time by 1-deamino-8-d-arginine vasopressin in various bleeding disorders. *Lancet* 1984;**1**:1145–1148.

42. Lethagen S, Rugarn P, Aberg M, Nilsson IM. Effects of desmopressin acetate (DDAVP) and dextran on hemostatic and thromboprophylactic mechanisms. *Acta Chir Scand* 1990;**156**:597–602.

43. Tiede A, Rand JH, Budde U, Ganser A, Federici AB. How I treat acquired von Willebrand syndrome. *Blood* 2011;**117**:6777–6785.

44. Rodeghiero F, Castaman G. Treatment of von Willebrand disease. *Semin Hematol* 2005;**42**:29–35.

45. Mannucci PM. Management of von Willebrand disease in developing countries. *Semin Thromb Hemost* 2005;**31**:602–609.

46. Lethagen S. Desmopressin in the treatment of women's bleeding disorders. *Haemophilia* 1999;**5**:233–237.

47. Powner DJ, Hartwell EA, Hoots WK. Counteracting the effects of anticoagulants and antiplatelet agents during neurosurgical emergencies. *Neurosurgery* 2005;**57**:823–831; discussion 823–831.

48. Cattaneo M, Tenconi PM, Alberca I, Garcia VV, Mannucci PM. Subcutaneous desmopressin (DDAVP) shortens the prolonged bleeding time in patients with liver cirrhosis. *Thromb Haemost* 1990;**64**:358–360.

49. Kobrinsky NL, Tulloch H. Treatment of refractory thrombocytopenic bleeding with 1-desamino-8-d-arginine vasopressin (desmopressin). *J Pediatr* 1988;**112**:993–996.

50. Despotis GJ, Levine V, Saleem R, Spitznagel E, Joist JH. Use of point-of-care test in identification of patients who can benefit from desmopressin during cardiac surgery: a randomised controlled trial. *Lancet* 1999;**354**:106–110.

51. Ozen SSU, Bakkaloglu A, Ozdemir S, Ozdemir O, Besbas N. Low-dose intranasal desmopressin (DDAVP) for uremic bleeding. *Nephron* 1997;**75**:119–120.

52. Crescenzi G, Landoni G, Biondi-Zoccai G, *et al.* Desmopressin reduces transfusion needs after surgery: a meta-analysis of randomized clinical trials. *Anesthesiology* 2008;**109**:1063–1076.

53. Suzuki S, Iwata G, Sutor AH. Vitamin K deficiency during the perinatal and infantile period. *Semin Thromb Hemost* 2001;**27**:93–98.

54. Zipursky A. Prevention of vitamin K deficiency in newborns. *Br J Haematol* 1999;**106**:256.

55. Alparin JB. Transfusion medicine issues in the practice of anesthesiology. *Transfus Med Rev* 1995;**9**:339.

56. Crowther MA, Douketis JD, Schnurr T, *et al.* Oral vitamin K lowers the international normalized ratio more rapidly than subcutaneous vitamin K in the treatment of warfarin-associated coagulopathy. A randomized, controlled trial. *Ann Intern Med* 2002;**137**:251–254.

57. Alperin JB. Estrogens and surgery in women with von Willebrand's disease. *Am J Med* 1982;**73**:367–371.

58. Mannucci PM. Hemostatic drugs. *N Engl J Med* 1998;**339**:245–253.

59. Heunisch C, Resnick DJ, Vitello JM, Martin SJ. Conjugated estrogens for the management of gastrointestinal bleeding secondary to uremia of acute renal failure. *Pharmacotherapy* 1998;**18**:210–217.

60. Tran A, Villeneuve JP, Bilodeau M, *et al.* Treatment of chronic bleeding from gastric antral vascular ectasia (GAVE) with estrogen-progesterone in cirrhotic patients: an open pilot study. *Am J Gastroenterol* 1999;**94**:2909–2911.

61. Coppola A, De Stefano V, Tufano A, *et al.* Long-lasting intestinal bleeding in an old patient with multiple mucosal vascular abnormalities and Glanzmann's thrombasthenia: 3-year pharmacological management. *J Intern Med* 2002;**252**:271–275.

62. Knudsen HE, Ott P. Treatment of chronic transfusion-requiring watermelon stomach with oral contraceptives. *Ugeskr Laeger* 2002;**164**:3364–3366.

63. Flordal PA. Pharmacological prophylaxis of bleeding in surgical patients treated with aspirin. *Eur J Anaesthesiol* 1997;**14** (Suppl):38–41.

64. Sedrakyan A, Treasure T, Elefteriades JA. Effect of aprotinin on clinical outcomes in coronary artery bypass graft surgery: a systematic review and meta-analysis of randomized clinical trials. *J Thorac Cardiovasc Surg* 2004;**128**:442–448.

65. Cole JW, Murray DJ, Snider RJ, Bassett GS, Bridwell KH, Lenke LG. Aprotinin reduces blood loss during spinal surgery in children. *Spine*, 2003;**28**:2482–2485.

66. Baldry C, Backman SB, Metrakos P, Tchervenkov J, Barkun J, Moore A. Liver transplantation in a Jehovah's Witness

with ankylosing spondylitis. *Can J Anaesth* 2000;**47**: 642–646.

67. Johansson T, Pettersson LG, Lisander B. Tranexamic acid in total hip arthroplasty saves blood and money: a randomized, double-blind study in 100 patients. *Acta Orthop* 2005;**76**:314–319.

68. Husted H, Blønd L, Sonne-Holm S, Holm G, Jacobsen TW, Gebuhr P. Tranexamic acid reduces blood loss and blood transfusions in primary total hip arthroplasty: a prospective randomized double-blind study in 40 patients. *Acta Orthop Scand* 2003;**74**:665–669.

69. Riewald M, Riess H. Treatment options for clinically recognized disseminated intravascular coagulation. *Semin Thromb Hemost* 1998;**24**:53–59.

70. Gai MY, Wu LF, Su QF, Tatsumoto K. Clinical observation of blood loss reduced by tranexamic acid during and after caesarian section: a multi-center, randomized trial. *Eur J Obstet Gynecol Reprod Biol* 2004;**112**:154–157.

71. O'Connell NM. Factor XI deficiency. *Semin Hematol* 2004;**41** (Suppl 1):76–81.

72. Daily PO, Lamphere JA, Dembitsky WP, Adamson RM, Dans NF. Effect of prophylactic epsilon-aminocaproic acid on blood loss and transfusion requirements in patients undergoing first-time coronary artery bypass grafting. A randomized, prospective, double-blind study. *J Thorac Cardiovasc Surg* 1994;**108**:99–106; discussion 106–108.

73. Florentino-Pineda I, Thompson GH, Poe-Kochert C, Huang RP, Haber LL, Blakemore LC. The effect of amicar on perioperative blood loss in idiopathic scoliosis: the results of a prospective, randomized double-blind study. *Spine* 2004;**29**:233–238.

74. Gunawan B, Runyon B. The efficacy and safety of epsilon-aminocaproic acid treatment in patients with cirrhosis and hyperfibrinolysis. *Aliment Pharmacol Ther* 2006;**23**:115–120.

75. Fuse I, Higuchi W, Mito M, Aizawa Y. DDAVP normalized the bleeding time in patients with congenital platelet TxA2 receptor abnormality. *Transfusion* 2003;**43**:563–567.

76. Nacul FE, *et al.* Massive nasal bleeding and hemodynamic instability associated with clopidogrel. *Pharm World Sci* 2004;**26**:6–7.

77. Frenette L, de Moraes E, Penido C, Paiva RB, Méier-Neto JG. Conjugated estrogen reduces transfusion and coagulation factor requirements in orthotopic liver transplantation. *Anesth Analg* 1998;**86**:1183–1186.

78. Verstraete M. Haemostatic drugs. In: Forbes CD, Bloom AL, Thomas DP, Tuddenham EGD (eds.) *Haemostasis and Thrombosis.* Churchill Livingstone, Edinburgh, Scotland, 1994, pp. 607–617.

79. Kahalley L, Dimick AR, Gillespie RW. Methods to diminish intraoperative blood loss. *J Burn Care Rehabil*, 1991;**12**: 160–161.

80. Rousou J, Levitsky S, Gonzalez-Lavin L, *et al.* Randomized clinical trial of fibrin sealant in patients undergoing rest-ernotomy or reoperation after cardiac operations. A multicenter study. *J Thorac Cardiovasc Surg* 1989;**97**:194–203.

81. Ismail S, Combs MJ, Goodman NC, *et al.* Reduction of femoral arterial bleeding post catheterization using percutaneous application of fibrin sealant. *Cathet Cardiovasc Diagn* 1995;**34**:88–95.

82. Mankad PS, Codispoti M. The role of fibrin sealants in hemostasis. *Am J Surg* 2001;**182** (2 Suppl):21S–28S.

83. Kohno H, Nagasue N, Chang YC, Taniura H, Yamanoi A, Nakamura T. Comparison of topical hemostatic agents in elective hepatic resection: a clinical prospective randomized trial. *World J Surg* 1992;**16**:966–969; discussion 970.

84. Rutgeerts P, Rauws E, Wara P, *et al.* Randomised trial of single and repeated fibrin glue compared with injection of polidocanol in treatment of bleeding peptic ulcer. *Lancet* 1997;**350**:692–696.

85. Harris WH, Crothers OD, Moyen BJ, Bourne RB. Topical hemostatic agents for bone bleeding in humans. A quantitative comparison of gelatin paste, gelatin sponge plus bovine thrombin, and microfibrillar collagen. *J Bone Joint Surg Am* 1978;**60**:454–456.

86. Seguin JR, Frapier JM, Colson P, Chaptal PA. Fibrin sealant improves surgical results of type A acute aortic dissections. *Ann Thorac Surg* 1991;**52**:745–748; discussion 748–749.

87. Levy O, Martinowitz U, Oran A, Tauber C, Horoszowski H. The use of fibrin tissue adhesive to reduce blood loss and the need for blood transfusion after total knee arthroplasty. A prospective, randomized, multicenter study. *J Bone Joint Surg Am* 1999;**81**:1580–1588.

88. Tredwell SJ, Sawatzky B. The use of fibrin sealant to reduce blood loss during Cotrel-Dubousset instrumentation for idiopathic scoliosis. *Spine* 1990;**15**:913–915.

89. McGill V, Kowal-Vern A, Lee M, *et al.* Use of fibrin sealant in thermal injury. *J Burn Care Rehabil* 1997;**18**:429–434.

90. Spotnitz WD, Dalton MS, Baker JW, Nolan SP. Reduction of perioperative hemorrhage by anterior mediastinal spray application of fibrin glue during cardiac operations. *Ann Thorac Surg* 1987;**44**:529–531.

91. Martinowitz U, Schulman S. Fibrin sealant in surgery of patients with a hemorrhagic diathesis. *Thromb Haemost* 1995;**74**:486–492.

92. Carless PA, Henry DA, Anthony DM. Fibrin sealant use for minimising peri-operative allogeneic blood transfusion. *Cochrane Database Syst Rev* 2003;(2):CD004171.

93. Holcomb JB, Pusateri AE, Harris RA, *et al.* Effect of dry fibrin sealant dressings versus gauze packing on blood loss in grade V liver injuries in resuscitated swine. *J Trauma* 1999;**46**:49–57.

94. Holcomb J, MacPhee M, Hetz S, Harris R, Pusateri A, Hess J. Efficacy of a dry fibrin sealant dressing for hemorrhage control after ballistic injury. *Arch Surg* 1998;**133**: 32–35.

95. Kheirabadi BS, Acheson EM, Deguzman R, *et al.* Hemostatic efficacy of two advanced dressings in an aortic

hemorrhage model in Swine. *J Trauma* 2005;**59**:25–34; discussion 34–35.

96. Poretti F, Rosen T, Körner B, Vorwerk D. [Chitosan pads vs. manual compression to control bleeding sites after transbrachial arterial catheterization in a randomized trial.] *Rofo* 2005;**177**:1260–1266.

97. Vournakis JN, Demcheva M, Whitson AB, Finkielsztein S, Connolly RJ. The RDH bandage: hemostasis and survival in a lethal aortotomy hemorrhage model. *J Surg Res* 2003;**113**:1–5.

98. Rowlands RG, Hicklin L, Hinton AE. Novel use of nebulised adrenaline in the treatment of secondary oropharyngeal haemorrhage. *J Laryngol Otol* 2002;**116**:123–124.

99. Sheridan RL, Szyfelbein SK. Staged high-dose epinephrine clysis is safe and effective in extensive tangential burn excisions in children. *Burns* 1999;**25**:745–748.

100. Beausang E, Orr D, Shah M, Dunn KW, Davenport PJ. Subcutaneous adrenaline infiltration in paediatric burn surgery. *Br J Plast Surg* 1999;**52**:480–481.

101. Bell MS. The use of epinephrine in breast reduction. *Plast Reconstr Surg* 2003;**112**:693–694.

102. Armour AD, Rotenberg BW, Brown MH. A comparison of two methods of infiltration in breast reduction surgery. *Plast Reconstr Surg* 2001;**108**:343–347.

103. O'Donoghue JM, Chaubal ND, Haywood RM, Rickard R, Desai SN. An infiltration technique for reduction mammaplasty: results in 192 consecutive breasts. *Acta Chir Plast* 1999;**41**:103–106.

104. Aysan E, Basak F, Kinaci E, Sevinc M. Efficacy of local adrenalin injection during sacrococcygeal pilonidal sinus excision. *Eur Surg Res* 2004;**36**:256–258.

105. Cheeseman GA, Chojnowski A. Use of adrenaline and bupivacaine to reduce bleeding and pain following harvesting of bone graft. *Ann R Coll Surg Engl* 2003;**85**:284.

106. Garrido Serrano A, Guerrero Igea FJ, Perianes Hernández C, Arenas Posadas FJ, Palomo Gil S. Local therapeutic injection in bleeding peptic ulcer: a comparison of adrenaline to adrenaline plus a sclerosing agent. *Rev Esp Enfer Dig* 2002;**94**:395–405.

107. Sorensen WT, Wagner N, Aarup AT, Bonding P. Beneficial effect of low-dose peritonsillar injection of lidocaine-adrenaline before tonsillectomy. A placebo-controlled clinical trial. *Auris Nasus Larynx* 2003;**30**:159–162.

108. Dunlevy TM, O'Malley TP, Postma GN. Optimal concentration of epinephrine for vasoconstriction in neck surgery. *Laryngoscope* 1996;**106**:1412–1414.

109. Bartos P, Popelka P, Adamcová P, Struppl D. Adrenalin versus terlipressin: blood loss and cardiovascular side-effects in the vaginal part of laparoscopically-assisted vaginal hysterectomy or vaginal hysterectomy. *Clin Exp Obstet Gynecol* 2000;**27**:182–184.

110. Lurie S, Appelman Z, Katz Z. Intractable postpartum bleeding due to placenta accreta: local vasopressin may save the uterus. *Br J Obstet Gynaecol* 1996;**103**:1164.

111. Yasim A, Asik R, Atahan E. Effects of topical applications of aprotinin and tranexamic acid on blood loss after open heart surgery. *Anadolu Kardiyol Derg* 2005;**5**:36–40.

112. Mand'ak J, Lonsky V, Dominik J. Topical use of aprotinin in coronary artery bypass surgery. *Acta Medica (Hradec Kralove)* 1999;**42**:139–144.

113. Carter G, Goss A. Tranexamic acid mouthwash—a prospective randomized study of a 2-day regimen vs 5-day regimen to prevent postoperative bleeding in anticoagulated patients requiring dental extractions. *Int J Oral Maxillofac Surg* 2003;**32**:504–507.

114. Seidman MD. Hot-water irrigation in the treatment of posterior epistaxis. *Arch Otolaryngol Head Neck Surg* 1999;**125**:1285.

115. Koperna T, Kisser M, Reiner G, Schulz F. Diagnosis and treatment of bleeding colonic diverticula. *Hepatogastroenterology* 2001;**48**:702–705.

116. Hongo F, Saitoh M. Intravesical instillation of Maalox for the treatment of bladder hemorrhage due to prostate cancer invasion: report of two cases. *Hinyokika Kiyo* 1999;**45**:367–369.

117. Kucuk M, Okman TK. Intrauterine instillation of trichloroacetic acid is effective for the treatment of dysfunctional uterine bleeding. *Fertil Steril* 2005;**83**:189–194.

118. Jetmore AB, Heryer JW, Conner WE. Monsel's solution: a kinder, gentler hemostatic. *Dis Colon Rectum* 1993;**36**:866–867.

119. Tujinaka S, *et al.* Formalin instillation for hemorrhagic radiation proctitis. *Surg Innov* 2005;**12**:123–128.

120. Fu LW, Chen WP, Wang HH, Lin AT, Lin CY. Formalin treatment of refractory hemorrhagic cystitis in systemic lupus erythematosus. *Pediatr Nephrol* 1998;**12**:788–789.

8 Recombinant Blood Products

Biotechnology is a promising science for blood management. It furnishes a variety of useful pharmaceuticals that avoid therapy with plasma-derived products. Among them are recombinant clotting factors, albumin, and recombinant hemoglobin (rHb). This chapter will address the chances and challenges biotechnology offers. Above all, it will discuss how biotechnologically manufactured blood proteins contribute to optimal blood management.

Objectives

1. To learn how biotechnology contributes to blood management.
2. To know how recombinant blood products are synthesized.
3. To list current and future recombinant products and how they relate to blood management.

Definitions

Biotechnology: The integration of natural sciences and engineering sciences in order to achieve the application of organisms, cells, parts thereof, and molecular analogs for products and science (European Federation of Biotechnology, 1989). Or, put simply, biotechnology is about adapting and using resources found in plants and animals.

Recombinant drugs: Medicines that are produced by employing recombinant DNA technology. In this process, DNA is altered, joining genetic material from two different sources.

A brief history

Honolulu, Hawaii is the birthplace of the recombinant sector of biotechnology. In 1972, during a conference on biochemistry, two professors reported the results of their research. Stanley Cohen told the audience that it was possible to introduce foreign DNA into *Escherichia coli*. Herbert Boyer described an enzyme that was able to split DNA in such a way that the strands have identical ends. Near Waikiki Beach, those men met and discussed the potential to combine their discoveries. Some months later, they were able to present their work. They had been able to introduce foreign DNA into the genome of *E. coli*. Recombinant DNA was invented and the recombinant sector of biotechnology took off [1].

Hemophilia patients were the first group of patients to benefit from recombinant blood proteins. Already in the 1970s, blood-derived coagulation products had aroused the hope that the crippling consequences of hemophilia could be prevented. However, blood products were obtained by pooling thousands of plasma sources, and hepatitis B and C were invariably detectable in antihemophiliac preparations. Almost all hemophilia patients were infected with hepatitis, which was considered acceptable in comparison with the benefits the clotting factors provided. In the 1980s, 60–70% of hemophilia patients were also infected with HIV. For this reason, recombinant technology seemed like another quantum leap in making factor concentrates safer. In 1984, the gene for factor VIII was cloned and the recombinant protein extracted. Four years later, recombinant factor concentrates were tested in clinical trials. The first generation of recombinant

Basics of Blood Management, Second Edition. Petra Seeber and Aryeh Shander.
© 2013 John Wiley & Sons, Ltd. Published 2013 by John Wiley & Sons, Ltd.

clotting factors still contained blood-derived albumin for stabilization, while this was eliminated in second-generation concentrates. Third-generation recombinant clotting factors do not contain human or animal products any more.

As recombinant antihemophilia preparations entered the market, other recombinant blood proteins were developed. Some are now being marketed, while others are still in different stages of investigation.

Basics of recombinant drugs

Producing a recombinant drug starts with the detection of the gene locus that encodes the protein of interest. By means of restriction enzymes, the DNA of interest is cut out. The isolated gene sequence is introduced into a vector, such as a virus or the plasmid of a bacterium. Via this vector, the DNA sequence is introduced into the genome of another organism. The organism will soon produce the protein that the DNA encodes, providing that vital factors, such as a promoter, are present. For some proteins, this is all that is required. For most drugs used in blood management, this is not enough though. Therapeutically used blood proteins often have a very complex structure. Vitamin K-dependent clotting factors, for instance, undergo a series of changes after their translation from DNA, such as γ-carboxylation, phosphorylation, and glycosylation. Post-translational changes are required to endow the proteins with their typical properties. Such changes are performed by enzyme systems in the medium that is used to extract the recombinant protein. Bacteria often lack vital enzyme systems for the post-translational changes, while mammalian cells may have what is needed. Baby hamster kidney cells and the Chinese hamster ovary (CHO) cells, for instance, are able to synthesize proteins that have their post-translational changes.

While today's recombinant drugs are often produced in the laboratory, in the future transgenic animals (e.g. sheep) may be used. Human genes encoding the required protein can be introduced into the genome of animals. Depending on where the genes are inserted, the recombinant drug can be secreted in the milk of animals, expressed in the blood, or found in their eggs. The synthesized protein can be purified and marketed. Animal farming for pharmacological purposes—also called pharming—is a lucrative business. The value of transgenic animals is immense. Additionally, the animals can breed, the number of stock can be adapted to the current

needs, and the maintenance of the herds is not as cumbersome as that of maintaining mammalian cell cultures. According to an interesting calculation, it takes only one transgenic cow to produce 2 kg of blood clotting factor IX per year [2].

A further step toward the production of an unlimited supply of blood proteins is the use of transgenic plants. Under the subtitle "Blood from a Plant," it was reported that thrombin, factor XIII, and coagulation factor VIII can be expressed in tobacco plants [2]. Although the mass production of blood proteins in transgenic plants still lies in the future, considerable progress has been made. It is already possible to produce immunoglobulins ("plantibodies") in soybeans. Tomato and tobacco plants can be used to produce human serum albumin [3, 4]. Hemoglobin can also be expressed in tobacco plants. The output of such transgenic plant systems needs to be increased further. Nevertheless, plants are an interesting alternative to allogeneic blood as a source of therapeutics.

Safety of recombinant blood proteins

Recombinant blood proteins are widely considered as safer than plasma-derived products. Nevertheless, there is still room for concern. Recombinant proteins may either lose their activity in the process of production, purification, transport, and storage, or they may be activated by it—both of which reduce their value. Additionally, it may even cause adverse effects if such proteins are used for therapeutic reasons. Proteins may become immunogenic or not perform the required activity. The smallest differences between human and recombinant proteins may have a large impact on the clinical use of the proteins.

The use of human or animal (plasma) components in recombinant clotting factors still holds the potential for disease transmission. They may be used in the culture medium and during the purification process. For instance, mouse monoclonal antibodies are used in the purification process of recombinant proteins and leave some remnants in the final product. Furthermore, cell lines used for protein synthesis can become infected by viruses. Another factor that threatens the safety of recombinant drugs is albumin. It is widely used to stabilize the final recombinant product and has been shown to be the source of viral contamination. Only the third-generation recombinant proteins are produced without the use of foreign proteins[5].

A comparison of recombinant and plasma-derived blood proteins is given in Table 8.1.

Table 8.1 Comparison of recombinant and plasma-derived blood proteins.

	Recombinant products	Blood-derived products
Safety	Third-generation products are made without blood proteins; therefore, there will be no transmission of blood-borne diseases First- and second-generation products are made with animal (and human) products in the production process; transmission of animal (and human) diseases is possible	Virus inactivation employed in some products, blood-borne diseases still transmissible, but undetected pathogens in products now unlikely
Efficacy	Depends on the quality of the product; less than blood-derived product when post-translational changes are inadequate; potentially higher than blood-derived products since protein is more homogenous than blood-derived product (no products of alternative splicing or mutant variations)	If not standardized, efficacy may vary with the factor content of the donor blood; product more heterogenous than recombinant product
Production of antibodies against protein	Possible	Possible (but immunosuppressive effects may alter antibody response compared to recombinant products)
Costs	Comparable to blood-derived products, occasionally higher; trend: costs will probably decrease due to mass production	Comparable to recombinant products, occasionally less; trend: costs will increase because of decreasing donor supply and increasing demand on safety
Use as standard treatment	Preferred over blood-derived products in most countries	Should be used only when recombinant products not available or indicated

Use of recombinant blood proteins in blood management

While there are many recombinant proteins available for clinical use, the following discussion is restricted to those that have promise in blood management.

Classical antihemophilia factors

Octocog: Recombinant factor VIII

As mentioned at the beginning of this chapter, patients with hemophilia A, i.e., patients lacking factor VIII (FVIII), were the first group to benefit from recombinant clotting factor concentrates, which now is first-line treatment for factor-dependent hemophilia A patients.

Initial recombinant clotting factor concentrates of FVIII resembled closely the natural pattern. The naturally occurring FVIII consists of a series of domains ([N-terminal]-A1-a1-A2-a2-B-a3-A3-C1-C2-[C-terminal]) [6], and some brands of recombinant FVIII mimic this [7]. However, the production process for full-length FVIII limits its availability. A variant of full-length FVIII, which is secreted more readily in cell cultures and is less sensitive to degradation, lacks the B-domain of the protein (B-domain deleted, BDD-FVIII); this is not mandatory for its hemostatic ability [7]. BDD-FVIII is available for the treatment of hemophilia A [8, 9]. Other variants of FVIII are designed to exclude domains A2 and C2, which tend to be more immunogenic. Nevertheless, antibody production to recombinant FVIII is still a major concern [10]. More recently, attempts have been made to prolong the half-life of the concentrates so that patients need fewer injections; this would release the strain on the supply chain [11].

Recombinant factor IX

Patients with hemophilia B are lacking factor IX (FIX). FIX concentrates are the treatment of choice. Currently, third-generation recombinant human FIX (rHuFIX) concentrates are available and are a safe alternative to serum-derived formulations. The high purity of the recombinant product eliminates unnecessary thrombotic complications that occur with crude plasma-derived therapeutics for hemophilia B therapy (such as prothrombin complex concentrates [PCC] and FIX concentrates). According to current recommendations, rHuFIX concentrates are the treatment of choice in patients with hemophilia B [5].

Eptacog: recombinant factor VIIa

Eptacog is a very special drug made from recombinant human factor VIIa (rHuFVIIa). Due to its unique properties, it was once termed the "universal hemostatic agent." There are two main hypotheses to explain why eptacog may be such a help to hemophilia patients. The first is that the action of rHuFVIIa depends on the presence of tissue factor to initiate clotting. Tissue factor, which is not normally present in blood, may limit the activation of rHuFVIIa to sites of injury exposing tissue factor locally. An alternative hypothesis claims that rHuFVIIa binds to platelet surfaces, activates FX, and enhances thrombin formation on the surface of platelets. Probably, rHuFVIIa works by a variety of modes of action.

rHuFVIIa was originally used in the therapy of hemophilia patients who developed inhibitors. In these cases it was shown to be effective for prophylaxis as well as for treatment of bleeding episodes, making it the treatment of choice in patients unresponsive to their respectively indicated specific factor concentrates [12].

The use of rHuFVIIa has shown encouraging results also in other coagulation deficiencies, such as in patients with a lack of vitamin K-dependent clotting factors (II, VII, IX, X), especially if the result of therapy with coumadins. Replacing the defective FVII with rHuFVIIa provides almost immediate hemostasis of bleeding caused by vitamin K antagonists [13]. For this indication, doses lower than 90 µg/kg (as low as 20 µg/kg) may provide adequate hemostasis [14, 15]. rHuFVIIa is also effective when reversal of anticoagulation prior to surgery is required. The drug, infused directly prior to surgery, acts within minutes. Given in sufficient doses, the clinical effect of rHuFVIIa lasts about 10–12 hours. During this time, surgery can be performed. After that, rHuFVIIa application can be repeated as needed, or the patient can return to the anticoagulated state.

In addition, rHuFVIIa can control bleeding due to thrombocytopenia and thrombasthenia. Since rHuFVIIa obviously also enhances the action of platelets, it has been used in a variety of settings where thrombocytes are either lacking or dysfunctional. The increased efficiency of thrombin generation by pharmacological doses of rHuFVIIa seems to compensate for the lack of functional platelets.

rHuFVIIA has been used in a variety of other settings. It was used successfully for achieving hemostasis in trauma and surgical patients, in postpartum hemorrhage, and in patients with congenital or acquired factor deficiencies or other coagulopathies, e.g., those elicited by the intake of antiplatelet drugs [16–18].

Although rHuFVIIa initially seemed to be almost omnipotent when it comes to arresting bleedings, this drug does have limitations. Hard evidence for outcome improvement has not been demonstrated. To date, rHuFVII has been shown to be capable of reducing blood product utilization in a wide variety of settings, but meaningful clinical endpoints, such as prolonged survival, have not been shown in the majority of studies. A reduced mortality was shown only when rHuFVIIa was given early. Especially responders, i.e., acutely bleeding surgical or trauma patients who react with an arrest or an obvious reduction of bleeding after rHuFVIIa therapy, seem to experience improved survival rates [19]. The high costs of the drug are prohibitive in many settings. Besides, certain conditions need to be met to ensure optimal results of rHuFVIIa therapy. Since hypothermia decreases the activity of rHuFVIIa (consistent with the common temperature dependence of enzymatic activity), normothermia should be maintained whenever possible. Acidosis drastically reduces the activity of rHuFVIIa. A drop of the pH from 7.4 to 7.0 virtually abolishes the activity of rHuFVIIa. Severely acidotic patients are therefore unlikely to benefit from rHuFVIIa. Additionally, as rHuFVIIa activates the endogenous clotting potential of fibrinogen, platelets, and other players in the clotting process, it seems prudent that rHuFVIIa is only given to patients who still have a residual endogenous clotting potential [16].

Practice tip Clinical use of rHuFVIIa

When rHuFVIIa is considered for a (formerly non-coagulopathic) patient with massive, uncontrollable bleeding, e.g., after severe trauma or postpartum hemorrhage, the drug is best given when as many of the following conditions as possible are met:

- Massive surgical bleeding has been controlled as much as possible.
- The patient has already received:
  - Tranexamic acid (1 g adult dose)
  - Calcium (if hypocalcemic)
  - Possibly DDAVP (0.3 µg/kg)
  - Fibrinogen concentrate, if indicated (level >0.5–1 g/L)
  - PCC in appropriate dose; best if guided by thrombelastogram.
- The patient:
  - Is normothermic
  - Has a pH >7.2 (if not, buffer)
  - Has a platelet count >20–50 × 10^9
  - Has a hemoglobin level of >5–7 g/dL.

Different dosing strategies for rHuFVIIa have been recommended: bolus injection (typically 90 µg/kg) or continuous infusion. The most commonly used regimen is bolus injection, but the more constant plasma level achieved by continuous infusion may decrease the total requirement of the drug. Pediatric patients tend to have a clearance of rHuFVIIa that is almost twice as high as that of adults and therefore, require higher doses or more frequent administration to achieve a satisfying hemostasis.

rHuFVIIa appears to have remarkably few side effects. Low-grade fever, anaphylactic and skin reactions, as well as hypertension have been reported. High doses (up to 300 µg/kg) have been given with no reported side effects. rHuFVIIa therefore seems to have a wide safety margin. There is concern about disseminated intravascular coagulation, thrombosis, and a possible increase of inhibitor titers. In clinical practice, thrombosis, pulmonary embolism or myocardial infarction are rare, but potentially life-threatening, complications [20].

US- as well as European-based recommendations have been published regarding the off-label use of rHuFVIIa [21, 22]. While the recommendations do not agree in all details, it seems that the following settings are appropriate for rHuFVIIa use:

• Bleeding patients with blunt trauma (grade B)
• Postpartum hemorrhage (grade E)
• Uncontrolled bleeding in surgical patients (grade E)
• Bleeding after cardiac surgery (grade D)
• Non-traumatic or expanding intracranial bleeding
• Patients on coumadin with intracranial bleeding
• Rescue therapy after clotting factor replacement has failed in severely bleeding patients in circumstances such as gastrointestinal bleeding in hepatic failure or in thrombocytopenia.

Other recombinant clotting factors

Recombinant factor XIII, fibrinogen, and thrombin
In addition to factors VII, VIII, and IX, many other blood proteins related to the clotting process have been synthesized in a recombinant fashion. Of special interest are recombinant human fibrinogen, recombinant human thrombin, and recombinant human factor XIII (rHuFXIII). Human recombinant fibrinogen can be expressed in the milk of transgenic animals and in yeast [23, 24]. Recombinant thrombin and its precursor prethrombin can be synthesized using CHO or E. coli cells [25], and rHuFXIII is produced in yeast [26] or plants [27].

Where available, they may have significant impact on blood management. The combination of the three recombinant factors fibrinogen, thrombin, and FXIII forms a stable clot, which makes the products a blood donation-independent fibrin glue. Even recombinant thrombin alone, when use topically, can reduce bleeding [28]. This is a viable alternative to the formerly used bovine or human plasma-derived thrombin. Patients with congenital or acquired deficiencies of the respective clotting factors may benefit as well from these recombinant proteins.

Of special interest is rHuFXIII. Naturally occurring FXIII stabilizes blood clots by cross-linking fibrinogen and protects them from destruction by plasmin. It also enhances wound healing and may modulate the immune system [29]. When it is lacking, blood clots remain fragile and patients tend to bleed. Congenital as well as acquired FXIII deficiencies may be treated with rHuFXIII. Patients undergoing cardiopulmonary bypass (CPB), for instance, typically have low levels of FXIII at the end of the CPB, so blood clot strength is reduced and postoperative bleeding may be pronounced. Treating these bleeding patients with rHuFXIII reduces further blood loss after CPB [30].

Recombinant human antithrombin
Antithrombin is an inhibitor of coagulation. It inhibits serine proteases (mainly thrombin and FXa) and probably also has some antiviral and immunomodulatory properties.

Antithrombin can be produced in a recombinant fashion (recombinant human antithrombin [rHuAT]) as well [31]. Certain animals transfected with the gene for human antithrombin excrete it in their milk or rHuAT is produced in yeasts or CHO cells.

Apart from spontaneously resolving skin hyperpigmentation at the injection site, no side effects are reported. Neither increased bleeding nor antibody formation has been observed [32].

Hereditary deficiency of antithrombin increases the risk of thrombosis, and once patients have had at least one thrombotic event, they are treated with oral anticoagulation. During pregnancy and in preparation for surgery, oral anticoagulation is stopped, theoretically increasing the risk of thrombosis. Although not evidence-based, plasma-derived antithrombin concentrates are given to prevent thrombosis. The advent of rHuAT may replace the use of plasma-derived antithrombin. rHuAT concentrates also seem to be useful in surgical patients who depend on heparin treatment, e.g., in CPB. When such patients develop heparin unresponsiveness, fresh frozen plasma (FFP) is sometimes used. rHuAT restores heparin responsiveness in such patients without exposing them to FFP [33].

Recombinant human serum albumin
About 60% of the protein in human serum is albumin. This is a globular protein that consists of three domains which can be produced in recombinant fashion in certain yeast cultures. Sixty-five to 300 mg of albumin can be yielded per liter of yeast solution [34]. After expression in the yeast, the recombinant human serum albumin (rHuSA) is purified to bring it to electrophoretic purity [35]. The resulting product is structurally equivalent to blood-derived albumin.

Plasma-derived albumin concentrate use is usually not evidence based, since only very few hard indications for its use exist; the same is true for rHuSA. However, recombinant clotting factors, vaccines, or other drug formulations need albumin for stabilization. Recombinant albumin is the first choice for this indication since it eliminates the risks inherent to plasma-derived products. For the same reason, rHuSA is also used as a coating for medical devices and to feed or stabilize cell cultures in the biotechnological environment [36]. Preliminary research has shown that rHuSA can also be used in humans in whom it is indicated [37].

Recombinant hemoglobin
The idea of hemoglobin as a source of infusible oxygen carriers is not new. A fully recombinant hemoglobin would have potential advantages over blood-derived hemoglobin: independence from blood donations; has no remnants of erythrocyte stroma (one reason for side effects); excludes blood-borne diseases; and the hemoglobin molecule could be custom-made for optimal oxygen delivery and use.

Recombinant human hemoglobin (rHuHb) can be expressed in different substrates, such as yeast, bacteria [38], milk, animal blood, tobacco plants, etc. None of the rHuHbs is currently available for clinical use as major problems have still to be overcome. For one thing, the production process is challenging since two different protein chains (alpha and beta) need to be co-expressed, assembled, and incorporated in the heme molecule in one single cell. *E. coli* can perform this miracle [39]. The resultant hemoglobin molecule has similar functional characteristics to human hemoglobin Ao. Nevertheless, modifications of the normal human hemoglobin

are needed to prevent rapid dissociation (which are unnecessary in naturally occurring hemoglobin as this is naturally protected from dissociation by the red cell membrane) and to decrease the oxygen affinity of hemoglobin to facilitate oxygen delivery (in naturally occurring red cells this is accomplished by the presence of 2,3-diphosphoglycerate).

Although some of the necessary modifications to rHuHb have been achieved, it still has severe side effects such as gastrointestinal upset and hypertension, which were thought to be due to nitric oxide scavenging and other mechanisms. Later generations of rHuHb seek to tackle these problems by synthesizing variants with more favorable characteristics. In these variants, the size, conformation, oxygen and carbon monoxide binding and release abilities of the hemoglobin molecule, the strength of globin chain association, susceptibility to oxidative damage, and nitric oxide-binding capacity all vary [40–42].

Vaccines, sera, and immunoglobulins
Several vaccines, sera, and immunoglobulins are derived from human or animal plasma. This comes with risks and side effects, allergic reactions to crude preparations being the most common. An interesting alternative to serum-derived immunoglobulins is avian antibodies, which are expressed and harvested in chicken eggs [43]. Hens are given injections of animal venom and they produce antibodies against it. As early as 12 days after injection, antibodies are detectable in the eggs and remain detectable for up to 100 days thereafter. Some simple steps of purification from the egg yolk (such as freezing and thawing) are needed to achieve a purified immunoglobulin that is ready for use. This method is an efficient and gentle means of preparing antivenoms. It has been reported that one egg may contain the same amount of antibodies as 300 mL of rabbit blood [44]. About 75–100 mg of antivenom can be yielded per egg.

While still in the experimental phase, it has been shown that transgenic tobacco plants, for instance, are another potential source of antibody production. When scaled-up and ready for use, recombinant sera may obviate the use of plasma-derived antibodies.

Key points
• Many blood-derived proteins can be synthesized by biotechnological methods.

- The safety of recombinant blood proteins is perceived to be greater than that of blood-derived products. However, blood-derived stabilizers added to the recombinant product, such as albumin, add risk to the product. Second- and third-generation products try to minimize or avoid this risk by reducing or eliminating human and animal protein from the manufacturing process.
- Whenever clinically possible, recombinant factor concentrates are preferred over plasma-derived concentrates.
- rHuFVIIa is considered a universal hemostatic agent, but certain conditions have to be met for optimal results.

Questions for review

1. What are rHuFVIII and rHuFIX used for?
2. What indication was rHuFVII originally developed for?
3. Which scenarios have been described where rHuFVII has been used off-label?
4. What factors influence the efficacy of rHuFVII? Which of them are treatable?
5. What other blood proteins are developed using biotechnology? What is their current use?

Suggestions for further research

What indications for albumin therapy are evidence-based?

Exercises and practice cases

A male patient with hemophilia A is undergoing liver surgery. He has a body weight of 70 kg, a hematocrit of 0.40, and a factor level of 1%.

Calculate the dose of recombinant clotting factor concentrate for this patient (see Table A.7).

How much clotting factor concentrate do you give initially? Would you repeat the therapy with clotting factors after the initial dose? If so, when and at what dose?

Imagine the same patient did not have hemophilia A, but hemophilia B. How would you now answer the above questions?

Homework

List all available recombinant blood proteins in your country. Record what animal or human proteins are used for their production. Record the product and the supplier contact details.

References

1. Special Report. *Nature* 2003;**421**:456–457.
2. Blood from a plant. http://biology.about.com/library/weekly/aa080599.htm accessed May 8, 1999.
3. Sijmons PC, Dekker BM, Schrammeijer B, Verwoerd TC, van den Elzen PJ, Hoekema A. Production of correctly processed human serum albumin in transgenic plants. *Biotechnology (NY)* 1990;**8**:217–221.
4. Fernandez-San Milan A. A chloroplast transgenic approach to hyper-express and purify human serum albumin, a protein hightly susceptible to proteolytic degradation. *Plant Biotechnol* 2003;**1**:71.
5. MASAC Recommendations concerning products licensed for the treatment of hemophilia and other bleeding disorders. MASAC Document #202, approved by the Medical and Scientific Advisory Council (MASAC) on, May 1, 2011, and adopted by the NHF Board of Directors on May 22, 2011. www.hemophilia.org
6. Mannucci PM, Tuddenham EG. The hemophilias–from royal genes to gene therapy. *N Engl J Med* 2001;**344**:1773–1779.
7. Lusher JM, Roth DA. The safety and efficacy of B-domain deleted recombinant factor VIII concentrates in patients with severe haemophilia A: an update. *Haemophilia* 2005;**11**:292–293.
8. Josephson CD, Abshire T. The new albumin-free recombinant factor VIII concentrates for treatment of hemophilia: do they represent an actual incremental improvement? *Clin Adv Hematol Oncol* 2004;**2**:441–446.
9. Kessler CM, Gill JC, White GC 2nd, *et al*. B-domain deleted recombinant factor VIII preparations are bioequivalent to a monoclonal antibody purified plasma-derived factor VIII concentrate: a randomized, three-way crossover study. *Haemophilia* 2005;**11**:84–91.
10. Francini M. Plasma-derived versus recombinant factor VIII concentrates for the treatment of haemophilia A: recombinant is better. *Blood Transfus* 2010;**8**:292–296.
11. Lillicrap D. Improvements in factor concentrates. *Curr Opin Hematol* 2010;**17**:393–397.
12. Valentino LA, Cooper DL, Goldstein B. Surgical experience with rFVIIa (NovoSeven) in congenital haemophilia A and B patients with inhibitors to factors VIII or IX. *Haemophilia* 2011;**17**:579–589.

13. Kessler C. Haemorrhagic complications of thrombocytopenia and oral anticoagulation: is there a role for recombinant activated factor VII? *Intensive Care Med* 2002;**28** (Suppl 2):S228–234.

14. Erhardtsen E, Nony P, Dechavanne M, Ffrench P, Boissel JP, Hedner U. The effect of recombinant factor VIIa (NovoSeven) in healthy volunteers receiving acenocoumarol to an International Normalized Ratio above 2.0. *Blood Coagul Fibrinolysis* 1998;**9**:741–748.

15. Deveras RAE, Kessler CM. Recombinant factor VIIa (rFVIIa) successfully and rapidly corrects the excessively high international normalized ration (INR) and prothrombin times induced by warfarin. *Blood* 2000;**96**:A2745.

16. Knudson MM, Cohen MJ, Reidy R, et al. Trauma, transfusions, and use of recombinant factor VIIa: A multicenter case registry report of 380 patients from the Western Trauma Association. *J Am Coll Surg* 2011;**212**:87–95.

17. Vavra KA, Lutz MF, Smythe MA. Recombinant factor VIIa to manage major bleeding from newer parenteral anticoagulants. *Ann Pharmacother* 2010;**44**:718–726.

18. Franchini M, Franchi M, Bergamini V, et al. The use of recombinant activated FVII in postpartum hemorrhage. *Clin Obstet Gynecol* 2010;**53**:219–227.

19. Grottke O, Henzler D, Rossaint R. Activated recombinant factor VII (rFVIIa). *Best Pract Res Clin Anaesthesiol* 2010;**24**:95–106.

20. Robinson MT, Rabinstein AA, Meschia JF, Freeman WD. Safety of recombinant activated factor VII in patients with warfarin-associated hemorrhages of the central nervous system. *Stroke* 2010;**41**:1459–1463.

21. Shander A, et al. *Consensus Recommendations for the Off-Label Use of Recombinant Human Factor VII (NovoSeven®) Therapy*. P&T®, November 2005, Vol 30, **No** 11, pp. 644–658.

22. Vincent JL, Rossaint R, Riou B, Ozier Y, Zideman D, Spahn DR. Recommendations on the use of recombinant activated factor VII as an adjunctive treatment for massive bleeding–a European perspective. *Crit Care* 2006;**10**:R120.

23. Butler SP, O'Sickey TK, Lord ST, Lubon H, Gwazdauskas FC, Velander WH. Secretion of recombinant human fibrinogen by the murine mammary gland. *Transgenic Res* 2004;**13**:437–450.

24. Tojo N, Miyagi I, Miura M, Ohi H. Recombinant human fibrinogen expressed in the yeast Pichia pastoris was assembled and biologically active. *Protein Expr Purif* 2008;**59**:289–296.

25. Soejima K, Mimura N, Yonemura H, Nakatake H, Imamura T, Nozaki C. An efficient refolding method for the preparation of recombinant human prethrombin-2 and characterization of the recombinant-derived alpha-thrombin. *J Biochem* 2001;**130**:269–277.

26. Bishop PD, Teller DC, Smith RA, Lasser GW, Gilbert T, Seale RL. Expression, purification, and characterization of human factor XIII in *Saccharomyces cerevisiae*. *Biochemistry* 1990;**29**:1861–1869.

27. Gao J, Hooker BS, Anderson DB. Expression of functional human coagulation factor XIII A-domain in plant cell suspensions and whole plants. *Protein Expr Purif* 2004;**37**:89–96.

28. Bowman LJ, Anderson CD, Chapman WC. Topical recombinant human thrombin in surgical hemostasis. *Semin Thromb Hemost* 2010;**36**:477–484.

29. Zaets SB, Xu DZ, Lu Q, et al. Recombinant factor XIII mitigates hemorrhagic shock-induced organ dysfunction. *J Surg Res* 2011;**166**:e135–142.

30. Chandler WL, Patel MA, Gravelle L, et al. Factor XIIIA and clot strength after cardiopulmonary bypass. *Blood Coagul Fibrinolysis* 2001;**12**:101–108.

31. Adiguzel C, Iqbal O, Demir M, Fareed J. European community and US-FDA approval of recombinant human antithrombin produced in genetically altered goats. *Clin Appl Thromb Hemost* 2009;**15**:645–651.

32. Konkle BA, Bauer KA, Weinstein R, Greist A, Holmes HE, Bonfiglio J. Use of recombinant human antithrombin in patients with congenital antithrombin deficiency undergoing surgical procedures. *Transfusion* 2003;**43**:390–394.

33. Avidan MS, Levy JH, van Aken H, et al. Recombinant human antithrombin III restores heparin responsiveness and decreases activation of coagulation in heparin-resistant patients during cardiopulmonary bypass. *J Thorac Cardiovasc Surg* 2005;**130**:107–113.

34. Dockal M, Carter DC, Ruker F. The three recombinant domains of human serum albumin. Structural characterization and ligand binding properties. *J Biol Chem* 1999;**274**:29303–39310.

35. Qiu RD, Li SY, Chen JG, Wu XF, Yuan ZY. High expression and purification of recombinant human serum albumin from *Pichia pastoris*. *Sheng Wu Hua Xue Yu Sheng Wu Wu Li Xue Bao (Shanghai)* 2000;**32**:59–62.

36. Chuang VT, Kragh-Hansen U, Otagiri M. Pharmaceutical strategies utilizing recombinant human serum albumin. *Pharm Res* 2002;**19**:569–577.

37. Kasahara A, Kita K, Tomita E, Toyota J, Imai Y, Kumada H. Repeated administration of recombinant human serum albumin caused no serious allergic reactions in patients with liver cirrhosis: a multicenter clinical study. *J Gastroenterol* 2008;**43**:464–472.

38. Fronticelli C, Koehler RC. Design of recombinant hemoglobins for use in transfusion fluids. *Crit Care Clin* 2009;**25**:357–371.

39. Hoffman SJ, Looker DL, Roehrich JM, et al. Expression of fully functional tetrameric human hemoglobin in *Escherichia coli*. *Proc Natl Acad Sci U S A* 1990;**87**:8521–8525.

40. Vasseur-Godbillon C, Sahu SC, Domingues E, et al. Recombinant hemoglobin betaG83C-F41Y. *FEBS J* 2006;**273**:230–241.

41. Wiltrout ME, Giovannelli JL, Simplaceanu V, Lukin JA, Ho NT, Ho C. A biophysical investigation of recombinant hemoglobins with aromatic B10 mutations in the distal heme pockets. *Biochemistry* 2005;**44**:7207–7217.

42. Choi JW, Lee JH, Lee KH, *et al.* Characteristic of aromatic amino acid substitution at alpha 96 of hemoglobin. *J Biochem Mol Biol* 2005;**38**:115–119.

43. Zhu L, van de Lavoir MC, Albanese J, *et al.* Production of human monoclonal antibody in eggs of chimeric chickens. *Nat Biotechnol* 2005;**23**:1159–1169.

44. Devi CM. Development of viper-venom antibodies in chicken egg yolk and assay of their antigen binding capacity. *Toxicon* 2002;**40**:857–861.

9   Artificial Blood

Recreating blood, the fluid of life, is a human dream that dates back thousands of years. However, myth and reality met when the first unsuccessful attempts were made to actually resuscitate patients. From the humble beginnings up to this day it has not been possible to even come close to recreating one of the main blood components, let alone whole blood. However, as the result of decades of research, several drugs have been developed that are able to mimic some of the properties of blood components. This chapter will give an overview of science's quest to recreate the fluid of life.

Objectives

1. To describe the main qualities of hemoglobin-based oxygen carriers (HBOCs).
2. To describe the main qualities of perfluorocarbons (PFCs).
3. To explain how different artificial blood components may substitute for platelets that are lacking.

Definitions

Artificial oxygen carriers (AOCs): Drugs that can bind, carry, and unload significant amounts of oxygen.

Perfluorocarbons: Inert chemical compounds consisting of carbon and fluorine that are able to dissolve gases. PFCs are the basis for artificial oxygen-carrying drugs.

Hemoglobin-based oxygen carriers: These are AOCs based on hemoglobin as the carrier entity.

A brief history

The first attempts to infuse solutions carrying oxygen were made at the beginning of the 20th century. In 1916, the British Dr Tunnicliffe used saline to infuse oxygen. He reported: "For some time it has been the practice, when using saline venous injections, either simple nutrient (glucose and lecithin) or medicated, to use oxygenated saline solution" [1]. Although this therapy seemed to work, Dr Tunnicliffe acknowledged the limitations of his approach: "We are quite aware that the quantity of oxygen introduced by this method is very small as compared with the oxygen requirement of the subject, nevertheless cyanosis is rapidly alleviated by the use of such solutions" [1]. These early attempts to use saline as an oxygen carrier proved that something different was needed to infuse oxygen, something that could carry much more oxygen than saline. Logical choices were hemoglobin solutions, i.e., solutions with a molecule designed especially to transport oxygen.

In the 1930s, experiments were undertaken to resuscitate a totally exsanguinated sheep with a hemoglobin solution made from cow's blood [2]. Human experiments with hemoglobin solutions started in the 1940s [3]. Amberson *et al.* infused cell-free hemoglobin into humans [3]. The solutions used by both research groups were hemoglobin from lysed red cells, and therefore contained considerable amounts of red cell membrane and stroma residues. The side effects of such solutions were tremendous, with renal failure and high blood pressure being the most prominent. In addition,

---

Basics of Blood Management, Second Edition. Petra Seeber and Aryeh Shander.
© 2013 John Wiley & Sons, Ltd. Published 2013 by John Wiley & Sons, Ltd.

coagulopathies were attributed to stromal contaminants. Therefore, purification was logical to reduce the risks of hemoglobin solutions.

After adding a purification step to the preparation of the early crude hemoglobin solutions, new experiments were performed on humans. In 1970, Rabiner treated hemorrhagic shock with stroma-free hemoglobin [4]. A test performed in 1978 by Savitsky [5] found only limited side effects after infusion of hemoglobin solutions into healthy volunteers. However, purified solutions also had major disadvantages, including renal toxicity and a short intravascular half-life.

To reduce the side effects further, hemoglobin was chemically altered. Modifications made in the 1980s aimed at making the solutions more stable and thus reduced the side effects resulting from hemoglobin chains that had disassembled.

Another group of compounds entered the race to become a usable AOC when in the 1960s, Dr Leland Clark started experiments with PFCs. Gollan and Clark demonstrated in 1966 that mice submerged completely in PFCs could survive for a prolonged time [6]. This was due to the oxygen-carrying capacity of the PFCs. After about two decades of research, the first chemically manufactured oxygen carrier entered the market. The first-generation PFC, Fluosol-DA—a product of the Green Cross in Japan—was approved in the United States for medical use in 1989. It was primarily used as an adjunct to percutaneous transluminal coronary angioplasty, but this ceased when catheter techniques improved. Fluosol-DA has also been used as an AOC. However, due to the low content of the PFC in the product and other properties, trials with the new drug in the therapy of severe anemia were disappointing.

As with many products used in blood management, the military had a keen interest in AOCs. Much was invested to have an AOC for the battlefield. Especially during the Vietnam War, efforts to provide such a product were intensified. However, no suitable product could be developed at that time. The military remains interested in AOCs and still drives research in this area [7].

While only a few marketable products have resulted from decades of intensive, costly research on artificial blood, this has generated a wealth of new information about red cell physiology, oxygen transport, and unloading. The development of AOCs can be viewed as an unprecedented basic science research effort. The research on AOCs has recently been sent back from the bedside to the bench. Following a review of clinical trials by Natanson et al. [8], the FDA stopped all clinical trials of hemoglobin-based oxygen carriers in 2008 until more basic research could improve the safety of clinical drug development.

Artificial oxygen carriers

AOCs were initially thought to serve as a "blood substitute" or as a substitute for red cells. They were designed to be an alternative to donor blood. It was hoped they would be simple, safe, and fast to apply. Besides, it was felt that such "artificial blood" should carry no infectious risks or other side effects, should have a sufficient intravasal half-life and a long shelf-life, and should be universally applicable, independent of blood group. Such AOCs were thought to provide an unlimited supply of medication to overcome blood shortages. However, decades of intensive research has not yielded a product that is even close to meeting the expectations of the early enthusiastic advocates of artificial blood. The early enthusiasm gave way to the notion that recreating blood is beyond the scope of human ability. At best, some of the features of blood can be mimicked, with more or less severe side effects.

Over the decades, two major groups of AOCs have been developed: hemoglobin-based oxygen carriers (HBOCs) and PFCs. Newer groups of AOCs are on the horizon, but are only in the very early phases of development.

Hemoglobin-based oxygen carriers

Sources of hemoglobin

Hemoglobin for infusion can be obtained in a variety of ways. Out-of-date human red cell concentrates can be used as a source. However, their supply is limited and blood shortages cannot be overcome by using human blood as a source of AOCs. It is also possible to use animal blood, e.g., from pigs or cows. This source of hemoglobin is potentially unlimited. Besides, bovine hemoglobin has some very favorable oxygen unloading characteristics (2,3-diphosphoglycerate [2,3-DPG] is not needed to unload oxygen; the P50 is about 30 mmHg, which is very similar to that of human hemoglobin in red cells). However, concerns include antigenicity and the transmission of animal diseases, such as bovine spongiform encephalitis.

Probably the best, yet most complicated, way to source hemoglobin is the recombinant route. Hemoglobin molecules can be expressed in yeast, *Escherichia coli*, plants, or transgenic animals [9]. The risk of disease transmission is very low, supply is potentially unlimited, and it is possible to modify the hemoglobin molecule to produce a product with the required qualities. However, even once a product has been developed and approved, there is as yet no technology that would provide enough hemoglobin to satisfy market demand.

Modification of hemoglobin

Native, cell-free hemoglobin is able to transport oxygen, but is not as antigenic as red cells (antigenic determinants are mainly embedded in the red cell membrane). However, the loss of the surrounding cell leaves the hemoglobin molecule "unprotected, helpless and too small for the job." The natural environment of the hemoglobin molecule provides it with everything it needs to do its assigned job. The cell protects the molecule from oxidative damage and provides systems to undo oxidation (superoxide dismutase, catalase, met-hemoglobin reductase, glutathione). The cell also provides 2,3-DPG, which hemoglobin needs to unload oxygen. Last but not least, the cell keeps hemoglobin molecules intact, as tetramers, and the individual hemoglobin tetramers together in a package that is large enough not to escape an intact circulation and to exert all its required effects to regulate blood flow and oxygen delivery, e.g., by exerting shear stress and by a graded interaction with nitric oxide. All these interactions of the red cell and the hemoglobin molecule are lost when hemoglobin is freed from the red cell. Free, native hemoglobin, therefore, comes with several problems:

• The hemoglobin tetramer rapidly disintegrates into its four protein chains. This leads to (a) nephrotoxicity, (b) escape into the extravascular space, and (c) a short intravascular half-life.
• Since there is no 2,3-DPG with the free hemoglobin, it cannot unload its oxygen normally and the hemoglobin's oxygen affinity is too high for it to be a clinically useful HBOC (P50 about 10–15 mmHg).
• Protective enzymes are lacking. The hemoglobin molecule is therefore easily auto-oxidized and met-hemoglobin is formed.
• Hemoglobin is far more reactive than when in a red cell. Therefore, it (a) easily scavenges NO (free hemoglobin reacts 1000 times faster with NO than does hemoglobin in a red cell) and (b) it may interchange oxygen with tissue more rapidly.

Clinically useful HBOCs must overcome the obstacles associated with the loss of the red cell environment. Different methods have been devised in an attempt to reduce the drawbacks associated with free hemoglobin. These produce basically two different kinds of HBOCs: HBOCs of the acellular (hemoglobin not embedded in a liposome) and of the cellular type (hemoglobin embedded in a liposome).

Acellular HBOCs

Most of the research on HBOCs has been done with acellular HBOCs. The following methods have been tried to overcome the above-mentioned drawbacks of free hemoglobin:

• **Surface modification (conjugation):** Surface-modified hemoglobins are combinations of hemoglobin molecules with large molecules like dextran, polyoxyethylene, or polyethylene glycol. This increases the size of the particle, amount of water bound to the molecule, and intravascular half-life. Besides, modified hemoglobin has a reduced antigenicity, a high oncotic pressure, and a high viscosity. Infusion of such HBOCs also results in plasma volume expansion.
• **Intramolecular cross-linking:** Cross-linking of the hemoglobin chains within a hemoglobin tetramer (e.g., by pyridoxylation or diacetylation) prevents the early dissociation of the hemoglobin tetramer into dimers. The size of the tetrameric hemoglobin molecule does not change considerably.
• **Polymerization:** Single hemoglobin molecules react with chemical cross-linkers and so hemoglobin polymers develop (polyHb). Sebacyl chloride and glutaraldehyde were first used in the 1960s to cross-link hemoglobin for polymerization [10]. *o*-Raffinose also serves this purpose. The size of the polyHb depends on how many single hemoglobin molecules are coupled to each other. The polymerized hemoglobins have a longer plasma half-life, but come with a higher antigenicity than naturally occurring hemoglobin molecules.
• **Adding antioxidants:** Free hemoglobin lacks the antioxidant systems that typically protect it in its natural environment, the red cell. To overcome this, certain antioxidants have been added to the hemoglobin molecules in the HBOCs. Enzymes such as superoxide dismutase (SOD), carbonic anhydrase, and catalase (CAT) can be added either by cross-linking the polyHb molecule (polyHb–SOD–CAT) or by encapsulation together with the hemoglobin molecule. In addition, the polynitroxylation of hemoglobin molecules improves the antioxidant status.

Cellular HBOCs

Following the research with acellular HBOCs, researchers found that a return to a more red cell-like compound would make for a potentially less hazardous hemoglobin-based oxygen carrier. Therefore, the encapsulation of hemoglobin into an artificial membrane-like structure to mimic the red cell was attempted. The result was a liposome-encapsulated hemoglobin solution (LEH; also called hemoglobin vesicles [HbVs], neo red cells [NRCs] or neohemocytes). Other developments lead to the advent of polymersome encapsulated hemoglobin (PEH, polymersomes).

Encapsulation of hemoglobin seemed to solve some of the problems encountered with acellular HBOCs. Encapsulated hemoglobin may have a decreased renal toxicity and decreased vasoactivity. It is possible to co-encapsulate antioxidants and compounds that modify oxygen unloading with the hemoglobin. The more corpuscular nature of the solution means that the oxygen unloading is more akin to that found in red cells. Also, the metabolism taking place in the reticuloendothelial system is more similar to that in naturally occurring red cells [7].

Unfortunately, there are also problems with cellular HBOCs. The challenges start during the production process. Initially, it was difficult to encapsulate clinically meaningful amounts of hemoglobin. This has been overcome by improvements is manufacturing. Also, the material used for encapsulation may cause side effects, such as cellular toxicity, platelet activation, or antigenicity. Therefore, over time, different encapsulation materials have been tested, including synthetic liposomes made from natural lecithin or synthetic phospholipids, biodegradable polyactide (used for resorbable surgical sutures) or polyglycolide [11, 12], and more recently CHHDA, an anionic non-phospholipid. The "ideal" material for encapsulation has still to be identified.

Effects of hemoglobin solutions

As outlined above, freeing hemoglobin from red cells changes its properties. Besides, during attempts to overcome these changes and to adapt the final drug to the needs of the patient, the HBOCs develop certain properties. Some of them are common to all or a group of HBOCs, while others are specific to one product.

Contaminants

Since highly purified hemoglobin is used in the production of HBOCs, theoretically stroma and endotoxins should not be a concern.

Oxygen affinity

Free hemoglobin molecules have a high oxygen affinity. To change this affinity to more physiological values,

hemoglobin has been modified. Pyridoxylation (adding pyridoxal-5-phosphate) or cross-linking (e.g., by 3,5-dibromosalicylate) decreases the oxygen affinity of hemoglobin [13]. The cross-linker, o-raffinose, modifies the 2,3-DPG pocket of the hemoglobin, resulting in a higher P50. However, it is not clear whether it is really beneficial to infuse hemoglobin with an oxygen affinity that is near to normal. It can be hypothesized that the more rapid reaction of oxygen with free hemoglobin compared to hemoglobin in the red cell may offset the effects of an increased oxygen affinity. However, a higher oxygen affinity may ensure that the microcirculation is not unduly affected by high oxygen levels and that oxygen is not unloaded too early in the circulation.

Oncotic effects

Red cell transfusions per se do not exert relevant oncotic pressure. In contrast, free hemoglobin does. This is a two-edged sword. To draw fluids from tissues into the circulation (plasma expansion) may be beneficial in hemorrhaging patients or in patients with ischemia due to tissue swelling. However, in cases where additional intravascular fluids are detrimental, the oncotic effects of HBOCs may be harmful. The extent of the oncotic effects encountered depends on the number and not on the size of the particles. Therefore, many small particles (as in intramolecularly cross-linked hemoglobins) exert a much greater oncotic pressure than fewer, yet larger particles containing the same amount of hemoglobin (as in LEH). Hypertonic saline has been added to modify the oncotic effects of HBOCs and produce a resuscitation fluid for trauma therapy. This may exploit the potentially beneficial effects of hypertonic saline together with those of an oxygen carrier [14].

Rheological properties, viscosity

A circulating viscous fluid in a vessel exerts a shear stress on the vessel wall. This results in the release of nitric oxide, a vasodilator. By this mechanism, whole human blood with a viscosity of about 4 cPoise (cP) is able to regulate the perfusion of the microvasculature. Artificial infusion solutions, including HBOCs, also exert certain effects on the microvascular system. However, since some HBOCs have a lower viscosity than blood, they may impair the microvascular blood flow. This effect is especially pronounced when a patient is so anemic that an increase in cardiac output cannot compensate for the decreased red cell level and viscosity. Since exactly that situation is the classical indication for HBOC therapy, the low viscosity of HBOCs may be detrimental. The rheological properties have to be taken into account when designing a solution [15]. Newer HBOCs do just that, such as the ultra-high molecular weight bovine hemoglobin polymer (polyHb) [16].

Vasopressor effects

Right from the early experiments with hemoglobin solutions, it was obvious that free hemoglobin has a strong vasopressor effect [17]. There are two theories to explain this phenomenon. The first relates to the vasoconstrictive response to the interaction of hemoglobin with nitric oxide (and endothelin, a strong vasoconstrictor). Hemoglobin in red cells can scavenge nitric oxide, but the extent of this is limited by the red cell membrane acting as a barrier. Free hemoglobin can scavenge nitric oxide as well. This capability is stronger when the red cell membrane—which normally acts as barrier to nitric oxide diffusion—is missing. Besides, small hemoglobin molecules can leave the vessels and interact directly with nitric oxide in the perivascular space. Modifications in the production of HBOCs can reduce the vasoconstrictive effect of hemoglobin. These modifications address the binding capacity of hemoglobin and nitric oxide, as well as the size of the hemoglobin molecules. Encapsulated hemoglobin may have a limited vasoactivity, since the neohemocytes mimic some effects of the red cells. The hemoglobin can no longer easily diffuse into the perivascular space and cannot react easily with nitric oxide [18]. The interaction of hemoglobin and nitric oxide has also been altered by chemical modification of the hemoglobin sites where nitric oxide is typically bound. Besides, recombinant hemoglobin can be designed in a way that reduces its nitric oxide-scavenging properties. The nitric oxide-binding site of the recombinant hemoglobin molecule can be modified, making it difficult for nitric oxide to bind to hemoglobin. In addition, tetrameric hemoglobin molecules, which are small and therefore diffuse outside the vasculature to scavenge nitric oxide, can be eliminated from the final HBOC. Vasoactive side effects of hemoglobin solution have been reduced in some products when tetrameric hemoglobin is removed. The less tetrameric hemoglobin, the lower the vasoconstrictive side effects and the more HBOC can be infused. Today, with only HBOC-201 left on the market as a "blood substitute," the clinician may use a low-dose nitro infusion together with the AOC to attenuate the vasoconstrictive effects of the drug. However, sodium nitrite ($NaNO_2$) infusion may cause increased pulmonary side effects [19].

The second theory used to explain the vasoconstrictive effects of HBOCs is inferred from the regulatory mechanisms of the microvasculature. Precapillary arterioles sense the oxygen level in the blood coming toward the capillaries and, depending on the oxygen content, constrict or dilate. Since free hemoglobin can react much faster than hemoglobin bound in red cells, oxygen may be released prematurely from the hemoglobin to the arterioles, giving the arterioles the illusion there is plenty of oxygen available. As a result, arterioles may not dilate as they would if red cells were arriving. This may impair the microcirculation. In this context, hemoglobin with a higher oxygen affinity than that of red cells may be beneficial [20].

Renal effects

Normal human hemoglobin is a tetramer. In the red cell it is stable, but it easily disassembles into dimers once it leaves the cell. The dimers pass through the glomeruli in the kidney and cause renal damage.

Intravascular half-life

Compared with red cells, the intravascular half-life of HBOCs is very short. Therefore, repeated infusions are needed to provide sufficient oxygen-carrying capacity. In order to prolong the stability and intravascular half-life of acellular hemoglobin, intramolecular cross-linking, polymerization, encapsulation, or conjugation with macromolecules has been employed in the current generation of HBOCs. Besides, recombinant hemoglobin does not disintegrate easily, prolonging its half-life. By these means, the plasma half-life of HBOCs is about 5–40 hours. Further work on HBOCs is attempting to increase the intravascular half-life even more.

Infectious risks and effects on the immune system

It is believed that the production process for HBOCs excludes every possibility of viral contamination from the original hemoglobin source. Moreover, since the cross-linking process for hemoglobin stabilizes the protein, heat sterilization is possible as well. HBOCs are therefore thought to be free from infectious agents.

Of greater concern is the effect of HBOCs on the immune system of the recipient. The high iron content of HBOCs may overload the reticuloendothelial system, impair bactericidal activities, and promote bacterial growth. Besides, these effects may potentiate the detrimental effects of endotoxin in the patients.

Antigenicity from red cell membranes does not occur with purified hemoglobins. Therefore, HBOCs can be administered independent of the blood group of the recipient. However, another form of antigenicity may evolve with the use of HBOCs. Reactions to polymerized hemoglobin molecules or to molecules from other species are of (theoretical) concern. During trials with the only bovine product, IgE production was not observed and only moderate levels of IgG were seen [21].

Oxidative damage

Superfluous delivery of oxygen may come with side effects. Oxygen may cause oxidative damage. Reperfusion injury may occur after therapy of conditions with prolonged ischemia, e.g., stroke, myocardial infarction, and severe prolonged hemorrhage. Also, blood cells are not immune to the damaging effects of oxygen. The iron of free hemoglobin is prone to oxidation and so met-hemoglobin builds up easily. Besides, peroxides and other oxidative products may accumulate and result in hemoglobin and endothelial damage. Red cells have enzymes that protect them from the influence of oxygen. SOD and CAT found in red cells may ameliorate the damaging effects of oxygen. The early HBOCs did not contain these enzymes. To control the oxygen-related damage to hemoglobin, these enzymes were added to the molecules, resulting in polyHb–SOD–CAT. These compounds were shown to remove free oxygen radicals and stabilize the hemoglobin molecule. Such protective enzymes can also be included in the liposomes of LEH [22]. Other approaches have been to add an antioxidant to hemoglobin (e.g., Tempol to form polynitroxylated α-α-Hb) as well. Simultaneous application of antioxidant agents (ascorbic acid, riboflavin) can protect against oxidative damage to the HBOCs [21].

Table 9.1 HBOCs and their properties.

	Class	Intravascular t1/2(h)	Oncotic pressure	Viscosity	Vasoactivity	Source of Hgb
MP4 (Hemospan), MP4OX, (Sangart)	Malemide-PEG-conjugated = MalPEG-Hb	c. 43	High (55 ± 20 mmHg)	High (2.5 ± 1 cP)	Low	Human
VTR-PHP, Hemoximer (Apex Bioscience, later VITARESC Biotech, then Curacyte and Ajinomoto)	Surface-modified polyoxyethylene-conjugated, pyridoxylated	c. 40	Moderate to high	Moderate to high	Mild	Human
PEG Hb (Enzon)	Surface-modified	44	Moderate to high	Moderate to high	Mild	Bovine
PEG-Hb in hypertonic saline (Aftershock, Prolong Pharmaceuticals)	Pegylated		2500 mOsm			bovine
Polyheme (Northfield)	GA-polymerized, pyridoxylated	24	Low (20–25 mmHg)	Low	Moderate to low	Human
Hemolink (Hemosol)	o-Raffinose polymerized	14–24	Low (COP 26 mmHg)	Low (1.15 cP)	Moderate	Human
Hemopure (Biopure) HBOC-201;Oxypure for veterinarian use approved (similar to HBOC-301 = Oxyglobin for veterinarian use approved)	GA-polymerized	9–24	Low (17 mmHg)	Low (1.3 cP)	Moderate	Bovine
Optro (Baxter, formerly Somatogen) (rHb 1.1); later rHb2.0	α-α-cross-linked recombinant hemoglobin from E. coli		Low	Low	Marked	Recombinant human, Presbyterian mutant of Hgb
HemAssist (Baxter)	Intramolecular cross-linked with diaspirin (DCLHb)	2–14 (dose-dependent)	Moderate to high (42 mmHg)	Low (1.0 cP)	Marked	Human

PEG, polyethylene glycol; GA, glutaralydehyde; Hb, hemoglobin; GI, gastrointestinal; COP, colloid osmotic pressure; AST, aspartate transaminase.

Hemostaseological alterations

Both thrombocytopenia and thrombocytopathy have been observed after infusion of certain HBOCs. These effects have been thought to be due to the nitric oxide-scavenging effects of hemoglobin. When scavenged, insufficient nitric oxide NO is available to exert its antiplatelet effects. Besides, activation of the complementary system may lead to thrombocytopenia, which is sometimes observed after HBOC infusion (especially after LEH).

Effects on erythropoiesis

It has been suggested that HBOCs stimulate erythropoiesis [23, 24].

Shelf-life

While red cells can be stored for a maximum of 49 days under standard conditions (about 4 °C), HBOCs can be stored for much longer. Some HBOCs can be refrigerated; others are stabile even at room temperature. Also, storage after lyophilization of the HBOC is possible. This prolongs their shelf life to 1–2 years or longer.

Other side effects

In healthy volunteers, infusion of HBOCs resulted in gastrointestinal upset (with increased motility and sphincter spasms) and flu-like symptoms (fever, chills, headaches, and backache) [25]. As a physiological response to infusion of hemoglobin, jaundice occurs. After administration of some HBOCs, liver enzyme levels increase.

Current products

Several types of HBOCs have been developed [26, 27] and their properties are summarized in Table 9.1. However, as regards blood management, only the most promising one has reached and remained on the market:

P50	Met-Hb%	% Hb tetramer	Hb (g/dL)	Use	Stability	Side effects	Status
6 ± 2	<0.5		4.2		Stable at −20 °C	GI and vasoactive effects very low to absent	Development of MP4 as red cell substitute halted; MP4OX as drug continued
20	3		10	NO-induced shock (sepsis)			In 2010 in phase III clinical trial for septic shock, interims analysis in March 2011 positive
15	<5		6	Cancer (radiosensitizer)			Trials suspended
				Trauma			Preclinical trials
28–30	<3	<1	10	Trauma, perioperative	At room temperature > 1 year	No GI, no vasoconstrictive	Development halted in 2009 since risk > benefit
39 ± 12	<10–25	30–36	10	Cardiac, general surgery, anemia		Marked GI, purification improved this, rise in blood pressure	Development stopped due to more myocardial adverse events
38–43	<10	<5	13	Perioperative, hemodilution, anemia	At room temperature stable	Chest pain (problem resolved), jaundice, mild increase in blood pressure, AST and lipase increased	Approved in South Africa in 2001; Biopure bankrupt in 2009, sold to OPK Biotech; manufacturing facility of Hemopure recommissioned in April 2011
30–33	<5		5	Surgery, trauma, hemodilution		Fever, headaches, rising blood pressure, purification has improved the situation, amylase, lipase increased	Pulled off market in 1998
30–32	4–18		10	Surgery, organ failure, trauma, stroke			Pulled off market in 1998

Hemopure [28]. Other HBOCs are marketed as therapeutic agents for ischemic lesions, and others, exploiting their vasoconstrictive activity, are used in the event of septic shock. Further products are used to preserve organs for transplantation or as contrast medium [29–31].

Other oxygen carriers

Albumin-based artificial oxygen carriers
Recombinant human albumin can be engineered so that it includes up to eight heme molecules or iron protoporphyrin. These conjugates have been shown to transport and release oxygen [32–34], and have an intravascular half-life of about 36 hours. Rats were able to survive a substantial exchange of their blood volume with albumin–heme conjugates, while the control group did not [35]. These early trials with albumin–heme conjugates show promise for a future generation of AOCs.

Hemoglobin aquasomes
Hemoglobin aquasomes consisting of hemoglobin molecules attached to a hydroxylapatite core have been synthesized [36]. These have been successfully tested in animals to transport oxygen and may represent another useful oxygen carrier.

Perfluorocarbons
The second group of artificial oxygen carriers is the PFCs. They are greenhouse gases that develop during the production of aluminum. Chemically, they are related to Teflon®. PFCs consist of carbohydrate chains with 8–10 carbon atoms, most of which are substituted by fluorine. Some of the carbon atoms may also be substituted by bromine.

PFCs can dissolve and thus carry gases. About 40–50 mL of oxygen can be dissolved in 100 mL of a PFC. The oxygen-carrying characteristics of PFCs are similar to those of saline or other liquids. They follow the physical principles described in Chapter 2 on oxygen physiology. The higher the partial pressure of a gas above the PFC, the more gas is dissolved in it. This characteristic is unlike hemoglobin which dissolves oxygen in a pH-dependent manner and cooperatively, as is depicted in hemoglobin's S-shaped oxygen-binding curve (see Figure 2.1). In contrast, the oxygen-binding curve of PFCs is a linear function. In clinical practice, this means that oxygen can be transported in relevant amounts in PFCs only when the inspiratory oxygen fraction is high enough. That is why patients on PFCs always need supplemental oxygen.

PFCs are insoluble in water. Therefore, they are provided as emulsions. The first-generation PFCs were dissolved in pluronic F-68. Since complement activation was associated with this compound, second-generation PFCs are now dissolved in a lecithin (and cholesterol) solution.

The intravasal half-life of PFCs is very short, some hours only. However, the biological half-life is much longer. PFC particles are chemically and physically inert. They are taken up by phagocytosis by components of the reticuloendothelial system (spleen, liver, and lung). There, the lecithin emulgator is metabolized and the PFCs remain inert and are slowly taken back into the bloodstream to be exhaled by the lung. There is concern that PFCs may block the reticuloendothelial system, which may immunocompromise the patient transiently. Furthermore, the PFC emulgator may be toxic to elements of the immune system. Therefore, there is a maximum dose of PFCs that should not be overstepped. Especially in patients with sepsis or an active infection, care must be taken. However, some beneficial effects of PFCs on the immune system have been postulated, since these may diminish the reperfusion damage in myocardial infarction or apoplexia. Overall, the clinical relevance of the immunomodulative effects is not yet clear.

Apart from immunosuppression, PFC administration may lead to fever 4–6 hours after infusion, shaking, nausea, and transient leukopenia. A transient thrombocytopenia is observed 2–3 days after infusion. It is usually not severe (<20% from baseline) and seems to be self-limiting after about 7 days. The thrombocytopenia occurs without proof of platelet function problems or prolongation of prothrombin time and partial thromboplastin time in healthy volunteers [37]. The second-generation PFCs do not show relevant immunogenic reactions or complement activation (Table 9.2) [21, 38, 39].

Oxygen delivery
Normal blood with a hematocrit of about 45% and at a PO_2 of 100 mmHg carries about 20 mL of oxygen/100 mL of blood. About 25%, i.e., 5 mL, is released during the blood's passage through a normal, resting organism. The venous blood that returns to the heart has about 75% of the oxygen left in it. When PFCs are given, the body first takes oxygen from the PFCs, since this is easier than taking oxygen from the "neatly packed" oxygen in the red cells. Before red cells can unload the oxygen and transfer it through their membrane, PFCs will have already filled the needs of the tissue. Therefore, if enough PFCs are in the blood, the blood may not need to unload

Table 9.2 Characteristics of perfluorocarbons.

	Fluosol-DA (Green Cross Corp., Osaka, Japan; later transferred to China)	Oxygent (Alliance)	Perftoran (Perftoran)	Oxycyte (Synthetic Blood International, now Oxygen Biotherapeutics Inc., Costa Mesa, Ca.)
Generation	First	Second	First	Third
Active constituents	14% perfluorodecalin and 6% perfluorotripropyl amine	58% perflubron (perfluorooctyl bromide, PFOB; C8F17 Br) and 2% perfluorodecyl bromide (PFDB, C10 F21 Br)	Perfluorodekalin (PFD) and perfluoromethylcyclohexylpiperidin (PFMCP) 2:1	60% F-tert-butyl cyclohexane (C10F20)
Emulgator	Pluronic F-68, egg yolk phospholipid	Lecithin (in phosphate-buffered aqueous electrolyte solution)	Proxanol	Egg yolk phospholipids
Size of particles (µm)	0.05–0.25	0.16–0.18	0,07	<0.2
Intravasal half-life (h)	12–18	4–15	About 24	20
Biological half-life (days)	7	4		
Dose	30 mL/kg	2.7 g PFC/kg (1.4 mL PFC/kg)	5–30 mL/kg	
Oxygen dissolved in the presence of pure oxygen and STPD (mL/dL)	6	17		
Viscosity (cP)	2.3	c. 4	2.3	3.2
Hemoglobin equivalency		4.0 ± 2.7 g/dL in a dose of 2.7 g/kg (recommended clinical dose)		
Use	As adjunct to percutaneous transluminal coronary angiography (PTCA), approved 1989, withdrawn from market after improvements in PTCA; not efficient as blood substitute	To reduce allogeneic transfusion through augmented intraoperative acute normovolemic hemodilution	As oxygen transporting plasma expander and oxygen therapeutic; limb ischemia, approved and currently in use in Russia	In preclinical and phase IIa tests
Storage	Frozen, mix before use	About 2 years with standard refrigeration or room temperature	Frozen for 3 years; at room temperature for 2 weeks	At room temperature

More PFCs have been developed, among them emulsified perfluorodichloro octane (Oxyfluor, HemaGEN), which was tested in phase II studies in the 1990s with the intent to improve the outcome in air embolism.
STPD, standard temperature and pressure, dry.

any oxygen and may return with nearly 100% of the oxygen it had when it left the lungs. In contrast, the PFCs deliver most of their oxygen. In fact, about 91% (under $PaO_2 = 500\,mmHg$) of the oxygen bound to PFCs is unloaded during one circulation [38].

The different characteristics of oxygen unloading make it difficult to compare hemoglobin and PFCs. Clinicians typically want to know how much oxygen is theoretically available to the patient. Since most clinicians are comfortable with knowing that the patient has a hemoglobin level sufficient to meet the oxygen needs, they have a problem when there is not enough hemoglobin, yet there is an agent that may mimic the hemoglobin's function. To make matters easier, the concept of "hemoglobin equivalency" has been developed. It tells how much of a PFC is equivalent to a certain amount of hemoglobin as regards to oxygen transportation ability. It relates the percentage of whole body oxygen consumption (VO_2) from PFC to that from hemoglobin. For example, a patient with a hemoglobin level of 8 g/dL uses 50% of oxygen from hemoglobin and 25% from the PFC. This means that the PFC contributes half the amount of oxygen to the tissue that is contributed by hemoglobin (25% is half of 50%). Therefore, the PFC is equivalent to 4 g/dL of hemoglobin (since half of 8 g/dL is 4 g/dL) [38]. Another term used in this connection is the "effective hemoglobin," which is the sum of the hemoglobin of the patient plus the hemoglobin equivalent of the PFC.

PFCs also have effects on oxygen delivery that are beyond that of increased intravascular oxygen transport. PFCs increase the availability of oxygen in the tissue, a phenomenon called "diffusion facilitation." It is not clear how this occurs. It is thought that PFCs can travel into very small vessels in the tissue which the red cells cannot reach. Besides, PFCs may help red cells to deliver their oxygen. Since the PFCs flow near the vessel wall, while the red cells are near the center of the vessel, PFCs may serve as a bridge between red cells and the tissue ("near wall phenomenon") [40].

Tested and potential indications
PFCs are promising in blood management (see below). Additionally, PFCs can be of potential benefit in other areas. PFC particles are many times smaller than red cells. This enables them to travel to tissues that are ischemic and where red cells can no longer travel, e.g., in myocardial infarction and ischemic limbs due to a tourniquet. PFCs are also used to avoid tissue ischemia during the repair of cerebral aneurysms and to improve the outcome of cardiopulmonary bypass (microbubbles, thought to

cause problems, can be readily absorbed by PFCs). PFCs augment tumor oxygenation and can preserve transplant organs [39]. PFCs were also proposed to be used in liquid ventilation in acute respiratory distress syndrome or acute lung injury, or as an ultrasound-imaging medium [21].

Artificial oxygen carriers in blood management

The original impetus to develop AOCs has been to provide a solution which substitutes for red cells. To a certain, limited extent, AOCs are able to do so. The following paragraphs outline how AOCs can be used in blood management

Perfluorocarbons

Severe anemia
Fluosol-DA, the first-generation PFC, has been used in severely anemic patients as an AOC. It was able to reverse the clinical signs of oxygen deficiency [40, 41]. However, the intravascular half-life was too short and, as a result, it was unable to improve the survival of these anemic patients. Therefore, it has not been developed further into an agent suitable for blood management [21, 30].

A second-generation PFC was shown in animal studies to be useful in resuscitation from hemorrhagic shock. Oxygen delivery can be maintained or re-established with PFCs, so that tissues submitted to severe anemia can continue with aerobic metabolism and organ function is preserved [42, 43]. A PFC first available in Russia has been used extensively in humans with severe anemia and it appears to improve tissue oxygenation under such circumstances [44].

Augmented acute normovolemic hemodilution
Oxygent, a second-generation PFC, is not an approved drug. However, several trials have been performed with it, many of which directly relate to blood management. As first learnt from the early trials with the first-generation PFCs in severe anemia, current PFC products are unable to remain in the circulation long enough to work until the patient's own erythropoiesis has made up the missing red cell mass. Many publications, therefore, discuss PFCs mainly in settings where short periods of decreased oxygen delivery are to be bridged. The most prominent indication in this connection is augmented acute normovolemic hemodilution (A-ANH™) [45]. Intraoperatively, PFCs have been shown to reverse signs of anemia ("the

transfusion trigger") more effectively than the infusion of autologous blood or colloids. Besides, when used in conjunction with A-ANH™, the transfusion rate for non-cardiac surgical patients with a high intraoperative blood loss (defined as >20 mL/kg) can be reduced [46, 47].

Despite the beneficial effect of reducing the transfusion of red cells, clinical trials with Oxygent™ were stopped in 2001 because of a higher incidence of stroke in the treatment group compared to the control group.

Sickle cell anemia
Patients with sickle cell anemia may benefit from PFCs when severe sickle cell-induced vaso-occlusion occurs. Since vaso-occlusion is often only partial and allows for a residual flow, small PFC molecules can still travel to the ischemic areas and ameliorate the effects of sickle cell crises. It was suggested that oxygenated PFCs could even unsickle and dislodge red cells, and thereby reduce the vaso-occlusion [48].

Hemoglobin-based oxygen carriers

Trauma and hemorrhagic shock
In theory, HBOCs are the ideal solutions for resuscitation of patients with trauma and in hemorrhagic shock [49]. In fact, in the emergency setting and in prehospital care, HBOCs can be used to treat anemia resulting from catastrophic blood loss [14]. However, trials with HBOCs demonstrated an increased mortality in severely hemorrhaging trauma patients. This was likely the result of the strong vasoactive properties of the product, resulting, amongst others, in myocardial infarction. It may also be due to impaired microcirculation, since the vasoconstrictive effects of the HBOC may prevent detection of hypovolemic shock, a situation similar to the administration of catecholamines in hypovolemic situations. The negative trial outcomes contrast with another study showing that up to 20 units of HBOCs can be given to trauma patients with a reduction in the 30-day mortality to 25%, compared with 64% in a control group [50]. Despite the encouraging results of animal trials, trials with HBOCs in trauma patients have not replicated a survival benefit. Currently, more animal studies are underway to gain more insight into the physiological and pathophysiological mechanisms behind the divergent results of HBOC use in trauma [51].

When red cells are not an option
HBOCs have also been used to treat patients with severe anemia who cannot be given donor blood transfusions [52, 53], mostly in a "compassionate use protocol." Anecdotal evidence from case reports suggests that the use of HBOCs may be beneficial, as witnessed by normalization of lactate and amelioration of signs of cardiac ischemia after the infusion of the HBOC. The highest-quality evidence for the use of HBOCs in severely anemic patients in whom transfusion is not an option probably comes from the recent large case series by Mackenzie et al in the setting of life-threatening anemia [54]. They conclude that earlier, compared with later, administration of HBOC-201 is associated with survival.

The inherent problem with the use of HBOCs in severe anemia is the short half-life of the HBOCs. Due to this, serial infusions over several days are necessary, until autologous erythropoiesis provides enough red cells. Initially, HBOCs were used for short periods only. Several case reports suggest that long-term survival is also possible by exclusively using HBOCs instead of red cells, as shown in reports of patients with sickle cell crisis [55], autoimmune hemolytic anemia [56], and leukemia [57].

Practice tip Trouble-shooting in HBOC-201 use

If you prescribe HBOC-201 for severe anemia and:
- Your patient develops methemoglobinemia: consider methylene blue.
- Your patient develops vasoconstrictive complications: consider therapy with nitro.
- Your patient needs laboratory assessment: inform your laboratory about your patient's therapy with HBOC-201, since it influences some measurements.

Acute normovolemic hemodilution
In analogy to A-ANH™ using PFCs, HBOCs have been used to perform A-ANH™. HBOCs can extend the tolerance of anemia during acute normovolemic hemodilution.

Surgical blood loss
Different HBOCs have been used to substitute surgical blood loss in the setting of general, cardiac, and vascular surgery [58–62]. As a result, red blood cell transfusions have been reduced [62, 63]. Hemopure™ (see Table 9.1), which has been approved in South Africa for the therapy of patients with major surgical blood loss, avoided red cell transfusions in 34%, 27%, 43%, and 60% of patients undergoing cardiopulmonary bypass, abdominal aortic reconstruction, general surgery, and orthopedic surgery,

respectively [64]. However, since HBOCs were put on clinical hold by the FDA, there have been no further studies regarding the use of HBOCs for surgical patients who can be transfused with donated blood.

Sickle cell anemia

In the event of ischemic complications of sickle cell disease, such as acute chest syndrome, HBOCs have been used in selected cases to treat anemia and other complications [55, 65].

Artificial platelet substitutes

Platelets are a very complex entity. Although much is known about the importance of platelets, their composition and modes of action are only partially understood. It is obvious, then, how difficult it is to produce platelet substitutes.

In analogy to human HBOCs, out-of-date platelets have been used as source material for platelet substitutes. Non-viable platelets, platelet microvesicles (membrane fragments), and even membrane phospholipids have been tested for their ability to support clotting [66]. Even tiny microvesicles have been shown to carry platelet receptors and enhance endogenous clotting or clotting processes induced by recombinant clotting factors [67].

Attempts have been made to use known elements of platelets to create a product that at least mimics some of the platelet's function. A plateletsome consisting of a liposome with a lipid bilayer has been employed as a carrier. Integrated in the lipid layer, platelet-derived receptors (e.g., for von Willebrand factor, fibrinogen, and thrombospondin) have been added. Infusion and topical application of the plateletsome solutions have been shown to decrease clinical bleeding in animals [68]. Such basic experiments aim to define which components of platelets are needed to trigger a favorable response in bleeding. With the prospect of being able to produce the necessary receptors in a recombinant fashion, the research is promising.

Another "artificial platelet substitute," called Synthocytes (Andaris Group Ltd., Quadrant Healthcare plc, Nottingham, UK), consists of albumin microcapsules with fibrinogen [69]. Since fibrinogen on the surface of Synthocytes can interact with receptors on platelets and activates platelets, Synthocytes, together with residual platelets in thrombocytopenia, may contribute to hemostasis [69]. It was hoped they would selectively target sites of hemorrhage. Indeed, in animal experiments, Synthocytes were shown to reduce bleeding.

Many other platelet substitutes, e.g., rehydrated, lyophilized platelets or thromboerythrocytes [70], are in development and are currently undergoing trials as to their usefulness as a clinically effective platelet substitute [71]. Another approach is to attach a peptide that mimics the carboxyl-terminal end of the fibrinogen molecule (which adheres to platelet receptors) to a nanoparticle such as a liposome or albumin. This entirely synthetic platelet substitute has been shown in vivo to enhance clotting in thrombocytopenic animals [72].

It was considered that in the "far future, procoagulant cell surface transformation may be influenced by topical application of inhaled thrombomodulin-loaded liposomes or by sense or antisense oligonucleotides inducing thrombomodulin expression or suppressing tissue factor expression, respectively" [73]. However, since research on platelet substitutes is at a very early stage, basic parameters have to be established to evaluate the final products as to their ability to reduce bleeding. To this end, the FDA has compiled recommendations for the testing of such products in humans [74].

Key points

• It is impossible for humans to recreate blood.
• First-generation AOCs have a very short half-life and unwanted side effects that make them unsuitable for general use as a blood substitute. Higher-generation AOCs are promising drugs with well-described indications and contraindications.

Questions for review

1. What are AOCs and what are their indications in blood management?
2. What are the sources of hemoglobin used for the production of HBOCs?
3. What are the differences between (a) hemoglobin in the viable red cell, (b) hemoglobin free after lysis of red cells, and (c) hemoglobin attached to polyethylene glycol?
4. What are common side effects of HBOCs and how have they been engineered to reduce these?
5. What is the source of PFCs?
6. How do PFCs transport oxygen?
7. What different platelet substitutes have been described?

Suggestions for further research

What is the current status of HBOCs and PFCs? Check the Internet and medical literature for more information.

Exercises and practice cases

Read the case report of Cothren and colleagues [75]. Discuss the management of the described patient. What indicators have there been to support the claim that (a) the patient benefited from HBOC and (b) the patient did not benefit from HBOC. What lessons do you learn from this report about the oxygen transport of HBOCs?

Homework

Find out whether there is somebody in your vicinity who uses AOCs. Record his/her contact information.

Is it possible in your country to get AOCs? If so, record the contact information of the provider(s).

References

1. Tunnicliffe FW, Stebbing GF. The intravenous injection of oxygen gas as a therapeutic measure. *Lancet* 1916;August 19:321–323.
2. Amberson W, *et al.* On the use of Ringer–Locke solutions containing hemoglobin as a substitute for normal blood in mammals. *J Cell Comp Physiol* 1937;**5**:359–382.
3. Amberson WR, *et al.* Clinical experience with hemoglobin-saline solution. *J Appl Physiol* 1949;**1**:469–489.
4. Rabiner SF, O'Brien K, Peskin GW, Friedman LH. Further studies with stroma-free hemoglobin solution. *Ann Surg* 1970;**171**:615–622.
5. Savitsky JP, Doczi J, Black J, Arnold JD. A clinical safety trial of stroma-free hemoglobin. *Clin Pharmacol Ther* 1978;**23**:73–80.
6. Clark LC Jr, Gollan F. Survival of mammals breathing organic liquids equilibrated with oxygen at atmospheric pressure. *Science* 1966;**152**:1755–1756.
7. Phillips WT, *et al.* Development of liposome encapsulated hemoglobin (LEH) and studies of hemorrhagic shock by use of imaging studies with oxygen-15 and other radiotracers. ftp://ftp.rta.nato.int/Pubfulltext/…///MP-HFM-109-P20.pdf, accessed June 2011.
8. Natanson C, Kern SJ, Lurie P, Banks SM, Wolfe SM. Cell-free hemoglobin-based blood substites and risk of myocardial infarction and death: a meta-analysis. *JAMA* 2008;**299**:2304–2312.
9. Looker D, Abbott-Brown D, Cozart P, *et al.* A human recombinant haemoglobin designed for use as a blood substitute. *Nature* 1992;**356**:258–260.
10. Chang TM. Hemoglobin-based red blood cell substitutes. *Artif Organs* 2004;**28**:789–794.
11. Sakai H, Tsuchida E. Performances of PEG-modified hemoglobin-vesicles as artificial oxygen carriers in microcirculation. *Clin Hemorheol Microcirc* 2006;**34**:335–340.
12. Chang TM. Oxygen carriers. *Curr Opin Investig Drugs* 2002;**3**:1187–1190.
13. Harris DR, Palmer AF. Modern cross-linking strategies for synthesizing acellular hemoglobin based oxygen carriers. *Biotechnol Prog* 2008;**24**:1215–1225
14. Leong B, Reynolds PS, Tiba MH, *et al.* Effects of a combination hemoglobin based oxygen carrier—hypertonic saline solution on oxygen transport in the treatment of traumatic shock. *Resuscitation* 2011;**82**:937–943.
15. Intaglietta M. Microcirculatory basis for the design of artificial blood. *Microcirculation* 1999;**6**:247–258.
16. Cabrales P, Zhou Y, Harris DR, Palmer AF. Tissue oxygenation after exchange transfusion with ultrahigh-molecular-weight tense- and relaxed-state polymerized bovine hemoglobins. *Am J Physiol Heart Circ Physiol* 2010;**298**:H1062–H1071.
17. Katz LM, Manning JE, McCurdy S, *et al.* Nitroglycerin attenuates vasoconstriction of HBOC-201 during hemorrhagic shock resuscitation. *Resuscitation* 2010;**81**:481–487.
18. Bucci E, Watts TL, Kwansa HE, *et al.* Cell-free hemoglobin, oxygen off-load and vasoconstriction. *Anasthesiol Intensivmed Notfallmed Schmerzther* 2001;**36** (Suppl 2):S123–S124.
19. Moon-Massat P, Scultetus A, Arnaud F, *et al.* The effect HBOC-201 and sodium nitrite resuscitation after uncontrolled hemorrhagic shock in swine. *Int J Care Injured* 2010, Nov 19 [Epub ahead of print].
20. Creteur J, Vincent JL. Hemoglobin solutions. *Crit Care Med* 2003;**31**(12 Suppl):S698–S707.
21. Dinkelmann S, Northoff H. Artificial oxygen carriers—a critical analysis of current developments. *Anasthesiol Intensivmed Notfallmed Schmerzther* 2003;**38**:47–54.
22. Chang TM. Future generations of red blood cell substitutes. *J Intern Med* 2003;**253**:527–535.
23. Lindahl SG. Thinner than blood. *Anesth Analg* 1995;**80**:217–218.
24. Hughes GS Jr, Francome SF, Antal EJ, *et al.* Hematologic effects of a novel hemoglobin-based oxygen carrier in normal male and female subjects. *J Lab Clin Med* 1995;**126**:444–451.
25. Viele MK, Weiskopf RB, Fisher D. Recombinant human hemoglobin does not affect renal function in humans: analysis of safety and pharmacokinetics. *Anesthesiology* 1997;**86**:848–858.

26. Weiskopf RB. Hemoglobin-based oxygen carriers: Compassionate use and compassionate clinical trials. *Anesth Analg* 2010;**110**:659–662.

27. Chen JY, Scerbo M, Kramer G. A review of blood substitutes. Examining the history, clinical trial results and ethics of hemoglobin-based oxygen carriers. *Clinics (Sao Paulo)* 2009;**64**:803–813.

28. Santry HP, Alam HB. Fluid resuscitation: Past, present and the future. *Shock* 2010;**33**:229–241.

29. Bone HG. Hemoglobin-based oxygen carriers in sepsis. *Anasthesiol Intensivmed Notfallmed Schmerzther* 2001;**36** (Suppl 2):S114–S116.

30. Kale PB, Sklar GE, Wesolowicz LA, DiLisio RE. Fluosol: therapeutic failure in severe anemia. *Ann Pharmacother*, 1993;**27**:1452–1454.

31. Strate T, Mann O, Standl T, Izbicki JR, Knoefel WT. The potential of HBOC in acute pancreatitis. *Anasthesiol Intensivmed Notfallmed Schmerzther* 2001;**36** (Suppl 2):S119–S120.

32. Komatsu T, Nakagawa A, Qu X. Structural and mutagenic approach to create human serum albumin-based oxygen carrier and photosensitizer. *Drug Metab Pharmacokinet* 2009;**24**:287–299.

33. Wang RM, Komatsu T, Nakagawa A, Tsuchida E. Human serum albumin bearing covalently attached iron(II) porphyrins as O_2-coordination sites. *Bioconjug Chem* 2005;**16**: 23–26.

34. Komatsu T, Ohmichi N, Nakagawa A, Zunszain PA, Curry S, Tsuchida E. O_2 and CO binding properties of artificial hemoproteins formed by complexing iron protoporphyrin IX with human serum albumin mutants. *J Am Chem Soc* 2005;**127**:15933–15942.

35. Komatsu T, Yamamoto H, Huang Y, Horinouchi H, Kobayashi K, Tsuchida E. Exchange transfusion with synthetic oxygen-carrying plasma protein "albumin-heme" into an acute anemia rat model after seventy-percent hemodilution. *J Biomed Mater Res A* 2004;**71**:644–651.

36. Khopade AJ, Khopade S, Jain NK. Development of hemoglobin aquasomes from spherical hydroxyapatite cores precipitated in the presence of half-generation poly(amidoamine) dendrimer. *Int J Pharm* 2002;**241**:145–154.

37. Leese PT, Noveck RJ, Shorr JS, Woods CM, Flaim KE, Keipert PE.. Randomized safety studies of intravenous perflubron emulsion. I. Effects on coagulation function in healthy volunteers. *Anesth Analg* 2000;**91**:804–811.

38. Faithfull NS. Fluorocarbon formulations and principles of oxygen delivery. *TATM* 2001;**3**:5–9.

39. Keipert PE. Perflubron emulsion (Oxygent(tm)): a temporary intravenous oxygen carrier. *Anasthesiol Intensivmed Notfallmed Schmerzther* 2001;**36** (Suppl 2):S104–S106.

40. Welte M. Current status of perfluorocarbons. *Anasthesiol Intensivmed Notfallmed Schmerzther* 2001;**36** (Suppl 2): S165–S168.

41. Spence RK, Norcross ED, Costabile J, *et al.* Perfluorocarbons as blood substitutes: the experience with Fluosol DA 20% in the 1980s. *Artif Cells Blood Substit Immobil Biotechnol* 1994;**22**:955–963.

42. Cabrales P, Carlos Briceño J. Delaying blood transfusion in experimental acute anemia with a perfluorocarbon emulsion. *Anesthesiology* 2011;**114**:901–911.

43. Kemming GI, Meisner FG, Wojtczyk CJ, *et al.* Oxygent as a top load to colloid and hyperoxia is more effective in resuscitation from hemorrhagic shock than colloid and hyperoxia alone. *Shock* 2005;**24**:245–254.

44. Maevsky E, Ivanitsky G, Bogdanova L, *et al.* Clinical results of Perftoran application: present and future. *Artif Cells Blood Substit Immobil Biotechnol* 2005;**33**:37–46.

45. Spahn DR, Willimann PF, Faithfull NS. The effectiveness of augmented acute normovolemic hemodilution (A-ANH). *Anaesthesist* 2001;**50** (Suppl 1):S49–S54.

46. Kemming G, Habler O, Zwissler B. Augmented acute normovolemic hemodilution (A-ANH(tm)) in cardiac and non-cardiac patients. *Anasthesiol Intensivmed Notfallmed Schmerzther* 2001;**36** (Suppl 2):S107–S109.

47. Spahn DR, Waschke KF, Standl T, *et al.* Use of perflubron emulsion to decrease allogeneic blood transfusion in high-blood-loss non-cardiac surgery: results of a European phase 3 study. *Anesthesiology* 2002;**97**:1338–1349.

48. Kaul DK, Liu X, Nagel RL. Ameliorating effects of fluorocarbon emulsion on sickle red blood cell-induced obstruction in an ex vivo vasculature. *Blood* 2001;**98**: 3128–3131.

49. Holly AD. Synthetic blood products: Science fiction of coming to an ICU near you? *Crit Care Resusc* 2008;**10**: 253–256.

50. Gould SA, Moore EE, Hoyt DB, *et al.* The life-sustaining capacity of human polymerized hemoglobin when red cells might be unavailable. *J Am Coll Surg* 2002;**195**:445–452; discussion 452–455.

51. Vazquez BY, Hightower CM, Martini J, *et al.* Vasoactive hemoglobin solution improves survival in hemodilution followed by hemorrhagic shock. *Crit Care Med* 2011;**39**: 1461–1466.

52. Mackenzie CF, Morrison C, Jaberi M, Genuit T, Katamuluwa S, Rodriguez A. Management of hemorrhagic shock when blood is not an option. *J Clin Anesth* 2008;**20**:538–541.

53. Fitzgerald MC, Chan JY, Ross AW, *et al.* A synthetic haemoglobin-based oxygen carrier and the reversal of cardiac hypoxia secondary to severe anemia following trauma. *MJA* 2011;**194**:471–473.

54. Mackenzie CF, Moon-Massat PF, Shander A, Javidroozi M, Greenburg AG. When blood is not an option: Factors affecting survival after the use of a hemoglobin-based oxygen carrier in 54 patients with life-threatening anemia. *Anesth Analg* 2010;**110**:685–693.

55. Lanzkron S, Moliterno AR, Norris EJ, *et al.* Polymerized human Hb use in acute chest syndrome: a case report. *Transfusion* 2002;**42**:1422–1427.

56. Mullon J, Giacoppe G, Clagett C, McCune D, Dillard T. Transfusions of polymerized bovine hemoglobin in a

patient with severe autoimmune hemolytic anemia. *N Engl J Med* 2000;**342**:1638–1643.

57. Agrawal YP, Freedman M, Szczepiorkowski ZM. Long-term transfusion of polymerized bovine hemoglobin in a Jehovah's Witness following chemotherapy for myeloid leukemia: a case report. *Transfusion* 2005;**45**:1735–1738.

58. Lamy ML, Daily EK, Brichant JF, *et al.* Randomized trial of diaspirin cross-linked hemoglobin solution as an alternative to blood transfusion after cardiac surgery. The DCLHb Cardiac Surgery Trial Collaborative Group. *Anesthesiology* 2000;**92**:646–656.

59. Hill SE, Gottschalk LI, Grichnik K. Safety and preliminary efficacy of hemoglobin raffimer for patients undergoing coronary artery bypass surgery. *J Cardiothorac Vasc Anesth* 2002;**16**:695–702.

60. Levy JH, Goodnough LT, Greilich PE, *et al.* Polymerized bovine hemoglobin solution as a replacement for allogeneic red blood cell transfusion after cardiac surgery: results of a randomized, double-blind trial. *J Thorac Cardiovasc Surg* 2002;**124**:35–42.

61. LaMuraglia GM, O'Hara PJ, Baker WH, *et al.* The reduction of the allogeneic transfusion requirement in aortic surgery with a hemoglobin-based solution. *J Vasc Surg* 2000;**31**: 299–308.

62. Schubert A, Przybelski RJ, Eidt JF, *et al.* Diaspirin-crosslinked hemoglobin reduces blood transfusion in noncardiac surgery: a multicenter, randomized, controlled, double-blinded trial. *Anesth Analg* 2003;**97**:323–332.

63. Anbari KK, Garino JP, Mackenzie CF. Hemoglobin substitutes. *Eur Spine J* 2004;**13** (Suppl 1):S76–S82.

64. Jacobs E. Clinical update: Hemopure(r)—a room temperature stable hemoglobin oxygen carrier. *Anasthesiol Intensivmed Notfallmed Schmerzther* 2001;**36** (Suppl 2):S121–S122.

65. Gonzalez P, Hackney AC, Jones S, *et al.* A phase I/II study of polymerized bovine hemoglobin in adult patients with sickle cell disease not in crisis at the time of study. *J Investig Med* 1997;**45**:258–264.

66. Alving B. Potential for synthetic phospholipids as partial platelet substitutes. *Transfusion* 1998;**38**:997–998.

67. Tonda R, Galán AM, Mazzara R, White JG, Ordinas A, Escolar G. Platelet membrane fragments enhance the procoagulant effect of recombinant factor VIIa in studies with circulating human blood under conditions of experimental thrombocytopenia. *Semin Hematol* 2004;**41** (Suppl 1):157–162.

68. Rybak ME, Renzulli LA. A liposome based platelet substitute, the plateletsome, with hemostatic efficacy. *Biomater Artif Cells Immobilization Biotechnol* 1993;**21**:101–118.

69. Davies AR, Judge HM, May JA, Glenn JR, Heptinstall S. Interactions of platelets with Synthocytes, a novel platelet substitute. *Platelets* 2002;**13**:197–205.

70. Coller BS, Springer KT, Beer JH, *et al.* Thromboerythrocytes. In vitro studies of a potential autologous, semi-artificial alternative to platelet transfusions. *J Clin Invest* 1992;**89**:546–555.

71. Fischer TH, Merricks E, Bellinger DA, *et al.* Splenic clearance mechanisms of rehydrated, lyophilized platelets. *Artif Cells Blood Substit Immobil Biotechnol* 2001;**29**:439–451.

72. Okamura Y, Takeoka S, Eto K, *et al.* Development of fibrinogen gamma chain peptide-coated, adenosine diphosphate-encapsulated liposomes as synthetic platelet substitute. *J Thrombos Haemostas* 2008;**7**:470–477.

73. Scherer RU. Haemostaseological aspects of perioperative blood management. *Zentralbl Chir* 2003;**128**:473–480.

74. US Department of Health and Human Services, Food and Drug Administration, Center for Biologics Evaluation and Research (CBER). *Guidance for Industry for Platelet Testing Evaluation of Platelet Substitute Products*, 1999.

75. Cothren CC, Moore EE, Long JS, Haenel JB, Johnson JL, Ciesla DJ.. Large volume polymerized haemoglobin solution in a Jehovah's Witness following abruptio placentae. *Transfus Med* 2004;**14**:241–246.

10 Oxygen Therapy

Medical oxygen is a drug. It exerts understood as well as yet unexplained effects on the human organism. Obviously, human life without oxygen is impossible. On the other hand, life is endangered when there is too much oxygen. Oxygen therapy, as a valuable adjunct to the prevention and therapy of anemic hypoxia and bleeding, has great benefits, but also side effects. It takes knowledgeable healthcare providers to make oxygen another life-saving piece in the armamentarium for blood management.

Objectives

1. To explain why patients in a blood management program may be candidates for inhalational or hyperbaric oxygen therapy.
2. To review the physiology, pathophysiology, and physics of oxygen.
3. To give basic advice on how to prescribe oxygen therapy, prepare the patient, and treat possible side effects of the therapy.

Definitions

Inhalational oxygen therapy: Inhalation of oxygen aimed at restoring normal oxygen exchange in the cardiopulmonary system and at the tissue level.

Hyperbaric oxygen therapy: Administration of oxygen with a pressure of greater than 1 atmosphere (atm). According to the Undersea and Hyperbaric Medical Society (UHMS), breathing 100% oxygen at 1 atm or the topical application of hyperbaric oxygen is not hyperbaric oxygen therapy.

A brief history

The use of gases for medical therapy dates back thousands of years. As with many other therapies, oxygen therapy was prescribed before even the basic mechanisms of action were known. Amazingly, oxygen therapy was used even before oxygen was discovered.

Medical use of oxygen initially built on the experience of divers. Since the lack of oxygen under water is the limiting factor for prolonged diving, the main challenge of diving is to make additional oxygen available. In 320 BC, Alexander the Great used a glass vessel to dive into the Bosporus Straits during the siege of Tyre. Much later, in 1620, Cornelius Drebbel developed a normobaric diving bell. It became the forerunner of today's medical hyperbaric chambers.

The first medical use of a hyperbaric environment was reported in 1662. Henshaw, a British clergyman, used compressed air for the treatment of pulmonary disease. Using a system of organ bellows, he could adjust pressure within a sealed chamber called a "domicilium." Valves were placed so that air could be either compressed into the chamber or extracted from it. In the domicilium, increased pressure was used for the treatment of acute diseases, and reduced pressure for the treatment of chronic diseases. Although this concept may not be accepted today, the treatment of anemia probably would have benefited from it. Patients with symptoms of acute anemia would have gained from the additional oxygen, while chronically anemic patients may have benefited from the increased erythropoietin production due to the lack of oxygen under hypobaric conditions.

Basics of Blood Management, Second Edition. Petra Seeber and Aryeh Shander.
© 2013 John Wiley & Sons, Ltd. Published 2013 by John Wiley & Sons, Ltd.

Scientific proof of the effectiveness of hyperbaric therapy was lacking at that time. The situation slowly changed. In 1670, Boyle gave the first description of decompression phenomena. Finally, oxygen, as a gas, was discovered independently by the Swedish apothecary Karl W. Scheele in 1772 and by the English chemist Joseph Priestley in 1774. Although Scheele was the first to discover oxygen, Priestley is credited with the discovery, since he published his findings in 1775, while Scheele published his work 2 years later. Priestley influenced a researcher named Lavoisier who eventually named the gas *oxygene*, meaning acid-former.

Priestley experimented with the new gas and published his findings in *Experiments and Observations on Different Kinds of Air*. Priestley appears to be the first person to inhale air with a greater concentration of oxygen than normal. He describes while breathing his "new air," he "fancied that (his) breast felt peculiarly light and easy for some time afterwards." He continued: "Hitherto only two mice and myself have had the privilege of breathing it" [1]. Priestley had already thought about the medical use of this gas, but added a warning, "From the greater strength and vivacity of the flame of a candle, in this pure air, it may be conjectured, that it might be peculiarly salutary to the lungs in certain morbid cases. But, perhaps, we may also infer from these experiments, that though (oxygen) might be very useful as a medicine, it might not be so proper for us in the usual healthy state of the body; for, as a candle burns out much faster in (oxygen) than in common air, so we might, as may be said, live out too fast."

Following Priestley's discovery, oxygen was employed for the treatment of many diseases. Quacks as well as scientists used this gas (or other gases supposed to be oxygen) for the cure of almost every disease, among them symptoms and diseases of the respiratory tract (tuberculosis, asthma, pneumonia, bronchitis, dyspnea), infectious conditions (cellulitis, pyemia, ulcers), and conditions possibly associated with shock (cholera, anemia, asphyxia, poisoning, eclampsia, septicemia). Curiously, oxygen was also used in conditions like indigestion, albuminuria, diabetes, spermatorrhea, rheumatism, gout, hysteria, and menstrual irregularities.

By the 1800s, hyperbaric medicine was fashionable and institutions offering it flourished throughout Europe. Famous medical journals like the *Lancet* [2] and the *British Medical Journal* reported on the topic. The interest in oxygen therapy was so great that societies were founded to further the use of oxygen. In 1798, the Pneumatic Institution for Inhalation Gas Therapy was founded by Thomas Beddoes. The engineer James Watt helped manufacture the gas. Low concentrations of oxygen were also thought to be beneficial. Patients with consumption, asthma, palsy, dropsy, obstinate venereal complaints, and others came to the institute for treatment and were treated for free. The institute closed in 1802.

In 1879, a French surgeon named Fontaine built a fully equipped mobile hyperbaric operating room. Therapeutically, he used the fact that the solubility of a gas in a liquid is proportional to the pressure of the gas over the solution. Under the hyperbaric conditions in the operating room, Fontaine increased the amount of oxygen in the patient's blood. It was claimed that patients did better when surgery was performed under hyperbaric conditions. They recovered from the anesthetic more rapidly, and cyanosis and asphyxia were reported to be less or absent. The chamber was also recommended for patients with anemia. Fontaine's work ended with a fatal accident at his work place.

Anemia was one of the indications for oxygen therapy. William Osler briefly recommended oxygen for anemia in his book *The Principles and Practice of Medicine*, published in 1892 [3]. J. Henry Davenport wrote: "Oxygen here acts as a tonic, increasing the weight and strength, and visibly restoring the natural ruddy hue of the face in health. It has in this way been found valuable in . . . anaemia . . . three or four gallons are inhaled daily" [4]. C.E. Ehinger confirmed these findings. However, the administered dose of oxygen was very low and oxygen was used only intermittently [5]. Therefore, the extent of the effects of oxygen therapy appear questionable from today's perspective.

By the end of the 19th century, oxygen therapy was becoming accepted by an ever-growing number of practitioners, although many still doubted its usefulness [6]. This is understandable when we see how oxygen was used. Oxygen was not only inhaled, but was also advocated as compound oxygen, i.e., bound in chemical compounds [7], as enema [8], for intra-abdominal and intrapleural insufflation [9], as well as injection into joints, veins [10], and the subcutis [11]. Oxygen was also used in shock, probably due to hemorrhage [9]. As Dr Howitt claimed, subcutaneous administration did not appear to help in urgent situations [11]. The described modes of oxygen application may indeed have looked strange to the prejudiced observer.

Despite all the ridicule, oxygen therapy was never completely devoid of advocates. In 1918, Dr Orval Cunningham studied the differences between people living through or dying due to the flu epidemic in the

Rocky Mountains. He noted people in the valley did better than people in the mountains. He reasoned that denser air in the valley helped people fight the infection. Cunningham used a small hyperbaric chamber, built next to his clinic, to test this hypothesis. He successfully treated a young colleague with influenza, who was near death due to restricted lung function and secondary hypoxia. Positive results in patients suffering from pneumonia encouraged him to build other oxygen chambers. After experiencing an amazing cure of his kidney disease after hyperbaric therapy, a grateful patient built a huge chamber for Cunningham in Kansas City in 1921. It looked like a hollow steel ball of approximately 20 meters in diameter. It was equipped with a smoking lounge, carpets, dining room, and private quarters. Seven years later, Cunningham built the world's largest functional hyperbaric chamber, a five-floor "hyperbaric hospital." However, Cunningham's hyperbaric hospital was closed during the Great Depression in the 1930s and was demolished for scrap metal for the impending war.

A turning point in the medical use of oxygen occurred after the First World War. Haldane described the use of oxygen in victims of gas poisoning. His article was a landmark in oxygen therapy [12]. A further impetus for hyperbaric medicine came from the Dutch Boerema in 1956. He demonstrated that pigs could survive in a hyperbaric environment without any red cells. His article "Life without blood" was another landmark in the scientific work-up of the age-old subject of hyperbaric medicine [13, 14]. In order to prolong operative time with a patient in cardiac arrest, Boerema and associates performed cardiac surgery in a hyperbaric chamber. Based on these experiences, in 1969, the (most probably) first case of hemorrhagic shock was reported to be treated successfully with hyperbaric oxygen therapy [15] instead of blood transfusions.

Widespread enthusiasm for hyperbaric medicine resulted in its use in cancer, stroke, and myocardial infarction. However, the scientific results were disappointing. In 1967, the UHMS was founded in the United States. During the 1970s, the practice of hyperbaric oxygen therapy decreased, probably due to the lack of improvement in many of the treatments for which hyperbaric oxygen was used. In 1976, the UHMS established a Committee on Hyperbaric Oxygen Therapy. It helped to lay the scientific basis for hyperbaric medicine. A set of approved indications were put together. Hyperbaric medicine gained renewed interest. In March 2000, the American Board of Medical Specialties approved undersea and hyperbaric medicine as a subspecialty of both emergency medicine and preventive medicine.

Physics and physiology of oxygen

Under the climatic conditions where human life is possible, oxygen is a gas. It obeys gas laws and other related physical principles. Do you remember the following laws?

Dalton's Law: The total gas pressure is the sum of all partial pressures of the gases in a gas mixture ($P_T = P1 + P2 + P3 + \ldots Pn$).

Henry's Law: The degree to which a gas is dissolved in a solution is directly proportional to the pressure of the gas.

Boyle's Law: When temperature remains constant, the volume of a gas is inversely proportional to its pressure.

Charles' law: When volume remains constant, pressure is directly proportional to temperature. For example, when the pressure increases from 1 to 3 atm, the temperature also increases three-fold.

Apart from knowing the above, it is also vital to know that the amount of gas dissolved in a liquid is determined by its solubility coefficient. This coefficient is specific for each fluid and is dependent on temperature. The lower the temperature, the more gas is dissolved. The solubility of oxygen in plasma at 37 °C is 0.0214 mL of oxygen/mL plasma per atmosphere partial pressure of oxygen (PO_2).

In our environment in ambient air, the gas we breathe consists of approximately 21% oxygen and 78% nitrogen, with trace amounts of other gases. Expressed in medical terms, we breathe with an inspiratory oxygen fraction (FiO_2) of 21%. At sea level, the gases exert a pressure of 1 atm, i.e., 760 mmHg (Table 10.1). The share exerted by each of the gases is proportional to their percentage in the gas mixture. Since about 21% of the gas in our atmosphere is oxygen, oxygen exerts a partial pressure (PO_2) of 21% of 760 mmHg, i.e., approximately 160 mmHg.

In the lung, the relationship of the gases changes. Carbon dioxide is added to the intrapulmonary gas. Carbon dioxide exerts a partial pressure of 40 mmHg. Water vapor is added as well. At normal body temperature (37 °C), the air in the lungs is saturated with water. The water exerts a pressure of 47 mmHg (= PH_2O, saturated water vapor pressure). Based on the alveolar gas equation (see below), on breathing room air, the PO_2 in the lung thus reduces from 160 mmHg in open air to about 100–110 mmHg in the alveoli.

Table 10.1 Units for barometric pressure.

1 atm (atmosphere)
760 mmHg (millimeters mercury) = Torr
1.470×10^1 psi (pounds per square inch = lbs/in^2)
1.033 kg/cm^2 (kilograms per square centimeter)
1.013 bar
3.305×10^1 fsw (feet or meters of seawater)
1.033×10^1 msw (meters of seawater)

How much oxygen finally reaches the blood stream is determined by the diffusion across the barrier between the alveoli and the vasculature. The alveolar-to-arterial gradient (A–a gradient) provides an assessment of this alveolar–capillary gas exchange and is the difference between the oxygen partial pressure in the alveoli (PAO_2) and the oxygen partial pressure in the arteries (PaO_2). The normal A–a gradient is estimated by adding 10 to the age of the patient and dividing this by 4. The A–a increases from 5 to 7 mmHg for every 10% increase in FiO_2. Values between 20 and 65 mmHg are normal. In severe respiratory distress, the A–a gradient may be more than 400. Another way to estimate how much oxygen is transferred across the barrier between alveoli and arterioles is to assume that for every six parts of oxygen in the lung, five parts are found in the vessels.

Alveolar gas equation

$$PAO_2 = (Pb - PH_2O \times FiO_2 - PACO_2$$
$$\times (FiO_2 \times [(1 - FiO_2)/R])$$

where Pb is barometric pressure; PH_2O is saturated water vapor pressure; $PACO_2$ is alveolar PCO_2, assumed to be equal to arterial PCO_2; and R is respiratory quotient, normally 0.8.

Oxygen—friend and enemy

Oxygen is the single most important substance for life. It is essential in the pathway leading from food intake to energy production. The cells, as electrical systems, depend on oxygen to perform the electron transfer that is needed to produce energy. Besides, oxygen combines with protons to form water, another essential substance. Since oxygen is such an important substance for life, it is not surprising that a severe lack of oxygen is fatal. Therefore,

the provision of oxygen to the tissue is the main goal of many therapies, and it proves lifesaving. However, oxygen also has effects that endanger life. Oxygen therapy therefore needs to be based on a thorough knowledge of oxygen's effects on the human body.

Effects of oxygen on the human body

Circulatory effects

Oxygen is a vasoconstrictor. Thus, inhalation of greater than normal oxygen concentrations modulates blood flow. Total peripheral resistance increases and with it the systemic blood pressure. A redistribution of blood flow from the skeletal muscles to areas of the splanchnic vasculature occurs [16]. Blood flow to the kidneys increases as well [17]. Hyperoxic ventilation in healthy persons with a normal hemoglobin level increases the systemic vascular resistance, and decreases the cardiac output (by decreasing both stroke volume and heart rate) and oxygen consumption [18, 19].

Oxygen also constricts myocardial vessels. This effect seems to be detrimental. Paradoxically, hyperoxia may subsequently lead to tissue hypoxia and increased mortality when compared to normoxia. This was proposed for patients with uncomplicated myocardial infarction [20] or after cardiac surgery [21]. Vasoconstriction may also play a role in the possibly worsened outcome after resuscitation of depressed newborns and adults with 100% oxygen ventilation [22, 23].

Interestingly, normovolemic anemia modulates the vascular effects of oxygen. Anemia increases the blood flow, and with it the shear stress on the vessel walls. NO is released and vessels dilate. Oxygen reverses this vasodilatation.

Immunological effects

Oxygen can act as an antibiotic [24]. It facilitates the clearance of bacteria from the tissue since it supports the work of neutrophils. Normally, neutrophils phagocytize bacteria, resulting in a respiratory (oxidative) burst—the creation of oxygen radicals, which play a role in bactericidal activity. This respiratory burst increases the oxygen consumption of the tissue 15–20 times. The PO_2 in the tissue containing the neutrophils is approximately 0–10 mmHg. The byproducts of the neutrophils' respiratory burst damage the tissue. Adding oxygen to this scenario (i.e., when the patient breathes more oxygen) facilitates the neutrophils' action, and the bacteria are cleared more effectively. Besides, tissue is provided with the required oxygen. Therefore, necrosis of the tissue is minimized and scars tend to be smaller when formed under oxygen therapy [24]. Oxygen thus promotes wound healing and angiogenesis.

Metabolic effects

Free oxygen radicals are needed for phagocytes to kill bacteria. But radicals and free oxygen itself may also damage cells. Sulfhydryl group-bearing enzymes are oxidized and the production of peroxides is increased [25]. Inhibition of these enzymes disturbs the metabolic activity. Excess oxygen may therefore damage tissues when enzyme levels are not allowed to recover.

Ocular effects

Preterm infants are often given oxygen to keep their arterial oxygen saturation above 90%. This causes side effects. Especially during the first weeks of life, supplemental oxygen may cause eye damage. Since oxygen accelerates angiogenesis, vessels may develop in the vitreous body, followed by fibrosis and retinopathy. This may lead to blindness (retrolental fibroplasia). The risk of such a serious retinopathy increases when the arterial oxygen saturation exceeds 80% [26].

Cerebral effects

Breathing oxygen either at a high FiO_2 or at a high ambient air pressure can cause cerebral damage. Generalized convulsions seen during hyperbaric therapy are a vivid expression of this damage. The combination of the direct toxic effect of oxygen, accumulation of carbon dioxide, and altered cerebral circulation may lead to this cerebral damage [27].

Oxygen therapy may also reduce the drive to breathe. The reduced breathing leads to hypercapnia and may result in carbon dioxide narcosis.

Pulmonary effects

Inhalation of higher than normal concentrations of oxygen results, primarily, in pulmonary damage (hyperoxia-induced lung injury [HALI]) [28]. First, an acute exudative phase, with interstitial and alveolar edema, hemorrhage, fibrinous exudate, formation of hyaline membranes, and the destruction of the capillary endothelial and type I alveolar epithelial cells results. This is followed by a second, subacute, proliferative phase. Interstitial fibrosis and proliferation of fibroblasts and type II alveolar epithelium cells follow, together with the partial resolution of the effects of the exudative phase.

Clinically, the first sign of oxygen toxicity is tracheobronchitis. Patients develop a cough and chest pain. The tracheal symptoms gradually spread through the pulmonary branches. Rales, ronchi, and bronchial breath sounds are heard on auscultation and the patients develop fever. Animal experiments with toxic levels of oxygen have shown that further development of pulmonary damage results in dyspnea and respiratory insufficiency with hypoxia and death [29].

Atelectasis is also typical of pulmonary exposure to oxygen. Since the inspired gas consists mainly of oxygen, nitrogen is washed out of the lung. Nitrogen is an inert gas, which is not absorbed by the lung. Its presence means that there is always gas in the alveoli. This serves as a "pneumatic splint" for the alveoli, preventing them from collapsing. When this inert gas is washed out by oxygen, problems arise. Oxygen is taken up from the alveoli into the body, the alveoli collapse, and atelectasis develops. Development of atelectasis is also facilitated by a lack of surfactant, which results from the damage exerted by toxic oxygen [29].

There are some factors that modify the effects of oxygen on the lungs. Probably, the most important factor is the adaptive response elicited by intermittent exposure to high oxygen levels. Intermittent exposure to a normal PO_2 is the most practical approach to minimize side effects of oxygen. Air breaks during hyperbaric oxygen therapy allow antioxidants to deal with free oxygen radicals and reduce oxygen toxicity.

A long list of drugs has been examined regarding their influence on the toxicity of oxygen. As a rule of thumb, factors that increase sympathetic influence enhance the toxic effects of oxygen, while increased vagal effects prove protective. Increased thyroid activity, cortisol, insulin, atropine, estrogen, hyperthermia, and catecholamines increase the detrimental effects of oxygen, while adrenergic blockers, antihistamines, antioxidants, cobalt, hypothermia, hypothyroidism, and starvation reduce the toxic effects of oxygen. Also, many general anesthetics protect against the toxic effects of oxygen on the lung as well as on the brain [29].

Hematological effects

A lack of oxygen, such as is seen in persons residing at high altitude, leads to the induction of erythropoietin gene expression and a subsequent increase in red cell mass. Whether or not the opposite is the case is a matter of debate. It has been claimed that it is not only the absolute lack of oxygen that leads to increased erythropoietin production; this can also occur with an artificial change in the oxygen partial pressure. Such an artificial change can be made when patients are breathing high oxygen concentrations for some time, followed by a return to normoxia. This intermittent increase and decrease in the PO_2 in the patient's blood, with its possible subsequent increase in erythropoietin levels and amelioration of anemia, is called the "normobaric oxygen paradox." Some researchers defend this theory, while others speak against it [30, 31].

Effects of pressurized oxygen on the human body

Hyperbaric oxygen therapy has two distinct beneficial effects: an increase in oxygen tension and an increase in pressure.

The effects of an increase in oxygen tension have already been discussed above. The effects of oxygen exposure in normobaric and hyperbaric environments are essentially the same. But, since the magnitude of the oxygen-related effects depends on the PO_2 in the body and not on the inspiratory oxygen fraction, hyperbaric conditions magnify the oxygen effects at a given FiO_2. Under hyperbaric conditions, decreases in heart rate (5–7%), stroke volume, and sympathetic tone have been observed [32]. This leads to a cardiac output decreased by 10–20% [32]. Hyperbaric oxygen therapy also leads to vasoconstriction, but the hyperbaric oxygenation of the tissues offsets any decrease in oxygen delivery by vasoconstriction [33].

Increased pressure drives more oxygen into the body fluids than the same FiO_2 at only 1 atm pressure. Resting tissues need 5–6 mL of oxygen/100 mL of blood to sustain life. Human life is generally not possible when oxygen is solely delivered by physical solution in plasma. Hemoglobin is needed to provide the major portion of oxygen required by the tissue. At 1 atm pressure, only 0.3 mL of oxygen is dissolved in 100 mL of plasma. When the FiO_2 is increased five times (by switching from inhalation of room air to inhalation of pure oxygen), the amount of oxygen dissolved in plasma is also five times greater, i.e. 1.5 mL/100 mL of plasma. Administering 100% oxygen at a pressure of 3 atm provides about 6 mL of oxygen/100 mL of blood. (At a PO_2 of 3.5 atm, the PaO_2 is 2100 mmHg.) This is enough to provide the tissue with the oxygen it requires, without depending on oxygen from hemoglobin [34].

Under hyperbaric and hyperoxic conditions, the carotid chemoreceptor activity is reduced. This reduces cerebral blood flow and the concentration of CO_2 in the brain tissue is increased [35]. Carbon dioxide is retained and a slight acidosis develops. Since hyperbaric oxygen fully saturates hemoglobin with oxygen, no reduced hemoglobin is left for the transport of CO_2. In case of hyperbaric oxygen therapy, other mechanisms are activated to transport CO_2. Under most conditions, these changes are not clinically significant. Only when other mechanisms add to CO_2 retention (in large right–left shunts and in inadequate ventilation) will hyperbaric oxygen therapy worsen an already precarious situation.

Effects exerted mainly by pressure follow Boyle's Law. According to this law, changes in pressure lead to changes in the volume of gas-filled cavities. When gas bubbles are at the root of a medical problem, such as in gas embolism, decompression sickness, and gas gangrene, hyperbaric therapy can be used to reduce the size of the gas collection and may speed recovery. On the other hand, abnormal gas collections, or normal gas collections that do not participate in pressure equalization (pneumothorax, emphysema, blocked middle ears, and paranasal sinuses), may cause problems and can cause barotrauma.

Normobaric oxygen inhalation therapy

Indications

Oxygen, as with all drugs, has its indications and contraindications. The indications for oxygen therapy have been summarized by the American College of Chest Physicians and the National Heart, Lung, and Blood Institute, and include the following:
- Cardiac and respiratory arrest
- Hypoxemia with an oxygen saturation below 90% or a PaO_2 of less than 59 mmHg
- Systolic blood pressure less than 100 mmHg
- A low cardiac output and a metabolic acidosis
- Respiratory distress with a respiratory rate of more than 24/min
- Anesthesia.

At the heart of all the indications is the prevention and treatment of hypoxemia (oxygen deficiency in arterial blood, PaO_2 <80 mmHg; arterial oxygen saturation, SaO_2 <90%) and hypoxia (the oxygen deficiency in the tissues). Hypoxia can be caused by hypoxemia (*hypoxic hypoxia*), low hemoglobin level (*anemic hypoxia*), and/or a diminished flow of blood with a normal amount of oxygen (*stagnant, ischemic hypoxia*). It can also be caused by a disruption of the use of oxygen in the cells (*toxic hypoxia*).

In blood management, oxygen therapy is warranted for the prevention and treatment of anemic hypoxia. In addition, other kinds of hypoxia may be present in anemic patients, contributing to the overall hypoxic state. These should be addressed by oxygen therapy as well, if appropriate. In addition, the vasoconstrictive effects of oxygen may be exploited as well, which may be beneficial in selected scenarios encountered in blood management.

Diagnostic measures

Since hypoxia is the main indication of oxygen therapy, it is important that this is recognized as early as possible and events that may lead to hypoxia are foreseen and prevented.

Clinical features of hypoxia include altered mental status and respiration, arrhythmia, blood pressure alterations, peripheral vasoconstriction with sweaty extremities, and gastrointestinal upset. Such non-specific findings often do not reliably indicate hypoxia. Cyanosis may also be unreliable as an indicator of hypoxia. Cyanosis appears when more than 1.5 g of hemoglobin/100 mL of blood is deoxygenated. In severely anemic patients, no cyanosis may develop.

Since clinical features are unreliable in detecting hypoxia, technical monitoring may be helpful. Measuring the SaO_2 helps to monitor the need for oxygen. Non-invasive pulse oximetry is an elegant method to do this and is available in many countries. Invasive monitoring of blood gases may give the PaO_2. Hypoxia may still exist when SaO_2 and PaO_2 are normal. This may be the case in patients with low cardiac output or in patients with anemia, and then the monitoring of the mixed venous oxygen partial pressure may be indicated in addition to SaO_2 and PaO_2 [36].

Although the above-mentioned monitoring tools may assist the diagnosis of hypoxia, the clinical response to oxygen therapy is still a valuable guide to the use oxygen in anemia. If the patient feels better with oxygen, his/her mind clears, and other clinical signs of hypoxia resolve, oxygen therapy is being applied correctly.

Technical background information

Oxygen supply

In most developed countries, therapeutic oxygen is readily available in tanks, either as a gas or as a liquid. Compressed gas systems use cylinder tanks containing compressed oxygen. The oxygen is stored in tanks as a gas at room temperature. For a hospital that needs much oxygen, the tank system is cumbersome, since the tanks need to be refilled frequently and maintenance is costly. On the other hand, small, portable oxygen tanks are handy and allow easy transportation of patients on continuous oxygen therapy.

When oxygen is cooled to less than −118 °C, it liquefies, thereby reducing the volume it occupies. The reduced volume under such conditions is helpful in transporting oxygen. Liquid oxygen can be stored at the facility prescribing oxygen. Special, usually stationary, containers, so-called vacuum insulated evaporators, are needed to keep the oxygen cooled. The stationary tank can be refilled with commercially available liquid oxygen. The liquid system can either be used to refill oxygen tanks, which contain compressed gaseous oxygen, or can be attached to the hospital wall system that distributes oxygen throughout the facility [37].

To guarantee a constant supply of oxygen for patients, a reliable source is mandatory. Where oxygen is not readily and reliably available, oxygen concentrators are a viable alternative for a hospital to provide patients with oxygen. Oxygen concentrators take oxygen from room air, which is drawn into the concentrator and pressurized to 4 atm. Then, the air is passed through a cylinder with zeolite (aluminum silicate). Nitrogen is bound to zeolite and 95% oxygen is available for inhalation. The zeolite cylinder is recovered by venting it to room air so that nitrogen is released. While the zeolite cylinder is recovering, the gas flow is switched to a second zeolite cylinder. A set of zeolite columns lasts approximately 20 000 hours [38]. Oxygen concentrators depend on electricity. Their use under conditions with frequent power cuts requires a back-up system for electricity supply. Apart from this requirement and the need for simple maintenance procedures, oxygen concentrators are a simple-to-use alternative to industrial oxygen.

Oxygen mixing

To receive the mix of gases needed to administer oxygen, two basic methods of air–oxygen mixing are available.

One method is jet mixing. It is widely used, but the FiO_2 is variable and changes with the atmospheric pressure. Jet mixing is performed with an injector (Venturi mechanism) or with a jet-mixing device. The Venturi mechanism uses the Bernoulli effect to draw in (= entrain) a second gas through a side arm. The first gas passes through a tube that narrows. This narrowing increases the speed the gas passes through it. Due to the increased speed, the pressure drops. A second gas is then drawn into the low-pressure area [37].

The alternative to jet mixing is the use of a high-pressure blender, which mechanically blends compressed air and oxygen. With this method, the FiO_2 is stable. Several valves ensure that air and oxygen mix at certain pressures, so that a chosen FiO_2 is reached.

Table 10.2 Oxygen delivery systems.

Method	Maximum achievable FiO_2
Nasal prong, catheter	0.45–0.50
Simple mask	0.35–0.50
Partial rebreathing mask	0.70–0.85
Non-rebreathing mask	0.8–0.95
Air entrainment mask	0.25–0.70
Oxygen tent	Near 1.0
Ventilator-assisted systems (endotracheal tube, larynx mask, etc.)	Near 1.0

Oxygen delivery systems (Table 10.2)

There is a great variety of systems delivering normobaric supplemental oxygen to the patient [36]. The FiO_2 delivered by some systems depends on the patient's breathing pattern (uncontrolled oxygen, non-capacitance systems), while in others, it does not (controlled oxygen, large-capacitance systems). In an uncontrolled system, the amount of gas delivered to the patient depends on the flow rate of oxygen and on the patient's breathing. A patient breathing with a low minute volume has a high oxygen concentration at a given flow, and vice versa. Non-capacitance systems do not influence the gas mixture just by exhalation, since the exhaled gas cannot be stored.

The simplest of all oxygen delivery systems are nasal tubes or catheters. Nasal tubes are held under the nostrils. Nasal catheters are inserted into the nose, down to the pharynx, and need to be taped to prevent migration into the esophagus. In emergencies, other soft fine catheters can be used as nasal catheters (e.g., nasogastric tubes, urinary catheters). Such simple oxygen delivery devices do not increase the amount of dead space. The FiO_2 increases by 3–4%/L of increased oxygen flow.

A more sophisticated method of oxygen delivery is the use of facemasks:

• A **simple facemask** acts like an increased anatomical reservoir from which the patient breathes. The mask does not have any valves or a reservoir. In order to reduce the rebreathing of exhaled gas, the oxygen flow must exceed the patient's ventilation volume/min. The FiO_2 depends on the respiratory activity of the patient.

• A **partial rebreathing mask** contains an oxygen reservoir from which the patient breathes. It provides a rela-

tively high FiO_2, while conserving oxygen. Oxygen flow is adapted so that about one-third (approximately the anatomical dead space of the patient) of the exhaled air distends the reservoir. After the first third of the exhaled volume has filled the reservoir, the remaining exhaled air escapes through holes in the sides of the mask. The mask reduces the oxygen flow requirement by about 30%.

• A **non-rebreathing mask** contains valves that direct oxygen flow. The valves ensure that exhaled gas is released into the room, while no room air is inhaled. Other valves prevent expired gas from entering the reservoir. The oxygen flow is adjusted so that the reservoir bag is constantly filled.

• A **high-flow oxygen-enrichment mask (air entrainment mask)** works with a high flow of oxygen. A high-flow velocity oxygen stream entrains room air and dilutes the oxygen stream. The gas stream exceeds the minute volume of the patient. Therefore, no valves and reservoirs are needed. FiO_2 depends on flow and the amount of air entrained.

Many more oxygen delivery systems are in use. Among them are face tents and whole body tents, tracheal cannulas, endotracheal tubes, larynx masks, and masks that are designed to deliver a very accurate amount of oxygen or pressure.

Practical recommendations

A safe prescription for oxygen includes the delivery system, flow rate of oxygen, and monitoring of the treatment. Usually, oxygen delivery should be titrated to reach a predefined target, such as oxygen saturation, arterial oxygen pressure or others.

As described above, there is a great variety of oxygen delivery systems available. The choice of delivery system depends on the intended duration of oxygen therapy, the acceptance and condition of the patient, and, most importantly, the maximal FiO_2 required. Short-term, low FiO_2 use of supplemental oxygen can be achieved by nasal tubes, cannulas, or simple masks. Some mask models not only administer oxygen, but can also maintain positive airway pressure. When oxygen therapy is used continuously, over an extended period or at a high flow rate in a conscious patient, a transtracheal oxygen catheter may be recommended.

The flow rate of oxygen or the FiO_2 have to be prescribed as well. In fact, most patients do not need controlled oxygen therapy, i.e., oxygen therapy with a limited, preset inspiratory oxygen fraction. Such strict control is only indicated in patients with chronic obstructive pulmonary disease, who have a hypoxic drive, and in premature infants. All other patients in need of oxygen may be adequately treated with uncontrolled oxygen therapy.

The duration of oxygen therapy depends mainly on the clinical condition. It is known that side effects of oxygen therapy occur with prolonged and high-concentration oxygen, and life-saving oxygen therapy cannot be denied solely on grounds of the potential hazards of oxygen. However, knowledge of the patient's resistance to oxygen toxicity and possible modifications of his/her oxygen tolerance is clinically important to minimize oxygen-related side effects. It is generally believed that prolonged exposure to an FiO_2 of 0.55–0.60 does not cause severe side effects. Others claim that a patient is only safe from oxygen toxicity when the FiO_2 is below 0.4. However, the oxygen resistance and tolerance of the individual patient are difficult to assess. Attempts have been made to modify oxygen tolerance pharmacologically. Most of the drugs tested need to be given in unacceptably high doses to achieve the desired clinical effects on oxygen tolerance [29]. Antioxidant vitamins are an exception, since they can be administered in the required dose without eliciting unacceptable side effects. Although their efficacy remains to be proven, antioxidant vitamins are used clinically to treat oxygen toxicity [32].

Hyperbaric oxygen

Indications

Hyperbaric oxygen therapy has a set of approved indications, issued by the Hyperbaric Oxygen Therapy Committee of the UHMS:
• Air or gas embolism
• Carbon monoxide poisoning (also in connection with cyanide poisoning)
• Gas gangrene (clostridial infection)
• Traumatic ischemias, such as crush injury and compartment syndrome
• Decompression sickness
• Wound healing for problem wounds
• Severe blood loss anemia
• Intracranial abscess
• Necrotizing soft tissue infections
• Refractory osteomyelitis
• Delayed radiation injury
• Skin grafts and flaps compromised in healing
• Thermal burns.

As the above list demonstrates, hyperbaric oxygen therapy plays a role in blood management (albeit a small

one). Increased pressure augments the effect of oxygen on the body. This effect is used as an adjunct in the therapy of severe anemia.

Contraindications

Untreated pneumothorax and bleomycin/doxorubicin or cisplatinum chemotherapy constitute contraindications for hyperbaric therapy.

Some other conditions are considered relative contraindications [35]. A history of a spontaneous pneumothorax or thoracic surgery may increase the likelihood of barotrauma to the lung. Infection of the upper respiratory tract as well as ear surgery may hinder pressure equalization in the middle ear, increasing the risk for barotrauma. Severe emphysema with hypercarbia may cause respiratory arrest in the chamber. A history of epilepsy may increase the seizure risk under hyperbaric conditions. Also, a high fever may predispose to convulsions. Patients with hereditary spherocytosis may experience exaggerated hemolysis under hyperbaric conditions, and a history of optical neuritis may be a risk factor for a pressure-associated recurrence of the visual disturbance.

Pregnancy does not constitute a contraindication for hyperbaric oxygen therapy.

Technical background information

Hyperbaric oxygen is administered in so-called hyperbaric chambers. The early chambers were "multiplace" chambers. These large tanks can hold more than one person. Usually, a transfer chamber allows persons to enter and leave without pressure in the main chamber being lost. The chambers are large enough to allow personnel to join patients and care for them under hyperbaric conditions. Specially modified medical equipment can be used in such chambers so that intensive care of the critically ill is possible. The chambers can build up a pressure of 6 atm or more. Oxygen is delivered directly to the patient, using masks or ventilators. To reduce fire hazards, the chamber itself is filled with compressed air rather than oxygen.

In contrast, "monoplace" chambers look like a bed surrounded by a tube made of metal and plastic. Only one person can be in the chamber at a time. The chambers are less costly than the large multiplace chambers and are often portable. Patients do not need to wear an oxygen mask. The whole chamber is filled with the gas that the patient is prescribed to breathe. Since the chamber is often filled with 100% oxygen, there is a high risk of explosion. Electronic equipment (ventilators and monitors) cannot be taken into the chamber, unless they are specifically designed for hyperbaric conditions. When intensive care is required for a patient in a monoplace chamber, non-collapsible intravenous tubes with unidirectional valves can be used, as well as ventilators and monitors. Pressure-sealed ports allow the treatment of the critically ill patient from outside the chamber [35].

Apart from the traditional monoplace and multiplace chambers, there is a wide variety of mobile monoplace chambers, designed for different uses [39]. An interesting example is the Gamow bag. The Gamow bag, which looks like a large sleeping bag, was designed as a portable hyperbaric chamber for use by mountain climbers who suffer from high-altitude sickness. The original bags were made of lightweight fabric, which did not withstand the standard pressures required for hyperbaric oxygen therapy. Modifications to the fabric mean the Gamow bag now withstands pressure of up to 2 atm [40]. Oxygen and pressure are provided to the bag, using oxygen cylinders, scuba tanks, or hospital wall ports. Gamow bags provide an affordable, portable alternative to conventional chambers. Patients with carbon monoxide poisoning, who report to a hospital that does not have a hyperbaric chamber, have successfully been treated with the Gamow bag [41]. To our knowledge, a Gamow bag has not been trialed in blood management therapy.

Patterns of therapy sessions

A very wide range of treatment patterns of hyperbaric oxygen are used, depending on the indications. When treatment of decompression sickness is required, initially patients may be treated with pressures up to 6 atm. Such high pressures are not needed for the therapy of severe anemia. The UHMS gives treatment protocols for its recommended indications. For exceptional blood loss anemia, the following recommendation is given: "Treatments are continued repetitively, as needed, at pressures dictated by clinical response. May be used in conjunction with erythropoietin, which has a lag time of 3–4 days. Average number of treatments: Until Hct >22.9% or based on clinical judgement" [35]. Whether this recommendation is of use to specialists in the field of blood management is debatable, but it does give a concept of hyperbaric oxygen therapy in blood management.

Severe anemia is usually treated with pressures up to a maximum of 2–3 atm. Pressurization lasts about 60–90 minutes. Depending on the clinical condition of the patient, the treatment is initially administered three times daily and the frequency is reduced as the patient becomes more stable. Other treatment modes are used at the discretion of the physician, depending on the clinical condition of the patient and his/her response to the treatment.

Practical recommendations

Before the therapy

As with all treatments, hyperbaric therapy requires the consent of the patient. Before therapy is commenced, an explanation, tailored to the needs of the patient, should be given and the patient needs to consent to the treatment.

If a patient is considered a candidate for hyperbaric therapy, he/she needs to be prepared, to avoid undue damage to his/her health [42]. A chest radiograph should rule out pneumothorax, severe obstructive lung disease, or other pathological gas-filled cavities. When a pneumothorax is present, a chest tube needs to be inserted and a water seal placed.

Patients must be checked regarding their ability to equalize pressure in their middle ears to prevent rupture of the eardrums. Vasoconstrictive drops may help. Pressure equalization tubes should be inserted into the eardrums when pressure equalization of the middle ears is not possible spontaneously. In emergencies, with a nonresponsive patient, paracentesis is required.

The pressure cuff of tubes, such as endotracheal tubes, changes in relation to the changes in the hyperbaric chamber. When the pressure increases, the volume of the cuff diminishes, no longer sealing the airway. This may lead to hypoventilation. When the pressure in the chamber is decreased, the cuff increases in size and may cause tracheal rupture. Therefore, saline should be used, rather than air, to fill the cuff tube. The same is true also for the balloons of bladder catheters.

Since the density of a gas increases as the pressure increases, patients in the hyperbaric environment have to use more exertion to breathe. When patients breathe through a tube or a tracheal stoma, the widest possible tubes should be employed to offset the density-induced increased workload. Patients with dyspnea, or those who cannot maintain adequate ventilation, need to be intubated and put on ventilatory support. The largest possible size of tube should be used.

In patients who are not hemodynamically stable, invasive monitoring with central lines, arterial lines, etc., should be established. On the other hand, any vascular accesses that are not needed should be discontinued to reduce the chance of air embolism.

If the patient is in a critical condition, monitoring or ventilation may be required. Equipment needs to be chosen that is fit for use under hyperbaric conditions.

Patients need adequate pain control and sometimes sedation for anxiety control. Opioids and diazepam or other suitable benzodiazepines are optimal.

The patient's current, or recent, medication needs to be revised. Steroids, thyroid hormones, and other drugs can increase the likelihood of oxygen toxicity and convulsions [43]. Patients receiving such drugs must be monitored closely for signs of convulsions. The medication of choice to treat and prevent convulsions is diazepam (or other suitable benzodiazepine). Patients on doxorubicin or cisplatinum must not receive hyperbaric treatment, since this may be fatal. This is probably due to hyperbaric oxygen increasing the cardiotoxic effects of the chemotherapeutics [44].

Diabetics need to have good control of their blood sugar. Availability of an adaptable insulin schedule and glucose helps to treat any disturbance of the blood sugar.

During the therapy

When the patient is in the chamber, the following measures may have to be taken to prevent and treat side effects of the therapy [42, 45].

When large amounts of pulmonary secretions are present, the patient needs to be suctioned to prevent air from being trapped in the lungs, leading to pulmonary barotrauma during ascent.

A seizure during therapy is mainly due to oxygen toxicity. It occurs in 1.3 of 10 000 cases and it usually does not have adverse consequences, since there is no hypoxia present [25]. Seizures during hyperbaric therapy can be resolved by reducing the oxygen concentration in the chamber, but not the pressure. Pharmacological therapy is not required in the majority of cases.

Physiological and pathological gas-filled cavities, in which pressure equalization cannot occur, are prone to develop barotrauma. The eardrums can rupture if it is not possible to equalize the pressure. To equilibrate the pressure, groaning, chewing, and swallowing or the valsalva maneuver may be encouraged. Barotrauma can also occur in the paranasal sinuses, teeth, gastrointestinal tract, and in pathological cavities like emphysema bullae or pneumothorax. The patient therefore needs to be monitored closely to detect any problems early enough to intervene.

Diabetics must be monitored closely during hyperbaric treatment, since blood glucose levels may fall rapidly under hyperbaric conditions, and hypoglycemia and insulin therapy dispose to increased oxygen toxicity and seizures.

After the therapy

Patients may complain about numb fingers and myopia after their treatment. Neither of these symptoms is permanent, usually resolving within weeks or months.

Oxygen in blood management

Supportive treatment in anemia and hemorrhagic shock

Oxygen has long been used for the supportive treatment of severe anemia and hemorrhagic shock. It augments oxygen delivery and may improve the outcome. This has been accredited to increased arterial oxygen content and improved arterial blood pressure, as well as to the redistribution of blood flow from the skeletal muscles to the splanchnic area [17]. Interestingly, animal data suggest that oxygen improves tissue oxygenation in hemorrhagic shock only after fluid resuscitation, but not before [46].

Interestingly, hyperoxic ventilation, but not red cell transfusion, improves tissue oxygenation [47]. Therefore, hyperoxic ventilation improves the safety of a therapeutic regimen for anemia. It was shown in animal experiments that switching from breathing room air to hyperoxic ventilation not only reversed signs of hypoxic myocardial dysfunction, but also allowed considerable further blood loss without recurrence of signs of myocardial dysfunction in the electrocardiogram (EKG) [48]. Besides, hyperoxic ventilation improves survival in hemorrhagic shock patients with controlled hemorrhage [49, 50]. It was shown that brain function and heart rate return to normal when severely anemic volunteers breathe oxygen [51].

Beneficial effects of oxygen therapy in hemorrhage are not always observed [52]. This may be due to the production of excess reactive oxygen species with resulting tissue damage. Also, while patients with controlled hemorrhage seem to benefit from the effects of oxygen, the same may not be true for those with uncontrolled hemorrhage [17]. Initially, the blood pressure rises, supposedly as an effect of the oxygen. The elevated blood pressure augments bleeding and the blood pressure drops soon afterward due to the increased blood loss. This is in line with the findings of other studies that have demonstrated that therapies administered to resuscitate patients (e.g., aggressive fluid resuscitation)—while beneficial when bleeding is controlled—may have adverse effects (increased total blood loss) when bleeding has not been controlled.

The oxygen-induced redistribution of blood to the splanchnic vasculature brings some theoretical benefit. In hemorrhagic shock, splanchnic perfusion is often impaired and ischemia may occur. This triggers a response that results in endothelial damage and a dysfunction of the epithelium and macrophages of the intestines. Bacterial translocation, endotoxinemia, and the resulting systemic response negatively affect the whole body. Oxygen may indeed be beneficial in reducing the ischemia that would develop during periods of hemorrhage.

Intraoperative hyperoxic ventilation

Oxygen therapy can reduce a patient's exposure to allogeneic blood. Hyperoxic ventilation in extreme hemodilution has been advocated [18]. Ventilating a patient with 100% oxygen rapidly increases the arterial oxygen content. The amount of oxygen dissolved in plasma is increased. This effect is enhanced in patients with anemia, since their plasma volume is expanded. Plasma, thus, becomes a significant source of oxygen. Using the concept of hyperoxic ventilation during acute normovolemic hemodilution helps to reduce allogeneic transfusions. Patients undergoing acute normovolemic hemodilution are hemodiluted down to the lowest acceptable hemoglobin level. When further blood loss occurs, mainly due to surgical losses, signs of impaired oxygen delivery may appear (e.g., a reduced mixed venous oxygen partial pressure, ST-segment changes in the EKG). When these occur, collected blood is given back. Autologous blood may then be depleted by the end of surgery and severe anemia cannot be treated quickly. Starting to retransfuse before surgical hemostasis is achieved may thus increase the likelihood of postoperative severe anemia. To minimize this anemia, the proposed approach in the event of signs of impaired oxygen delivery is to switch from a low oxygen concentration in the ventilated gas to 100% oxygen. Now, enough oxygen is available to reverse the signs of impaired oxygen delivery and the surgery can continue. An average of 30 minutes can be bought by this approach [18]. This may bridge the time until surgical hemorrhage is stopped. Afterward, the autologous blood is returned.

Hyperbaric oxygen in severe anemia

High oxygen content in the plasma can supplement or supplant the oxygen delivery by hemoglobin. Since the amount of a gas dissolved in a liquid is proportional to the pressure of the gas above the liquid, an increase in the ambient air pressure can greatly increase the amount of oxygen dissolved in plasma. When the hemoglobin-bound oxygen is unable to meet the needs of the body, hyperbaric oxygen therapy can dissolve enough oxygen into the plasma. In this way, hyperbaric oxygen therapy can maximize oxygen dissolved in the plasma while the patient synthesizes hemoglobin.

Hyperbaric oxygen therapy is a therapeutic option for patients with severe symptomatic anemia. Multiple case reports and case studies [15, 32, 53–55], but no controlled trials, testify to this. Besides, a review of the available literature on the use of hyperbaric oxygen therapy in severe anemia summarized that "all publications report a positive result when HBO$_2$ [hyperbaric oxygen therapy] is delivered as treatment for severe anemia" [56]. In particular, it has been shown that ischemic changes in the EKG (ST-segment changes), and corresponding clinical signs, such as angina pectoris, heart failure with pulmonary edema, metabolic acidosis, impaired mental status, and diminished kidney and bowel function, rapidly resolve after exposure to hyperbaric oxygen. Often, the beneficial effects of the temporarily increased oxygen delivery last for minutes to several hours after the therapy.

Hyperbaric oxygen in sickle cell crisis

Hyperbaric oxygen therapy has also been used in sickle cell crisis [57]. Patients with sickle cell disease experience vaso-occlusive crisis when hemoglobin S is polymerized and sickling occurs. This is seen under conditions that expose red cells to low oxygen tensions. Some of the red cells are irreversibly sickled, while others are desaturated but not irreversibly sickled. Sickled, stiff cells block the microcirculation and cause tissue ischemia and infarction. In patients with a developing crisis, hyperbaric oxygen can reduce the number of sickle cells in peripheral blood. Hyperbaric treatments, when started within the first 24 hours after the onset of symptoms, may shorten total hospital stay of patients compared with those receiving conventional treatment [57].

More recent experiments have not demonstrated a direct effect of hyperbaric oxygen on the number of sickle cells in blood samples. It was thought that other effects might, in vivo, contribute to the beneficial effect of hyperbaric oxygen in sickle cell crisis [58]. Due to the lack of evidence, the UHMS does not list sickle cell crises as a recommended indication for hyperbaric oxygen therapy.

Oxygen therapy to reduce blood loss

Several preliminary studies on the use of oxygen, either normobaric or hyperbaric, suggest it has hemostatic effects. It may be hypothesized that these effects are exerted via induction of vasoconstriction, enhancement of healing, or other, as yet unknown, measures. It has been suggested that short-term preoperative hyperbaric oxygen administration may reduce blood loss during and after cardiac surgery [59]. Inhalation of high-flow oxygen after birth was suggested to reduce postpartum blood loss [60]. Also, hyperbaric oxygen therapy seems to reduce or eliminate hemorrhagic episodes in post-radiation hemorrhagic proctitis [61].

Oxygen therapy to induce erythropoiesis

Some studies have suggested an erythropoiesis-stimulating effect of intermittent oxygen breathing [62, 63]. The normobaric oxygen paradox was suggested to be the basis for this effect. Whether or not further research substantiates or refutes the existence of the normobaric oxygen paradox, the idea that oxygen induces erythropoiesis in intriguing.

Key points

• Oxygen therapy can be life-saving in the case of anemia.
• Severe cases of anemia can be treated with hyperbaric oxygen.
• The choice of the right oxygen delivery device influences how much oxygen the patient finally breathes.

Questions for review

1. What laws govern the physical behavior of oxygen?
2. How does the body react to oxygen in anemic and non-anemic states?
3. What information is needed to safely prescribe inhalational oxygen therapy?
4. What preparations are needed for a patient who is to be treated with hyperbaric oxygen?
5. What are the side effects of oxygen therapy?

Suggestions for further research

• What role does oxygen play in reperfusion injury?
• How does the position of the patient while breathing oxygen influence his/her arterial oxygen content (sitting, supine, prone, head-down, on his/her side)?

Exercises and practice cases

Calculate the oxygen partial pressure in the lung of a normal healthy young man who breathes room air at sea level. Do the same when he is breathing 100% oxygen.

You are asked to teach interns about oxygen therapy. How would you go about it? What information do you think will benefit them? How would you present the information? What demonstration material would you take along with you? Is there an article you would recommend to the students for further reading?

Homework

Obtain the contact details of the nearest hyperbaric chamber and consider how to transfer a patient there, if necessary.

Find out how oxygen is provided to the patients in your facility:

• What color are the oxygen tanks?
• Where does the hospital get the oxygen from?
• What safety precautions are there:
  ○ To prevent explosion?
  ○ To prevent errors in administration (to make sure that oxygen is administered and not another gas)?

References

1. Priestley J. *Experiments and Observations on Different Kinds of Air and Other Branches of Natural Philosophy Connected with the Subject*, in three volumes. Printed by Th. Pearson, sold by J. Johnson, St. Paul's Church-Yard: Birmingham, London, 1790.
2. Birch SB. On the therapeutic use of oxygen. *Lancet* 1857;August 1:112.
3. Osler W. *The Principles and Practice of Medicine*. D. Appleton & Co., New York, 1892.
4. Davenport JH. Oxygen as a remedial agent. *Boston Med Surg J* 1872;**10**:61–64.
5. Ehinger CE. *Oxygen in Therapeutics: A Treatise Explaining the Apparatus, the Material and the Processes Used in the Preparation of Oxygen and Other Gases with Which It May Be Combined, Also, Its Administration and Effects, Illustrated by Clinical Experience of the Author and Others*. W.A. Chatterton & Co., Chicago, 1887.
6. Conklin WL. The therapeutic value of oxygen. *N Y State Med J* 1899;September 2:338–341.
7. Starkey P. *Compound Oxygen—Its Origin and Development*. 1529 Arch Street, Philadelphia, PA, 1888.

8. Kellogg JH. Oxygen enemata as a remedy in certain diseases of the liver and the intestinal tract. *JAMA* 1888;**11**: 258–262.

9. Bainbridge WS. Oxygen in medicine and surgery—a contribution, with report of cases. *N Y State J Med* 1908;**8**: 281–295.

10. Tunnicliffe FW, Stebbing GF. The intravenous injection of oxygen gas as a therapeutic measure. *Lancet* 1916;August 19:321–323.

11. Howitt HO. The subcutaneous injection of oxygen gas. *CMAJ* 1914;**4**:983–985.

12. Haldane JS. The therapeutic administration of oxygen. *BMJ* 1917;February 10:181–183.

13. Boerema I, Meyne NG, Brummelkamp WH, *et al.* [Life without blood.] *Ned Tijdschr Geneeskd* 1960;**104**: 949–954.

14. Boerema I, Meyne NG, Brummelkamp WK, *et al.* Life without blood. A study on the influence of high atmospheric pressure and hypothermia on dilution of blood. *J Cardivasc Surg* 1960;**13**:133–146.

15. Amonic RS, Cockett ATK, Lorhan PH, Thompson JC. Hyperbaric oxygen therapy in chronic hemorrhagic shock. *JAMA* 1969;**208**:2051–2054.

16. Meier J, Pape A, Kleen M, Hutter J, Kemming G, Habler O. Regional blood flow during hyperoxic haemodilution. *Clin Physiol Funct Imaging* 2005;**25**:158–165.

17. Sukhotnik I, Krausz MM, Brod V, *et al.* Divergent effects of oxygen therapy in four models of uncontrolled hemorrhagic shock. *Shock* 2002;**18**:277–284.

18. Habler O, Kleen M, Kemming G, Zwissler B. Hyperoxia in extreme hemodilution. *Eur Surg Res* 2002;**34**:181–187.

19. Neubauer B, Tetzlaff K, Staschen CM, Bettinghausen E. Cardiac output changes during hyperbaric hyperoxia. *Int Arch Occup Environ Health* 2001;**74**:119–122.

20. Conti CR. Is hyperoxic ventilation important to treat acute coronary syndromes such as uncomplicated myocardial infarction? *Clin Cardiol* 2011;**34**:132–133.

21. Perz S, Uhlig T, Kohl M, *et al.* Low and "supranormal" central venous oxygen saturation and markers of tissue hypoxia in cardiac surgery patients: a prospective observational study. *Intens Care Med* 2011;**37**:52–59.

22. Rabi Y, Rabi D, Yee W. Room air resuscitation of the depressed newborn: A systematic review and meta-analysis. *Resuscitation* 2007;**72**:353–363.

23. Liu JQ, Saugstad OD, Cheung PY. Using 100% oxygen for the resuscitation of term neonates until evidence of spontaneous circulation: More investigations needed. *Resuscitation* 2010;**81**:145–147.

24. Knighton DR, Halliday B, Hunt TK. Oxygen as an antibiotic. A comparison of the effects of inspired oxygen concentration and antibiotic administration on in vivo bacterial clearance. *Arch Surg* 1986;**121**:191–195.

25. Jaeger K, Juttner B, Franko W. Hyperbaric oxygen therapy—options and limitations. *Anasthesiol Intensivmed Notfallmed Schmerzther* 2002;**37**:38–42.

26. Tin W. Oxygen therapy: 50 years of uncertainty. *Pediatrics* 2002;**110**:615–616.

27. Lambertsen CJ, Douch RH, Cooper DY, Emmel GL, Loeschcke HH, Schmidt CF. Oxygen toxicity; effects in man of oxygen inhalation at 1 and 3.5 atmospheres upon blood gas transport, cerebral circulation and cerebral metabolism. *J Appl Physiol* 1953;**5**:471–486.

28. Gore A, Muralidhar M, Espey MG, Degenhardt K, Mantell LL. Hyperoxia sensing: from molecular mechanisms to significance in disease. *J Immunotoxicol* 2010;**7**:239–254.

29. Clark JM, Lambertsen CJ. Pulmonary oxygen toxicity: a review. *Pharmacol Rev* 1971;**23**:37–133.

30. De Bels D, Corazza F, Germonpré P, Balestra C. The normobaric oxygen paradox: A novel way to administer oxygen as an adjuvant treatment for cancer? *Med Hypoth* 2011;**76**: 467–470.

31. Debevec T, Keramidas ME, Norman B, Gustafsson T, Eiken O, Mekjavic IB. Acute short-term hyperoxia followed by mild hypoxia does not increase EPO production: resolving the "normobaric oxygen paradox". *Eur J Appl Physiol* 2011 Jul 7 [Epub ahead of print].

32. Greensmith JE. Hyperbaric oxygen reverses organ dysfunction in severe anemia. *Anesthesiology* 2000;**93**:1149–1152.

33. Bassett BE, Bennett BP. Introduction to the physical and physiological bases of hyperbaric therapy. In: Davis JC, Hunt TK (eds.) *Hyperbaric Oxygen Therapy*. Undersea Medical Society, Betheseda, 1977, p. 20.

34. Tibbles PM, Edelsberg JS. Hyperbaric-oxygen therapy. *N Engl J Med* 1996;**334**:1642–1648.

35. Hancock DL. Hyperbaric oxygen therapy. *Am J Anesthesiol* 1997;**24**:297–307.

36. Bateman NT, Leach RM. ABC of oxygen. Acute oxygen therapy. *BMJ* 1998;**317**:798–801.

37. Varvinski AM, Hunt S. Acute oxygen treatment. *Update Anesth* 2000;**12**:Article 3.

38. Dobson MB. Oxygen concentrators for district hospitals. *Update Anesth* 1999;**10**:Article 11.

39. Bouak F. Lightweight portable hyperbaric chambers. *Technical Memorandum DRDC Toronto TM 2003–157.* Defence R&D Canada—Toronto, 2003.

40. Shimada H, Morita T, Kunimoto F, Saito S. Immediate application of hyperbaric oxygen therapy using a newly devised transportable chamber. *Am J Emerg Med* 1996;**14**: 412–415.

41. Jay GD, Tetz DJ, Hartigan CF, Lane LL, Aghababian RV. Portable hyperbaric oxygen therapy in the emergency department with the modified Gamow bag. *Ann Emerg Med* 1995;**26**:707–711.

42. Matos LA. Hyperbaric medicine. In: Civetta JM, Taylor RW, Kirby R (eds.) *Critical Care*. Lippincott-Raven, Philadelphia, 1997, pp. 777–785.

43. Leifer G. Hyperbaric oxygen therapy. *Am J Nurs* 2001;**101**:26–34; quiz 34–35.

44. Sauerstoffü berdrucktherapie (Hyperbare Oxygenationstherapie; HOT). In: Wiemann, K. (ed.) *MSD-Manual der*

Diagnostik und Therapie, 5th edn. Urban u. Fischer, Munich, 1993, pp. 3228–3236.

45. Strelow H. Die hyperbare Medizin—Mö glichkeiten und Grenzen der Sauerstoff-Ü berdrucktherapie: 8. Folge: Komplikationen und Grenzen der OHP. *Die Schwester/Der Pfleger* 1986;**25**:96–101.

46. Takasu A, Iwamoto S, Ando S, *et al*. Effects of various concentrations of inhaled oxygen on tissue dysoxia, oxidative stress, and survival in a rat hemorrhagic shock model. *Resuscitation* 2009;**80**:826–831.

47. Suttner S, Piper SN, Kumle B, *et al*. The influence of allogeneic red blood cell transfusion compared with 100% oxygen ventilation on systemic oxygen transport and skeletal muscle oxygen tension after cardiac surgery. *Anesth Analg* 2004;**99**:2–11.

48. Meier J, Kemming G, Meisner F, Pape A, Habler O. Hyperoxic ventilation enables hemodilution beyond the critical myocardial hemoglobin concentration. *Eur J Med Res* 2005;**10**:462–468.

49. Meier J, Kemming GI, Kisch-Wedel H, Wölkhammer S, Habler OP. Hyperoxic ventilation reduces 6-hour mortality at the critical hemoglobin concentration. *Anesthesiology* 2004;**100**:70–76.

50. Meier J, Kemming GI, Kisch-Wedel H, Blum J, Pape A, Habler OP. Hyperoxic ventilation reduces six-hour mortality after partial fluid resuscitation from hemorrhagic shock. *Shock* 2004;**22**:240–247.

51. Weiskopf RB, Feiner J, Hopf HW, *et al*. Oxygen reverses deficits of cognitive function and memory and increased heart rate induced by acute severe isovolemic anemia. *Anesthesiology* 2002;**96**:871–877.

52. Knight AR, Fry LE, Clancy RL, Pierce JD. Understanding the effects of oxygen administration in haemorrhagic shock. *Nurs Crit Care* 2011;**16**:28–35.

53. McLoughlin PL, Cope TM, Harrison JC. Hyperbaric oxygen therapy in the management of severe acute anaemia in a Jehovah's Witness. *Anaesthesia* 1999;**54**:891–895.

54. Hart GB, *et al*. Hyperbaric oxygen in exceptional acute blood-loss anemia. *J Hyperb Med* 1987;**2**:205–210.

55. Hart GB. Exceptional blood loss anemia. Treatment with hyperbaric oxygen. *JAMA* 1974;**228**:1028–1029.

56. Van Meter KW. A systematic review of the application of hyperbaric oxygen in the treatment of severe anemia: an evidence-based approach. *Undersea Hyperb Med* 2005;**32**:61–83.

57. Hart GB, *et al*. Amelioration of sickle cell crises with intensive hyperbaric oxygen. *J Hyperb Med* 1991;**6**:75–85.

58. Mychaskiw G II, Woodyard SA, Brunson CD, May WS, Eichhorn JH. In vitro effects of hyperbaric oxygen on sickle cell morphology. *J Clin Anesth* 2001;**13**:255–258.

59. Yogaratnam JZ, Laden G, Guvendik L, Cowen M, Cale A, Griffin S. Hyperbaric oxygen preconditioning improves myocardial function, reduces length of intensive care stay, and limits complications post coronary artery bypass graft surgery. *Cardiovasc Revasc Med* 2010;**11**:8–19.

60. Sekhavat L, Firuzabadi RD, Karimi Zarchi M. Effect of postpartum oxygen inhalation on vaginal blood loss. *J Matern Fetal Neonatal Med* 2009;**22**:1072–1706.

61. Girnius S, Cersonsky N, Gesell L, Cico S, Barrett W. Treatment of refractory radiation-induced hemorrhagic proctitis with hyperbaric oxygen therapy. *Am J Clin Oncol* 2006;**29**:588–592.

62. Burk R. Oxygen breathing may be a cheaper and safer alternative to exogenous erythropoietin (EPO). *Med Hypoth* 2007;**69**:1200–1204.

63. Balestra C, *et al*. The "Normobaric Oxygen Paradox": a simple way to induce endogenous EPO production and concomitantly Hb in anemic patients. *Transfu Altern Transfu Med* 2010;**11**:39–42.

11 Preparation of the Patient for Surgery

The outcome of a patient's surgery is likely to be more favorable if suitable preparations are made. Once a specific goal has been established—in our case improving the outcome of treatment by appropriate blood management—advance preparation is required. Preoperative planning is essential to optimize the patient's condition before surgery, reduce perioperative blood loss, increase anemia tolerance, and smooth postoperative recovery. This chapter will introduce the reader to an algorithm for preoperative blood management.

Objectives

1. To review how to take a history and perform a physical examination while focusing on the patient's blood management.
2. To be able to calculate a patient's blood volume and allowable blood loss.
3. To practice how to draw up a care plan.
4. To know how to prepare patients with commonly encountered diseases for surgery in a blood management program.

Definitions

Preparation: The English words "preparation" or "to prepare" have their roots in the Latin *paratus* and *praeparare*, meaning "prepared," "ready," "equipped," and "skilled." Closely related is the word "apparatus," meaning not only "equipment" but also "exertion" and "effort." Another Latin word for "prepared" is *promptus*, meaning

"ready at hand." It also denotes persons who are prepared, resolute, or prompt. The full scope of the word "preparation" therefore means to be ready, have the required equipment, be skilled, and be prompt in taking action. Preparation also means exertion and effort.

The algorithm

This chapter gives an overview of how to prepare a patient for surgery in a blood management program. Help is given on how to integrate the various drugs and methods into a whole treatment concept. The algorithm (Figure 11.1) is discussed step by step. Practice using this algorithm, even if a patient initially presents for minor surgery only. Commit the lines of the algorithm to memory so that you always think along these lines. In time, even patients presenting as complex cases will be easy to prepare.

Step 1: History and physical examination

It has been said that taking a good history and performing a physical examination are 90% of the diagnosis [1]. It could also be said that it is 90% of the basis for a patient's blood management plan. A skilled history and physical examination are the basis for preparing the patient for surgery, and informing the surgeon of the equipment required and the approach to be taken. A thorough preoperative work-up serves to identify the problems unique to the patient and helps spot potential obstacles to a favorable outcome related to blood

Basics of Blood Management, Second Edition. Petra Seeber and Aryeh Shander.
© 2013 John Wiley & Sons, Ltd. Published 2013 by John Wiley & Sons, Ltd.

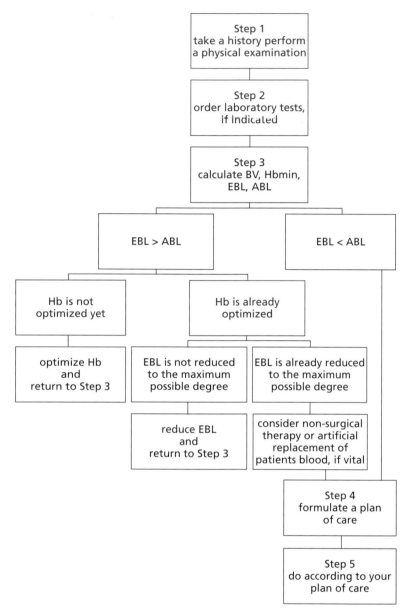

Figure 11.1 Algorithm: preparing a patient for surgery in a blood management program. BV, blood volume; EBL, expected blood loss; ABL, allowable blood loss; Hb, hemoglobin; Hbmin, minimum tolerable hemoglobin.

management. The first step in the algorithm is therefore to take a focused history and perform a physical examination [2].

Taking a focused history

A healthcare provider surely needs no explanation of how to take a history. There are, of course, different approaches, each with advantages and disadvantages. No matter how history taking is structured, all the information required has to be obtained in as convenient a manner as possible. A systematic approach to history taking makes it easier and helps avoid overlooking important issues. Some suggestions as to what to include in the history, in the style you prefer, are given below. The facets of the patient's history relevant to blood management are also included.

> **Practice tip Simplifying documentation**
>
> As a reminder of what information needs to be gathered
> from a patient in preparation for surgery, a form can be
> developed. This may be used to record the findings of the
> history taking and the physical examination, as well as the
> required preparations (e.g., work-up of anemia, availability
> of equipment). Such a form can be kept in the patient's file
> where it will be available for any necessary review.

Begin as usual with the patient's demographic data. This will provide the first pieces of the puzzle that finally constitute the individual picture presented by the patient. Interestingly, there are a number of studies that use demographic data to predict the likelihood of major blood loss or of a patient receiving a transfusion.

• **Age:** Tolerance of anemia is age-dependent. Young children tolerate anemia much better than the elderly. There are also age-dependent differences in the probability of the patient presenting with morbidities relevant to blood management. Increasing age itself is a significant predictor for transfusions [3, 4].

• **Gender:** There are differences between genders relevant to blood management. Women are more likely to receive transfusions than men [3–5]. They have a lower average red blood cell count and are prone to regular blood loss via menses and childbirth. Both may precipitate iron loss and deficiency. Hormonal differences between genders exist and account, at least partially, for the different hemoglobin levels. The decision as to what therapy to use for anemia may also be influenced by the gender of the patient (e.g., whether to use recombinant human erythropoietin [rHuEPO] or androgens for the therapy of renal anemia).

• **Weight and height:** To calculate drug dosage, blood volumes, and allowable blood loss, note the patient's height and weight. The patient's size may also provide indications as to whether he/she will usually be considered a transfusion candidate. Low body weight and a small size are predictors for transfusions in some procedures [3, 4], while obesity contributes to the risk of receiving transfusions in other surgeries [6].

• **Race, ethnic background, religion, and a long-term stay abroad** are also relevant. Some types of anemia and coagulation disorders are more common in certain races. For instance, there is a high prevalence of factor XI deficiency in Ashkenazi Jews. Inhabitants of Mediterranean regions often suffer from anemia due to favism. The nutritional status may also be affected by the background of the patient, influenced by the lifestyle and foods prohibited by religion.

Areas of specific inquiry related to blood management

When taking the history of a patient, most healthcare providers would first inquire about the chief complaint. The same approach is taken for patients whose blood management is the responsibility of the healthcare provider. In addition to inquiring about the condition that brought the patient to the office, continue asking about the five main patient-related obstacles to transfusion-free therapy, namely, anemia, hemostatic disturbances, medical conditions that may increase perioperative blood loss, obstacles to surgical hemostasis, and factors that decrease anemia tolerance. These issues should be evaluated in detail. The following questions and hints serve as a reminder of what to ask about.

First, some simple questions help elucidate a possible *history of anemia*. Has the patient been anemic in the past? How did the anemia manifest itself? What was the reason for the anemia? When did it occur and how long did it last? What treatment was used and did the treatment help? Has the patient ever received transfusions of red blood cell concentrates? Why was the transfusion given? Were there any side effects? Who treated the patient? The latter is important because the patient may not know the details of the anemia and it might be useful to ask the patient's former healthcare provider for medical records. Patients may be heterozygous for an inherited anemia that may manifest itself only under severe (surgical) stress, drugs, and disease, and the patient may as yet be unaware of any such problem. A family history may help identify such inherited disorders.

Often, the patient is unaware of whether he/she is or ever has been anemic. Therefore, ask about signs and symptoms that may indicate anemia. Moderate or severe anemia produces symptoms such as decreased exercise tolerance, dyspnea, palpitations, headache, dizziness, vertigo, fainting, anorexia, nausea, intolerance to cold, amenorrhea, menorrhagia, loss of libido, and impotence. In persons with atherosclerosis, symptoms of angina pectoris or intermittent claudication may be more easily provoked than normal. Also, difficulty swallowing (Plummer Vinson syndrome) and eating of indigestible items such as earth, paper, or ice (pica) may be indicative of anemia. Patients with such symptoms should raise your index of suspicion; further evaluation is needed.

Second, assessment of the patient's bleeding history is the most sensitive way to identify patients with impaired hemostasis and those at increased risk for perioperative hemorrhage [7]. Inquire about a *history of coagulation problems*. Ask directly about any known coagulation disorder. Has the patient ever had a problem with hemostasis? How did this manifest? What was the reason for the disorder? When did it occur and how long did it last? What treatment was given and did the treatment help? Has the patient ever received a transfusion of coagulation products? If so, for what reason and did the transfusion achieve the desired goal? And once again, who treated the patient?

Occasionally, patients are unaware of impaired coagulation. Therefore, ask directly about signs of hemorrhage obvious to a layman (e.g., Do you bleed or bruise easily?). In cases of injury or surgical intervention, ask about prolonged hemorrhage or a return of bleeding either immediately following or some hours after the insult. Minor cuts and dental extractions may serve as examples of hemostatic challenges. Bleeding disorders may be disguised if there has been no previous surgical challenge, but there are subtle signs that should arouse suspicion. A defect in hemostasis is suspected when spontaneous hemorrhage occurs or when hemorrhage exceeds the amount expected after injury. Nose bleeds, especially bilateral ones, gums that bleed for more than 3 minutes after teeth brushing, easy bruising, and prolonged bleeding after cuts all occur if hemostasis is impaired. Ask about the sites of bleeding, timing in relation to the insult, duration, and frequency. Also, ask about the severity of hemorrhage, e.g., by comparing the size of a bruise with a coin. Often, however, the only sign of a coagulation disorder is a heavy menses. A substantial proportion of women with menorrhagia and a normal pelvis examination have an inherited bleeding disorder [8]. To standardize questioning about a possible history of bleeding disorders it has been proposed that patients fill out a supplementary questionnaire before they see their healthcare provider. Table 11.1 gives examples of questions for such a questionnaire [7, 9].

It is easy to determine whether a clotting problem is related more to defects or deficiencies in the platelets or to clotting factors. In platelet disorders bleeding occurs immediately after the injury and occurs mainly in the skin and mucosa. If the problem is mainly fibrin clot formation (as in factor deficiencies), hemorrhage occurs some time, even hours, after initial injury. It tends to affect deep tissue and the joints.

Table 11.1 Questions to be asked in a screening questionnaire to evaluate a patient's hemostatic system.

Have you ever suffered from prolonged bleeding?

Do you develop bruises or "black spots" without being able to remember when or how you injured yourself?

What was the longest time you bled after having a tooth extracted? Did bleeding ever start again after it had stopped?

Was it hard to stop the bleeding?

Have you ever bled excessively after surgery or during labor?

Have you ever bled from the gums or nose without any apparent reason?

In your opinion, do you bleed excessively during menstruation?

Within the past 5 years have you ever had a medical problem requiring a doctor's care? Do you have any disorders of the liver or kidneys?

What medications have you taken during the last 14 days?

Has any blood relative ever had a problem with unusual bruising or bleeding?

Have you or a blood relative ever had transfusions?

Third, medical conditions associated with increased perioperative blood loss should be identified. The association between liver diseases and impaired coagulation is well established. Renal failure leading to uremia is also known to impair hemostasis, lead to anemia and perioperative bleeding complications, and increase the likelihood of the patient being transfused. Patients with musculoskeletal disorders often have impaired hemostasis, potentially leading to increased perioperative blood loss. This has been described for patients with scoliosis and various types of muscular dystrophy [10, 11]. Patients with thyroid diseases may also occasionally have impaired hemostasis [12].

Fourth, *obstacles to surgical hemostasis* are also of interest. The surgeon's main aim is to operate skillfully and cause the least possible blood loss. However, there are some conditions that make this a challenge. What are they? Clearly, a procedure differs depending on whether it is being done for the first time in a patient or if it is a repeat procedure in the same patient. Reoperations tend to cause greater blood loss and have a higher transfusion rate than first-time procedures [13]. Vascular supply may be altered by a previous procedure in the same area as the proposed operation. Ask explicitly about previous surgery. Prior infection in the area of the operation may cause abnormalities. For example, after pelvic inflammation, adhesions may make patients more prone to bleeding after further surgery. Congenital alterations in anatomy may be a cause of unusual blood supply and should prompt further evaluation.

Fifth, the general condition of the patient determines how well anemia is tolerated.

Review of systems with respect to blood management

A review of body systems is a systematic way to take a history. Go through the systems from head to toe and double-check for any complaint that may have been forgotten. While not directly related to anemia and hemostasis, disturbances in almost every part of the body can have an impact on blood management. To determine the lowest acceptable hemoglobin level, find out about the patient's comorbidities.

Neurological system

A history of stroke may indicate arteriosclerosis that may decrease the patient's ability to tolerate anemia. Syncope may be a sign of anemia.

Respiratory system

The lung is essential for oxygenation and diseases of the lung may impair this process. Lung diseases such as chronic obstructive pulmonary disease may also increase the likelihood of the patient being transfused [13]. Do not forget to ask if the patient suffers from shortness of breath, asthma, chest pain, bloody sputum, or any lung diseases.

Cardiovascular system

While healthy hearts often tolerate very low hemoglobin levels, those with coronary artery disease do not tolerate anemia to the same extent. Symptoms such as ankle edema, claudication, angina pectoris, orthopnea, paroxysmal nocturnal dyspnea, dyspnea on exertion, palpitations, dizziness, etc. may all be indicators for heart (or vascular) disease.

Urogenital tract

The kidneys are the site of synthesis of erythropoietin. Therefore, dialysis-dependent as well as non–dialysis-dependent patients with kidney disease may develop renal anemia. The urinary tract and female genitalia are sites where bleeding may be visible in coagulopathy, e.g., via hematuria. As a natural form of blood loss, menstruation can also cause anemia.

Gastrointestinal tract

Occult bleeding in the gastrointestinal tract may lead to anemia. A history of peptic ulcers and gastritis indicates that the patient is prone to a recurrence of this in the perisurgical period. Further, blood loss via the gastrointestinal tract can often be prevented by prudent intervention. Worm infestations are often found in tropical countries and precipitate blood loss and vitamin deficiency with consequent anemia. Ask about the appearance of the stool. Is it dark (melena), indicating bleeding in the gastrointestinal tract? Are there indicators for worm infestations? Is there any hematemesis or abdominal pain? The liver synthesizes coagulation factors and albumin and these may be diminished if the liver is diseased. Diabetes mellitus, another disorder related to the gastrointestinal tract, is often accompanied by silent cardiovascular disease.

Skin and connective tissues

Signs of autoimmune disorders often present with skin changes. Bones and joints may be the sites of chronic disorders such as rheumatism. Diseases of the connective tissues may indirectly indicate anemia of chronic disease or hematological derangements due to autoimmune processes. In rheumatic patients, cardiopulmonary disease involvement of the serosa must not be overlooked. Some diseases of connective tissue, such as those associated with "weak tissue" (e.g., in Ehlers–Danlos syndrome, Marfan syndrome, scoliosis syndromes), are associated with a platelet disorder.

Other

Malignancies and infections often cause anemia; therefore it is beneficial to look for signs of them. Ask about any recent weight loss, night sweats, fever, shivers, rashes, lumps or masses.

The nutritional status of the patient is also of concern because this affects hematopoiesis, synthesis of factors involved in hemostasis, and the patient's general condition. A lack of vitamins K and C may cause coagulopathy.

A deficiency in B vitamins and iron can cause anemia. Both under- or mal-nutrition decrease the patient's ability to tolerate anemia, heal wounds, synthesize clotting factors, etc.

Closely related to nutrition are allergies, which should be asked about explicitly. They may cause loss of red cells and platelets. Some foods may cause hemolysis, as in favism, and should therefore be avoided.

Drugs taken by patients may hinder optimal blood management. Some drugs may cause anemia either by inducing bleeding (non-steroidal anti-inflammatory drugs [NSAIDs], coumadin), causing hemolysis, or suppressing erythropoiesis (chemotherapeutics). Other drugs may cause coagulopathies. This may be the desired effect, such as with heparin and aspirin, or the coagulopathy may be a side effect. Long-term antibiotics damage the intestinal flora, which normally synthesize vitamin K. If this is lacking, coagulopathies result. If aspirin or NSAIDs are taken, occult blood loss via the gastrointestinal tract may occur, causing anemia and iron deficiency.

It is therefore very important to have a complete list of drugs taken currently and in the recent past. This list should include non-prescription drugs, nutritional supplements, and so-called alternative medicines. A patient may not readily report on all drugs, especially if he/she fears the doctor would disapprove or because of the general perception that such drugs are harmless. Asking specifically about all drugs helps obtain a complete drug list.

Perform a physical examination

After having taken a history, continue with the physical examination of the patient. Look for signs and symptoms that support and supplement the information already obtained and keep in mind all the symptoms related to the patient's blood management.

In particular, look for signs of anemia. Pallor is the leading sign of anemia. It is most obvious on mucous membranes, conjunctivae, and nail beds. An icterus may also be indicative of anemia since it may be caused by hemolysis. A maxillary overgrowth is associated with chronic hemolytic anemia. Decubital ulcers are often associated with anemia [14]. Tachycardia is sometimes present, especially when anemia is accompanied by hypovolemia.

Further, look for signs of coagulation disorders. Ecchymosis and large deeper hematomas are signs of impaired humoral hemostasis. Petechiae are suspect for a defect or deficiency of platelets or a problem with the vessel wall.

Multiple small red spots on the lips (dilated capillaries), as found in hereditary hemorrhagic telangiectasia, bleed easily when traumatized. Patients with this disease frequently have nose bleeds and bleed from the gastrointestinal tract. Indirectly related to coagulation disorders are signs of liver disease, which may cause clotting factor deficiencies. Spider angioma, palmar erythema, dilated veins on the abdomen (caput medusae), light pink or silver colored nails, a bright, shiny, red tongue, and glossy lips are indicators for liver disease that should be evaluated further.

Signs of infections and chronic illness (e.g., rheumatic arthritis) should also be noted since such conditions may cause anemia, impair coagulation, and influence the overall condition of the patient. Hypersplenism is especially suspect since thrombocytopenia and anemia are often present. Especially before surgery in the elderly, assessment of the nutritional and volume status is mandatory.

Step 2: Laboratory and other tests

The second step in our algorithm is to order tests as indicated. Judicious use of laboratory tests adds to the evaluation. However, care must be taken to avoid undue preoperative iatrogenic blood loss. As described in Chapter 12, blood loss due to phlebotomy may be significant and may even lead to severe anemia in certain patient groups. Therefore, diagnostic phlebotomy needs to be restricted. There should be no routine order for complete laboratory work-up of patients. Order laboratory tests only if they provide potentially valuable information that will influence the treatment. The earlier history taking and physical examination will inform which laboratory values are needed. Based on the findings, decide now which tests are most likely to contribute to the therapy.

Preoperative work-up of anemia

The hemoglobin value is of central importance to the patient's blood management. In contrast to other laboratory studies, a hemoglobin level should be obtained routinely for all patients unless they present for minor surgery with little blood loss. However, if there are indications of cardiovascular or renal disease, malignancy, diabetes mellitus, aspirin or NSAIDs use, or full anticoagulation, a hemoglobin value should be obtained even in patients with only minimal expected blood loss. To reduce iatrogenic blood loss and to speed up the medical work-up, a fingerstick hemoglobin can be obtained in the office on the patient's first visit. In areas where laboratory work-up is beyond a patient's means or otherwise unavailable, the Haemoglobin Color Scale [15] recommended by the World Health Organization (WHO) can aid in estimating a patient's hemoglobin.

Once it has been established that the patient is anemic, the reason for the anemia must be found. Algorithms such as the one shown in Figure 11.2 may be used to guide the anemia work-up. A systematic search for the cause of anemia can be performed based on a complete blood count, preferably performed more than 30 days before elective surgery.

Preoperative work-up of impaired clotting

It is tempting to rely on global coagulation laboratory tests to screen for the risk of intra- and post-operative hemorrhage. Unfortunately, there is no such laboratory test that can predict this. The most common bleeding disorders cannot be detected with Quick, international normalized ratio (INR), activated partial thromboplastin time (aPTT), template bleeding time, and platelet count [16–21]. However, this is no reason to despair. A detailed history has already been taken and a physical examination has been performed. These are the most important steps in determining whether or not the patient is at risk for a coagulation problem. If the history and physical examination are negative in this respect, then it is very unlikely that the patient has a surgically relevant coagulation disorder [7]. "Patients without historical risk factors or physical findings suggestive of an increased bleeding risk are unlikely to have congenital or acquired coagulopathies that will result in increased postoperative bleeding and do not require testing" [22].

Laboratory testing is warranted for patients with a positive history of coagulation disorder or physical findings suggesting this. If the underlying disorder is already known, then laboratory testing is straightforward. Refer to Table 11.2 for the indicated tests [23].

If a thorough coagulation history of the patient is unobtainable, a set of coagulation tests may be indicated ahead of surgery with potential major blood loss. It has been suggested that Quick, aPTT, fibrinogen, platelet count, and a global platelet function test [24] be used.

If the history and physical examination reveal a bleeding disorder and there is no obvious underlying disease, start with a set of global coagulation tests. For instance, use the combination of Quick, aPTT, fibrinogen, von Willebrand factor test(s), factor XII, platelet count, and a global test for platelet function [24]. Depending on the

results of the tests, refer to Table 11.3 for patient follow-up. If diagnosis of the bleeding disorder is not straightforward or if the suggested tests are unavailable, consider sending the patient to a specialist, if available.

Preoperative work-up of accompanying disorders

Preoperative blood tests other than for hemoglobin level and coagulation profile are seldom recommended if neither the history nor physical examination gives sound reason to believe something is wrong. In certain situations, creatinine, glucose, and a pregnancy test are recommended.

Since tolerance of anemia depends on the ability of the heart to compensate for decreased red cell mass by increasing cardiac output, the heart should also be focused on in the work-up.

Step 3: Some mathematics

With the history, physical examination, and results of the tests ordered, everything reasonably possible has been done to elucidate the patient's key problems. As the third step in the algorithm, make various calculations using the variables found in the work-up. Four things are particularly important: the expected blood loss of the patient's proposed procedure, the patient's blood or red cell volume, the minimum tolerable hemoglobin or hematocrit, and the allowable blood loss.

Expected blood loss

To prepare the patient, anticipate how much blood loss can be reasonably expected. The literature abounds with reports about average blood losses for a specific surgery [25–28], but these vary widely [29]. Therefore, a blood manager must obtain estimates of average blood losses for a given procedure performed at his/her own institution. Since the blood loss with a certain procedure depends greatly on the skills of the surgeon, it is not only important to know *what* procedure will be done, but also *who* will do it. Do not hesitate to ask the surgeon for the expected blood loss. Estimating the blood loss for a certain surgical procedure is difficult and is typically underestimated. Collecting blood in graduated containers, measuring the amount of lavage fluid, and weighing sponges and drapes help, but it is still difficult because losses by evaporation and spillage onto the floor are not easy to estimate.

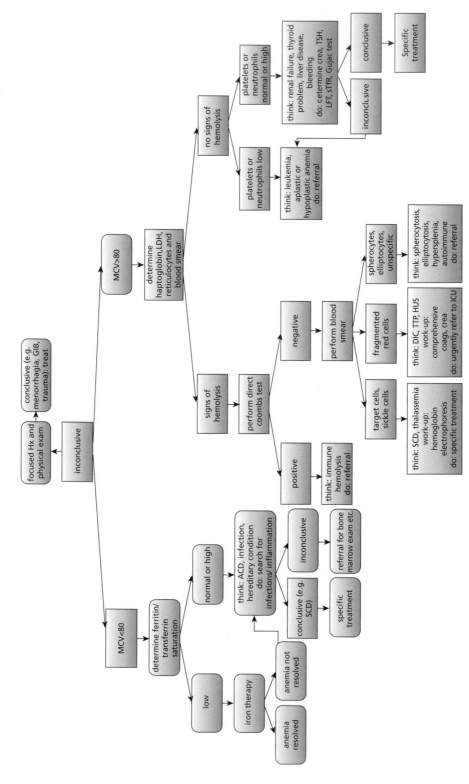

Figure 11.2 Clinical care pathway for identification and evaluation of anemia in elective surgical patients. Hx, history; GIB, gastrointestinal bleeding; MCV, mean cell volume; LDH, lactate dehydrogenase; ACD, anemia of chronic disease; SCD, sickle cell disease; TSH, thyroid stimulating hormone; LFT, liver function test; sTfR, soluble transferrin factor; DIC, disseminated intravascular coagulation; TTP, thrombotic thrombocytopenic purpura; HUS, hemolytic-uremic syndrome; ICU, intensive care unit.

Table 11.2 Laboratory tests in relation to a known or highly likely coagulation disorder.

Known or probable cause of coagulation disorder	Indicated tests
Dysfibrinogenemia	Fibrinogen level
Factor VII deficiency	Factor VII
Hemophilia A	Factor VIIIc
Hemophilia B	Factor IX
Factor XI deficiency	aPTT, factor XI
Factor XIII deficiency	Factor XIII
Von Willebrand disease	von Willebrand factor antigen, ristocetin cofactor, factor VIII activity
Patient with liver disease	Platelet count, Quick, aPTT, fibrinogen, hematocrit (possibly factors II, V, VII, IX, X, protein C, protein S, antithrombin III)
Patients with kidney disease	Quick, aPTT, platelet count, hematocrit, global platelet function test

aPTT, activated partial thromboplastin time.

Table 11.3 Follow-up of patients with a pathological coagulation test result.

Pathological test	Differential diagnosis	Further tests to confirm diagnosis
Quick	Vitamin K deficiency or therapy with vitamin K antagonist (factor V normal)	Factors II, V, VII, X, fibrinogen
	Factor synthesis in disturbed liver or loss of coagulation factors (factor V reduced)	
	Congenital deficiency of factors II, V, VII, IX, X, hypo- or dys-fibrinogenemia	
aPTT	Measure thrombin time:	
	If thrombin time is prolonged: heparin effect	
	If thrombin time is normal: factor deficiency of factors V, VIII, IX, XI, XII (also in vitamin K deficiency due to lack of factor IX)	
	Autoimmune diseases causing inhibitors	
	Factor XII deficiency does not cause increased blood loss during or after surgery	Thrombin time, factors V, VIII, IX, XI, XII
Von Willebrand test(s)	Congenital or acquired deficiency (e.g., drug-induced)	
Factor XIII assay	Acquired or congenital factor XIII deficiency	
Platelet count	Pseudothrombocytopenia, drug-related thrombocytopenia, hypersplenism, bone marrow diseases	Repeat platelet count to check for pseudothrombocytopenia, ultrasound of spleen, antiplatelet antibodies
Global platelet function test		Platelet aggregation tests

aPTT, activated partial thromboplastin time.

Methods based on the average amount of blood usually transfused can also be used to calculate how much blood a patient loses. Models to estimate blood loss are based on one, two, or three variables (uni-, bi-, tri-variate) [30]. For univariate analysis, units of blood transfused to all patients undergoing a certain procedure are recorded over a period of time. Then a calculation is made of how many units are needed so that in 80–90% of cases enough blood is available to meet the perceived need. In bivariate analysis, the units of blood transfused to patients with certain admission hematocrits are used to predict further requirements of patients with the same admission hematocrit. In trivariate analysis, the patient's blood and red cell volumes are used as the third variable. To estimate red blood cell (RBC) loss during surgery and in following 5 days, use an equation such as:

$$\text{Estimated RBC loss (mL)} = \text{BV} \times \text{Hct before surgery}$$
$$- \text{Hct on day 5 postop})$$
$$+ \text{mL of RBC transfused}$$

where Hct is the hematocrit and BV the blood volume.

In addition to variables dependent on the surgeon's skill, patient variables also influence perioperative blood loss and must be kept in mind when estimating expected blood loss. As shown above, smaller patients, females, and the elderly are at higher risk for transfusion than larger patients, males, and the young. Low preoperative hemoglobin is a predictor for transfusions. Apart from those general characteristics, procedure-specific variables may influence blood loss. Consider cardiac surgery as an example. It has been shown that cardiac patients undergoing heart surgery who are smokers, insulin-dependent diabetics with circulatory or renal manifestations, or who present with a new episode of myocardial infarction have a higher risk for transfusions than other patients. Patients who have undergone reoperations or emergency surgery, who have had a heart catheterization during the same hospitalization, who have been on cardiac bypass at low body temperature for long periods, and who have been on a low-dose heparin regimen have greater blood losses than other patients. The number of bypass grafts is a predictor for transfusions as well [3, 31–34]. Other surgeries have other risk factors for bleeding. The amount of blood loss in burn patients depends on the area of burns to be excised [35], and that in patients undergoing hip replacement depends on the way the prosthesis is fixed [36]. The presence of metastasis in surgery for colorectal cancer is associated with a higher likelihood

Table 11.4 Methods to estimate the blood volume of a patient.

EBV men [L] = (3.29 × BSA [m^2]) − 1.229

EBV women [L] = (3.47 × BSA [m^2]) − 1.954

EBV men = 2740 mL/m^2 BSA

EBV women = 2370 mL/m^2 BSA

EBV [mL] = factor for gender × body weight (kg)

Factor for men: 66 mL/kg; factor for women: 60 mL/kg (according to the American Association of Blood Banks)

Allen's formulas:

EBV men [L] = (0.417 × height [m]^3) + (0.0450 × weight [kg]) − 0.030

EBV women [L] = (0.414 × height [m]^3) + (0.0328 × weight [kg]) − 0.030

Note: Blood volume based on lean body mass tends to be more accurate than that based on actual body weight. EBV, estimated blood volume; BSA, body surface area. *Source*: The Medical Algorithm Project (www.medal.org).

for transfusions [37]. The size of a liver resection is also a predictor for the transfusion rate [38].

Estimate the blood volume of the patient

There are many methods that can be used to estimate a person's blood volume (Table 11.4). For our purposes we assume that a male has 66 mL of blood/kg ideal body weight and a female has 60 mL of blood/kg ideal body weight.

Minimum tolerable hemoglobin

Unfortunately, there is no simple calculation for the minimum tolerable hemoglobin level. To set a reasonable limit, use clinical judgment from the information from the history. A child or a healthy youth easily tolerates a hemoglobin of 5 mg/dL or less, while a sickly, elderly person may experience problems if the hemoglobin drops below 9 g/dL. Taking into consideration any comorbidities and how historical patient populations with a certain comorbidity were able to handle anemia serves as guideline. However, one must keep in mind that anemia itself is a risk factor for adverse outcomes. While most patients tolerate even severe anemia, it will reduce the patient's overall strength and his/her ability to survive any complication that may arise. Anemia may increase wound infections, cardiac events, and respiratory events, and may prolong length of hospital stay and reduce the patient's ability to recover smoothly. Therefore, if at all possible, the minimum tolerable hemoglobin should be the level that is reasonably tolerable without causing adverse outcome. It is not the point where the patient's life is threatened, nor the point at which procedures are stopped, staged or postponed, nor is it an excuse not to use blood-sparing techniques. It is the hemoglobin that is the best compromise between the benefit of the procedure and blood-sparing techniques on the one hand, and the risks of the procedure and of anemia on the other hand.

Allowable blood loss

Finally, calculate how much blood loss the patient can reasonably tolerate. Use the following equation:

$$\text{Allowable RBC loss} = (\text{blood volume} \times \text{Hct}_{actual}) - (\text{blood volume} \times \text{minimum tolerable Hct})$$

(To convert hemoglobin to hematocrit, multiply by 3. A hemoglobin of 10 mg/dL equals a hematocrit of about 30%.)

Step 4: The care plan

After completing the first three steps of the algorithm, all the information needed is available. It is now time to tailor an individual treatment concept for the patient. Having a detailed care plan is the basis for successful blood management [39, 40]; the lack of a plan may result in disaster [41].

Take a sheet of paper and begin by listing the key features of the patient and make an inventory of all obstacles to blood management, e.g., relevant drugs, malnutrition, comorbidities. This will be the problem list. A brief glance at the list will show whether care of the patient can be continued or whether support is needed. An experienced colleague may be asked to assist if there are only a limited number of problems for which help is needed. If a case is anything other than simple and straightforward, a multidisciplinary approach to the patient's blood management is the best approach. The care plan needs to be developed by a decision-making and planning team

including the patient, surgeon, anesthesiologist, hematologist, and transfusion specialist [42].

Since the patient's problems have already been listed, awareness of them should mean they can be handled with the appropriate treatment. As a team, decide how to handle the problems. Determine not only the treatment but also set therapy goals and time limits for re-evaluation, and arrange for consultations with specialists as indicated.

How much preparation and how much blood conservation is needed depend a great deal on the expected blood loss and allowable blood loss. Understandably, proceed as usual with preparation if the allowable blood loss is greater than the expected blood loss, e.g., as in a young, healthy adult undergoing a procedure with an expected blood loss of only 50 mL. On the other hand, if expected blood loss greatly exceeds the allowable blood loss or if the patient does not have sufficient reserves to compensate for blood loss, more intensive preparation is needed. The hematocrit is the strongest predictor for perioperative transfusions [3, 43]. Patients with high-normal or slightly supranormal hematocrits are less likely to receive transfusions than anemic patients. Therefore, first plan how to increase the patient's hematocrit. In any case, therapy of any bleeding disorder should also have high priority in the care plan.

Once the patient's hemoglobin level has been optimized, a new calculation is warranted. If the estimated blood loss still exceeds the allowable blood loss, measures to reduce estimated blood loss should be added to the treatment concept. In some cases it may be prudent to prepare the patient for surgery by reducing the volume of tissue to be operated on. Tumors can be downstaged by chemotherapeutic pretreatment or radiation therapy. For hypervascular tumors or organs that present a high risk of bleeding, vessels can be selectively embolized [44, 45]. Surgical and anesthetic measures to reduce blood loss should be included in the plan as well as methods using autologous blood. Decisions about the method of surgical cutting, and the use of a cell salvaging device and hemodilution should be made. Several treatment options can be combined to gain the desired effect. The blood-saving effects add up.

Procedures with expected major blood loss may at times be staged. Staged procedures (also called planned reoperation) are performed by dividing the surgery into two or more steps performed one at a time at intervals. This allows the patient to recover from the blood loss experienced in one surgical step, giving him/her time to recuperate before the next step of the procedure is performed. Proper care and especially suitably adapted alimentation facilitate the recovery. The total blood loss (and the complications) of all steps of the procedure combined may even be less than the blood loss of the same procedure performed in one step [46].

The duration of surgery is directly related to the amount of blood transfused [47]. Measures to shorten the operating time also reduce a patient's exposure to allogeneic blood. Two instead of one surgeon or other reasonable increases in team size can shorten the duration of surgery.

In recent years, computer-based planning has been advocated by some specialists. The basis for such planning is usually imaging of the area under consideration. A spiral computerized tomography (CT) scan or magnetic resonance imaging (MRI) provides details of the patient's anatomy. A three-dimensional image can be computer generated. The surgeon can study the blood supply and use a simulation program to trial different approaches to surgery. It is not clear whether this rather sophisticated method will help avoid transfusions, but it is an interesting approach to the planning of complicated procedures.

At times reducing the estimated blood loss below the allowable blood loss may seem difficult. In such a case, continue developing the care plan by re-evaluating the method for the planned surgical intervention. Often there is more than one surgical approach to the treatment of the patient. The procedure first chosen may be modified or replaced by another method. The decision on the surgical method is an important step in reducing blood loss. At times, minimally invasive techniques are superior to traditional procedures with respect to minimizing blood loss, but occasionally, expected blood loss may still exceed allowable blood loss. Under such circumstances it may be wise to consider other treatment for the patient rather than a surgical procedure. Radiation therapy may offer as good a prognosis as surgery. Chemotherapy and interventional radiology may be reasonable alternatives when there appear to be no methods available that avoid allogeneic transfusions. By taking a broader look at the therapeutic options open to patients, successful therapy may still be possible without resorting to allogeneic transfusions.

While pondering over which procedure to recommend to the patient, think also about possible emergencies that may complicate treatment. This anticipatory, provident approach to surgery leads to questions such as "What preparations need to be taken to handle such emergencies?" The care plan should include the equipment actually needed as well as the equipment to handle emergencies. If there is any uncertainty about caring for emergencies alone, back-up from a colleague is helpful.

Once decision-making has advanced to the stage where a certain approach to treatment has been decided on, put the plans down in writing. Record:
• How the patient's medical problems are to be treated, e.g., coagulation problems.
• How to optimize the hemoglobin level.
• What surgery is to be done and how it will be prepared for.
• What measures will be taken to reduce blood loss.
• What emergencies can be expected and how they will they be dealt with.

Also, list all the additional personnel, items, and drugs needed.

While trying to formulate a care plan it may become clear that certain equipment is not available in the institution or that insufficient willingness or experience is available to take care of the patient. It may not be possible to handle a potential emergency correctly. Pride on the part of the surgeon in such a situation may endanger the life of the patient. The patient's best chance of a favorable outcome may be forfeited by his/her insistence on taking care of the patient when another doctor may be in a much better position to do so. In such a situation, transfer of the patient is the only ethically and medically correct decision. Gather information about other physicians and centers where patients could be transferred in anticipation of this situation arising.

Step 5: Preparation

Prepare the patient

Treating adverse conditions

Preoperative anemia and polycythemia
Preoperative anemia is a strong predictor for perioperative transfusions [3, 13]. A considerable proportion of patients presenting for surgery with anemia develop it during hospitalization while waiting for surgery [48]. Blood sampling, recent angiography and other invasive procedures, and the effect of drugs may be the cause. It is imperative in blood management to optimize hemoglobin preoperatively and avoid further blood loss. Conditions causing anemia, such as infection, inflammation, and malignancies, should be under control whenever possible. By using rHuEPO and hematinics as described

in Chapters 3 and 4, respectively, anemia can be treated appropriately and the recommendations given in Chapter 12 will help prevent iatrogenic anemia.

Some patient populations are prone to preoperative transfusions. Among them are patients with sickle cell disease, a genetic disorder that presents with abnormal hemoglobin (HbS) that aggregates when deoxygenized and cause rigidity and sickling of the red cells. This results in hemolytic anemia and tissue injury due to vaso-occlusive diseases. Sickling of the hemoglobin and vaso-occlusive crises can be caused by surgery and anesthesia, and occur when pain, hypoxia, hypoperfusion, acidosis, dehydration, and hypothermia are present. Up to 30–40% of surgical patients with sickle cell disease develop complications such as vaso-occlusive crises or acute chest syndrome. These are reported even for minor surgery. In an attempt to reduce these incidences, exchange transfusion has been performed before surgery. However, it was shown that in comparison to simple top-up transfusion, this does not reduce the development of sickle cell complications but does increase transfusion complications. Currently, a trial is underway to clarify whether there is a difference between the outcomes of preoperatively transfused versus non-transfused sickle cell patients [49]. Based on clinical experience, but without solid scientific proof, some measures should be taken to prevent unnecessary sickling and hemolysis in the perioperative period. These measures include giving oral liquids as close to the surgery as possible, administering intravenous fluids, maintaining normocapnia and normothermia, and avoiding any undue pain and surgical stress by using the least invasive surgical approach possible. Besides, patients for elective surgery should be in the best possible condition. Some drugs may help in this regard. Hydroxyurea, an antineoplastic agent that increases fetal hemoglobin, improves anemia in sickle cell patients, and is also used to reduce their exposure to donor blood and improve their survival [50]. Other promising therapies include butyrate compounds and antiadhesion agents. Preoperatively, hydroxyurea or another suitable therapy should be initiated to increase the safety margin for patients with sickle cell disease. Close cooperation between the patient, his/her hematologist, and the surgeon is needed to choose the best available preparation method for surgery.

Patients with polycythemia have a high risk of perisurgical hemorrhage. Untoward effects are also due to hyperviscosity. Treatment before surgery is preferable. Phlebotomies, hydroxyurea, radioactive phosphorus, interferon, anagrelide, and antiplatelet medications are all used and the best choice is the subject of debate. No matter what treatment approach is used, elective surgery should be postponed until the red cell and platelet counts are normalized. In an emergency, phlebotomy is the treatment of choice.

Coagulation disorders

Functional hemostatic processes are vital for minimum blood loss. Preoperative optimization of the patient's capability for hemostasis includes treatment as well as prevention of coagulation disorders.

Treat coagulopathies

Now that the patient's work-up has been completed, the cause of any bleeding disorder should be apparent and can be treated.

Von Willebrand disease is a relatively common inherited bleeding disorder. Desmopressin is the treatment of choice in most patients. In selected cases, a factor concentrate may be indicated. Cryoprecipitate would work as well, but is no longer recommended due to the risks involved [42].

Hemophilia A and B are inherited coagulation disorders with well-defined sequelae. Even if no major bleeding episodes have occurred so far, surgery may be a sufficient trigger to cause excessive intra- and postoperative bleeding if no treatment is given. The treatment typically is administration of desmopressin or replacement of the missing coagulation factor. For the latter, a variety of products are available, both derived from human blood and recombinant products. Keeping the kinetics of the factors in mind, replacement therapy is best started just prior to surgery and continued until wound healing has progressed sufficiently.

Chronic renal failure causes a uremic bleeding disorder characterized by thrombocytopathy, altered plasma coagulation, anemia, and vessel wall abnormalities [51]. If there is still time for preparation, anemia should be corrected with erythopoietin. Patients with end-stage renal disease should be intensively dialyzed on the day before surgery. If the patient is dialyzed on the day of surgery, it may be prudent to wait at least 12 hours to be sure the dialysis heparin has been metabolized and therefore avoid excessive bleeding during surgery [52, 53]. Peritoneal dialysis seems to be superior to conventional dialysis in reducing bleeding risk. To further treat uremic coagulopathy, desmopressin, conjugated estrogens, low-dose transdermal estrogens or estrogen–progesterone combinations can be used. Cryoprecipitate may also be administered in selected cases [23]. The algorithm found in the article by Hedges *et al.* [51] can guide the use of the above mentioned therapeutics in different clinical settings of uremic bleeding.

Patients whose coagulopathy is due to an underlying liver disease may present with a multifactoral bleeding disorder comprising thrombocytopathy and thrombocytopenia, lack of plasma coagulation factors, and accelerated fibrinolysis. Depending on the leading coagulation problem, antifibrinolytics, factor concentrates, or conjugated estrogens may be indicated [54].

Some patients with dysproteinemias and myeloproliferative syndromes sometimes have excessive bleeding that appears to be caused by abnormal platelet function. In these patients, bleeding symptoms usually respond to appropriate therapy, such as plasmapheresis or cytoreductive therapy [55].

Thrombocytopenia in patients with rheumatic or other autoimmune diseases is often caused by increased platelet destruction. Steroids, danazol, intravenous immunoglobulin, or splenectomy are treatment options that should be considered before surgery.

Manage anticoagulation

Therapeutic anticoagulation is a common treatment for a variety of disorders. When patients under anticoagulation present for surgery, anticoagulation drugs may increase the surgical blood loss [56, 57]. Whenever safely possible, these should be substituted for an agent that is easily reversible, stopped, or antagonized. The risk of thrombosis or embolism may increase when medications for anticoagulation are stopped and this should be taken into consideration. Weighing the competing risks of thromboembolism and bleeding is therefore prudent. Skillful surgery may avoid major bleeding complications even in anticoagulated patients.

Vitamin K antagonism is a common treatment principle to induce anticoagulation. In elective surgery, time

Table 11.5 Monitoring and reversal of common anticoagulants.

Agent	Coumarin and derivatives	Unfractionated heparin	Low-molecular-weight heparin	Fondaparinux pentasaccharide	Dabigatran	Danaparoid	Hirudin	Lepirudin	Bivalirudin
Mode of action	Antagonism of vitamin K	Binds to AT III for indirect thrombin inhibition	Activates AT III to inhibit FIIa and FXa	Binds to AT to neutralize FXa	Inhibits thrombin	Inhibits FXa and to lesser degree FIIa	Direct thrombin inhibitor	Direct thrombin inhibitor, almost irreversible	Thrombin inhibitor, reversible
Monitoring	INR, Quick	aPTT, platelet count for HIT detection	Anti-Xa-test	May be not needed	May not be needed	Anti-Xa-activity	aPTT thrombin time, ecarin clotting time	aPTT [76] thrombin time, ecarin clotting time	ACT
Reversal	Prothrombin complex concentrate, FEIBA, rHuFVIIa [60, 61], vitamin K	Specific antidote; protamine sulfate; consider: PEG-modified protamine heparinase I, certain peptides	Protamine reverses about 60% of anti-Xa activity	No specific antidote; try rHuFVIIa	Not available	No specific antidote; protamine reverses slightly; certain peptides	Dialysis with specialized equipment	Dialysis with specialized equipment	Case report: mix of hemodialysis, modified ultrafiltration, rFVIIa, FFP, Cryo-ppt

Note: The "Reversal" column lists not only well-established methods of reversal of anticoagulants or treatment of anticoagulant-induced bleeding, but also therapies whose value is not yet fully understood.
AT, antithrombin; FIIa, factor IIa; FXa, factor Xa; rHuFVIIa, recombinant human factor VIIa; HIT, heparin-induced thrombocytopenia; aPTT, activated partial thromboplastin time; FEIBA, factor eight inhibitor bypassing activity; FFP, fresh frozen plasma; Cryo-ppt, cryoprecipitate; GPIIb/IIa, glycoprotein IIb/IIa; TEG, thromboelastography.

can be built into the care plan for the effect of the vitamin K antagonists to wear off. Vitamin K administration speeds up this process. Emergency reversal is at times indicated. If patients are at significant risk of developing embolic complications when anticoagulation is interrupted, oral anticoagulation should be stopped temporarily, and for the briefest of intervals, to allow surgery to be performed. Perioperatively, such patients on vitamin K antagonists should be treated with full-dose heparin instead of vitamin K antagonists. This permits emergency reversal with protamine if bleeding occurs.

Another common anticoagulant is aspirin, an antiplatelet agent. It has been documented as a reason for an increased risk of perioperative bleeding [56], although this effect has not been demonstrated in other studies. The antiplatelet effect of aspirin is pronounced if the patient has taken other anticoagulants, has a pre-existing problem with hemostasis, or if alcohol is taken concurrently [53]. Since aspirin irreversibly inhibits thromboxane synthesis in platelets, it is best stopped several days before surgery and the surgeon should wait until functional platelets are produced.

Nowadays many other anticoagulants are used in clinical practice. Table 11.5 provides an overview of the available drugs and potential reversal methods if reversal becomes necessary [58–79].

Avoid pharmacological coagulopathies

Many drugs are not used for anticoagulation but nevertheless affect hemostasis (Table 11.6) [53, 80, 81]. Whether all such drug effects translate into increased perioperative bleeding has not yet been determined. However, if at all possible, such pharmacologically-induced coagulopathies should be avoided. Often it is possible to switch from one drug to another or to stop

Argatroban	Prasugrel	Clopidogrel	Tirofiban	Abciximab	Dipyridamole	Aspirin	Ticlopidine	Rivaroxaban	Eptifibatide
Direct thrombin inhibitor	Inhibits $P2Y_{12}$ platelet ADP receptor	Irreversible blockage of platelet ADP receptor	GPIIb/IIIa inhibitor	Blocks GPIIb/IIIa receptor of platelets		Thromboxane inhibition	Irreversible blockage of platelet ADP receptor	Direct FXa inhibitor	GPIIb/IIIa inhibitor
aPTT	Possibly by light transmission aggregometry (VN-P2Y12)	Specific platelet function tests (aggregometry or platelet count ratio) using ADP as an activator, platelet count		Hemodyne analysis, modified TEG	Platelet function assay			Not necessary	
	Not available		Dialysis, possibly desmopressin or rHuFVIIa, fibrinogen/cryo-ppt		Aprotinin, desmopressin, rHuFVIIa, plasmapheresis	Desmopressin	Desmopressin, fibrinogen/cryo-ppt	Not available	Desmopressin

Table 11.6 Examples of drugs and herbs that can cause coagulopathies and may increase perioperative blood loss.

Non-steroidal anti-inflammatory drugs
Penicillin
Some cephalosporins such as cefotaxime, moxalactam
Quinidine
Alteplase
Protamine
Nifedipine
Nitroglycerine
Paroxetine, fluvoxamine (vitamin C)
High-dose vitamin C
Valproate
St John's wort
Ginger
Garlic
Certain hydroxyethyl starches (desmopressin)

Note: The agents in parenthesis may be used to counteract pharmacological coagulopathies.

the drug altogether. Drug-induced coagulopathies can be antidoted occasionally.

Cardiopulmonary and general condition

In coronary artery disease, the ability to increase the cardiac output is impaired, thus limiting the patient's ability to tolerate anemia. It is important to avoid cardiac ischemia. Perioperative analgesia, anxiolytic medications, normothermia, judicious beta-blockade, and close monitoring for cardiac events are recommended [82]. If the patient has had beta-blockers before surgery, these should be continued to prevent withdrawal, which may otherwise cause ischemia. The perioperative risk for ischemia can also be reduced by preoperative coronary revascularization.

There are several measures available to optimize a patient's pulmonary function prior to surgery. Incentive spirometry before and after surgery should be encouraged in patients with pulmonary problems. Medical therapy is at times indicated, such as bronchodilators for wheezing, and beta-agonists and atropine analogs in patients with asthma and chronic obstructive pulmonary disease.

Optimizing the surgical field

In certain situations it seems prudent to optimize the surgical field. There are several methods for reducing

the surgical field, e.g., reducing the size of a tumor by preoperative chemotherapy or radiation. The vascularity of the surgical field can also be reduced. Preoperative embolization for primary tumors and metastases, as well as for whole organs, can reduce perfusion and thus blood loss [83–85]. Pharmacological therapy may be equally effective in selected cases. For instance, finasteride given before benign prostate hyperplasia operations reduces both angiogenesis in the prostate and bleeding [86–88].

Patient education

By definition, blood management is patient centered. This means that at all times the patient is the center of all efforts. It is crucial, therefore, to actively include him/her in the preparations for surgery or any other treatment. This is essential for a good patient–doctor relationship and improves patient compliance. The patient can do much to reduce exposure to donor blood. All patients should be advised not to take drugs on their own initiative. Patients need to understand that a single aspirin for a headache or menstrual discomfort can increase blood loss. Sound habits such as healthy nutrition, sufficient sleep, and abstinence of noxae are very basic measures, but these improve a patient's general condition. Moderate physical exercise may improve not only the overall condition of the patient but may also improve anemia [89]. An information booklet may be handed to the patient detailing the planned blood management procedures. It may also include a summary of what the patient can do during the treatment and perisurgical period. Such a booklet may remind the patient of the need to adhere to the prescribed schedule of therapy.

Prepare the equipment

Hours before the battle of Waterloo, Napoleon Bonaparte told his generals: "This affair will be no more serious than eating one's breakfast." Shortly thereafter, however, he was proven wrong. It was raining. The raindrops rendered the weapons useless, made the roads muddy and impassable for war wagons, blocked the vision of the combatants, and left the soldiers soaked to the skin. The battle at Waterloo was lost, at least in part, because proper, water-proof equipment was lacking. Something as insignificant as raindrops defeated Napoleon. Experience gained in years of campaigning was rendered useless due to the presence of rain. This drives home an important point. The most sophisticated equipment is of little use if it is damaged or unavailable. Therefore, make sure all devices and drugs are to hand before surgery. When it starts pouring and vision is obscured, equipment must be readily available to master the situation. Always prepare the equipment and have the required drugs available to ensure the patient does not meet his/her Waterloo.

Preparation should not only involve getting ready for the intended procedure; emergency equipment should also be made ready. One suggestion is to prepare an emergency tray with all that is required to treat sudden massive bleeding [90]. The contents of such a tray can be tailored to the specialty and skills of the surgeon. It may contain tourniquets, tamponade materials, catheters to block vessels, special clamps, glues, mashes, balloons, etc. It may also contain copies of algorithms that guide the management of emergency or heavy bleeding [90]. Having such a tray ready saves time in an emergency and may reduce the total blood loss.

Be prepared

The duration of a surgical procedure influences the degree of blood loss. Independent of other factors, long operation times increase blood loss. However, speeding up a procedure at the expense of quality does not reduce blood loss. Rehearsing the procedure before going to the operating theater is wise, because the surgeon will then have the steps of the procedure fresh in his/her mind. This may not only shorten the duration of the procedure but also improve the quality of the operation, both of which reduce blood loss.

Key points

- Algorithm for preparation of a patient for surgery:
  1. Take a thorough history and perform a physical examination, paying special attention to obstacles to transfusion avoidance and matters pertaining to blood management; review test results already available.
  2. Order laboratory and other tests if these are clearly indicated, but beware of iatrogenic blood loss.
  3. Based on the findings of 1 and 2, calculate the allowable blood loss, blood volumes, and determine the lowest tolerable hematocrit.
  4. Formulate a care plan (with a timetable). It should include the allowable blood loss and the expected blood loss. Record:
     ◦ How the patient's medical problems will be treated, e.g., coagulation problems
     ◦ How to optimize the hemoglobin level

◦ What surgery is to be done and what preparations are necessary
◦ What measures will be taken to reduce blood loss
◦ What emergencies can be expected and how these will be dealt with.
   Further, list all additional personnel, items, and drugs required.
  5. Prepare the patient and the equipment, and make personal preparation in accord with the care plan.

Questions for review

1. What are the vital steps to prepare a patient for surgery in a blood management program?
2. How do drugs influence the blood management of patients?
3. What measures need to be taken to work-up a patient with anemia and a patient with a coagulopathy?
4. What preparations are required for surgery in a blood management program?

Suggestions for further research

Compile a list of drugs that have an impact on surgical blood loss.

   List the laboratory tests for coagulation and evaluate their value as predictors for surgical blood loss.

Exercises and practice cases

Answer the following questions:
1. A patient does not complain of any signs of a bleeding disorder. During the physical examination petechiae and a splenomegaly are found. Which laboratory tests should be ordered for the patient?
2. Last week, a patient presented with a Quick of 28%. He was treated with appropriate doses of vitamin K. Today, he presents with a Quick of 35%. What needs to be done?
3. A female patient complains of heavy menstrual bleeding, although no obvious anatomical pathology is found in a gynecological exam. Otherwise, she is healthy. Her Quick is 114%, her aPTT is 24 seconds, her platelet count is 250, and her hematocrit is 28%. What tests should be ordered?
4. A male patient presents for elective hip replacement. He is scheduled for surgery in 3 weeks. On questioning,

he states that he usually takes up to 2.5 g of aspirin/day about once a week for tension headache. Otherwise he is healthy. What tests should be ordered?

> Miss B is 70 years old; she has been sent by her family doctor for bilateral hip replacement. She suffers from a long-standing arthrosis. She has never had an operation before.
>
> Miss B lives alone on the third floor of an apartment building and has increasing difficulty climbing stairs. Her friend Millie used to have the same trouble. Once she received artificial joints, Millie says she was again able to go for extended walks in the park. Miss B wants to join her friend and asks for the same procedure.
>
> Among other information the letter from Miss B's doctor contains the following:
>
> Her height is 1.60 m and weight 55 kg
>
> Miss B takes the following drugs:
> - Amiodarone tablets 200 mg per os 1-0-0-0
> - Coumarin tablets 3 mg per os depending on the INR
> - Ibuprofen tablets 400 mg per os 1-1-1-1.
>
> Current laboratory test results:
> - Hematocrit 30%
> - Hemoglobin 10 g/dL (red cell indices: mean corpuscular volume and mean corpuscular hemoglobin content decreased)
> - Leukocytes 8000
> - Platelets 250 000
> - Electrolyte profile, liver and kidney panel unremarkable.
>
> Experience shows that implanting a single artificial hip joint causes the loss of 1000 mL of whole blood.

Introduce Miss B to a colleague. Discuss in a multidisciplinary fashion how her treatment should be continued and write a care plan for Miss B.

What is the allowable blood loss for patients with the following characteristics:

1. A 66-kg male with a minimum tolerable hematocrit of 20% and a current hematocrit of 45%?
2. A 100-kg male with a minimum tolerable hematocrit of 30% and a current hematocrit of 33%?
3. A 40-kg female with a minimum tolerable hematocrit of 25% and a current hematocrit of 37%?

Homework

Take a focused history from three surgical patients in the hospital; be sure to obtain all the data required for the patients' blood management.

Go to the hospital laboratory and find out whether platelet function tests are available. If so, obtain more information on them.

Find out what the three most common congenital and three most common acquired bleeding disorders in your field of practice are.

Following the example of Table 11.7, draw up a list of contents for an emergency hemorrhage tray or chart for at least one of the following departments: Emergency department (acute trauma care), gastroenterology, urology, operating room for unexpected major bleeding, pediatrics, ENT, or any other you prefer.

Table 11.7 Proposal for emergency hemorrhage equipment used in obstetrics and gynecology.

Drugs/glues	Equipment	Laminated emergency information	Remarks
Tranexamic acid, desmopressin, conjugated estrogens, aprotinin, oxytocin, ergot derivative, prostaglandin analogs (Carboprost, Misoprostol), anticoagulant for cell salvage (heparin, citrate), vasopressin and glues for enhancement of packing, other topical hemostatics (gelatin, collagen, etc.)	Packing (5-yard roll), balloon device for uterine tamponade (Foley, Sengstaken- Blakemore, Bakri), straight (10 cm) eyed-needles and large curved eyed-needles for use with No. 1 suture, 3 Heaney vaginal retractors, 4 sponge forceps, container and suction for cell salvage	Diagrams + instructions for the various types of compression sutures and tamponade techniques; algorithm for non-blood management of postpartum hemorrhage, phone number of radiology dept. (embolization), pharmacy (rHuFVIIa), dosage and indications for mentioned drugs	Determine storage time, sterilization, responsible persons, intervals of checks, training

References

1. Drager LF, Abe JM, Martins MA, Lotufo PA, Benseñor IJ. Impact of clinical experience on quantification of clinical signs at physical examination. *J Intern Med* 2003;**254**: 257–263.
2. Keating EM. Preoperative evaluation and methods to reduce blood use in orthopedic surgery. *Anesthesiol Clin North Am* 2005;**23**:305–313, vi–vii.
3. Scott BH, Seifert FC, Glass PS, Grimson R. Blood use in patients undergoing coronary artery bypass surgery: impact of cardiopulmonary bypass pump, hematocrit, gender, age, and body weight. *Anesth Analg*, 2003;**97**: 958–963.
4. Khanna MP, Hebert PC, Fergusson DA. Review of the clinical practice literature on patient characteristics associated with perioperative allogeneic red blood cell transfusion. *Transfus Med Rev* 2003;**17**:110–119.
5. Scott BH, Seifert FC, Glass PS. Does gender influence resource utilization in patients undergoing off-pump coronary artery bypass surgery? *J Cardiothorac Vasc Anesth* 2003; **17**:346–351.
6. Tzilinis A, Lofman AM, Tzarnas CD. Transfusion requirements for TRAM flap postmastectomy breast reconstruction. *Ann Plast Surg* 2003;**50**:623–627.
7. Liumbruno GM, Bennardello F, Lattanzio A, Piccoli P, Rossetti G; Italian Society of Transfusion Medicine and Immunohaematology (SIMTI) Working Party. Recommendations for the transfusion management of patients in the perioperative period. I. The pre-operative period. *Blood Transfus* 2011;**9**:19–40.
8. Kadir RA, Economides DL, Sabin CA, Owens D, Lee CA. Frequency of inherited bleeding disorders in women with menorrhagia. *Lancet* 1998;**351**:485–489.
9. Rapaport SI. Preoperative hemostatic evaluation: which tests, if any? *Blood* 1983;**61**:229–231.
10. Saito T, Takenaka M, Miyai I, *et al.* Coagulation and fibrinolysis disorder in muscular dystrophy. *Muscle Nerve* 2001;**24**:399–402.
11. Noordeen MH, Haddad FS, Muntoni F, Gobbi P, Hollyer JS, Bentley G. Blood loss in Duchenne muscular dystrophy: vascular smooth muscle dysfunction? *J Pediatr Orthop B* 1999;**8**:212–215.
12. Franchini M. Hemostasis and thyroid diseases revisited. *J Endocrinol Invest* 2004;**27**:886–892.
13. Ouattara A, Niculescu M, Boccara G, *et al.* [Identification of risk factors for allogeneic transfusion in cardiac surgery from an observational study.] *Ann Fr Anesth Reanim* 2003;**22**:278–283.
14. Bergquist S, Frantz R. Pressure ulcers in community-based older adults receiving home health care. Prevalence, incidence, and associated risk factors. *Adv Wound Care* 1999;**12**: 339–351.
15. Dobson M. World Health Organization Haemoglobin Colour Scale: a practical answer to a vital need. *Anesthesia* 2002;**15**:Article 18.
16. Asaf T, Reuveni H, Yermiahu T, *et al.* The need for routine pre-operative coagulation screening tests (prothrombin time PT/partial thromboplastin time PTT) for healthy children undergoing elective tonsillectomy and/or adenoidectomy. *Int J Pediatr Otorhinolaryngol* 2001;**61**:217–222.
17. Gewirtz AS, Kottke-Marchant K, Miller ML. The preoperative bleeding time test: assessing its clinical usefulness. *Cleve Clin J Med* 1995;**62**:379–382.
18. Gewirtz AS, Miller ML, Keys TF. The clinical usefulness of the preoperative bleeding time. *Arch Pathol Lab Med* 1996;**120**:353–356.
19. Peterson P, Hayes TE, *et al.* The preoperative bleeding time test lacks clinical benefit: College of American Pathologists' and American Society of Clinical Pathologists' position article. *Arch Surg* 1998;**133**:134–139.
20. Zwack GC, Derkay CS. The utility of preoperative hemostatic assessment in adenotonsillectomy. *Int J Pediatr Otorhinolaryngol* 1997;**39**:67–76.
21. Derkay CS. A cost-effective approach for preoperative hemostatic assessment in children undergoing adenotonsillectomy. *Arch Otolaryngol Head Neck Surg* 2000;**126**:688.
22. Eckman MH, Erban JK, Singh SK, Kao GS. Screening for the risk for bleeding or thrombosis. *Ann Intern Med* 2003;**138**: W15–W24.
23. DeLoughery TG. Management of bleeding with uremia and liver disease. *Curr Opin Hematol* 1999;**6**:329–333.
24. Dempfle CE. Perioperative Gerinnungsdiagnostik. *Anaesthesist* 2005;**54**:167–177.
25. Hu SS. Blood loss in adult spinal surgery. *Eur Spine J* 2004;**13** (Suppl 1):S3–S5.
26. Senthil Kumar G, Von Arx OA, Pozo JL. Rate of blood loss over 48 hours following total knee replacement. *Knee* 2005;**12**:307–309.
27. Yuasa T, Niwa N, Kimura S, *et al.* Intraoperative blood loss during living donor liver transplantation: an analysis of 635 recipients at a single center. *Transfusion* 2005;**45**:879–884.
28. Cushner FD, Scott WN, Scuderi G, Hill K, Insall JN. Blood loss and transfusion rates in bilateral total knee arthroplasty. *J Knee Surg* 2005;**18**:102–107.
29. Surgenor DM, Churchill WH, Wallace EL, *et al.* The specific hospital significantly affects red cell and component transfusion practice in coronary artery bypass graft surgery: a study of five hospitals. *Transfusion* 1998;**38**:122–134.
30. NATA. *TAB: Transfusion Medicine and Alternatives to Blood Transfusion.* 2000 Edition. Available on http://www.nataonline.com/CONNATTex2.php3.
31. Surgenor DM, Churchill WH, Wallace EL, *et al.* Determinants of red cell, platelet, plasma, and cryoprecipitate transfusions during coronary artery bypass graft surgery: the Collaborative Hospital Transfusion Study. *Transfusion* 1996;**36**:521–532.

32. Despotis GJ, Filos KS, Zoys TN, Hogue CW Jr, Spitznagel E, Lappas DG. Factors associated with excessive postoperative blood loss and hemostatic transfusion requirements: a multivariate analysis in cardiac surgical patients. *Anesth Analg* 1996;**82**:13–21.

33. Parr KG, Patel MA, Dekker R, *et al.* Multivariate predictors of blood product use in cardiac surgery. *J Cardiothorac Vasc Anesth* 2003;**17**:176–181.

34. Moskowitz DM, Klein JJ, Shander A, *et al.* Predictors of transfusion requirements for cardiac surgical procedures at a blood conservation center. *Ann Thorac Surg* 2004;**77**:626–634.

35. Criswell KK, Gamelli RL. Establishing transfusion needs in burn patients. *Am J Surg* 2005;**189**:324–326.

36. Grosflam JM, Wright EA, Cleary PD, Katz JN. Predictors of blood loss during total hip replacement surgery. *Arthritis Care Res* 1995;**8**:167–173.

37. Nilsson KR, Berenholtz SM, Dorman T, *et al.* Preoperative predictors of blood transfusion in colorectal cancer surgery. *J Gastrointest Surg* 2002;**6**:753–762.

38. Mariette D, Smadja C, Naveau S, Borgonovo G, Vons C, Franco D. Preoperative predictors of blood transfusion in liver resection for tumor. *Am J Surg* 1997;**173**:275–279.

39. Hunt PS. Bleeding ulcer: timing and technique in surgical management. *Aust N Z J Surg* 1986;**56**:25–30.

40. Forest RJ, Groom RC, Quinn R, Donnelly J, Clark C. Repair of hypoplastic left heart syndrome of a 4.25-kg Jehovah's Witness. *Perfusion* 2002;**17**:221–225.

41. Lawry K, Slomka J, Goldfarb J. What went wrong: multiple perspectives on an adolescent's decision to refuse blood transfusions. *Clin Pediatr (Phila)* 1996;**35**:317–321.

42. Bolan CD, Rick ME, Polly DW Jr. Transfusion medicine management for reconstructive spinal repair in a patient with von Willebrand's disease and a history of heavy surgical bleeding. *Spine*, 2001;**26**:E552–E556.

43. de Andrade JR, Jove M, Landon G, Frei D, Guilfoyle M, Young DC. Baseline hemoglobin as a predictor of risk of transfusion and response to Epoetin alfa in orthopedic surgery patients. *Am J Orthop* 1996;**25**:533–542.

44. Hansen ME, Kadir S. Elective and emergency embolotherapy in children and adolescents. Efficacy and safety. *Radiologe* 1990;**30**:331–336.

45. Chou MM, Hwang JI, Tseng JJ, Ho ES. Internal iliac artery embolization before hysterectomy for placenta accreta. *J Vasc Interv Radiol* 2003;**14**:1195–1199.

46. Tsirikos AI, Chang WN, Dabney KW, Miller F. Comparison of one-stage versus two-stage anteroposterior spinal fusion in pediatric patients with cerebral palsy and neuromuscular scoliosis. *Spine (Phil PA 1996)* 2003;**28**:1300–1305.

47. Matin SF, Abreu S, Ramani A, *et al.* Evaluation of age and comorbidity as risk factors after laparoscopic urological surgery. *J Urol* 2003;**170**:1115–1120.

48. Karski JM, Mathieu M, Cheng D, Carroll J, Scott GJ. Etiology of preoperative anemia in patients undergoing scheduled cardiac surgery. *Can J Anaesth* 1999;**46**:979–982.

49. Firth PG, McMillan KN, Haberkern CM, Yaster M, Bender MA, Goodwin SR. A survey of perioperative management of sickle cell disease in North America. *Pediatr Anesth* 2011;**21**:43–49.

50. Steinberg MH, McCarthy WF, Castro O, *et al.*; Investigators of the Multicenter Study of Hydroxyurea in Sickle Cell Anemia and MSH Patients' Follow-Up. The risks and benefits of long-term use of hydroxyurea in sickle cell anemia. A 17.5 year follow-up. *Am J Hematol* 2010;**85**:403–408.

51. Hedges SJ. Evidence-based treatment recommendations for uremic bleeding. *Nat Clin Pract Nephrol* 2007;**3**:138–158.

52. Krishnan M. Preoperative care of patients with kidney disease. *Am Fam Physician* 2002;**66**:1471–1476, 1379.

53. George JN, Shattil SJ. The clinical importance of acquired abnormalities of platelet function. *N Engl J Med* 1991;**324**:27–39.

54. Chou R, DeLoughery TG. Recurrent thromboembolic disease following splenectomy for pyruvate kinase deficiency. *Am J Hematol* 2001;**67**:197–199.

55. Papers to Appear in Forthcoming Issues. *Gynecol Oncol* 1998;**68**:218.

56. Ferraris VA, Ferraris SP, Lough FC, Berry WR. Preoperative aspirin ingestion increases operative blood loss after coronary artery bypass grafting. *Ann Thorac Surg* 1988;**45**:71–74.

57. Chu MW, Wilson SR, Novick RJ, Stitt LW, Quantz MA. Does clopidogrel increase blood loss following coronary artery bypass surgery? *Ann Thorac Surg* 2004;**78**:1536–1541.

58. Kessler CM. Current and future challenges of antithrombotic agents and anticoagulants: strategies for reversal of hemorrhagic complications. *Semin Hematol* 2004;**41** (Suppl 1):44–50.

59. van Aart L, Eijkhout HW, Kamphuis JS, *et al.* Individualized dosing regimen for prothrombin complex concentrate more effective than standard treatment in the reversal of oral anticoagulant therapy: an open, prospective randomized controlled trial. *Thromb Res* 2006;**118**:313–320.

60. Levi M, Bijsterveld NR, Keller TT. Recombinant factor VIIa as an antidote for anticoagulant treatment. *Semin Hematol* 2004;**41** (Suppl 1):65–69.

61. Freeman WD, Brott TG, Barrett KM, *et al.* Recombinant factor VIIa for rapid reversal of warfarin anticoagulation in acute intracranial hemorrhage. *Mayo Clin Proc* 2004;**79**:1495–1500.

62. Hanslik T, Prinseau J. The use of vitamin K in patients on anticoagulant therapy: a practical guide. *Am J Cardiovasc Drugs* 2004;**4**:43–55.

63. Baker RI, Coughlin PB, Gallus AS, *et al.*; Warfarin Reversal Consensus Group. Warfarin reversal: consensus guidelines, on behalf of the Australasian Society of Thrombosis and Haemostasis. *Med J Aust* 2004;**181**:492–497.

64. Chang LC, Lee HF, Chung MJ, Yang VC. PEG-modified protamine with improved pharmacological/pharmaceutical properties as a potential protamine substitute: synthesis and in vitro evaluation. *Bioconjug Chem* 2005;**16**:147–155.

65. Stafford-Smith M, Lefrak EA, Qazi AG, et al. Efficacy and safety of heparinase I versus protamine in patients undergoing coronary artery bypass grafting with and without cardiopulmonary bypass. Anesthesiology 2005;103: 229–240.

66. Schick BP, Gradowski JF, San Antonio JD, Martinez J. Novel design of peptides to reverse the anticoagulant activities of heparin and other glycosaminoglycans. Thromb Haemost 2001;85:482–487.

67. Warkentin TE, Crowther MA. Reversing anticoagulants both old and new. Can J Anaesth 2002;49:S11–S25.

68. Stratmann G, deSilva AM, Tseng EE, et al. Reversal of direct thrombin inhibition after cardiopulmonary bypass in a patient with heparin-induced thrombocytopenia. Anesth Analg 2004;98:1635–1639.

69. Bodendiek I, Lentz S, Seeger M, Bruhn HD. [Chromogenic substrate as antidote against the thrombin inhibitor Melagatran.] Hamostaseologie 2003;23:97–98.

70. Elg M, Carlsson S, Gustafsson D. Effect of activated prothrombin complex concentrate or recombinant factor VIIa on the bleeding time and thrombus formation during anticoagulation with a direct thrombin inhibitor. Thromb Res 2001;101:145–157.

71. Reiter RA, Mayr F, Blazicek H, et al. Desmopressin antagonizes the in vitro platelet dysfunction induced by GPIIb/IIIa inhibitors and aspirin. Blood 2003;102:4594–4599.

72. Li YF, Spencer FA, Becker RC. Comparative efficacy of fibrinogen and platelet supplementation on the in vitro reversibility of competitive glycoprotein IIb/IIIa (alphaIIb/beta3) receptor-directed platelet inhibition. Am Heart J 2001;142:204–210.

73. Akowuah E, Shrivastava V, Jamnadas B, et al. Comparison of two strategies for the management of antiplatelet therapy during urgent surgery. Ann Thorac Surg 2005;80:149–152.

74. Nacul FE, de Moraes E, Penido C, Paiva RB, Méier-Neto JG. Massive nasal bleeding and hemodynamic instability associated with clopidogrel. Pharm World Sci 2004;26:6–7.

75. Samama MM, Gerotziafas GT, Elalamy I, Horellou MH, Conard J. Biochemistry and clinical pharmacology of new anticoagulant agents. Pathophysiol Haemost Thromb 2002;32:218–224.

76. Lubenow N, Greinacher A. Drugs for the prevention and treatment of thrombosis in patients with heparin-induced thrombocytopenia. Am J Cardiovasc Drugs 2001;1:429–443.

77. Dyke CM, Koster A, Veale JJ, Maier GW, McNiff T, Levy JH. Preemptive use of bivalirudin for urgent on-pump coronary artery bypass grafting in patients with potential heparin-induced thrombocytopenia. Ann Thorac Surg 2005;80:299–303.

78. Greilich PE, Alving BM, Longnecker D, et al. Near-site monitoring of the antiplatelet drug abciximab using the Hemodyne analyzer and modified thrombelastograph. J Cardiothorac Vasc Anesth 1999;13:58–64.

79. Tanaka KA, Szlam F, Kelly AB, Vega JD, Levy JH. Clopidogrel (Plavix) and cardiac surgical patients: implications for platelet function monitoring and postoperative bleeding. Platelets 2004;15:325–332.

80. Tielens JA. Vitamin C for paroxetine- and fluvoxamine-associated bleeding. Am J Psychiatry 1997;154:883–884.

81. Winter SL, Kriel RL, Novacheck TF, Luxenberg MG, Leutgeb VJ, Erickson PA. Perioperative blood loss: the effect of valproate. Pediatr Neurol 1996;15:19–22.

82. Nierman E, Zakrzewski K. Recognition and management of preoperative risk. Rheum Dis Clin North Am 1999;25:585–622.

83. Wirbel RJ, Roth R, Schulte M, Kramann B, Mutschler W. Preoperative embolization in spinal and pelvic metastases. J Orthop Sci 2005;10:253–257.

84. Chatziioannou AN, Johnson ME, Pneumaticos SG, Lawrence DD, Carrasco CH. Preoperative embolization of bone metastases from renal cell carcinoma. Eur Radiol 2000;10:593–596.

85. Layalle I, Flandroy P, Trotteur G, Dondelinger RF. Arterial embolization of bone metastases: is it worthwhile? J Belge Radiol 1998;81:223–225.

86. Li GH, He ZF, Yu DM, Li XD, Chen ZD. [Effect of finasteride on intraoperative bleeding and irrigating fluid absorption during transurethral resection of prostate: a quantitative study.] Zhejiang Da Xue Xue Bao Yi Xue Ban 2004;33:258–260.

87. Hagerty JA, Ginsberg PC, Harmon JD, Harkaway RC. Pretreatment with finasteride decreases perioperative bleeding associated with transurethral resection of the prostate. Urology 2000;55:684–689.

88. Crea G, Sanfilippo G, Anastasi G, Magno C, Vizzini C, Inferrera A. Pre-surgical finasteride therapy in patients treated endoscopically for benign prostatic hyperplasia. Urol Int 2005;74:51–53.

89. Dimeo F, Knauf W, Geilhaupt D, Böning D. Endurance exercise and the production of growth hormone and haematopoietic factors in patients with anaemia. Br J Sports Med 2004;38:e37.

90. Baskett TF. Surgical management of severe obstetric hemorrhage: experience with an obstetric hemorrhage equipment tray. J Obstet Gynaecol Can 2004;26:805–808.

12 Iatrogenic Blood Loss

Anemia largely develops during or after surgery or major trauma, or due to an underlying medical condition. However, anemia may also develop in hospital, secondary to common medical practice (hospital-acquired anemia). Typically, a series of small iatrogenic blood losses add up, resulting in patients becoming anemic. This chapter will address seven of the major causes of such iatrogenic blood loss and describe methods to minimize these losses.

Objectives

1. To list the different ways in which a medical caregiver inadvertently causes blood loss.
2. To describe methods to minimize iatrogenic blood loss.
3. To explain the vital role of minimizing iatrogenic blood loss for a comprehensive blood management.

Definitions

Iatrogenic blood loss: The word "iatrogenic" stems from the word "*iatros*," which is Greek for "physician," and "*genesis*," which translates as "origin" or "cause." "Iatrogenic" therefore means "caused by a physician." All blood losses that are directly or indirectly caused by a physician's intervention are summarized under the phrase "iatrogenic blood loss." Actually, iatrogenic blood loss is not caused by physicians alone. Every member of the care team can cause blood loss. In turn, every member of the medical care team can also help to reduce iatrogenic blood loss.

Causes of iatrogenic blood loss

You may ask: "How can a medical caregiver be the culprit?" and, "In what ways is iatrogenic blood loss caused?" Well, almost everything a medical team does has the potential to cause blood loss—directly or indirectly. This is true of every medical specialty, not just surgery. Blood loss may be caused simply by the fact that a patient has to see a physician. The patient may be so stressed by the very thought of seeing a doctor that he/she develops a stress ulcer and bleeds internally. Patients prescribed bed rest soon show a lowered red cell count. Many diagnostic procedures cause blood loss, some of them to such an extent that clinically significant anemia develops. Also, many therapeutic interventions cause blood loss. This holds true for drug therapy as well as for more invasive approaches, such as dialysis and other forms of extracorporeal circulation (ECC). Nevertheless, all of these interventions can be adapted so that iatrogenic blood loss is minimized.

Problem 1: Phlebotomy—laboratory testing causes blood loss

Blood loss by phlebotomy is not a new phenomenon. For ages, phlebotomy in the form of blood letting was a legitimate "cure" for all kinds of ailments, including anemia. While beneficial in selected cases, phlebotomy to the extent of blood letting more often than not harmed the patient, even resulting in his/her death. Blood losses by today's phlebotomists are more subtle, yet clearly detectable as well. They have a great impact on patient care and

Basics of Blood Management, Second Edition. Petra Seeber and Aryeh Shander.
© 2013 John Wiley & Sons, Ltd. Published 2013 by John Wiley & Sons, Ltd.

outcome. Since laboratory results are an important tool to achieve a diagnosis and to guide medical care, a certain amount of blood usually is required to get the required information. However, a great quantity of blood drawn for laboratory testing is drawn needlessly. It is frequently drawn without good reason, drawn too often, or drawn even when not indicated. Some members of the care team ordering blood tests are not aware of the significance of the results obtained. Often, laboratory results do not influence a patient's care at all. What then is the point of obtaining them? Another problem with phlebotomy is that excessive blood volumes are drawn. A study in a pediatric intensive care unit (ICU), for instance, indicated that more than half of the blood drawn was not needed for the requested tests [1].

When blood is drawn from indwelling arterial or venous lines, a certain amount of blood ("dead space volume") is withdrawn to clear the line, before the actual phlebotomy volume is drawn. This is done in order to reduce the mixing of the catheter flushing solution with the blood sample. The drawn dead space volume is usually discarded. Depending on local custom, the discarded volume varies between 2 and 10 mL per blood draw [2].

The total daily amount of blood drawn for laboratory tests varies, depending on the patient's pathology and length of stay. Sicker patients experience more blood loss than those who are less sick, placing the sicker patients at higher risk for anemia. Table 12.1 demonstrates how sub-

Table 12.1 Average phlebotomy-induced blood loss in critically ill patients.

Reporting country	Setting	Average phlebotomy-induced blood loss (mL/day)
United States	Cardiothoracic ICU	377
United States	General surgical ICU	240
United States	Medical surgical ICU	41.5
Great Britain	First day in ICU	85.3
Great Britain	Following days	66.1
Europe	Medical ICUs	41.1

ICU, intensive care unit.

stantial the total daily amounts of blood drawn from one patient can be [2].

Possible solution: Reduction of phlebotomy-induced blood loss

Strategies to reduce phlebotomy-induced blood loss are usually employed in patients at high risk for anemia, such as neonates, pediatric patients, the critically ill, and patients for whom transfusions are not an option.

Reduction of the amount of phlebotomy

Reducing the amount of blood for phlebotomy starts with the simple avoidance of unnecessary phlebotomy. Thoughtless ordering of a variety of tests does not contribute to your value as a caregiver, nor does it help your patient. Ask yourself: What would change in the care of the patient if I do or do not have the result? If there is no clear indication for a blood test, it is most probably not indicated and a waste of blood and money. Standing orders (e.g., "Mr Miller is going to have his liver function test every other day, no matter what") should be reconsidered and in many instances eliminated.

When you know which laboratory values are required, consider if batching the requests is possible. One specimen is often sufficient to obtain several values at a time. Then, make sure that you know how much blood is needed to perform the requested tests. Phlebotomy overdraw can be substantial. Especially in small children, small amounts of blood, drawn unnecessarily, matter. Collection tubes with fill lines should help in this regard. Drawing the blood up to the fill line prevents overdraw, either caused by drawing too much blood for one sample or by drawing blood for the same test twice. The latter may be the case when insufficient blood is drawn into the container, resulting in an incorrect mixing ratio of blood and the additive provided in the container (e.g., anticoagulant). In this case, blood has to be drawn again, resulting in unnecessary blood loss.

Patients at high risk for anemia will probably benefit from further measures to reduce blood draws. The use of neonatal tubes with a smaller fill volume reduces blood loss but still provides the required results (Table 12.2). A switch from adult- to pediatric-sized tubes may reduce the diagnostic blood loss by over 40% [3]. A method that saves even more blood is microsampling. Only a few microliters of blood are required to obtain certain information, e.g., 150 μL for blood gases, electrolytes, hemoglobin and hematocrit, and blood sugar. Devices for point-of-care testing [4] often require only small blood volumes. Some point-of-care devices are even able to

Table 12.2 Phlebotomy volumes of commercially available blood tubes.

	Regular (mL)	Pediatric (mL)	Neonatal/ microsampling (μL)
Hematology	3.5–9	2.6–3.0	
Serology	4.9–10	2–2.7 mL	250–1000
Coagulation	4–10	2.9–3.0 mL	
Blood sugar	2.6–3.0		20–50 (or less)
Sedimentation rate	2		
Blood gases	1–3		100–500

return the drawn blood directly back to the patient after it has been analyzed [5]. In areas where rather expensive point-of-care devices are not available, color scales may help to obtain fairly accurate laboratory results from only one drop of the patient's blood [6].

Keeping track of the amount of blood taken is especially helpful in high-risk patients (neonates, the severely anemic). It sensitizes the healthcare personnel (physicians, nurses, phlebotomists, laboratory technicians) to take great care in their efforts towards blood conservation. Therefore, it may be beneficial to flag the notes of such high-risk patients in order to alert the team to be especially careful. Getting every member of the care team to sign a special sheet when ordering or executing phlebotomy may also be of help, especially in the initial phase of establishing blood saving techniques.

Practice tip

Place a sheet of paper next to all patients in the ICU and have all persons who draw blood list the total volume of blood drawn from them. After the patient leaves the unit, add all losses up and present this information to the healthcare team for discussion.

Reduction and elimination of the discard volume

The dead space volume drawn before obtaining the blood sample is usually discarded. It was shown that a volume of only twice the catheter dead space is sufficient to gain the required accuracy of the drawn laboratory values [7]. Whatever goes beyond this volume is a wasted resource.

To avoid discard volume as a source of iatrogenic blood loss altogether, several methods are used. The simplest one is probably just to return the sterile dead space volume once the blood sample is drawn. Discard volume is completely eliminated when a passive extracorporeal arteriovenous backflow is used [8]. For this technique, a double-stopcock system connects the central line and arterial line. When the appropriate stopcocks are opened, blood from the arterial line flows back, through the tubing, toward the venous line. The blood is allowed to flow a certain distance (which equals the usual discard volume) past a sampling port. Then, the blood sample is drawn through the sampling port and the remaining blood is directed back to the patient.

Additionally, special systems that use a reservoir in an arterial line are available for the withdrawal of dead space volume and subsequent retransfusion. Adapting arterial blood draws by using a closed system may reduce the blood loss by about 50% [9].

If the dead space volume cannot be returned to the patient, then the choice of the blood sampling site may reduce discard volumes. Direct venipuncture produces no discard volume, blood drawn from peripheral venous and arterial lines a small discard volume, and central lines typically the largest discard volume [1].

Replacement of phlebotomy by "bloodless" monitoring

Blood draws are unnecessary if "bloodless" methods are used to provide the required information. Some values (e.g., pH, partial pressure of carbon dioxide, partial pressure of oxygen, arterial oxygen saturation, bicarbonate, base excess) can be obtained with satisfactory accuracy using indwelling measuring catheters with photochemical sensors [10]. The catheter can either be inserted into an extracorporeal circulation or directly into the vascular system [11]. Photochemical sensors can be placed intravascularly for continuous measurement, or extravascularly for on-demand measurement.

To obtain some blood values, direct contact between blood and a measuring device is not always necessary. Skin sensors may be placed on patients who are at high risk for iatrogenic blood loss. The sensors may measure, for instance, the partial pressures of carbon dioxide and oxygen, bilirubin, hemoglobin, and glucose transcutaneously, obviating the need for serial blood draws.

Education

Educating members of the team on techniques for reducing unnecessary blood loss, e.g., ordering only essential blood tests, exercising the greatest care in infants, practicing drawing blood samples into syringes, etc., may also help. While studies to evaluate the effect of education on the appropriate use of phlebotomy have not shown a significant change in practice, the introduction of mandatory policies and guidelines for laboratory use have.

Problem 2: Resting patients lose blood

Even patients who do nothing at all may lose blood. One reason for this is that inactivity and bed rest elicit physiological responses that lead to anemia [12]. This anemia is termed the "anemia of inactivity." In contrast to anemia of inflammation, there is no detectable increase in inflammatory makers. It seems that bone marrow is replaced by adipocytes, which either occupy space usually required for bone marrow or actively produce substances that inhibit bone marrow activity. This anemia of inactivity seems to be related to bed rest per se, i.e., taking weight off the legs [13].

Another problem in bed-resting patients may be the development of decubital ulcers, leading to so-called "pressure sore anemia" [14]. Anemia due to decubital ulcers is characterized by mild-to-moderate anemia with low serum iron and normal or increased ferritin in combination with hypoproteinemia and hypoalbuminemia. Anemia probably develops because of the chronic inflammatory state caused by the presence of pressure ulcers.

Possible solution: Keep them moving

Since resting patients may experience a gradual decrease in their blood count, unnecessary bed rest in hospitalized patients should be avoided. There is no evidence that ambulation of patients decreases their transfusion exposure, but there is some evidence that it reduces postoperative pneumonia, length of stay in hospital, and psychological changes [15]. Moderate physical training has been shown to reduce anemia [16–18]. The reasons for this phenomenon are not clear. One hypothesis is that exercise increases hormones that stimulate erythropoiesis and leukopoiesis. Growth hormones, granulocyte colony-stimulating factor (G-CSF), and a variety of other cytokines are produced during exercise. Besides, cytokines, which are typically produced in an inflammatory state and inhibit hematopoiesis (e.g., interleukin 6), seem to diminish during exercise [19, 20].

Whatever the reason, exercise may ameliorate anemia. This can be used to the good of the patient. Educating the patient and his/her family that moderate exercise is very beneficial is essential. Also, physical therapy may be prescribed. This may be especially beneficial for patients with chronic anemia (such as dialysis patients). These patients should be advised to exercise regularly. A dialysis patient presenting for elective surgery should be started on an exercise program. Certain types of anemia react very well to exercise. Through an exercise routine, the blood levels of preoperative anemia patients can be optimized. Thirty minutes per day of interval training, on a stationary ergometer, for 3 weeks may be sufficient for a substantial improvement in the patient's blood count. Patients who experience prolonged periods of chemotherapy-induced anemia may start with moderate exercise immediately after chemotherapy. Preferably, the exercise should be out of bed, with the patient bearing weight. This is recommended since the anemia of immobility cannot be treated by exercise undertaken in bed [13]. If it is not possible for the patient to get out of bed, exercise in the supine position, using a "bed bike" or cycling in the air, may be recommended. Most medical and surgical patients will benefit from being mobilized as early as possible. Adequate pain management, nutrition, and a schedule for mobilization and exercise may enhance patient compliance with the prescribed program [16–19].

As already mentioned, pressure ulcers, which can develop during bed rest, contribute to anemia as well. Diligent nursing staff know how to avoid the development of such sores. If ulcers are already present, appropriate therapy is warranted. Pressure sore anemia needs to be taken seriously. Iron therapy is said to be useless. Instead, it has been recommended to treat the serum protein alterations, prescribing a diet rich in protein and calories [21]. Both anemia and hypoproteinemia disappear once the pressure ulcers heal.

Problem 3: Stressed patients lose blood

It is not only resting patients who suffer from iatrogenic blood loss and anemia. Stressed patients share the same fate, but due to completely different underlying mechanisms. Critically ill patients regularly (40–100%) develop alterations in the mucosa of the gastrointestinal tract. This may contribute to the development of stress "ulcers" in the gastrointestinal tract. Up to 90% of ventilated patients admitted to an ICU suffer from stress ulcers by the third day of their stay [22, 23]. These may lead to occult gastrointestinal hemorrhage. About 1–2% of these patients even experience severe hemorrhage, leading to severe anemia. Such blood loss is aggravated by antico-agulant use and coagulopathy.

While all pediatric and adult patients may develop stress ulcers, there are a variety of conditions that obviously predispose patients to stress ulcers. The classical conditions are head and brain trauma, major burns, emergency or major surgery, major trauma, shock, coagulopathies, mechanical ventilation for more than 2 days, therapy with drugs that may cause ulcers, and a history of gastrointestinal ulcers.

Possible solution: Ulcer prophylaxis

Stress ulcer prophylaxis is an integral part of a strategy to avoid iatrogenic blood loss. The first and most important method is to attempt to maintain adequate mucosal perfusion. Unfortunately, specific measures to do so are limited. Maintaining sufficient cardiac output and giving sufficient oxygen in hypoxia enhance the mucosal integrity, and are the basis for ulcer prophylaxis.

A simple, yet often overlooked, measure to protect the integrity of the gastrointestinal mucosal lining is enteral feeding. This is thought to be due to the food's neutralizing effect on the acid in the stomach as well as the nutritional effect on the mucosa. Patients should be asked to eat. If this is not possible, enteral tube feeding has the same effect.

If enteral feeding is not possible, or the patient is at high risk of developing stress ulcers, medical prophylaxis is indicated. Histamine-2-receptor antagonist therapy aims at reducing the gastric acid levels in the stomach, but tolerance develops rapidly. It was shown to decrease the incidence of gastrointestinal hemorrhage. There is a trend toward decreased hemorrhage when antacids are used for the same purpose (compared with no therapy). Sucralfate may be as effective in reducing hemorrhage as gastric pH-altering drugs. Advantages of sucralfate include a lower rate of pneumonia and mortality, as well as lower costs [24]. Proton pump inhibitors may be even more effective than histamine-2-receptor 2 antagonists. They reduce severe hemorrhage in patients with peptic ulcers and effectively decrease rebleeding [25].

Problem 4: Diagnostic interventions cause blood loss

Diagnostic and therapeutic interventions at times cause blood loss. Among them are the placement of arterial and central lines, as well as interventions such as tracheos-tomy [26] and angiography or percutaneous coronary interventions.

The impact of blood loss caused by the insertion of a central line is obvious when an untrained individual performs the insertion. Often, blood flows back freely, pouring out on to the drapes, and is lost. Quantifying such blood losses is difficult. One study on iatrogenic blood loss did mention the insertion of arterial and central venous catheters as a source of blood loss, but did not determine the amount of blood lost [27]. Though the magnitude of blood loss is not clearly defined, obtaining vascular access and a variety of other procedures doubtless cause blood loss.

Also, the presence of arterial lines causes blood loss. This happens when blood is drawn freely using this easy access to the patient's blood [28].

Possible solution: Practice

A certain amount of skill is needed to obtain vascular access. It seems that unskilled healthcare providers, such as trainees, lose on average more blood than skilled persons. In patients at high risk of anemia, it may be more appropriate that a skilled healthcare provider places lines, rather than a trainee.

Also, the location and choice of technique to obtain vascular access may influence the amount of blood lost during the procedure. The risk for major bleeding seems higher in femoral than in radial cannulation. Obtaining central vascular access guided by ultrasound reduces bleeding compared to landmark-guided insertion [29]. Inserting an arterial line using the open Seldinger technique causes more blood loss than the same procedure performed using the modified Seldinger technique (closed system) or by direct cannulation. Slight changes in the method of using the guidewire may also reduce blood loss. One article describes this as follows [30]: "The method entails inserting the guide wire through a previously created side hole in a standard 5 mL plastic syringe. The problems of needle dislodgement, air embolism and blood loss are virtually eliminated with this technique." The use of valves in the introducer sheaths for large vascular catheters may help reduce blood loss as well [31]. Besides, some types of arterial closure devices used after cannulation for percutaneous coronary intervention reduce bleeding compared with manual compression [32].

Another way to minimize blood loss associated with placed arterial or central venous lines is to remove them soon as possible. This will also reduce easy access to the patient's blood [28].

The method used to perform some interventions can result in higher or lower than average blood loss. Tracheostomy, for instance, can be performed as a conventional surgical procedure or as a percutaneous dilatational tracheostomy. The latter was shown to have a lower peri- and post-operative blood loss than the conventional approach. The reason may be that "following percutaneous placement, the stoma fits snugly around the tracheostomy tube. This lack of dead space conceivably serves to tamponade bleeding vessels" [26]. There are also different methods for the insertion of a permanent pacemaker, some of which cause less blood loss than others [33].

Problem 5: Medications may cause blood loss

Medications may cause blood loss by many different mechanisms. Over-anticoagulation may contribute to the blood loss, as may the side effects of medications given during hospitalization. Commonly encountered mechanisms that increase iatrogenic blood loss are discussed below (Table 12.3). It goes beyond the scope of this chapter to engage in an in-depth discussion of all possible effects of drugs on blood loss, and consultation of a reference book is often tremendously helpful.

Possible solution: *"Medica mente, non medicamente"*

Since medications have the potential to increase iatrogenic blood loss, care must be taken in their choice. If the patient's comorbidities reveal a "sensitivity," allergy or intolerance to drugs, such medications should be avoided, if possible.

If anticoagulation or antiplatelet drugs are required, judicious use is warranted. Before patients are started on the drugs, they should be assessed for their individual risk for major bleeding, e.g., by the HAS-BLED score [34]. For several anticoagulants, monitoring is prudent, and should be employed to prevent over-anticoagulation, which may lead to undue blood loss. When a patient is at high risk of hemorrhage, e.g., when he/she has a very low platelet count, anticoagulation may not be the wisest choice. Thrombosis prophylaxis may be more appropriate using non-drug methods such as compression stockings or intermittent pneumatic compression [35], or in selected cases, the placement of a vena cava filter.

Other drug regimens with impact on the hematological system may also be amendable for adaptation. Chemotherapy can be varied to reduce the impact it has on hematopoiesis. Antibiotics can be chosen so as not to unnecessarily aggravate coagulopathy. Hemolysis due to hypotonic solutions and other medications is also preventable.

Table 12.3 Drug effects that may increase iatrogenic blood loss.

Examples of drugs	Effect
Aspirin and other non-steroidal anti-inflammatory drugs, glucocorticoids	(Occult) gastrointestinal hemorrhage
Heparin, aspirin, heart glycosides, thyrostatics, histamine-2-receptor antagonists	Thrombocytopenia
Metamizol, allopurinol, indapamide	Agranulocytosis or aplastic anemia
Chloramphenicol, cis-platinum and other chemotherapeutics, gold derivatives, neuroleptics, pyrimethamine	Blunted hematopoiesis
Some cephalosporins	Toxic changes in the blood count, e.g., leukopenia, thrombocytopenia
Ajamlin, L-asparaginase, carbamazepine, rifampicin, thiazides, rapid infusion of hypotonic solutions	Hemolysis
High-dose penicillins, aspirin, valproic acid, serotonin antagonists	Impairment of coagulation

Problem 6: Blood loss caused by extracorporeal circulation

Patients with end-stage renal failure, undergoing open heart surgery, or with potentially reversible heart or lung failure all have something in common: they have a good chance of needing therapy that includes an extracorporeal circulation (ECC), such as hemodialysis, cardiopulmonary bypass, ventricular assist devices, or extracorporeal membrane oxygenation. The basic principle of an ECC is the same, regardless of the specific purpose of the device. All these devices have the potential to cause iatrogenic blood loss. Additionally, other devices being introduced into the blood stream of a patient (such as intra-aortic balloon pumps, ventricular assist devices, and prosthetic heart valves) may cause hemolysis [36].

ECC is a non-physiological approach to blood circulation that takes its toll on the blood. The blood in the ECC comes into contact with air and foreign surfaces, and the shear stress within the blood increases. Furthermore, the flow pattern in the circulation changes from a pulsatile to a non-pulsatile flow. All of this leads to alterations in the corpuscular elements of the blood, activation of the coagulation and complement cascade, and activation and adherence of a variety of other blood proteins. As a result, red cells hemolyze, platelets are activated and change in number, shape, and functionality, clotting ability is disturbed, and blood proteins are reduced in the circulation.

Anticoagulation is needed for the successful use of ECC. However, it contributes to blood losses as well. Over- and under-anticoagulation may lead to intra- and post-operative coagulopathies and unnecessary blood loss. If the patient is exposed to excess amounts of an anticoagulant, he/she may hemorrhage due to the action of the anticoagulant. If he/she is not sufficiently anticoagulated, clotting factors and platelets are activated and will be used up during the ECC, leaving the patient coagulopathic after ECC. Besides, reversal of anticoagulation in excess of the anticoagulant present may also add to coagulopathies.

Other factors, directly or indirectly related to the use of an ECC, influence the magnitude of iatrogenic blood loss as well. Blood remaining in the tubing after discontinuation of the procedure adds to the blood loss. Also, coagulopathy induced by anticoagulation and patient-specific factors (e.g., a disturbed erythropoiesis in renal insufficiency) contribute to the fact that patients requir-

ing an ECC are at higher risk for anemia than other patients. According to one study, daily blood loss in patients requiring dialysis or hemofiltration in an ICU was 5.8 times higher than the blood loss in intensive care patients not requiring such therapy [27].

Possible solution: Minimizing blood loss due to extracorporeal circulation

The use of an ECC inevitably causes blood loss and with it anemia and coagulopathy. To avoid it, an ECC should be used only when therapeutic measures without ECC are not possible. For instance, off-pump coronary artery bypass surgery (OPCABG) is associated with less derangement of the blood than on-pump heart surgery. Unfortunately, complete avoidance of an ECC is not always possible, but the time during which it is used can be reduced by the perfusionist or the attending physician [37].

In former times, patients on an ECC, such as cardiopulmonary bypass, were transfused with considerable amounts of blood. Even the ECC was primed with donor blood. Today, this is obsolete in most instances. Priming with crystalloid solutions is sufficient to start the pump but this leads to hemodilution. While hemodilution is of benefit to patients undergoing hypothermia and who experience the accompanying increase in blood viscosity, most patients do not benefit. In such instances, retrograde autologous priming is a method that reduces the hemodiluting effect of the ECC. The use of autologous blood to prime the circuit not only reduces hemodilution but also the extent of intraoperative and postoperative anemia [38]. Since it does not require additional disposables, retrograde autologous priming is a very inexpensive technique. Several techniques for retrograde autologous priming have been advocated. Basically, the circuit is partially primed with asanguinous fluids such as crystalloids. The patient's own blood, draining from the venous tube, is used to further fill the circuit. Another way to reduce hemodilution on cardiopulmonary bypass is to use microplegia. It adds less crystalloids to the circulation than conventional amounts of cardioplegic solutions.

Preoperative normovolemic hemodilution and blood component pheresis

Since the contact of blood with the ECC causes a variety of changes, one method to avoid this is to take some blood from the patient's circulation before the ECC is initiated. Such procedures are performed mainly before on-pump cardiac surgery. Acute normovolemic hemodilution and the fractionation of whole blood to provide platelet-rich and platelet-poor plasma are methods to spare blood contact with the ECC.

Platelet anesthesia

The term "platelet anesthesia" refers to a concept that is still in the experimental stage. It is a strategy to minimize platelet activation and adhesion during the period the blood is circulating via ECC (usually during cardiopulmonary bypass). Short-acting platelet inhibitors (such as ticlopidine, tirofiban or argatroban) are used during the ECC period; they temporarily inhibit platelet activation and adhesion. When the action of the inhibitor wears off after the end of the ECC, a larger number of functionally adequate platelets are still available. This is thought to reduce postoperative blood loss and normalize *in vitro* coagulation parameters.

Adaptation of the extracorporeal circuit

Technical details of the ECC influence the magnitude of the changes in the blood components.

Blood contact with artificial surfaces leads to activation of humoral and cellular elements of the blood. The contact activation or its effects can be reduced by using biocompatible circuits and avoiding leukocyte depletion filters. In turn, blood loss may be reduced [39].

The choice of an appropriate oxygenator in ECCs used to oxygenate the blood is also important. In general, membrane oxygenators tend to influence *in vitro* markers of protein activation and blood cell alterations less than bubble oxygenators (the latter have a larger blood–surface interface). *In vivo*, membrane oxygenators seem to be superior to bubble oxygenators in patients undergoing long perfusion periods. During shorter perfusion times, *in vivo* experiments have not shown a reduction in blood loss with membrane oxygenators.

Minimized extracorporeal circulation (MECC), preferably with vacuum-assisted venous drainage, may also reduce iatrogenic blood loss and unnecessary hemodilution [40]. An MECC consists of a biocompatible tubing system with a pump and oxygenator. A venous reservoir and a vent are not included. The priming volume is much lower than in conventional extracorporeal circuits (about 450 mL instead of about 1500 mL [40]). MECCs cause less hemodilution and hemolysis when compared to the conventional ECC for cardiopulmonary bypass [39]. For very small children and neonates, the cardiopulmonary bypass system can be minimized so that the priming volume is as low as 130–160 mL [41]. This enables surgeons to perform cardiac surgery even in children without the use of allogeneic transfusions.

The type of ultrafiltration chosen may affect iatrogenic blood loss as well. Conventional ultrafiltration, which is used throughout the time of cardiopulmonary bypass, does not seem to reduce blood loss. In contrast, modified ultrafiltration used at termination of the cardiopulmonary bypass, reduces blood loss. Therefore, the latter is currently recommended for blood conservation [39].

Retransfusion of blood left in the extracorporeal circuit

Blood left in the tubing after termination of the ECC would be wasted if not given back to the patient. There are different ways to return the remaining blood to the patient. It can simply be reinfused or it can be processed and then given back. Blood can be centrifuged using a cell saving device or it can be hemoconcentrated with a filter. The use of the centrifuge removes platelets and plasma components, and allows mainly the concentrated red cells to be given back to the patient. It has the advantage that heparin is not given back to the patient. In contrast, while ultrafiltration and the return of unprocessed blood do return heparin to the patient, plasma components and platelets are preserved [42]. Ultrafiltrated blood may be more hemolyzed than unprocessed blood, but the hemoconcentration achieved by ultrafiltration prevents the return of large amounts of fluids [43]. The right choice of method to return residual blood after ECC seems to have an impact on the red cell mass, degree of hemodilution, and extent of coagulopathy. The 2011 recommendations of the Society of Thoracic Surgeons and the Society of Cardiovascular Anesthesiologists prefer centrifugation of pump salvage volume over direct reinfusion since it has the potential to reduce transfusions [39].

Monitoring and reversal of anticoagulation

Since inadequate heparinization as well as excessive or insufficient reversal of heparin may cause coagulopathies and blood loss, anticoagulation calls for close monitoring. The individual patient's response to heparin is variable. A variety of laboratory values and tests are instrumental in monitoring anticoagulation. Among them are thrombin time, prothrombin time (PT), activated partial thromboplastin time (aPTT), activated coagulation time (ACT), and heparin concentration monitoring, as well as the use of the thrombelastogram. However, no single test is able to monitor anticoagulation reliably. The combination of two or more tests seems to increase the reliability when the clinical picture is added to the assessment (e.g., ACT and heparin concentration). Some studies have demonstrated a reduced blood product use when appropriate monitoring techniques are employed [44].

Appropriate reversal of anticoagulation also contributes to a reduced blood loss. The preferred antidote for heparin is protamine, a positively charged compound binding to the negatively charged heparin, whereby it neutralizes the anticoagulant effect of heparin. Excess protamine, however, also impairs coagulation and reduces the platelet count. Since protamine can cause such abnormalities itself, it is only beneficial when the amount required to neutralize the heparin is used. Current recommendations prefer titration or low-dose protamine. The best method to avoid undue protamine use is still the appropriate use of heparin.

Problem 7: Timing influences blood loss

If a patient bleeds, immediate intervention to prevent further blood loss is mandatory. Blood loss is like a bucket with a hole. To keep it filled, you can pour in more fluid (in our case, by transfusing blood), or you can fix it by closing the hole. If hemorrhaging patients are not treated immediately, blood loss increases. All blood loss that can potentially be stopped is, strictly speaking, iatrogenic blood loss.

On the other hand, rushing an unprepared patient into a surgical or medical intervention may also increase blood loss and the likelihood for adverse outcome.

Possible solution: *Carpe diem*

Time is a precious commodity, especially for patients who bleed. Achieving timely hemostasis must be of uppermost importance in a blood management program. This should be reflected in the way trauma and other surgical and medical teams prepare for bleeding patients. Up-to-date algorithms for hemorrhage, appropriate training, trauma drills, and equipment readily available and fully functional contribute to the minimization of the time that elapses until definite hemostasis is achieved. Depending on the severity of the ongoing blood loss, diagnostic measures should be expedited. Such rapid treatment of patients not only reduces blood loss and subsequent anemia and coagulopathy, but may even improve survival. This has been shown for different kinds of hemorrhage, such as early endoscopy for gastroin-

testinal hemorrhage [45] and early tranexamic acid for trauma patients [46]. Similarly, patients who develop anemia or coagulopathy in a more gradual fashion also benefit from early recognition and appropriate treatment of their condition. This is especially true for patients who develop anemia while suffering from cardiovascular disease or renal insufficiency [47]. Waiting under "transfusion protection" for a possible spontaneous resolution of bleeding is futile and dangerous. A "wait and see attitude" definitely does not have a place in the therapy of an acutely hemorrhaging patient.

In contrast, elapsing time may also be beneficial. It provides a patient with the opportunity to recover from blood loss. Patients who have undergone angiography, for instance, may need surgery. If this surgery can be postponed safely for some days, the time may be sufficient for hematopoiesis to synthesize blood components lost during the diagnostic procedure [48]. Another example where allowing time to elapse may be beneficial is cord clamping after delivery of a baby. Waiting just 30–120 seconds before the cord is clamped increases the hematocrit of the baby and minimizes neonatal anemia [49].

Role of iatrogenic blood loss in blood management

After discussing common sources of iatrogenic blood loss, you may ask yourself: "Does iatrogenic blood loss really matter?", and "Does avoiding such small and probably seemingly insignificant blood losses enhance patient care and improve outcome?"

Unquestionably, medical personnel cause substantial blood losses in their patients. Among them, phlebotomy is the most extensively studied example. It seems that there is a substantial overdraw of blood for laboratory testing. In the United States, hospitals caring for adults draw 2.5–10 times more blood for standard laboratory panels than pediatric hospitals [50]. A study performed in Great Britain showed that attempts to reduce the blood loss stemming from phlebotomy were rare. In adult ICUs, dead space volume was returned in only 18.4% of units and pediatric tubes were used in only 9.3%. In contrast, pediatric ICUs returned the dead space volume in 67% of cases [51]. This demonstrates that there is still room for improvement. Diagnostic blood loss is a major determinant of anemia in adult and neonatal ICUs, accounting for substantial amounts of transfused blood [52, 53]. In fact, in the ICU setting, the total amount of diagnostic blood loss is a significant predictor of allogeneic transfusion [27]. As shown above, comprehensive blood management effectively reduces phlebotomy-induced blood loss [54, 55] and such attempts reduce the patient's degree of anemia [5, 56].

Apart from phlebotomy, there are many other items under the control of a medical care team that affect the blood count of a patient. In many instances, attention to detail helps to avoid unnecessary blood loss [57, 58]. Even if there are not many randomized controlled studies demonstrating that attention to all the above-mentioned details translates into a predictable outcome improvement, they still appear to be good clinical practice for blood management.

Key points

- Blood loss occurs directly and indirectly from the practices of medical caregivers, e.g., due to:
  - Diagnostic phlebotomy
  - Bed rest
  - Occult gastrointestinal hemorrhage and stress ulcers
  - Invasive monitoring (arterial lines, etc.)
  - Drugs, including anticoagulants
  - Extracorporeal circulation
  - Unnecessarily wasting time while the patient bleeds
  - Blunted erythropoiesis due to iatrogenic malnutrition.
- Iatrogenic blood loss accounts for increased use of transfusions.
- Iatrogenic blood loss, and with it the development of iatrogenic anemia and coagulopathy, can be minimized.
- Ways to minimize iatrogenic blood loss include:
  - Reduction of the frequency of phlebotomy and the volume of blood drawn
  - Return of dead space volume
  - Ulcer prophylaxis
  - Attention to detail in diagnostic or therapeutic interventions, including the choice of a skilled practitioner and a suitable technique
  - Judicious use of drugs, including anticoagulants
  - Adaptation of procedures involving an ECC
  - Expedited hemostasis in all hemorrhaging patients.

Questions for review

1. What can be done to reduce blood loss induced by phlebotomy?

2. What diagnostic procedures are available that reduce iatrogenic blood loss?
3. How can ECC be adapted to minimize blood loss?
4. Does timing play a role in avoiding iatrogenic blood loss?
5. How do sports influence iatrogenic blood loss?

Suggestions for further research

1. What different methods are available for autologous retrograde priming of a cardiopulmonary bypass? (http://perfline.com/textbook/local/rap/rap.html)
2. What is the suggested effect of leukocytes in the development of coagulopathies after ECCs and how is this affected by the use of leukocyte filtration during ECC?
3. How does thrombelastography work and how do the tracings change with changes in amount and functionality of plasma clotting factors, platelets, red cells, and reduced temperature?

Exercises and practice cases

A 65-year-old diabetic man is admitted to the ICU with pneumonia and partial respiratory insufficiency. His weight is 70 kg, height is 170 cm, and initial hematocrit is 0.34. He is monitored with a central venous catheter and an arterial line.

All blood draws are taken from the central line, except the ones for the blood cultures, which are taken directly from the vein. Before a blood sample is drawn into the sampling tubes from the central line, 10 mL of the blood is discarded. Before blood is drawn from the arterial line, 5 mL of the blood is discarded. The blood tubes used are the standard tubes in the ICU with the following volumes: hematology 9 mL, serology 10 mL, coagulation profile 10 mL, blood glucose levels 3 mL, erythrocyte sedimentation rate 2 mL, blood gases 2 mL, and blood cultures 10 mL each for aerobic, anaerobic, and fungal cultures.

The order "ICU complete" means complete blood count with differential, erythrocyte sedimentation rate, blood glucose level, INR, aPTT, D-dimer, troponin, C-reactive protein, sodium, potassium, calcium, chloride, lactate, liver panel, and kidney panel.

The order "ICU small" means complete blood count, blood glucose level, INR, aPTT, C-reactive protein, sodium, potassium, calcium, and chloride.

Continued

Since the hospital laboratory is small, some blood is sent to specialized laboratories. One blood sample is sent for serology of HIV and hepatitis, another to determine the procalcitonin (PCT).

On the first day, intensive diagnosis is made. Therefore, the attending physician orders: "ICU complete, blood cultures now and in 2 hours, blood glucose levels × 5, PCT, HIV/hepatitis serology, central venous oxygen saturation every 6 hours, arterial blood gases every 6 hours."

On the second and following 6 days, the attending physician orders: "ICU small, blood glucose levels × 5, central venous oxygen saturation every 6 hours, arterial blood gases every 6 hours."

Use the above information to estimate the blood loss this patient suffers during his stay in the ICU.

Homework

Practice giving back the dead space volume when you next draw blood.

Check the volumes of the blood tubes you currently use. Explore whether there are alternative tubes with smaller volumes.

References

1. Valentine SL, Bateman S. Identifying factors to minimize phlebotomy-induced blood loss in the pediatric intensive care unit. *Pediatr Crit Care Med* 2012;**13**:22–27.
2. Fowler RA, Berenson M. Blood conservation in the intensive care unit. *Crit Care Med* 2003;**31** (12 Suppl):S715–720.
3. Smoller BR, Kruskall MS, Horowitz GI. Reducing adult phlebotomy blood loss with the use of pediatric-sized blood collection tubes. *Am J Clin Pathol* 1989;**91**:701–703.
4. Guiliano KK. Blood analysis at the point of care: issues in application for use in critically ill patients. *AACN Clin Issues* 2002;**13**:204–220.
5. Widness JA, Madan A, Grindeanu LA, Zimmerman MB, Wong DK, Stevenson DK. Reduction in red blood cell transfusions among preterm infants: results of a randomized trial with an in-line blood gas and chemistry monitor. *Pediatrics* 2005;**115**:1299–1306.
6. Lewis SM, Stott GJ, Wynn KJ. An inexpensive and reliable new haemoglobin colour scale for assessing anaemia. *J Clin Pathol* 1998;**51**:21–24.
7. Rickard CM, Couchman BA, Schmidt SJ, Dank A, Purdie DM. A discard volume of twice the deadspace ensures clinically accurate arterial blood gases and electrolytes and

prevents unnecessary blood loss. *Crit Care Med* 2003;**31**: 1654–1658.
8. Weiss M, Fischer J, Boeckmann M, Rohrer B, Baenziger O. Evaluation of a simple method for minimizing iatrogenic blood loss from discard volumes in critically ill newborns and children. *Intensive Care Med* 2001;**27**:1064–1072.
9. Gleason E, Grossman S, Campbell C. Minimizing diagnostic blood loss in critically ill patients. *Am J Crit Care* 1992;**1**: 85–90.
10. Rais-Bahrami K, Rivera O, Mikesell GT, Short BL. Continuous blood gas monitoring using an in-dwelling optode method: clinical evaluation of the Neotrend sensor using a luer stub adaptor to access the umbilical artery catheter. *J Perinatol* 2002;**22**:367–369.
11. Meyers PA, Worwa C, Trusty R, Mammel MC. Clinical validation of a continuous intravascular neonatal blood gas sensor introduced through an umbilical artery catheter. *Respir Care* 2002;**47**:682–687.
12. Krasnoff J, Painter P. The physiological consequences of bed rest and inactivity. *Adv Ren Replace Ther* 1999;**6**:124–132.
13. Payne MW, Uhthoff HK, Trudel G. Anemia of immobility: caused by adipocyte accumulation in bone marrow. *Med Hypoth* 2007;**69**:778–786.
14. Turba RM, Lewis VL, Green D. Pressure sore anemia: response to erythropoietin. *Arch Phys Med Rehabil* 1992;**73**: 498–500.
15. Kamel HK, Iqbal MA, Mogallapu R, Maas D, Hoffmann RG. Time to ambulation after hip fracture surgery: relation to hospitalization outcomes. *J Gerontol A Biol Sci Med Sci* 2003;**58**:1042–1045.
16. Goldberg AP, Geltman EM, Gavin JR 3rd, *et al.* Exercise training reduces coronary risk and effectively rehabilitates hemodialysis patients. *Nephron* 1986;**42**:311–316.
17. Hagberg JM, Goldberg AP, Ehsani AA, Heath GW, Delmez JA, Harter HR. Exercise training improves hypertension in hemodialysis patients. *Am J Nephrol* 1983;**3**:209–212.
18. Dimeo F, Fetscher S, Lange W, Mertelsmann R, Keul J. Effects of aerobic exercise on the physical performance and incidence of treatment-related complications after high-dose chemotherapy. *Blood* 1997;**90**:3390–3394.
19. Dimeo F, Knauf W, Geilhaupt D, Böning D. Endurance exercise and the production of growth hormone and haematopoietic factors in patients with anaemia. *Br J Sports Med* 2004;**38**:e37.
20. Dimeo FC, Thomas F, Raabe-Menssen C, Pröpper F, Mathias M. Effect of aerobic exercise and relaxation training on fatigue and physical performance of cancer patients after surgery. A randomised controlled trial. *Support Care Cancer* 2004;**12**:774–779.
21. Fuoco U, Scivoletto G, Pace A, Vona VU, Castellano V. Anaemia and serum protein alteration in patients with pressure ulcers. *Spinal Cord* 1997;**35**:58–60.
22. Raynard B, Nitenberg G. [Is prevention of upper digestive system hemorrhage in intensive care necessary?] *Schweiz Med Wochenschr* 1999;**129**:1605–1612.

23. Reveiz L, Guerrero-Lozano R, Camacho A, Yara L, Mosquera PA. Stress ulcer, gastritis, and gastrointestinal bleeding prophylaxis in critically ill pediatric patients: a systematic review. *Pediatr Crit Care Med* 2010;**11**:124–132.

24. Cook DJ, Reeve BK, Guyatt GH, *et al*. Stress ulcer prophylaxis in critically ill patients. Resolving discordant meta-analyses. *JAMA* 1996;**275**:308–314.

25. Leontiadis GI, Sharma VK, Howden CW. Systematic review and meta-analysis: proton-pump inhibitor treatment for ulcer bleeding reduces transfusion requirements and hospital stay–results from the Cochrane Collaboration. *Aliment Pharmacol Ther* 2005;**22**:169–174.

26. Freeman BD, Isabella K, Lin N, Buchman TG. A meta-analysis of prospective trials comparing percutaneous and surgical tracheostomy in critically ill patients. *Chest* 2000; **118**:1412–1418.

27. von Ahsen N, Müller C, Serke S, Frei U, Eckardt KU. Important role of nondiagnostic blood loss and blunted erythropoietic response in the anemia of medical intensive care patients. *Crit Care Med* 1999;**27**:2630–2639.

28. Smoller BR, Kruskall MS. Phlebotomy for diagnostic laboratory tests in adults. Pattern of use and effect on transfusion requirements. *N Engl J Med* 1986;**314**:1233–1235.

29. Fragou M, Gravvanis A, Dimitriou V, *et al*. Real time ultrasound-guided subclavian vein cannulation versus the landmark method in critical care patients: a prospective randomized study. *Crit Care Med* 2011;**39**:1607–1612.

30. Kiell C, Curtas S, Meguid MM. Refinement of central venous cannulation technique. *Nutrition* 1989;**5**: 37–38.

31. Vesely TM, Fazzaro AG, Gherardini D. Preliminary evaluation of a valved introducer sheath for the insertion of tunneled hemodialysis catheters. *Semin Dial* 2004;**17**: 65–68.

32. Allen DS, Marso SP, Lindsey JB, Kennedy KF, Safley DM. Comparison of bleeding complications using arterial closure device versus manual compression by propensity matching in patients undergoing percutaneous coronary intervention. *Am J Cardiol* 2011;**107**:1619–1623.

33. Liu KS, Liu C, Xia Y, Li YH, Du W, Wei QM, Zhao WJ. Permanent cardiac pacing through the right supraclavicular subclavian vein approach. *Can J Cardiol* 2003;**19**:1005–1008.

34. Lip GY, Frison L, Halperin JL, Lane DA. Comparative validation of a novel risk score for predicting bleeding risk in anticoagulated patients with atrial fibrillation: the HAS-BLED (Hypertension, Abnormal Renal/Liver Function, Stroke, Bleeding History or Predisposition, Labile INR, Elderly, Drugs/Alcohol Concomitantly) score. *J Am Coll Cardiol* 2011;**57**:173–180.

35. Lippi G, Favaloro EJ, Cervellin G. Prevention of venous thromboembolism: focus on mechanical prophylaxis. *Semin Thromb Hemost* 2011;**37**:237–251.

36. Scharte M, Fink MP. Red blood cell physiology in critical illness. *Crit Care Med* 2003;**31**(12 Suppl):S651–657.

37. Zelinka ES, Brevig J, McDonald J, Jin R. The perfusionist's role in a collaborative multidisciplinary approach to blood transfusion reduction in cardiac surgery. *J Extra Corpor Technol* 2010;**42**:45–51.

38. Zelinka ES, Ryan P, McDonald J, Larson J. Retrograde autologous prime with shortened bypass circuits decreases blood transfusion in high-risk coronary artery surgery patients. *J Extra Corpor Technol* 2004;**36**:343–347.

39. Society of Thoracic Surgeons Blood Conservation Guideline Task Force, Ferraris VA, Brown JR, Despotis GJ, *et al*. 2011 update to the Society of Thoracic Surgeons and the Society of Cardiovascular Anesthesiologists blood conservation clinical practice guidelines. *Ann Thorac Surg* 2011;**91**: 944–982.

40. Remadi JP, Marticho P, Butoi I, *et al*. Clinical experience with the mini-extracorporeal circulation system: an evolution or a revolution? *Ann Thorac Surg* 2004;**77**:2172–2175; discussion 2176.

41. Ugaki S, Honjo O, Nakakura M, *et al*. Transfusion-free neonatal cardiopulmonary bypass using a TinyPump. *Ann Thorac Surg* 2010;**90**:1615–1621.

42. Boldt J, von Bormann B, Kling D, Jacobi M, Moosdorf R, Hempelmann G. Preoperative plasmapheresis in patients undergoing cardiac surgery procedures. *Anesthesiology* 1990;**72**:282–288.

43. Smigla GR, Lawson DS, Shearer IR, Jaggers J, Milano C, Welsby I. An ultrafiltration technique for directly reinfusing residual cardiopulmonary bypass blood. *J Extra Corpor Technol* 2004;**36**:231–234.

44. Despotis GJ, Joist JH, Hogue CW Jr, *et al*. The impact of heparin concentration and activated clotting time monitoring on blood conservation. A prospective, randomized evaluation in patients undergoing cardiac operation. *J Thorac Cardiovasc Surg* 1995;**110**:46–54.

45. Strate LL, Naumann CR. The role of colonoscopy and radiological procedures in the management of acute lower intestinal bleeding. *Clin Gastroenterol Hepatol* 2010;**8**:333–343; quiz e344.

46. CRASH-2 collaborators, Roberts I, Shakur H, Afolabi A, *et al*. The importance of early treatment with tranexamic acid in bleeding trauma patients: an exploratory analysis of the CRASH-2 randomised controlled trial. *Lancet* 2011;**377**: 1096–1101, e1–2.

47. McCullough PA, Lepor NE, The deadly triangle of anemia, renal insufficiency, and cardiovascular disease: implications for prognosis and treatment. *Rev Cardiovasc Med* 2005;**6**: 1–10.

48. Karski JM, Mathieu M, Cheng D, Carroll J, Scott GJ. Etiology of preoperative anemia in patients undergoing scheduled cardiac surgery. *Can J Anaesth* 1999;**46**:979–982.

49. Rabe H, Reynolds G, Diaz-Rossello J. A systematic review and meta-analysis of a brief delay in clamping the umbilical cord of preterm infants. *Neonatology* 2008;**93**:138–144.

50. Hicks JM. Excessive blood drawing for laboratory tests. *N Engl J Med* 1999;**340**:1690.

51. O'Hare D, Chilvers RJ. Arterial blood sampling practices in intensive care units in England and Wales. *Anaesthesia* 2001;**56**:568–571.

52. Lin JC, Strauss RG, Kulhavy JC, *et al.* Phlebotomy overdraw in the neonatal intensive care nursery. *Pediatrics* 2000;**106**: E19.

53. Corwin HL, Parsonnet KC, Gettinger A. RBC transfusion in the ICU. Is there a reason? *Chest* 1995;**108**:767–771.

54. MacIsaac CM, Presneill JJ, Boyce CA, Byron KL, Cade JF. The influence of a blood conserving device on anaemia in intensive care patients. *Anaesth Intensive Care* 2003;**31**: 653–657.

55. Dech ZF, Szaflarski NL, Nursing strategies to minimize blood loss associated with phlebotomy. *AACN Clin Issues* 1996;**7**:277–287.

56. Madan A, Kumar R, Adams MM, Benitz WE, Geaghan SM, Widness JA. Reduction in red blood cell transfusions using a bedside analyzer in extremely low birth weight infants. *J Perinatol* 2005;**25**:21–25.

57. Enk D, Palmes AM, Van Aken H, Westphal M. Nasotracheal intubation: a simple and effective technique to reduce nasopharyngeal trauma and tube contamination. *Anesth Analg* 2002;**95**:1432–1436.

58. Singer AJ, Blanda M, Cronin K, *et al.* Comparison of nasal tampons for the treatment of epistaxis in the emergency department: a randomized controlled trial. *Ann Emerg Med* 2005;**45**:134–139.

13 Physical Methods of Hemostasis

Achieving expedited hemostasis after any kind of bleeding is vital to reduce mortality and morbidity. There is a vast array of methods to achieve this goal. A basic knowledge of these methods is essential to enable a blood manager to critically appraise them and to use them appropriately. Therefore, this chapter explores some of the physical methods available to achieve hemostasis, their indications, contraindications, and value in reducing blood loss.

Objectives

1. To relate the basic principles of surgical cutting and hemostasis.
2. To explore alternatives to a scalpel.
3. To learn about surgical maneuvers to reduce blood loss.
4. To describe the different methods to achieve hemostasis in a variety of hemorrhages.

Definitions

Cautery: The word cautery is derived from the Greek word "*causis*," meaning "to burn," or the Latin word "*cauterium*" for "searing iron." Cautery means the act of coagulating blood and destroying tissue with a hot iron, by freezing, or with a caustic agent. The term cautery is also used for the instrument used to perform cauterization. *Electrocautery* means cauterization (cutting or hemostasis) achieved by bringing an electrically heated metal instrument into contact with the tissue.

Diathermy: The word diathermy is derived from the Greek "*dia*" for "through" and "*thermos*" for "heat." Diathermy means the generation of heat in the tissue by means of electrical current. Medical diathermy is used for the therapeutic heating of tissue. Surgical diathermy (synonymous with *electrosurgery*) means the localized heating of tissue for cutting and hemostasis (*electrocoagulation*) by absorption of a high-frequency electrical current.

Desiccation: Coagulation resulting in dehydrated cells. Desiccation is sometimes used synonymously with fulguration.

Thermal knife: Refers to any surgical cutting device that uses heat as the acting physical principle for cutting.

Surgical coagulation: The disruption of tissue by physical means to form an amorphous residuum. With respect to blood vessels, two forms are distinguished:

• *Obliterative* coagulation occurs by direct electrode contact with or electrical arching to the tissue. Vessel walls shrink and the lumen is occluded by contracted tissue and thrombosis. It is the best method for vessels smaller than 1 mm in diameter.
• *Coaptive* coagulation occurs by mechanically apposing the edges of the vessel with a hemostat or forceps and applying current to the hemostat or forceps. The adventitia of the vessel is destroyed, the muscular layer shrinks, and the intima fuses.

A brief history

Surgical cutting and attempts to achieve hemostasis are not new. Ayurvedic medicine, which claims to be about

Basics of Blood Management, Second Edition. Petra Seeber and Aryeh Shander.
© 2013 John Wiley & Sons, Ltd. Published 2013 by John Wiley & Sons, Ltd.

6000 years old, mentions the use of sharp bamboo splinters for surgical cutting. In early human history, all kinds of knives were used as scalpels, not without problems. Hemorrhage and death occurred as a result of injury or surgical interventions. King Hammurabi of Babylon (1955–1912 BC) therefore introduced laws that dealt with surgical cutting for wound care. The *Code of Hammurabi* contains the paragraph: "If a physician makes a wound and cures a freeman, he shall receive ten pieces of silver . . . However it is decreed that if a physician treats a patient 'with a metal knife for a severe wound and has caused the man to die—his hands shall be cut off'". This decree placed much emphasis on the proper use of a scalpel and achieving hemostasis, and imposed a severe penalty on the physician who was unfortunate to lose a surgical patient.

As testified to by ancient papyri, such as the Edwin Smith Papyrus (circa 1600 BC) and the Eber Papyrus (circa 1500 BC), the ancient Egyptians used the sharp blade of a papyrus reed as a scalpel. They also used heated scalpels, the precursors of the modern hemostatic scalpel. Attempts to achieve hemostasis included cautery and tamponade with linen. The Edwin Smith Papyrus also makes the first mention of sutures for wound care.

Greek physicians, among them Hippocrates (466–377 BC), tapped Egyptian medical wisdom. Hippocrates recommended the use of compressive bandages. About 700–800 BC, Homer's *Iliad* described detailed means of surgical hemostasis for wounds.

The Romans learned from the Greeks. Celsus reported the use of a hemostatic forceps [1]. Galen (131–201), one of the most influential physicians in the Roman world, gained experience in wound care and trauma surgery while working with gladiators. Galen's most important contribution to surgery is the first mention of ligature of vessels to halt bleeding. In turn, Paul of Aegina (6th century) was the first to recommend ligature of blood vessels *before* a surgical procedure in a wound.

In the Islamic realm, the physician Al-Razi (841–926) was famous for his work. He used silk sutures and alcohol for hemostasis. The Persian physician Avicenna (Ibn-Cina) (980–1037) described vessel ligature in his work *Canon*.

During the Middle Ages (circa 400–1400), some Christian clergymen, who were able to read and had access to old writings, often worked as surgeons. However, in 1131, the Council of Reims issued a papal decree forbidding clerics to do surgical work. For a long time, the edict: *"Ecclesia abhorrent a sanguine!"* (Church abhors blood!) proved to be a death blow to surgery. It meant that literate men were no longer allowed to practice surgery. Important knowledge was lost, e.g., the knowledge about ligature of blood vessels. Illiterate laymen, e.g., barbers, were now in charge of wound care. They could not benefit from the knowledge accumulated by their ancestors.

Guy de Chauliac (1300–1368), one of the most influential surgeons of the 14th and 15th centuries, revived surgical hemostasis and, as documented in his surgical textbook (*Collectorium cyrurgie*, 1363) he considered hemostasis to be the central issue of surgery. He built on the work of Al-Zahrawi (circa 930–1013), who practiced near Cordoba and used special cotton, cautery, and ligature of blood vessels to achieve hemostasis. Guy de Chauliac quoted Al-Zahrawi over 200 times. De Chauliac's writings remained influential in Europe until the publications of the Frenchman Ambrose Paré (1510–1590). He was originally a barber and advanced to become a surgeon on the battle field. Using traditional methods such as treating wounds with hot oil and the searing iron to stop bleeding, he observed in 1537, during a battle in Italy, that—because of a lack of oil—"untreated" soldiers did better than those treated with hot oil. Paré stopped the use of hot oil and the searing iron for wound care and hemostasis. Instead, he reinvented ligature of vessels and used it for amputations.

About 1700, a new technique for hemostasis appeared— the tourniquet. Pelet coined the actual term "tourniquet" in 1718. The use of a tourniquet was accompanied by Esmarch's limb exsanguination technique in 1873. In 1904, Cushing developed a pneumatic tourniquet [2], similar to the one used today.

The 19th century brought a drastic change in surgical cutting and hemostasis. In 1854, the surgeon Albrecht Theodor Middeldorpf published a monograph on galvanocautery. He described a platinum wire that was caused to glow by connecting it to an electrical battery [3]. Although not his invention, Middeldorpf was the first to develop galvanocautery into a usable surgical method. This was one of the earliest uses of electrical current for surgery. Modern surgical diathermy with high-frequency alternating current was introduced in 1909 by the dermatologist Franz Nagelschmidt from Berlin [3]. The electrosurgical instrument, introduced by WT Bovie and H Cushing in 1928, became such a ubiquitous instrument that even today's surgeons refer to the electrosurgical knife as "the Bovie." At the time of invention, the explosive anesthetics made electrosurgery a hazardous undertaking. It was therefore not widely used. In the 1950s and 1960, non-explosive anesthetics were introduced. This accelerated the spread of electrosurgery into the operating room.

The 20th century brought the advent of countless equipment for surgical cutting and concomitant hemostasis. As early as the 1920s, Irving Langmuir worked with the flow of highly ionized gases in a closed atmosphere. He laid the groundwork for the surgical use of plasma. Experiments with plasma as a surgical cutting tool started in the 1960s. In 1976 Russian scientists reported the clinical use of a plasma scalpel. The argon plasma coagulator was invented by Dr Jerome Canady, who applied for a US patent for this in July 1991 and it was granted in May 1993. In 1960, the first laser was built and it was used shortly thereafter in surgery. The microwave tissue coagulator was introduced by Tabuse in 1979 [4]. In 1982, Papachristou reported on the first use of a water jet in surgery. The Filipino surgeon Wilmo Orejola invented the harmonic scalpel that was introduced commercially in 1993. Many more cutting and coagulation methods have been invented or modified since.

Basics of surgical techniques

The amount of blood loss during surgery has a profound impact on morbidity and mortality. In fact, patient outcome is more dependent on intraoperative blood loss than preoperative hemoglobin level [5]. Although inadvisable in elective surgery, patients with low hemoglobin levels can safely undergo surgery if precautions are taken to minimize blood loss. Therefore, learning how to operate without causing unnecessary blood loss is a major contribution to improved patient outcome. To fulfill this important role, a surgeon must demonstrate expertise in reducing blood loss where possible.

Before surgery, some basic issues should be kept in mind: the choice of surgeon and choice of surgical technique. The surgeon needs to consider his/her own expertise, skills, and experience. Referral to an experienced surgeon seems to be appropriate in situations where blood loss is a predominant issue. Fast, but not careless, hands are needed. Accurate hemostasis and the speed with which it is achieved are crucial. The choice of an appropriate surgeon is therefore the first and most vital step in reducing blood loss.

Long before transfusions were in vogue, surgeons realized that hemostasis is a *sine qua non* of professional patient care. This is mirrored in the principles of Dr Halsted who formulated the "Tenets of Halsted," namely:

- Gentle tissue handling
- Aseptic technique
- Sharp anatomical dissection of tissues
- Careful hemostasis (using fine, non-irritating suture material in minimal amounts)
- Obliteration of dead space in the wound
- Avoidance of tension
- Importance of rest.

Although in parts controversial, these tenets are the basis for modern surgical craftsmanship [7]. They also form the basis of expert surgical blood management. Certain aspects, derived from Halsted's tenets, deserve special consideration when it comes to surgical blood management [8]:

- **Attention to detail:** Any bleeding, major or minor, needs to be stopped. Even small losses add up and constitute major bleeding if left unattended.
- **Partial dissection:** Incising a portion of a wound, achieving hemostasis, and continuing by incising another portion.
- **Avoid stripping:** Stripping the fat layer off fascia makes identification of layers for closure easier, but increases blood loss.
- **Anatomical dissection:** Cutting along anatomical, avascular planes requires a thorough knowledge of anatomy. It reduces uncontrolled vessel injury.
- **Gentle tissue handling:** A "rip and tear" approach to surgery increases tissue damage and blood loss, and should be avoided.

The choice of surgical technique or surgical access reportedly influences the amount of blood loss. Some surgical techniques make less demand on hemostasis than other approaches to the same problem. For example, modified methods for aortic surgery may translate into reduced blood loss. Minor changes in surgical technique—the addition of some strategically placed sutures—reduce blood loss [6]. The chosen route of access to the surgical site can also influence blood loss. Open transabdominal access is the most widely accepted in the treatment of infrarenal abdominal aortic aneurysms, but this approach may cause significant intraoperative blood loss. Alternative approaches, such as with minimal access procedures, may be as effective as the transperitoneal approach, but causes less intraoperative blood loss in well-selected cases.

As adjuncts to surgical craftsmanship, there are many surgical devices that reduce blood loss. However, reduction of blood loss is more dependent on the surgeon's skill than the use of sophisticated equipment. Nevertheless, in the hands of a skilled surgeon, such devices can be employed beneficially. No surgeon can master every method and not every method suits all surgeons. It is better to master a limited number of techniques that fit the procedures performed than to have a whole array of gadgets without really mastering any of these.

Surgical tools

The ideal cutting device combines a number of different characteristics [9]. It can cut at least as well as a scalpel and coagulate at least as well as monopolar electrosurgery, while causing minimal tissue injury, producing little or no smoke to obscure the visual field, and posing no danger either to the patient or personnel. No special patient preparation is needed for its use, and surgeons can handle it without special training. It also incurs no great costs. It is easily perceived that this is the "ideal," as yet non-existent, device. Every cutting method has its advantages and disadvantages that make it best suited for one procedure or another. It is up to the surgeon to determine from the equipment available which is best suited for the case.

Scalpel

The oldest means of cutting still in use is the scalpel "cold steel". Despite the overwhelming flood of new surgical instruments, the scalpel has kept its prominent position. Its universal availability, independence from electricity for use, and low cost make it the method of choice in many surgical interventions.

A plain scalpel is most frequently used for the skin incision. It gives a clean cut, which is associated with a small scar and relatively rarely with wound infections. Although it has been shown that thermal techniques for skin incision (such as diathermy; see below) reduce blood loss when compared to the scalpel, these techniques are currently recommended only in selected circumstances, e.g., in patients who have a coagulopathy or who will receive anticoagulation during surgery [10], but may gain wider acceptance soon.

Heat in surgery

Heat transferred to tissue can either benefit or harm the patient. Knowledge of the basic characteristics and effects of heat in tissue helps to get the best out of equipment that uses heat for surgery while minimizing the associated risks.

Heat can be transferred to and within tissue by conduction (increased molecular energy that occurs with increased temperatures), convection (through movement of matter, e.g., blood), and radiation. Distribution of heat in tissue will increase tissue temperature and cause changes in the tissue. The extent of such changes not only depends on the temperature, but also on the time the tissue is influenced by the temperature, and on the characteristics of the tissue itself. The extent to which tissue is perfused also influences the effect of the heat. Blood flow diverts heat away from the site of thermal injury (i.e., cutting or coagulation).

Heat alters tissue elements in a temperature-dependent fashion. Proteins coagulate at about 60°C. Tissue temperatures between 60 and 80°C cause shrinkage of Type I collagen in the walls of blood vessels, airways, and bile ducts. Collagen shrinkage closes the lumen and seals the vessel. Cellular changes occur at temperatures up to 100°C. Cell wall and membrane damage as well as DNA denaturation and enzyme deactivation occur. Above 100°C, the water content of the tissue vaporizes and the remains of the cells pyrolyse (i.e., the primary structure of the compound dissociates). Temperatures from 300 to 400°C are needed to pyrolyse triglycerides and at about 600°C proteins pyrolyse.

Surgical methods that use heat to cut are often used to achieve coagulation as well. Hemostasis is provided simultaneously with cutting. It is also possible to either cut or coagulate exclusively with these methods. Both the cutting and coagulating cause some degree of tissue damage. If the heat is decreased, so is the effect on hemostasis.

Exposure of tissue to thermal energy for cutting or coagulation also has some clinical effects. Epithelium migration and wound healing are delayed. Wounds made with a thermal knife are thought to be less resistant to bacterial infection than those made with "cold steel."

Thermocoagulator

The thermocoagulator (hot-jet coagulator) uses a stream of hot air to coagulate bleeding surfaces. Temperatures of up to 500°C develop at the tip of the instrument. The tip can be held just above the bleeding tissue to coagulate the tissue surface [11].

Hot water

Hot water, applied manually or with the aid of technical devices, can be useful in selected surgical situations for blood management. When hot water is applied with a surgical sponge onto a bleeding surface, it may be able to reduce diffuse bleeding. But care must be taken not to harm adjacent nerves or other delicate tissues. Hot water applied in the uterine cavity may be used for endometrial ablation in the treatment of menorrhagia, a method called hydrothermal ablation [12]. Hot water irrigation may also stop epistaxis.

Electrical current for surgery

Two basic methods using electrical current, each with many variations, have been introduced into surgery: electrocautery and electrosurgery (= diathermy or "cold caustic"). In electrocautery, a metal applicator is heated by means of an electrical current. The cautery effect is restricted to the site where heat is transferred from the metal to the tissue. No current enters the patient's body. In electrosurgery, heat is created at the metal–tissue interface through tissue–current interactions.

Depending on the frequency, electrical currents affect tissue in a distinct way. If tissue is exposed to up to 3000 Hz, nerves and muscles are stimulated in a dose-dependent fashion. Between 3000 and 5000 Hz, a plateau is reached. At currents between 5000 and 10 000 Hz, neuromuscular effects decrease. At frequencies of more than 10 000 Hz, neuromuscular reaction no longer occurs. At this point, body tissue works as an electrical conduction path. Conduction is limited by the tissue resistance to the flow of current (also called impedance). Resistance can be expressed as follows:

$$\text{Resistance} = \text{Resistivity} \times (\text{Length}/\text{Area})$$

Resistivity, the biological impedance (ohm cm), depends on tissue characteristics and on the frequency of the electrical current. The larger the area to which the current spreads, the lower the resistance to a specific electrical current will be. Applied to surgical cutting, this means the smaller the area touched by the electrode, the hotter the tissue. The small active electrode in the wound touches only a small area of tissue. There is a high current density. Heat will develop as this current has to struggle against the resistance of the tissue in contact with the electrode. The tissue is heated locally. As the current spreads throughout the body, however, there is a large mass of tissue (i.e., a larger surface area) and no significant heating occurs. The current leaves the body (in monopolar surgery) by way of a grounding pad, which has a large surface area. Again, no significant heat develops at this large exit for the current.

The degree of coagulation and the speed or depth of cutting with an electrical current depend on the power delivered. Power is the product of current squared multiplied by the resistance. This means that, if the current is doubled, four times the heat is generated in the tissue. The higher the power, the faster and deeper the cutting, and the more coagulation and tissue damage. The mode of operation, cutting and/or coagulation, depends also on the waveform of the current:
- Strictly cutting, no coagulation: undamped continuous sinus wave
- Coagulation, no cutting: damped, intermittent sinus wave
- Combined, cutting and coagulation: interrupted sinus wave.

Method 1: Electrocautery: the hemostatic scalpel

A hemostatic scalpel unit consists of a controller, a handle, and a disposable scalpel blade similar to a conventional scalpel blade [13]. The blade consists of various metal layers. Between the layers there is an electrical microcircuit that heats the blade. The blade temperature range is adjustable from 110 to 270 °C. Skin is usually incised at a temperature of 110 °C and vessels with a diameter of up to 2 mm are sealed at temperatures between 210 and 270 °C. When the scalpel blade touches the tissue, hemostasis is achieved by direct transmission of heat to the tissue. Since no electrical current is transmitted into the tissue, there is no interference with electrically powered monitoring. Muscles do not contract or fibrillate.

A variation of electrocautery was introduced in 1994. A procedure termed "muscle fragment welding" uses electrocautery through a rectal muscle fragment. A piece of muscle is applied to the bleeding area and then cautery forms a coagulum from the muscle fragment. This provides seemingly immediate and permanent hemostasis. Rectal muscle fragment welding is an effective and practical method of controlling presacral and other hemorrhage [14, 15].

Method 2: Electrosurgery

In electrosurgery, a closed electrical circuit is created of which the patient is a part [16]. Alternating high-frequency current travels through tissue. This causes ionized molecules in the tissue to oscillate and the tissue heats up (up to 300 °C). A pure cutting current produces a small line of tissue destruction at the edges of the incision. The upper layer consists of carbon particles, beneath is a layer of desiccated or coagulated tissue. The current also desiccates the tissues, forms scars, and produces smoke.

Surgical diathermy has three adjustable variables: (a) power, (b) frequency (which provides the choice between coagulation and cutting), and (c) polarity (monopole *vs* bipole, referring to the distance between the electrical poles).

In monopolar electrosurgery ("the Bovie"), the active electrode is in the wound. The current returns to the large return electrode, which is placed elsewhere on the patient, far away from the active electrode. The current flows through the patient. Heat develops in the tissue around the active electrode.

In bipolar electrosurgery, an instrument that looks like a pair of forceps is used. One arm of the forceps is the active electrode, the other the return electrode. The active and return electrodes are only millimeters apart. Both are in the wound. The current flows through the tissue that is grasped between the forceps and coagulation takes place. Cutting is not possible in bipolar electrosurgery.

While electrosurgery is very safe, some hazards must be kept in mind and measures taken to prevent them. Current follows the path of least resistance. In monopolar surgery, this may cause problems, namely, electrical burns in the area of the return electrode or any area used to ground the patient (grounding injury). Since the electrical current flows directly through the body, pacemakers and monitoring may be disturbed and cardiac arrhythmias induced. Some disadvantages are shared by bipolar and monopolar electrosurgery. While there is no longer any danger of explosion from anesthetic gases, other gases still pose a hazard. Bowel gases (methane, hydrogen) are explosive and can cause injury if they come into contact with electrosurgical equipment. Electrosurgery also generates smoke, which may delay healing and promote infection [10].

Electrosurgery is used in almost all kinds of procedures. It is especially practical for surgery in densely vascularized areas. However, it is relatively ineffective in treating areas of diffuse or heavy bleeding and cumbersome if used to treat a broad bleeding surface. When vessels are coagulated in electrosurgery, the desired effects are a change in color (tanning) and retraction of the tissue. A typical popping sound is heard when tissue is cauterized, leaving a charcoal coating. Overzealous use of the device creates unnecessary tissue damage [9]. Sticking of tissue debris to the active electrode is a further disad-

vantage. A scratch pad helps to rid the blade of charcoaled tissue.

Method 3: Radiofrequency ablation

High frequency electrical current can be used not only to cut or achieve hemostasis, but also to denature tissue. To that end, one of more electrodes is inserted into the tissue that needs to be treated. Radiofrequency electrical current is applied and the tissue around the electrode is heated up. This leads to desiccation and denaturation of the surrounding tissue. If this tissue is a tumor, then tumor necrosis is induced, which may halt the tumor progress. In some instances, this approach has even proven curative. In other instances, it has been used with palliative intent. Finely-tuned application of radiofrequency electrodes can also be used to dissect soft tissue, such as liver or spleen. The electrode or a set of electrodes are introduced into the tissue along the plane of intended resection and heated. Within a few seconds, surrounding tissue, i.e., the resection margin, is denatured and hemostasis is promoted. Then, the resection margin can be divided with a scalpel or other means [17].

Variations in the use of electrical current in surgery

Saline-enhanced thermal sealing

Saline-enhanced thermal sealing uses a combination of electrosurgery with a cooling flow of saline applied directly at the tip of the active electrode. When connected to a conventional electrosurgical generator, set at 40–140 W, the tip of the device transmits electrical energy to the tissue. This energy heats the tissue (as in normal electrosurgery). The continuous flow of saline (4–8 mL/min) reduces the heat developing in the tissue. The tissue temperature is kept below 100 °C. This prevents desiccation, eschar, smoke, and sticking of tissue debris to the electrode [18].

Different types of devices allow for either monopolar or bipolar use of saline-enhanced thermal sealing. The monopolar device, called "floating ball", uses continuous infusion of saline through the tip of a ballpoint pen-like device. A similar device can be used in the bipolar mode. A bipolar device (sealing forceps, resembling an endoscopic stapler) is also available. During operation, tissue is grasped in the forceps, which are activated until tissue adjacent to the forceps blanches.

Indications for saline-enhanced thermal sealing include lung surgery, where the technique not only provides hemostasis but also aerostasis, trauma surgery (splenic and hepatic lacerations), partial nephrectomy, radical prostatectomy, as well as laparoscopic myomectomy [19].

Electrothermal bipolar vessel sealer

Electrothermal bipolar vessel sealing uses a combination of pressure and radiofrequency to achieve hemostasis [16]. A generator senses the density of the tissue held between a forceps-like device and adjusts the energy delivered. It employs high currents (4 A) and low voltage (<200 V) bipolar radiofrequency. The high current fuses collagen and elastin, and forms a plastic-like sealed zone. This produces a permanent and translucent seal that obliterates the vessel lumen.

Electrothermal bipolar vessel sealing can be used for vessel diameters of 1–7 mm and for bundles of tissue. It takes 2–5 seconds to seal a vessel. Heat spread is less than 2 mm. Electrothermal bipolar vessel sealing is a suitable measure for hemostasis in tight and deep spaces. It saves time compared to hemostasis by suture ligature. It has been shown to be usable in a wide variety of laparoscopic and open surgeries, such as hemorrhoidectomy, hepatectomy, hysterectomy, splenectomy, prostatectomy, cystectomy, and nephrectomy [20, 21].

Microwaves in surgery

That microwaves can be used to heat and cook food is well known. They can also be used to heat tissue, making them suitable for use in coagulation in surgery.

Microwave coagulation

Microwaves are generated at a frequency of 2450 MHz. The energy is transmitted from a generator through a cable to a handle, which holds a needle probe. Probes of varying lengths are inserted into the tissue and are activated. This denatures the surrounding tissue. A further few seconds are allowed for dissociation of tissue from the probe. The probe may be reinserted to coagulate more tissue. This may be all that is needed to devitalize tumor tissue. Alternatively, the technique may be used to coagulate an intended resection margin in a soft tissue such as the kidney, liver or spleen. Afterward, the tissue can be dissected using a normal scalpel or scissors. Because the tissue is sealed before it is cut, bleeding should not occur. If bleeding does occur, however, the vessels are difficult to ligate using regular sutures, because

coagulated tissue is brittle. In such a case, gentle handling, careful suturing, and the use of glue provide the needed hemostasis [22, 23].

Light in surgery

Similar to electrical current, light can be used for cutting. It interacts with tissue and can heat it. Targeted light in the form of lasers can be used for surgery.

Infrared contact coagulator

The infrared contact coagulator uses a beam of infrared light in order to coagulate bleeding surfaces. A halogen light beam is modified by various optical devices (reflectors, quartzes) and can be targeted at the site of bleeding. Using this means, bleeding in the spleen, liver, kidney, lungs, or cancer sites can be stopped [24–27].

Laser

Laser is in fact an acronym for Light Amplification by Stimulated Emission of Radiation. Light is an electromagnetic wave that is generated by atomic processes. Laser light is generated when an atom with a high energy state is struck by a photon of a precise frequency. This results in the emission of two photons of the same frequency and direction. These photons stimulate others so that the light is amplified exponentially in a manner similar to a chain reaction. The resulting light is monochromatic (of the same color and thus wavelength) and the beam can be focused on a very small spot.

When light touches tissue, it can either be reflected, travel through the tissue, or be absorbed. Absorbed light heats up tissue. Light that is not absorbed travels through deeper tissue layers and does not create the energy density needed for tissue vaporization.

Absorption of light in the visible electromagnetic range is influenced by the color of the tissue. Non-pigmented tissue does not absorb much light energy. However, if wavelengths longer than 1 μm are used, the absorption becomes independent of the tissue color. The longer the wavelength, the more independent the absorption becomes in relation to tissue color.

Laser can be used in two different ways. First, it can be used as a heat source for an instrument. The instrument heats up and upon contact with the tissue, the tissue is coagulated. This is equivalent to electrocauterization. Second, the laser can be directed right into tissue and heat it to achieve the effects described above [28].

Table 13.1 Examples of lasers in medicine.

Ruby laser	Visible wavelength, pulsed mode	Remarks
Argon laser	Blue–green light, therefore strongly influenced by the tissue color; preferentially absorbed by red tissues	Most suitable for coagulation due to the wave length being readily absorbed by hemoglobin; used to (endoscopically) photocoagulate gastrointestinal bleeding
Neodymium:YAG laser (neodymium: yttrium–aluminum garnet laser)	Invisible, near infrared beam, relatively independent of tissue color; most powerful surgical laser (up to 100 W)	High initial costs, stringent safety requirements
CO_2 laser	Invisible, far infrared beam; completely independent of tissue color	Vaporizes skin/tissue for cutting or coagulation. Cuts if in focus, coagulates if defocused

One of the inherent problems of laser surgery is fluid. If fluids impede the laser, its cutting ability is diminished substantially.

The use of lasers is associated with complications and calls for stringent safety measures. Laser can easily perforate tissue, e.g., the bowel, and hemorrhage may occur. CO_2 gas, when absorbed (e.g., from the gastrointestinal tract), can cause respiratory distress [29]. Laser beams or their reflections (e.g., from metal instruments in the wound) may cause eye and skin lesions. Spectacles need to be worn. Fire and explosion may result if unsuitable materials are exposed to the beam, e.g., drapes, clothing (unless kept moist), plastics, flammable anesthetics, and skin preparations.

Lasers have been used in a variety of clinical settings (Table 13.1). Depending on how they are used, they may increase or decrease blood loss [30–33].

Lightning

Plasma (not to be confused with blood plasma) is a partially ionized hot gas. It is generated by creating an electrical arc between two electrodes and then passing a gas (e.g., argon, helium) between them under high pressure. The electrical energy is converted to heat in the gas, causing the gas to become extremely hot. The heat frees electrons from the atoms of the gas (partial ionization). After the gas leaves the electrical field it cools down and the free electrons recombine with the atoms, releasing a photon.

Plasma scalpel

If a hot plasma stream is directed at tissue, it can be used for cutting [34]. A fine, hot gas jet (3000 °C) delivered from a nozzle performs the cutting. Some energy diffuses through the edges of the incision so that the tissue is also coagulated. When the plasma stream is used for cutting, the handle is placed directly on the tissue. For coagulation, the handle is held 1–2 cm above the tissue. The jet of hot gas both clears the tissue of blood and coagulates at the same time. The tip of the handle will still work even when submerged in fluid. As it cuts, the plasma scalpel effectively cauterizes blood vessels of up to 3 mm in diameter [35].

Argon beam coagulation

Argon is a colorless, odorless, inert gas that does not support combustion. It is readily available and inexpensive. At room temperature, ionized argon gas transmits electrical current. It can therefore be used to transfer electricity to tissue.

An argon beam coagulator (= argon plasma coagulator) has a pen-like handle that emits a gentle coaxial flow of argon gas at room temperature. This gas blows away blood and debris to optimize visualization. When the tip of the nozzle is within 1 cm of the tissue surface, radiofrequency energy is transferred through the stream to the tissue. Electrical energy is "sprayed," "painting" the surface of the bleeding tissue. The beam leaves a 1–2-mm eschar (consisting of small, consolidated, coagulated blood vessels) firmly attached to the tissue surface and this provides hemostasis. The hemostatic effect may be enhanced if albumin is applied to the bleeding tissue just before the argon beam coagulator is applied [36]. There is no contact between any metal or nozzle and the tissue. Therefore, less tissue adhesion occurs, less tissue damage results, and no debris sticks to the electrode.

Argon beam coagulation has been used for a wide range of procedures, in particular, liver, spleen, head and neck, and urological surgery (kidneys, bladder, prostate) [37, 38]. It can also be used in endoscopy [39]. The argon beam coagulator is not designed to cut but is suitable for use in areas where diffuse bleeding occurs. It is especially helpful in coagulating bleeding from the surface of parenchymal organs.

Kinetic energy in surgery

Water jet

Water that has been pressurized and then focused into a small jet has long been used to cut metal. The same principle can be used to cut tissue in surgery. Water is delivered under pressure through a variety of nozzle sizes. Both the diameter of the nozzle and the water pressure have an effect on blood loss, speed of dissection, and degree of tissue necrosis. No thermal damage occurs in surrounding tissue.

Hepatic surgery is the classical indication for a water jet [40, 41]. Liver parenchyma are washed away by high-pressure water, leaving vessels and nerves intact. The exposed intrahepatic vessels stand out clearly for accurate ligation or coagulation. A water jet can also be used for other types of tissue, such as the kidney [42], brain [43], and gastrointestinal tract. It can even be used in laparoscopy [44].

High-frequency water jet

A variation of the water jet combines the properties of a water jet and of electrosurgery. A high-frequency electrical current is applied to the water stream and current is transmitted to the patient. Using this combination, cutting and coagulation can be combined [45] so that smaller vessels are coagulated and larger ones remain for separate ligation.

Vibration for surgical cutting

Vibration can cause tissue damage. If harnessed, vibration can be used for surgical interventions. Mechanical energy is transferred to the tissue and cavitational bubbles result from pressure differentials, causing vacuolization in the cells. The vacuoles expand and collapse, leading finally to fragmentation of tissue. The rate of cavitational activity is proportional to the water content of the cells. Soft, fleshy tissue with a high water content is fragmented readily.

Two cutting methods use vibrations: the ultrasonic scalpel and the cavitron ultrasonic surgical aspirator (CUSA).

Ultrasonic scalpel (harmonic scalpel)

The harmonic scalpel uses ultrasound technology to facilitate both cutting and coagulation. An ultrasound generator creates a natural harmonic frequency of 55.5 kHz [25]. The acoustic wave sets the tip in vibration, causing cavitational fragmentation and cutting rather than electrical coagulation. An ultrasonic scalpel provides a focused area of dissection with excellent hemostasis. Since the tip vibrates, it becomes warm. The temperatures that develop (50–100 °C) are lower than those used in electrosurgery or with lasers. Coagulation occurs as a result of protein denaturation when the vibrating blade sticks to proteins, forming a coagulum that seals small vessels. When the effect is prolonged, secondary heat is produced that seals larger vessels. If increased hemostasis is desired, the cutting speed is reduced.

The harmonic scalpel has distinct advantages. Much less heat is transferred into the tissue, causing less tissue damage and smoke. Since there is no smoke, the harmonic scalpel can be used favorably in laparoscopy [46]. A harmonic scalpel also functions in fluids, which makes it useful for cutting submerged tissue.

Cavitron ultrasonic surgical aspirator

CUSA is a dissecting tool that consists of a hollow titanium tip that vibrates along its length at 23 or 36 kHz. The excursion of the tip (amplitude) is set to remove tissue within a 1–2-mm radius. Tissue damage is confined to an area of about 25–50 µm surrounding the tip, with minimal thermal injury and protein denaturation.

The CUSA simultaneously executes three functions: ultrasonic fragmentation, irrigation, and aspiration. The irrigant helps to emulsify tissue and cools the shaft and tip of the tool, which may become warm with extended use. Aspiration through the center of the unit removes dissected tissue and any debris or blood.

The rate of cavitational activity is proportional to the water content of the cells, i.e., soft, fleshy tissues with a high-water content are fragmented more readily than other tissues. Therefore, different types of tissue fragment at different rates, with the result that dissection will leave blood vessels, ureters, and connective tissue skeletonized and intact. Blood vessels then need to be ligated or coagulated separately with techniques other than the CUSA.

The CUSA has been used in neurosurgery, general and oncological surgery, heart surgery, and in gynecology, both in open as well as laparoscopic procedures [47].

Impact of surgical cutting on blood loss

Surgery almost invariably causes blood loss. Reducing this is one of the main goals of blood management. Compared to the use of conventional scalpel and ligature, many of the more modern techniques described above have the potential to reduce blood loss and to enhance surgical hemostasis [10, 48–50]. Comparing the modern techniques, some appear to be superior to others in certain procedures or surgical areas [47]. However, the amount of blood loss during any particular surgery still depends mainly on the forethought, skill, and willingness of the surgeon to restrict blood loss as far as is possible. The right choice of technique may only enhance the surgeon's abilities when used in the right place, in the right manner, and with the correct intent. The unavailability of a technique must never be an excuse not to apply the basic principles of hemostasis.

Apart from the sophisticated equipment available for cutting and coagulation, there are many manual or low-cost measures to stop bleeding or to reduce blood loss. The methods involve selectively occluding vessels, applying pressure to whole organs and bleeding surfaces, or lowering hemostatic pressure in vessels leading to the surgical field.

Selective occlusion of vessels—externally and internally

Classical methods: Sutures and clips

Bleeding from injured vessels can be stopped by ligation with a suture. This is an efficient, yet tedious and time-consuming, task. Metal or plastic clips are available to make vessel ligation easier. Clips are easily placed and staplers help to reach even deep vessels. Some forms of clips can be used for endoscopic hemostasis. However, staplers are expensive and clips can dislodge. The use of sutures as well as clips for hemostasis leaves foreign material in the body. Nevertheless, sutures and clips are still the mainstay of hemostasis in many surgical interventions.

Vascular maneuvers

One of the most feared operative hazards of parenchymal surgery is hemorrhage. Ligation of vessels supplying the parenchyma may help to reduce blood loss.

The liver is a delicate organ and bleeds easily. About 20–30% of the cardiac output flows through the liver. During hepatic surgery, blood loss is almost invariably high, unless specific techniques are used to prevent and stop bleeding. It is not surprising that many variations of liver vessel occlusion have been described. Reducing blood flow prevents excessive hemorrhage during dissection of the parenchyma, e.g.:

• **Pringle maneuver** (pedicle ligation technique; Pringle 1908): A soft clamp—or better, a banding, or just the fingers—are used to temporarily occlude the portal triad. By means of this maneuver, the arterial and portal vein inflow to the liver is stopped, but the back flow from the hepatic veins is still active.

• For **total vascular exclusion**, the vena cava is isolated above and below the liver and occluded. Additionally, the portal vein and hepatic artery are occluded. This technique provides the best possible vascular control. It is used for large tumors close to the vena cava. A severe side effect may be significant hemodynamic derangement.

• **Selective hepatic vascular exclusion:** To control inflow and outflow to major hepatic veins only, without occlusion of the caval blood flow, hemihepatic vascular clamping and occlusion of the corresponding hepatic vein or clamping of the hepatic pedicle with occlusion of the three hepatic veins is possible. It is much more effective than the Pringle maneuver for controlling intraoperative bleeding (prevention of backflow bleeding), and it may be associated with better postoperative liver function and shorter hospital stay [51]. Another advantage is that the caval blood flow is not interrupted, avoiding grave hemodynamic changes. But this method is much more sophisticated to use and needs an experienced team of surgeons.

• **Makuuchi's maneuver** [52] (hemihepatic vascular clamping): During this procedure, vascular clamping selectively interrupts the arterial and venous inflow to the right or left hemiliver. This avoids both splanchnic blood stasis and ischemia or ischemia–reperfusion injury to the whole liver. The negative aspect is that bleeding of the resection plane cannot be completely avoided.

Temporary clamping of vessels may damage them. Clamp trauma, i.e. intimal denudation and medial arterial wall damage, may lead to postoperative stenosis and spasm of the vessels. Occlusion of vessels leading to the liver may also lead to ischemic damage to this organ. Ischemic and reperfusion damage is usually negligible when surgical time is kept short. Nevertheless, transient elevations in hepatic enzymes may be seen, but this does not result in increased morbidity when compared to control groups. Patients with cirrhotic and fatty livers may experience more damage since they do not tolerate ischemia as well. To prolong the tolerable ischemia time, several modifications have been proposed. Ischemic preconditioning of the liver and intermittent inflow occlusion are examples. Good results were observed when the vessel occlusion was released every 5–20 minutes. Some concerns have been voiced regarding frequent reperfusion periods, which may have a worse outcome than only one reperfusion period. Intermittent release of the vessel occlusion may not be necessary since ischemic injury is usually not a problem. A third method to reduce ischemic damage is cooling of the liver. Fortner and colleagues described this technique for the first time in 1974. Such cooling is only necessary when long periods of liver ischemia are expected, e.g., in liver transplant procedures.

Liver surgery is not the only surgery in which vascular occlusion is beneficial. The kidney, spleen, uterus, and other organs can be handled similarly [53].

Endovascular grafts

Occluding vessel walls from within while preserving blood flow through a vessel is the principle behind endovascular grafts. Via vessel puncture, a wire is inserted into a vessel and is guided under radiological control to the damaged part of the vessel. There, a graft is applied through the vessel puncture to tape the vessel wall from within. It is used to stop or prevent surgical or traumatic hemorrhage and has been advocated for a variety of indications [54]. If life-threatening hemorrhage occurs from a large, yet difficult-to-reach or inaccessible vessel, an endoluminal stent–graft can be used to manage the bleeding [55]. It can also be used as a blood-conserving, alternative approach to repair of an abdominal aortic aneurysm [56] or for the treatment of aortobronchial or other vessel fistulae.

Embolization

Another way to occlude vessels from within is embolization. Via a catheter inserted through a fitting vessel, the vessel can be occluded. This can be performed to occlude a vessel temporarily or permanently. A great variety of embolizing agents have been proposed, among them contrast media like lipiodol, sclerosing agents, cyanoacrylate, various particulate substances, or coils.

Embolization can be used in emergency situations to treat bleeding in the brain, nose (epistaxis), uterus, bladder, liver, spleen, gastrointestinal tract (e.g., peptic ulcers), chest wall, pelvic fractures, extremities, etc. [57–60]. However, care must be taken that necessary surgical interventions are not delayed. This may lead to further unnecessary blood loss.

Non-bleeding vessels can be prophylactically embolized (temporarily or permanently) to prevent major blood loss during surgery or rebleeding. This has been described for a variety of cancer and metastatic surgeries, myoma resection of the uterus, uterine bleeding expected during delivery when mothers have errant placentation, and recurrent gastrointestinal bleeding [61–64]. It is also possible to simply place catheters for embolization preoperatively, and then proceed with the surgery; if major blood loss should occur, the vessels can be embolized through the catheters that are already correctly placed.

Also, embolization can be employed as an alternative to surgery. This has been described for the therapy of uterine fibroids or for tumors and metastases, and may avoid blood loss that would have been associated with surgery.

Tourniquet

A more indirect way to achieve temporary vascular occlusion, mainly of the extremities, is the use of a tourniquet. This results in an almost bloodless surgical field. In this instance, occlusion is gentler than direct vessel clamping. A tourniquet minimizes the amount of vessel dissection required, and improves visualization and mobilization of vessels in the surgical field. It avoids the trauma to vessels associated with temporary clamping. Using a tourniquet also avoids postoperative stenosis and spasms of vessels that occur if vessels are clamped.

Before a tourniquet is applied, the limb should be protected by soft cotton padding. Limb elevation for 1–2 minutes before inflation of the tourniquet is also beneficial to reduce the amount of blood in the extremity. Proper wrapping with a rubber bandage (Esmarch) just before tourniquet inflation is crucial to completely exsanguinate the extremity. If there is still oozing after application of a tourniquet, poor exsanguination is usually the cause, not inadequate pressure of the tourniquet. Esmarch bandage techniques should not be used in patients with infected wounds (to prevent dissemination of bacteria) and in patients with deep vein thrombosis.

A pneumatic tourniquet can be inflated with a prede-termined pressure [2]. The pressure used for inflation depends on the limb circumference, systolic blood pressure, tourniquet width, limb shape, cuff design, and vascular status of the limb. The optimal pressure should be kept as low as possible. As a rule of thumb, arterial occlusion pressure plus 50 mmHg is recommended. About 140–320 mmHg is used. Wide cuffs require less pressure than narrower cuffs and reduce the potential for damage to underlying nerves and muscles.

The complications of tourniquet use are nerve compression and ischemic muscle damage. A complete nerve conduction block develops from 15 to 45 minutes after inflation of the tourniquet and is restored within 30 minutes after deflation, providing the total tourniquet time does not exceed 2 hours. By the same token, ischemia times of less than 2 hours do not seem to cause lasting muscle damage. The metabolism of the muscle recovers within 20 minutes after deflation of the cuff. Tourniquet times of more than 2 hours may be associated with irreversible changes in nerve and muscle tissues. The "safe" ischemic interval can be prolonged by the use of heparin (100 mg/kg i.v. 3–5 minutes before the tourniquet is inflated). Cooling the extremity of the limb may also prolong the safe ischemia time.

A full-blown "post-tourniquet syndrome" consists of tissue edema, muscle weakness without paralysis, stiffness, and dysesthesia with pain or numbness. The syndrome usually resolves within 1 week, though the recovery period may be prolonged. Complications associated with tourniquets can be avoided if two tourniquets are applied simultaneously and inflated alternately. Placing good padding beneath the tourniquet is also important to prevent any fluids from running under the tourniquet.

Some surgeons favor release of the tourniquet before the wound is closed. They argue that this enables them to visualize vessels that bleed after tourniquet release and these vessels can be ligated or cauterized before the wound is closed. Others release the tourniquet only after the wound is closed and compressive bandages are applied. The latter approach may cause less blood loss.

A tourniquet is used mainly on limbs, such as in localized endarterectomy, arteriovenous fistula creation, joint replacement, and many other procedures that potentially lead to heavy hemorrhaging from the limbs. Application of tourniquets is not restricted to the extremities; they can be applied to some whole organs. Uterine bleeding, for instance, can be treated temporarily by application of a tourniquet around the cervix [65].

Extremity trauma as well as extremity surgery may be an indication for tourniquet use. In recent years, the use of tourniquets for immediate hemorrhage control after extremity trauma has been advocated. The reason for the recommendation was that heavily bleeding casualties in a combat setting seem to have a higher survival rate than those not receiving a tourniquet. This effect is even more pronounced when the tourniquet is applied immediately, i.e., before the onset of shock [66].

Compression

Manual wound compression

Direct manual compression of bleeding wounds, arteries leading to the wound or whole organs is a recognized technique of first aid [67]. It helps prevent exsanguination and buys some time until complete hemostasis is achievable. Manual compression is also helpful in the surgical setting. It may prevent hematoma formation and permits clotting or the initiation of other hemostatic measures.

Traditionally, manual compression is applied directly over the area of an injured vessel, such as after vessel puncture and especially after arterial puncture. Manual compression of the aorta is also often a life saver and can be used for uterine bleeding, ruptured aortic aneurysm [68], or any injury below a compressible aortic area, e.g., in massive pelvic hemorrhage. Such compression may bridge the time until a patient can be taken to a facility where definite hemostasis can be achieved.

Whole organs can also be compressed to prevent exsanguination. The liver is compressible when the abdomen is open. The uterus can be compressed in an open abdomen as well as from the outside. Uterine massage may also help to reduce postpartum hemorrhage [69].

Compressive bandaging

The use of compressive bandaging is often preferred over extended manual compression, since it frees the hands of the healthcare provider to continue administering further care. It also increases patient comfort. Compressive bandages are applied in emergencies, as well as in the perioperative period, to achieve temporary hemostasis at the site of injury. A prerequisite is that bandaging of the bleeding wound is possible. This may be difficult at some locations. Elastic adhesive bandages may broaden the spectrum of wounds that can be bandaged while applying compression [67]. Addition of hemostatic agents to the bandage may further add to its hemostatic actions [70].

Antishock garment

While something of a misnomer, an antishock garment is still a valuable tool for blood management. Antishock garments look like a pair of pants that fit tightly around a patient's legs and pelvis. Such garments exert pressure on the lower extremities and the pelvis, and hasten hemostasis in lower extremity and traumatic or postpartum bleeding. Antishock garments come in different versions. Some are pneumatic, exerting their effect by inflation of the device. Others are made of elastic neoprene. Where such sophisticated antishock garments are not available, they can be improvised with bicycle tubes and sheets, as described previously [71].

Antishock garments reduce blood flow to the lower extremities and the pelvis, and may therefore reduce fatal hemorrhage. The garments are typically worn until definite hemostasis can be achieved. Application times of more than 2 days have been described.

Packing

Direct control of bleeding is the most desirable choice. However, in some instances this is not possible. Diffuse bleeding ("oozing") may make surgical hemostasis difficult or impossible. Topical hemostasis may be achieved with glues, mesh, argon beam, etc., or by correcting an underlying coagulation defect intraoperatively. At times, hemostasis cannot be achieved by these measures. Hemodynamic stabilization as well as the correction of any underlying coagulopathy is required beforehand. Packing the wound or the bleeding body cavity with sterile towels and tamponades slows the bleeding and allows time to correct the coagulopathy (hypothermia, acidosis, and pre-existing coagulopathy) by reversing the underlying cause. This is part of the damage-control technique that is associated with improved survival in a variety of settings.

Abdominal packing is a life-saving technique for temporary control of severe injury. It is used in the pelvic area and for liver and spleen lacerations [72, 73]. Control of bleeding from the abdominal cavity can be achieved by applying controlled pressure with several large abdominal packs. The packing must exert enough pressure to tamponade the bleeding, but must not stop blood flow through the organ. Skin is closed loosely or by interposing surgical mesh to give room for expansion—to prevent increased intra-abdominal pressure leading to respiratory and perfusion problems. Packing is usually removed 48–72 hours later in the operating room, but no increased infection rate has been observed even after 7–10 days of packing.

Packing is also possible in the nose to treat epistaxis, in wounds, and in the uterus, all in an attempt to stop bleeding.

Mesh wrap

Since intra-abdominal packing increases intra-abdominal pressure and may provoke complications, it has been proposed that a damaged organ be selectively compressed rather than compressing the whole abdomen. An absorbable mesh tailored to a lacerated organ can be applied (Figure 13.1) instead of the usual packing with surgical towels. Pressure is applied to the organ by varying the tension applied while suturing the mesh around the organ. Tamponade is self-contained and does not impair the flow through the vessels leading to the organ. Intra-abdominal pressure is not increased by this method. It is

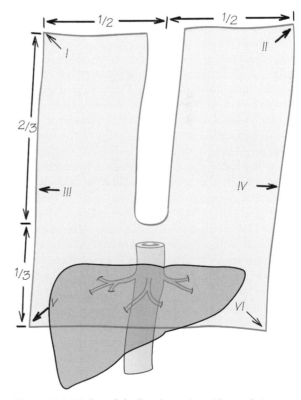

Figure 13.1 Mesh graft for liver lacerations. The mesh is wrapped around the liver and sutured together along the line made by points I–II and V–VI, respectively. Point I is sutured to V and II to VI; then, beginning from point III, the mesh is closed by suturing from III to the point where I and V unite. The same is done with the opposite side.

not necessary to reopen the abdomen. Mesh wraps are applied around the liver [74], kidney, and spleen [75].

Balloon tamponade

Self-made or commercially available balloons are a very valuable adjunct to achieving hemostasis in a great variety of settings.

Hepatic injuries are associated with high morbidity and mortality. Many techniques have been devised to stem bleeding. Balloon tamponade is among the armamentarium of the surgeon and is especially helpful when the injury is near the hilus of the liver, when the caudate lobus is involved or when central wounds are present. The technique of balloon tamponade is easy and has been described as follows: "The balloon tamponade is accomplished by the use of a 1×12-inch Penrose drain and a 16-French red rubber Robinson catheter. One end of the Penrose drain is ligated with a 2-0 silk suture. The red rubber catheter is placed into the open end of the Penrose, and this end is then ligated with a second 2-0 silk suture, making it air and water tight. This is then passed through the wound, allowing 2–3 cm on each side. The Penrose drain is inflated with sterile normal saline, using an Asepto syringe (gastrographin may be added to make it radio-opaque). The amount of inflation depends on the size of the defect. Normal saline is added until it is clear that tamponade has been achieved" [76]. The balloon inflation time can be between 24 hours and 10 days.

Various balloons specifically designed to stop hemorrhage are on the market [77–79]. The Sengstaken–Blakemore tube was designed for use in bleeding esophageal varices. The tube has two inflatable balloons, a round one at the distal end and a cone-shaped one in the middle. With the balloons deflated, the tube is inserted into the stomach and the distal balloon is inflated in the stomach. Then the tube is drawn back until the inflated balloon reaches the cardia and increased resistance to withdrawal of the tube is encountered. At that point, the second balloon is inflated. It is now situated in the esophagus and compresses the bleeding varices. The tube is kept under slight tension until the balloon is inflated. After about 12 hours, the balloon is deflated and after 12 more hours, the tube can be gently removed. Bleeding should have stopped by then.

A similar device is the Linton–Nachlas tube. It has only one balloon, which is pear-shaped and situated at the distal end of the tube. The tube is inserted into the stomach, the balloon is inflated, and the tube is pulled back slightly until it meets the resistance of the cardia.

Since the balloon is pear-shaped, it fits well into the cardia and compresses bleeding at that point. The Linton tube is mainly used for Mallory–Weiss tears.

Foley catheters are simple, safe, and effective tools to stop hemorrhage in a wide variety of settings and are also usable in emergencies. Many different bleeding sites can be compressed by the balloons of such catheters. Examples are the retropubic space [80], prostatic urethra after transurethral resection of the prostate, cervix [81], non-pregnant, pregnant or postpartal uterus [82, 83], nasopharynx [84], nose in epistaxis [85], colon [86], neck and supraclavicular fossae [87], in bleeding from extraperitoneal pelvic bullet tracks [88], rectum [89], maxillofacial wounds [90], and liver [91]. Foley catheter tamponade has even been employed in unusual situations such as in intercostal hemorrhage in preterm infants [92] and penetrating left ventricular wounds [93]. The catheter can be filled with saline. The balloon may be deflated after a few hours to check whether bleeding has stopped. If this is not so, the catheter can be blocked again by reinjecting saline. Radio-opaque fluid may also be used instead of saline. This permits radiological control of the position of the balloon.

Use of drains

The use and misuse of drains in surgery is an ongoing topic in the medical literature. There are not many evidence-based indications for drains. However, drains can increase postoperative blood loss [94, 95].

Complete avoidance of wound drains is sometimes favored over their use. When blood or other fluids collect in a closed wound cavity, they cause compression and may reduce further blood loss. At times, suction drains are clamped for a certain period after surgery to achieve the same compressive effect, e.g., after knee replacement. This may effectively reduce postoperative bleeding after total knee replacement [96].

An advanced method of drain use is retrograde infusion of saline into the wound. After knee arthroplasty, about 50 mL of saline is injected via the suction drain. When surgery is finished and compressive bandages are applied, saline is infused. To enhance the effect of the saline infusion, a low concentration of epinephrine (1:200 000) or tranexamic acid can be added [97]. After the saline is injected, the drain is clamped and left for a few hours, after which it is unclamped and then suctioned in the routine fashion. Clamp times vary from 1 to 24 hours.

Positioning

Appropriate positioning of the patient prior to surgery sometimes improves hemostasis and access to vessels. A lateral position, for instance, may support the surgeon in performing a splenectomy [46]. Elevating the area operated on reduces perfusion in the surgical area and blood loss. Such elevation can easily be accomplished by adjusting the position of the operating table or by using pillows. For further details of intraoperative positioning, refer to Chapter 14.

Positioning is also important in the postsurgical period. After knee surgery, tension on the wound can be increased by positioning the leg appropriately. This tension aids in hemostasis and decreases blood loss. A pillow to flex both hip and knee joints at a 90-degree angle helps. The position should be maintained for 24 hours after surgery. Elevation of the knee reduces postoperative hyperemia in the wound and the anatomical dead space within the knee. There are also mechanical components that partially compress the flow in the popliteal vessels [98].

Key points

• Low intraoperative blood loss facilitates surgery in anemic patients.
• The faster appropriate hemostasis is achieved, the better the patient's outcome.
• Even the most sophisticated equipment is useful only if the surgeon is capable and willing to avoid any undue blood loss.
• The choice of an appropriate hemostatic device can reduce intraoperative blood loss and postoperative anemia.
• Pay attention to the "tenets of bloodless surgery": (a) attention to detail, (b) partial dissection, (c) avoid stripping, (d) anatomical dissection, and (e) gentle tissue handling.

Questions for review

1. What are the Halstedian principles?
2. What devices are there to make a surgical incision? How do they work? What are the advantages and disadvantages of each of the methods?

3. How can vessels be occluded to provide hemostasis?
4. What are the means to exert compression on a bleeding wound?
5. How do drains influence blood loss?

Suggestions for further research

1. What safety measures are taken in an operating room to prevent hazards potentially caused by surgical methods to cut?
2. What measures are required to maintain equipment for cutting and coagulation to make a surgical incision and to stop bleeding functioning, respectively?

Exercises and practice cases

Using the following exercises, practice the skills required for hemostasis and improve your ability to improvise.
• Imagine you are the first at the site of a car accident and the patient is bleeding heavily from his knee; jot down five ways to stop the bleeding.
• Gather all the materials needed to make a balloon tamponade as described in this chapter.
• Take a piece of tissue and tailor it to fit around a lacerated liver. Then suture it accordingly.

Homework

Research the availability of the devices listed below in your hospital. List the manufacturer and its contact information. Note the departments in which the device is used, and the persons who are trained in their use.

Scalpel, thermocoagulator, hemostatic scalpel, electrosurgery (mono- and bi-polar), saline-enhanced thermal sealing, electrothermal bipolar vessel sealing, microwave coagulation, infrared contact coagulator, laser, plasma scalpel, argon beam coagulation, water jet, high-frequency water jet, harmonic scalpel, cavitron ultrasonic surgical aspirator (CUSA), sutures, clips, endovascular grafts, tourniquets (pneumatic, manual), bandages (non-adhesive *vs* adhesive), anti-shock garment, packing with towels, absorbable mesh, Foley catheter, Sengstaken–Blakemore tube, Linton–Nachlas tube, drains + epinephrine, pillows for positioning.

References

1. Sachs M, Auth M, Encke A. Historical development of surgical instruments exemplified by hemostatic forceps. *World J Surg* 1998;**22**:499–504.
2. Snyder SO Jr. The pneumatic tourniquet: a useful adjunct in lower extremity distal bypass. *Semin Vasc Surg* 1997;**10**:31–33.
3. Sachs MSH. Aus der Geschichte des chirurgischen Instrumentariums: 7. Das erste elektrochirurgische Instrumentarium: Galvanokauter und elektrische SChneideschlinge (1854). *Zentralbl Chir* 1998;**123**:950–954.
4. Naito S, Nakashima M, Kimoto Y, *et al.* Application of microwave tissue coagulator in partial nephrectomy for renal cell carcinoma. *J Urol* 1998;**159**:960–962.
5. Spence RK, Costabile JP, Young GS, *et al.* Is hemoglobin level alone a reliable predictor of outcome in the severely anemic surgical patient? *Am Surg* 1992;**58**:92–95.
6. Pratali S, Milano A, Codecasa R, De Carlo M, Borzoni G, Bortolotti U. Improving hemostasis during replacement of the ascending aorta and aortic valve with a composite graft. *Tex Heart Inst J* 2000;**27**:246–249.
7. Guis JA. *Fundamentals of General Surgery.* Chicago, Yearbook Medical Publishers, 1962.
8. Spence RK, Cernaianu AC, Carson J, DelRossi AJ. Transfusion and surgery. *Curr Probl Surg* 1993;**30**:1101–1180.
9. Amaral JF. Laparoscopic cholecystectomy in 200 consecutive patients using an ultrasonically activated scalpel. *Surg Laparosc Endosc* 1995;**5**:255–262.
10. McHugh SM, Hill AD, Humphreys H. Intraoperative technique as a factor in the prevention of surgical site infection. *J Hosp Infect* 2011;**78**:1–4.
11. Aagaard J, Skov BG, Hjelms E. An experimental study of hot air thermocoagulation in cardiac surgery. *Eur J Cardiothorac Surg* 1991;**5**:546–548.
12. Pennix JPM. Bipolar radiofrequency endometrial ablation compared with hydrothermablation for dysfunctional uterine bleeding: A randomized controlled trial. *Obstet Gynecol* 2010;**116**:819–826.
13. Pilnik S, Steichen F. The use of the hemostatic scalpel in operations upon the breast. *Surg Gynecol Obstet* 1986;**162**:589–591.
14. Ayuste E Jr, Roxas MF. Validating the use of rectus muscle fragment welding to control presacral bleeding during rectal mobilization. *Asian J Surg* 2004;**27**:18–21.
15. Xu J, Lin J. Control of presacral hemorrhage with electrocautery through a muscle fragment pressed on the bleeding vein. *J Am Coll Surg* 1994;**179**:351–352.
16. Brill AI. Bipolar electrosurgery: convention and innovation. *Clin Obstet Gynecol* 2008;**51**:153–158.
17. Bong JJ, Kumar R, Spalding D. A novel technique of partial splenectomy using radiofrequency ablation. *J Gastrointest Surg* 2011;**15**:371–372.
18. Yim AP, Rendina EA, Hazelrigg SR, *et al.* A new technological approach to nonanatomical pulmonary resection: saline enhanced thermal sealing. *Ann Thorac Surg* 2002;**74**:1671–1676.
19. Pearson M. Saline enhanced thermal sealing of tissue: Potential for bloodless surgery. *Min Invas Ther Allied Technol* 2002;**11**:265–270.
20. Hao P. A single institution experience using the LigaSure vessel sealing system in laparoscopic nephrectomy. *Chin Med J* 2011;**124**:1242–1252.
21. Gehrig T, Müller-Stich BP, Kenngott H, *et al.* LigaSure versus conventional dissection technique in pancreatoduodenectomy: a pilot study. *Am J Surg* 2011;**201**:166–170.
22. Castle SM, Salas N, Leveille RJ. Initial experience using microwave ablation therapy for renal tumor treatment: 18-month follow-up. *Urology* 2011;**77**:792–797.
23. Zhou XD, Tang ZY, Yu YQ, *et al.* Microwave surgery in the treatment of hepatocellular carcinoma. *Semin Surg Oncol* 1993;**9**:318–322.
24. Angerpointner TA, Lauterjung KL, Holschneider AM, Hecker WC. Infrared-contact coagulation of parenchymatous organs—report of three cases. *Z Kinderchir* 1983;**38**:356–358.
25. Angerpointner TA, Lauterjung KL, Hoffecker A. Haemostasis in injuries of parenchymatous organs by infrared contact coagulation. *Prog Pediatr Surg* 1990;**25**:32–38.
26. Hofstetter A, Staehler G, Mellin HE, *et al.* [The infrared contact coagulator for hemostasis in the renal parenchyma (author's transl)]. *MMW Munch Med Wochenschr* 1976;**118**:1537–1540.
27. Welter H, Seifert J, Nath G, Kreitmair A, Eberhardt H, Gokel JM. [Hemostasis in the liver, lungs, and spleen using an infra-red contact coagulator]. *Zentralbl Chir* 1980;**105**:94–101.
28. van Melick HH, van Venrooij GE, Boon TA. Laser prostatectomy in patients on anticoagulant therapy or with bleeding disorders. *J Urol* 2003;**170**:1851–1815.
29. Dwyer R. The history of gastrointestinal endoscopic laser hemostasis and management. *Endoscopy* 1986;**18** (Suppl 1):10–13.
30. Corbitt JD Jr. Laparoscopic cholecystectomy: laser versus electrosurgery. *Surg Laparosc Endosc* 1991;**1**:85–88.
31. Pearlman NW, Stiegmann GV, Vance V, *et al.* A prospective study of incisional time, blood loss, pain, and healing with carbon dioxide laser, scalpel, and electrosurgery. *Arch Surg* 1991;**126**:1018–1020.
32. Wyman A, Rogers K. Radical breast surgery with a contact Nd:YAG laser scalpel. *Eur J Surg Oncol* 1992;**18**:322–326.
33. Wyman A, Rogers K. Randomized trial of laser scalpel for modified radical mastectomy. *Br J Surg* 1993;**80**:871–873.
34. Link WJ, Incropera FP, Glover JL. The plasma scalpel. *Med Prog Technol* 1976;**4**:123–131.
35. Link WJ, Incropera FP, Glover JL. A plasma scalpel: comparison of tissue damage and wound healing with electrosurgical and steel scalpels. *Arch Surg* 1976;**111**:392–397.

36. Mueller GR, Wolf RF, Hansen PD, Gregory KW, Prahl SA. Hemostasis after liver resection improves after single application of albumin and argon beam coagulation. *J Gastrointest Surg* 2010;**14**:1764–1769.

37. Quinlan DM, Naslund MJ, Brendler CB. Application of argon beam coagulation in urological surgery. *J Urol* 1992;**147**:410–412.

38. Ward PH, Castro DJ, Ward S. A significant new contribution to radical head and neck surgery. The argon beam coagulator as an effective means of limiting blood loss. *Arch Otolaryngol Head Neck Surg* 1989;**115**:921–923.

39. Eickhoff A, Enderle MD, Hartmann D, Eickhoff JC, Riemann JF, Jakobs R. Effectiveness and Safety of PRECISE APC for the treatment of bleeding gastrointestinal angiodysplasia–a retrospective evaluation. *Z Gastroenterol* 2011;**49**:195–200.

40. Baer HU, Stain SC, Guastella T, Maddern GJ, Blumgart LH. Hepatic resection using a water jet dissector. *HPB Surg* 1993;**6**:189–196; discussion 196–198.

41. Rau HG, Meyer G, Jauch KW, Cohnert TU, Buttler E, Schildberg FW. [Liver resection with the water jet: conventional and laparoscopic surgery]. *Chirurg* 1996;**67**:546–551.

42. Basting RF, Djakovic N, Widmann P. Use of water jet resection in organ-sparing kidney surgery. *J Endourol* 2000;**14**:501–505.

43. Oertel J, Gaab MR, Piek J. Waterjet resection of brain metastases—first clinical results with 10 patients. *Eur J Surg Oncol* 2003;**29**:407–414.

44. Shekarriz H, Shekarriz B, Kujath P, et al. Hydro-Jet-assisted laparoscopic cholecystectomy: a prospective randomized clinical study. *Surgery* 2003;**133**:635–640.

45. Rau HG, Buttler ER, Baretton G, Schardey HM, Schildberg FW. Jet-cutting supported by high frequency current: new technique for hepatic surgery. *World J Surg* 1997;**21**:254–259; discussion 259–260.

46. Rothenberg SS. Laparoscopic splenectomy using the harmonic scalpel. *J Laparoendosc Surg* 1996;**6** (Suppl 1): S61–63.

47. El Moghazy WM, Hedaya MS, Kaido T, Egawa H, Uemoto S, Takada Y. Two different methods for donor hepatic transection: cavitron ultrasonic surgical aspirator with bipolar cautery versus cavitron ultrasonic surgical aspirator with radiofrequency coagulator-A randomized controlled trial. *Liver Transpl* 2009;**15**:102–105.

48. Kajja I, Bimenya GS, Eindhoven B, Jan Ten Duis H, Sibinga CT. Blood loss and contributing factors in femoral fracture surgery. *Afr Health Sci* 2010;**10**:18–25.

49. Levy B, Emery L. Randomized trial of suture versus electrosurgical bipolar vessel sealing in vaginal hysterectomy. *Obstet Gynecol* 2003;**102**:147–151.

50. Miller E, Paull DE, Morrissey K, Cortese A, Nowak E. Scalpel versus electrocautery in modified radical mastectomy. *Am Surg* 1988;**54**:284–286.

51. Lau WY, Lai EC, Lau SH. Methods of vascular control technique during liver resection: a comprehensive review. *Hepatobiliary Pancreat Dis Int* 2010;**9**:473–481.

52. Makuuchi M, Mori T, Gunvén P, Yamazaki S, Hasegawa H. Safety of hemihepatic vascular occlusion during resection of the liver. *Surg Gynecol Obstet* 1987;**164**:155–158.

53. Kwawukume EY, Ghosh TS. Extraperitoneal hypogastric artery ligation in control of intractable haemorrhage from advanced carcinoma of cervix and choriocarcinoma. *East Afr Med J* 1996;**73**:147–148.

54. Erzurum VZ, Shoup M, Borge M, Kalman PG, Rodriguez H, Silver GM. Inferior vena cava endograft to control surgically inaccessible hemorrhage. *J Vasc Surg* 2003;**38**: 1437–1439.

55. Boufi M, Bordon S, Dona B, et al. Unstable patients with retroperitoneal vascular trauma: an endovascular approach. *Ann Vasc Surg* 2011;**25**:352–358.

56. Kapma MR, Verhoeven EL, Tielliu IF, et al. Endovascular treatment of acute abdominal aortic aneurysm with a bifurcated stentgraft. *Eur J Vasc Endovasc Surg* 2005;**29**: 510–515.

57. Bae SH, Han DK, Baek HJ, et al. Selective embolization of the internal iliac arteries for the treatment of intractable hemorrhage in children with malignancies. *Korean J Pediatr* 2011;**54**:169–175.

58. Cherry RA, Goodspeed DC, Lynch FC, Delgado J, Reid SJ. Intraoperative angioembolization in the management of pelvic-fracture related hemodynamic instability. *J Trauma Manag Outcomes* 2011;**5**:6.

59. Liu PP, Lee WC, Cheng YF, et al. Use of splenic artery embolization as an adjunct to nonsurgical management of blunt splenic injury. *J Trauma* 2004;**56**:768–772; discussion 773.

60. Ding X, Zhu J, Zhu M, et al. Therapeutic management of hemorrhage from visceral artery pseudoaneurysms after pancreatic surgery. *J Gastrointest Surg* 2011;**15**:1417–1425.

61. Wirbel RJ, Roth R, Schulte M, Kramann B, Mutschler W. Preoperative embolization in spinal and pelvic metastases. *J Orthop Sci* 2005;**10**:253–257.

62. Ngeh N, Belli AM, Morgan R, Manyonda I. Pre-myomectomy uterine artery embolisation minimises operative blood loss. *BJOG* 2004;**111**:1139–1140.

63. Weinstein A, Chandra P, Schiavello H, Fleischer A. Conservative management of placenta previa percreta in a Jehovah's Witness. *Obstet Gynecol* 2005;**105**:1247–1250.

64. Tesdal IK, Filser T, Weiss C, Holm E, Dueber C, Jaschke W. Transjugular intrahepatic portosystemic shunts: adjunctive embolotherapy of gastroesophageal collateral vessels in the prevention of variceal rebleeding. *Radiology* 2005;**236**: 360–367.

65. Ikeda T, Sameshima H, Kawaguchi H, Yamauchi N, Ikenoue T. Tourniquet technique prevents profuse blood loss in placenta accreta cesarean section. *J Obstet Gynaecol Res* 2005;**31**:27–31.

66. Kragh JF Jr, Littrel ML, Jones JA, et al. Battle casualty survival with emergency tourniquet use to stop limb bleeding. *J Emerg Med* 2011;**41**:590–570.

67. Naimer SA, Anat N, Katif G. Evaluation of techniques for treating the bleeding wound. *Injury* 2004;**35**:974–979.

68. Kin N, Hayashida M, Chang KH, Uchida K, Hanaoka K. External manual compression of the abdominal aorta to control hemorrhage from a ruptured aneurysm. *J Anesth* 2002;**16**:164–166.

69. Hofmeyr GJ, Abdel-Aleem A, Abdel-Aleem MA. Uterine massage for preventing postpartum haemorrhage. *Cochrane Database Syst Rev* 2008;(3):CD006431.

70. Poretti F, Rosen T, Körner B, Vorwerk D. [Chitosan pads vs. manual compression to control bleeding sites after transbrachial arterial catheterization in a randomized trial]. *Rofo* 2005;**177**:1260–1266.

71. Hauswald M, Williamson MR, Baty GM, Kerr NL, Edgar-Mied VL Use of an improvised pneumatic anti-shock garment and a non-pneumatic anti-shock garment to control pelvic blood flow. *Int J Emerg Med* 2010;**3**:173–175.

72. Burlew CC, Moore EE, Smith WR, *et al.* Preperitoneal pelvic packing/external fixation with secondary angioembolization: optimal care for life-threatening hemorrhage from unstable pelvic fractures. *J Am Coll Surg* 2011;**212**:628–635; discussion 635–637.

73. Allard MA, Dondero F, Sommacale D, Dokmak S, Belghiti J, Farges O. Liver packing during elective surgery: an option that can be considered. *World J Surg* 2011;**35**:2493–2498.

74. Luchtman M. Mesh wrap in severe pediatric liver trauma. *J Pediatr Surg* 2004;**39**:1485–1489.

75. Leemans R, van Mourik JB. A new surgical, splenic salvage technique: the Vicryl net. *Neth J Surg* 1987;**39**:197–198.

76. Seligman JY, Egan M. Balloon tamponade: an alternative in the treatment of liver trauma. *Am Surg* 1997;**63**:1022–1023.

77. Burcharth F, Malmstrom J. Experiences with the Linton-Nachlas and the Sengstaken-Blakemore tubes for bleeding esophageal varices. *Surg Gynecol Obstet* 1976;**142**:529–531.

78. Panés J, Terés J, Bosch J, Rodés J. Efficacy of balloon tamponade in treatment of bleeding gastric and esophageal varices. Results in 151 consecutive episodes. *Dig Dis Sci* 1988;**33**:454–459.

79. Teres J, Cecilia A, Bordas JM, Rimola A, Bru C, Rodés J. Esophageal tamponade for bleeding varices. Controlled trial between the Sengstaken-Blakemore tube and the Linton-Nachlas tube. *Gastroenterology* 1978;**75**:566–569.

80. Aungst M, Wagner M. Foley balloon to tamponade bleeding in the retropubic space. *Obstet Gynecol* 2003;**102**:1037–1038.

81. Bowen LW, Beeson JH. Use of a large Foley catheter balloon to control postpartum hemorrhage resulting from a low placental implantation. A report of two cases. *J Reprod Med* 1985;**30**:623–625.

82. Georgiou C. Intraluminal pressure readings during the establishment of a positive "tamponade test" in the management of postpartum haemorrhage. *BJOG* 2010;**117**:295–303.

83. Marcovici I, Scoccia B. Postpartum hemorrhage and intrauterine balloon tamponade. A report of three cases. *J Reprod Med* 1999;**44**:122–126.

84. de Figueiredo DG, de Carvalho FF. Balloon tamponade of the pharynx in transnasophenoidal operations: technical note. *Neurosurgery* 1981;**8**:567–568.

85. Wurtele P. How I do it: emergency nasal packing using an umbilical cord clamp to secure a Foley catheter for posterior epistaxis. *J Otolaryngol* 1996;**25**:46–47.

86. Ganchrow MI, Facelle TL. Control of hemorrhage from a mucous fistula with Foley catheter tamponade. *Dis Colon Rectum* 1992;**35**:1001–1002.

87. Gilroy D, Lakhoo M, Charalambides D, Demetriades D. Control of life-threatening haemorrhage from the neck: a new indication for balloon tamponade. *Injury* 1992;**23**:557–559.

88. Gonzalez RP, Holevar MR, Falimirski ME, Merlotti GJ. A method for management of extraperitoneal pelvic bleeding secondary to penetrating trauma. *J Trauma* 1997;**43**:338–341.

89. Khan SA, Hu KN, Marder C, Smith NL. Hemorrhoidal bleeding following transrectal prostatic biopsy. Etiology and management. *Dis Colon Rectum* 1982;**25**:817–819.

90. Shuker S. The management of hemorrhage from severe missile injuries using Foley catheter balloon tamponade. *J Oral Maxillofac Surg* 1989;**47**:646–648.

91. Thomas SV, Dulchavsky SA, Diebel LN. Balloon tamponade for liver injuries: case report. *J Trauma* 1993;**34**:448–449.

92. McElroy SJ, Pietsch JB, Reese J. Foley catheter tamponade of intercostal hemorrhage in preterm infants. *J Pediatr* 2004;**145**:241.

93. McQuillan RF, McCormack T, Neligan MC. Penetrating left ventricular stab wound: a method of control during resuscitation and prior to repair. *Injury* 1981;**13**:63–65.

94. Parker MJ, Roberts CP, Hay D. Closed suction drainage for hip and knee arthroplasty. A meta-analysis. *J Bone Joint Surg Am* 2004;**86-A**:1146–1152.

95. Walmsley PJ, Kelly MB, Hill RM, Brenkel I. A prospective, randomised, controlled trial of the use of drains in total hip arthroplasty. *J Bone Joint Surg Br* 2005;**87**:1397–1401.

96. Ryu J, Sakamoto A, Honda T, Saito S. The postoperative drain-clamping method for hemostasis in total knee arthroplasty. Reducing postoperative bleeding in total knee arthroplasty. *Bull Hosp Jt Dis* 1997;**56**:251–254.

97. Sasanuma H, Sekiya H, Takatoku K, Takada H, Sugimoto N, Hoshino Y. Efficient strategy for controlling postoperative hemorrhage in total knee arthroplasty. *Knee Surg Sports Traumatol Arthrosc* 2010;**19**:921–925.

98. Timlin M, Moroney P, Collins D, Toomey D, O'Byrne J. The 90/90 pillow reduces blood loss after knee arthroplasty: a prospective randomised case control study. *J Arthroplasty* 2003;**18**:765–768.

14 Anesthesia—More than Sleeping

The anesthesiologist plays an important role in the peri-operative blood management of patients. His/her work is not just inducing hypnosis, relaxation, and pain control, but also includes many facets of blood management. These include preparing the patient for surgery, reducing blood loss during surgery, and caring for the patient after surgery. This chapter will outline some of the basics of how an anesthesiologist can give anesthesia in a way that reduces the patient's blood loss and enhances his/her outcome.

Objectives

1. To explain the role of the anesthesiologist in a blood management team.
2. To identify a variety of methods an anesthesiologist can use to reduce blood loss.
3. To describe the impact of these measures on the overall blood management of the patient.

Definitions

Anesthesiology: The medical specialty of preparing patients for anesthesia, rendering patients insensitive for painful surgical, obstetric, diagnostic, and other therapeutic procedures, and monitoring, maintaining or restoring homeostasis in perioperative and critically ill patients.

The anesthesiologist in a blood management team

Anesthesiologists are vital in a blood management team. They should be included in the planning team for a patient's procedure right from the beginning. Anesthesiologists contribute to the success of the team with their experience in preparing patients for surgery. Also, the various intraoperative and postoperative activities they perform, as well as their knowledge of the therapy of severely sick patients, are of great benefit to the team.

Preoperatively, anesthesiologists are in a good position to coordinate the optimization of the patient's condition. In many hospitals around the world, the anesthesiologist meets with the patient well before surgery and performs an initial assessment during this preoperative visit. He/she can therefore detect obstacles to optimal blood management at an early stage. Typically, anesthesiologists aim at optimizing the cardiopulmonary function of the patient. They may also be able to assess the hematological status of the patient and resolve any derangements (coagulopathy or anemia) if present. In cooperation with the surgeon, he/she can adapt anticoagulatory regimens or change other drug regimens if necessary, and initiate specialist consultations when needed. The best anesthetic procedure can be chosen. Besides, logistical decisions can be made by the anesthesiologists, e.g., ordering drugs or special monitoring or cell salvage devices for use in the operating room.

Intraoperatively, the anesthesiologist is responsible for the well-being of the patient. This includes not only administering anesthesia, but also monitoring the cardiopulmonary and hematological status, administration of fluids and drugs, performing autologous transfusion, and stabilizing the cardiopulmonary condition of the patient. The anesthesiologist works closely with the surgical team to position the patient.

Postoperatively, the anesthesiologist is responsible for the care of the patient in the recovery room, and sometimes for some time after the patient has returned to the

Basics of Blood Management, Second Edition. Petra Seeber and Aryeh Shander.
© 2013 John Wiley & Sons, Ltd. Published 2013 by John Wiley & Sons, Ltd.

ward. There, he/she can oversee the return of autologous blood, administer further drugs, and continue monitoring the patient.

In the intensive care unit and the emergency room, anesthesiologists often care for severely sick patients. Such patients are often eligible for blood management measures. As such, they benefit also from the anesthesiologist's expertise in the various aspects of blood management.

All this shows that it is vital for a blood management team to include anesthesiologists from the beginning of patient care. Besides, it demonstrates that all anesthesiologists should be aware of the immense role they can play in blood management and should therefore continue to educate themselves to keep pace with modern blood management rather than limping behind on the crutches of outdated transfusion therapy.

Specific intraoperative anesthetic measures to reduce blood loss

Positioning

Before surgery starts, the patient is usually positioned to meet the needs of the surgery. Positioning allows a good view of the body part being operated on. It also allows for comfortable access to the surgical site and minimizes the risk of nerve and compression damage due to a certain position. Another aspect of positioning is its ability to reduce blood loss. For many types of surgery, there are different positions that are suitable for the intended operation. Some of these may increase blood loss, while others decrease it. The choice of a patient's position must take reduction of blood loss into consideration.

Some basic mechanisms explain how blood loss can be influenced by the position of the patient. Blood flow and pressure in various vascular sections vary with the position of the patient. In the venous system, the blood pressure is determined by hydrostatic pressure (as determined by hydration status and position) and by transmural pressure. When the patient stands, approximately 500–800 mL of blood follows gravity and is found in the lower parts of the body. This effect is reversed when the patient is brought into the supine position. In the arteries, the blood flow and pressure are much less dependent on volume and position. Arterial blood pressure is actively regulated by humoral factors (e.g., epinephrine) and autonomous reflex mechanisms. The global blood pressure is maintained by reflex mechanisms that also react

to changes in posture so that perfusion pressure of vital organs is maintained.

Also, surgical position affects blood pressure and flow. When a patient is positioned on his/her abdomen, blood is squeezed into the extremities and the venous return flow is hindered. The preload and cardiac output are reduced. Besides, when the vena cava is compressed, blood pressure therein rises [1] and blood flows increasingly through anastomoses found peri- and intravertebrally. This increases the perfusion of the spinal region.

When the patient is positioned with his/her legs positioned higher than the head (Trendelenburg position, lithotomy position), blood returns readily to the trunk and preload increases. In this position, baroreceptor reflexes are normally elicited, and blood pressure increases, but cardiac output decreases. On the other hand, when the patient's feet are positioned below the level of the head (reverse Trendelenburg position, sitting position), venous return is decreased. When the patient's legs and hips are flexed, the venous return flow is hindered even further. Again, this decreases preload and cardiac output. However, if baroreceptors are intact, peripheral vascular resistance increases and blood pressure returns near to normal.

These physiological reactions of the body in response to a change in position can be used effectively to reduce blood loss. It must be taken into consideration, though, that reflex mechanisms that would normally allow a hemodynamic response to the position may be blunted by anesthetics.

Two basic principles should guide the preoperative positioning of the patient:
• **Elevate the surgical field.** If possible, the surgical field should be elevated above the level of the heart. This decreases the perfusion pressure in the vessels of the surgical area. Some examples may illustrate this. For prostatectomy, a patient can be kept at a 25–30% Trendelenburg position to reduce blood loss [2]. Orthognathic procedures can be performed in the head-up position to reduce blood loss [3]. Patients undergoing intracranial surgery can often be positioned in the sitting posture. Sitting up of the patient seems to be associated with a reduced blood loss and fewer transfusions when compared with horizontal positioning [4].
• **Do not compress the venous drainage of the surgical field.** This means that unnecessary flexion of the extremities should be avoided. Besides, the patient's body or positioning tools should not be placed so as to compress the venous plexus or other main routes of venous drain-

Table 14.1 Positions proposed to reduce blood loss in spinal surgery.

Positions without frames	Positions with frames
Use of chest rolls	Canadian frame (Hastings 1969)
Kneeling position (Ecker 1949)	Relton-Hall frame (1969)
Mohammedan praying position (Lipton 1950)	Andrews frame
Knee–chest position (Tarlov 1967)	Wilson bank
Tuck position (Wayne 1967)	Jackson table
	Cloward surgical saddle
	Heffington frame

age. The following are examples. In head surgery, the head should not be turned to one side or the other in order not to hinder venous drainage of the surgical field. If the patient is positioned supine for abdominal surgery, compression of the vena cava should be avoided and pressure should be taken off the cava. This is easily accomplished by slightly rotating the operating table to the left. When the patient is in the prone position, e.g., for spinal or other back surgery, pressure should be taken off the abdomen and especially the vena cava. This can be done by supporting the hips and shoulders with pillows or other devices (frames) (Table 14.1). The blood can now follow under gravity and collect in the abdomen, rather than in the surgical area [1]. Blood loss decreases.

While it is prudent to avoid blood loss during surgery, at times it may also be wise to provoke bleeding, namely at the end of surgery when the adequacy of hemostasis needs to be checked. Typically, the surgeon is content with the extent of hemostasis he/she has achieved at the end of surgery, but knows that a rise in blood pressure during wake-up or a change in the position of the patient may provoke further bleeding due to undetected open vessels. To prevent this, the quality of hemostasis is challenged before wound closure and any further bleeding vessels are closed. This can be done by positioning the potentially bleeding surgical field under the level of the heart. Vessels that are still open start bleeding, the surgeon ties them quickly, and then the wound can be closed with a good conscience. For head and neck surgery, for instance, this means bringing the patient into the Tren-

delenburg position shortly before closing the wound. This is even more effective than the Valsalva maneuver to detect bleeding [5].

Intraoperative positioning may also serve purposes that are only tangentially associated with reducing blood loss. Liver resection may be performed in 15-degree head-down position. This may seem contrary to the principle of positioning patients with elevated surgical fields. However, when liver surgery is performed in controlled hypotension, tilting the head down may improve renal perfusion and aid in maintaining a marginal urine output during surgery [6]. Thus, this position may allow for reduction of blood loss by means of the reduced systemic blood pressure without unduly compromising renal perfusion.

The patient's posture not only influences intraoperative blood loss, but may also be important in the postoperative period. In the recovery room, patients can be positioned to reduce blood loss from a variety of sites. The same basic principles of intraoperative positioning apply here as well. After knee surgery, the leg can be elevated in the hip (35-degree flexion) and kept straight in the knee, or the knee (70–90 degrees) and the hip (90 degrees) can be flexed. Both measures seem to reduce blood loss significantly [7].

Controlled hypotension

Surgical bleeding is a result of many factors, ranging from the number and size of dissected blood vessels, time until bleeding vessels are closed, coagulation profile of the patient, and blood pressure in the opened blood vessels. Reducing the latter—in the form of controlled hypotension—is a simple and effective means to reduce blood loss.

The concept of controlled hypotension (also called induced hypotension or deliberate hypotension) means purposely reducing the blood pressure during surgery in which major blood loss is expected. This translates into reduced hydrostatic pressure in the vessels in the wound and this reduces blood loss. This kind of hypotension is typically induced by reducing the peripheral vascular resistance. The aim is to maintain the cardiac output despite reduced blood pressure.

It is not only a low blood pressure that reduces blood flow to the wound. Blood flow is also a result of the cardiac output. If cardiac output is very high, blood flow can be increased despite the pressure being low. It has been claimed that the cardiac output (and especially the heart rate) needs to be normalized in order to reduce blood loss. Otherwise, controlled hypotension was thought to be ineffective [8]. However, it has also been claimed that despite an increased cardiac output, with hypotension there is reduced blood loss [9].

While low blood pressure may be beneficial to reduce blood loss, too low a pressure may also be detrimental. A basic understanding of the pathophysiology of hypotension is needed to get this right. Hypotension may be divided into two types. The first is induced by volume or blood loss. This results in vasoconstriction and a reduced cardiac output with low blood flow. This reduction in blood flow reduces the blood pressure and causes hypotension, which is potentially detrimental due to ischemic complications. The second type is caused by vasodilatation and results in a compensatory increased cardiac output. The latter form of hypotension does not pose such a high risk for ischemia as the former.

Practically speaking, there are three ways to induce controlled hypotension: fluid restriction, vasodilating drugs, and regional anesthesia. Restricting fluid administration seems to be effective for selected patients undergoing procedures with a limited duration. However, restricting volume infusion during surgery only in the interest of inducing hypotension comes with the increased risk of regional ischemia. Therefore, fluid restriction is usually not an option. This is especially true when a procedure is expected to be prolonged and/or severe blood loss is anticipated.

The second way to induce hypotension is more practical. It uses drugs to induce vasodilatation. A variety of agents have been proposed for this purpose [10–12] (Table 14.2). It has not yet been determined which drug is best for a given situation. Some of the drugs primarily

Table 14.2 Agents for induction of controlled hypotension.

Agent	Group/mechanism of action	Remarks
Adenosine	Endogenous purine analog	Potent vasodilator, acts more on arteries than on veins, very short half-life, continuous infusion required
Esmolol	Beta-receptor blocker, negative inotrope, vasodilatation	Rapid acting
Nitroprusside	Direct vasodilatation, forms nitric oxide	Caveat: Cyanide poisoning may occur in prolonged use, relaxes arterial and venous smooth muscles
Nitroglycerin	Smooth muscle relaxation, forms nitric oxide	Venous dilatation more pronounced than arterial dilatation
Trimetaphan	Ganglion blocker, direct smooth muscle relaxation	Arterial and venous dilatation, decreases cardiac output
Nicardipine	Calcium channel blocker, negative inotrope, vasodilatation	Rapid acting
Fenoldopam	Dopamine D1 receptor agonist	May preserve renal and splanchnic perfusion in hypotension
Prostaglandin E1 (PGE1)	Vasodilator	Mechanism of action mainly unknown
Labetalol	Sympathetic receptor blocker (alpha 1, beta 1, beta 2)	Lowers blood pressure without reflex tachycardia
Isoflurane, desflurane	Inhalational anesthetics	Arterial dilatation more pronounced than venous dilatation
Propofol	Intravenous anesthetic	
Morphine	Opioid	Arterial and venous pressure decrease (histamine release, vascular tone reduced)
Fentanyl, remifentanil	Opioids	

reduce venous pressure, others predominantly the arterial pressure. A common way to induce hypotension is by using anesthetics, such as gases (desflurane, sevoflurane, and isoflurane), which induce mainly vasodilatation. Intravenous anesthetics (propofol or thiopental) also induce hypotension, but mainly by reducing cardiac output, a less desirable effect. High-dose fentanyl (30 μg/ kg) has been used for the induction of controlled hypotension [13]. Remifentanil is also used to induce hypotension and may be easily titrated. Another group of drugs are those not used for anesthesia but for the sole purpose of inducing hypotension [14].

The third way to induce hypotension resorts to regional or epidural anesthesia. These types of anesthesia induce vasodilatation in the anesthetized parts of the body by reducing sympathetic activity. The required degree of hypotension is achievable with a combination of bolus or continuous epidural infusion, possibly with a vasopressor to counteract any excessive hypotension [15]. Epidural anesthesia combines the blood-saving properties of regional anesthesia with those of controlled hypotension.

Controlled hypotension is a very old and time-proven technique. When only moderate degrees of hypotension are used (80–90 mmHg systolic), it is very safe for the majority of patients. However, some patients may experience side effects and therefore need to be excluded from induction of (marked) hypotension. Patient selection is therefore essential. Patients who have an impaired vascular response (as in untreated hypertension, atherosclerosis, or diabetes mellitus) or those who are susceptible to ischemia (severe ischemic heart or brain disease) must not undergo induction of hypotension or at least not to the same degree as healthy patients; it may be possible to use mild hypotensive anesthesia in some of these patients as well.

In surgery using hypotensive anesthesia, a target level of hypotension must be set. On the one hand, the blood pressure must be reduced to an extent that blood loss decreases; on the other, perfusion of vital organs must be maintained [16]. Controlled hypotension is usually targeted to a certain mean arterial or systolic pressure. Different levels of hypotension have been described: mild hypotension with a mean arterial pressure of 70–80 mmHg, moderate hypotension with a mean arterial pressure of 55–70 mmHg, and marked hypotension with a mean arterial pressure of 45–55 mmHg. In other instances, the central venous pressure, rather than the mean arterial pressure, is used as a guide. This is the case in liver surgery, since blood loss during such procedures depends more on the central venous rather than on the arterial blood pressure. Low central venous pressure, e.g., of not more than 5 mmHg, may be a reasonable target to reduce blood loss in liver surgery [6, 17].

Intraoperative monitoring also contributes to the safety of controlled hypotension. For safe monitoring of controlled hypotension, a continuous arterial blood pressure reading is desirable. Signs of hypoperfusion and cardiac impairment must be recognized (serum lactate, acidosis, reduced urine output, ST-segment changes, and arrhythmia on the electrocardiogram [EKG]). If the pulse oximeter does not show a reading, systemic hypoperfusion may have developed. For some indications, such as spinal surgery, evoked electroencephalogram (EEG) potentials are used to monitor the progress of surgery. These may also be used to monitor the controlled hypotension. When the latency or amplitude of the potentials increases, hypotension may be the cause and should be abandoned. When anemia reaches below a certain hematocrit level, controlled hypotension should be abandoned [18].

When the above-mentioned precautions are taken, side effects are extremely rare. When they occur, then they are usually the result of regional hypoperfusion. Rare occasions of myocardial ischemia or infarction have been reported. A very rare, yet much feared, complication of controlled hypotension is ischemic optic neuropathy, resulting in postoperative blindness. This has been described in cardiac surgery patients who were severely anemic and also in patients who have undergone spinal surgery, especially when performed in the prone position. Although it is not proven that hypotension is the cause of this blindness, it seems to contribute to its development.

Controlled hypotension can be used for many surgeries, such as joint arthroplasty [19], spinal surgery [18], prostatectomy [20], cystectomy [21], burn surgery, orthognathic surgery [22], and gynecological surgery. It may be used in adults as well as in children. Studies report reductions of blood loss of about 50% compared to that of the control group. In addition, reductions of transfusion volume have been reported to range from 20% to 83% [9].

Hypotensive anesthesia is most useful when combined with other measures, such as cell salvage, surgical techniques for hemostasis, and anesthetic measures to reduce blood loss. While somewhat controversial, controlled hypotension has also been successfully used in combination with moderate acute normovolemic hemodilution [23]. Hypotensive anesthesia may be a suitable measure for reducing blood loss when other blood-sparing techniques are deemed contraindicated, e.g., in infected prosthesis after hip replacement.

Warming

The human body is designed to work best at 37 °C. This is particularly true of the many enzymatic reactions that are vital for health, including those participating in the clotting process. Additionally, the platelet count in peripheral blood is higher in normothermic individuals compared with hypothermic patients. When a patient becomes hypothermic, he/she develops a profound, yet reversible, hemostatic defect. This is caused by platelet dysfunction (platelet thromboxane A2 and glycoprotein IB decrease). The humoral clotting factor activity is reduced. Fibrinolysis is increased [24]. It comes as no surprise that blood loss increases when patients get cold. Patients who are at special risk of becoming chilled are those undergoing surgery. A marked reduction in the core temperature can be seen after induction of general anesthesia. This is due to a redistribution of cold blood from the periphery to the core, as well as reduced metabolic heat production during anesthesia. In addition, infusing fluids at room temperature reduces the core temperature. During surgery, the patient loses even more heat in the cold environment of the operating room.

It was shown that patients with lower than optimal body temperature lose more blood. Therefore, in an attempt to reduce blood loss, an anesthesiologist needs to keep patients warm. Several methods have been described. Patients should be covered with warm blankets on arrival in the preoperative holding area or in the operating theater. Air conditioners should be switched off and room ambient air temperature should be set high. Patients should be actively warmed for about 30 minutes before induction of anesthesia (prewarming). The idea behind this procedure is that patients who are actively warmed to have warm extremities do not suffer from a drop in their core temperature when anesthesia causes a redistribution of blood flow. This prevents the aforementioned drop in core temperature. In addition to prewarming, active warming should continue throughout the surgery and, if needed, in the recovery room. All fluids given to the patient need to be warmed, including the intravenous fluids and fluids needed for wound irrigation. Active warming should be guided by continuous measurement of the patient's core temperature, so that the patient ideally is kept at the normal temperature of 37 °C.

Table 14.3 Hypothermia-related adverse outcomes.

Increased blood loss (perioperative, in trauma)
Increased mortality in trauma patients
More surgical wound infections
Delayed wound healing
More cardiac events (arrhythmia)
Longer stay in recovery room and in hospital
Higher costs of treatment

Simply by keeping the patient's core temperature at normal levels or rewarming the patient, the patient's outcome can be improved (Table 14.3). He/she not only loses 20–25% less blood, but has also improved wound healing, fewer postoperative cardiac complications, and reduced mortality. Such beneficial effects have been shown in trauma patients, and in gastrointestinal [25] and orthopedic surgery [26, 27].

Choice of ventilation patterns and blood loss

How a patient is ventilated influences the amount of blood lost during surgery. Essentially, two mechanisms have been postulated: changes in intravascular pressure and reflex vasoconstriction or vasodilatation induced by ventilation.

Mechanical ventilation with positive pressure, typically used during general anesthesia, has profound hemodynamic effects. These effects are pronounced when large tidal volumes are used, as well as during the application of positive end-expiratory pressure (PEEP). Due to the resulting increase in intrathoracic pressure, the pressure in intrathoracic vessels increases. When the patient is in the prone position, an increased intra-abdominal pressure may add to the increased pressure that results from high pressure ventilation. The venous return is reduced. This may lead to increased venous bleeding (especially in caval anastomoses).

Ventilation of the patient influences the level of blood gases. When a patient is hypoventilated, i.e., hypercapnic and/or hypoxic, sympathetic stimulation and other reflex mechanisms change the vascular tone. The systemic arterial pressure rises. On the contrary, when a patient is hyperventilated, only intracranial (intact) vessels constrict, while vessels in the periphery dilate. Such effects have been used in an attempt to reduce blood loss. It has been established that ventilation with high pressures during hepatic surgery contributes to an increased blood loss. Therefore, it may be wise to reduce the PEEP or to avoid it entirely during phases of surgery where blood loss from the liver usually occurs. It has also been proposed that the use of increased PEEP in postoperative cardiac patients may reduce blood loss. However, this seems not to be the case [28]. It was also proposed to use spontaneous ventilation during general anesthesia in order to reduce blood loss, since spontaneous ventilation does not increase blood pressures, unlike general anesthesia with mechanical ventilation [29].

As a general rule, normoxia and normocapnia using normoventilation should be achieved during anesthesia. Hypoventilation must be avoided. When local anesthesia is used together with sedation, care must be taken that the level of sedation does not induce hypoventilation, leading to hypercapnia with resulting increased blood loss. It was proposed, though, that mild hyperventilation may theoretically aid in reducing blood loss when surgery is performed on body parts that vasoconstrict during hyperventilation (brain, uterus), but this effect has not been demonstrated in clinical practice.

Related to the ventilation pattern is the choice of airway management. It seems that the use of the laryngeal airway mask is associated with reduced blood loss during head and neck surgery when compared with the use of an endotracheal tube.

Choice of drugs

Anesthetics exert a variety of effects which may contribute to the amount of blood loss during surgery. Generally, anesthesia must be deep enough to prevent sympathetic stimulation in reaction to surgical activities. Such stimulation would increase the blood pressure and with it the blood loss.

As was shown decades ago, blood loss varies with the chosen drugs. Table 14.4 gives blood loss in uterine evacuation under different anesthetic regimens [30].

The reasons for the differences in blood loss in relation to the chosen anesthetic drug are not clear. One reason may be that many anesthetics impair coagulation [31]. Halothane seems to be the most potent platelet inhibitor among inhalational agents. Sevoflurane also seems to have clinically important inhibitory actions on platelets, while this seems not to be true for isoflurane and desflurane. The inhibitory effects of inhalational agents on platelets seem to last for 1–6 hours postoperatively. Nitrous oxide also seems to have inhibitory effects on coagulation, but its role is controversial. Propofol in clinically used doses also inhibits platelets, while barbiturates,

Table 14.4 Blood loss in relation to the chosen anesthetic regimen for uterine evacuation.

Drug regimen	Blood loss (mL)
1% halothane	283
0.5% halothane + 75% nitrous oxide	169
0.5% halothane + 75% nitrous oxide + thiopental + meperidine	286
5% fluroxene	233
80% nitrous oxide + thiopental + meperidine	58
Paracervical block with 1% lidocaine	25

benzodiazepines, opioids, clonidine, and muscle relaxants do not seem to affect clotting. There are no data available as to whether or not etomidate or ketamine affect bleeding. Local anesthetics exert an antithrombotic effect and inhibit platelets, but only in higher than clinically used concentrations. Many of the drugs used as anesthetic adjuvants also impair coagulation, among them starch and dextran solutions, as well as a variety of antibiotics. Avoiding such platelet inhibitors may be clinically significant when patients have reduced levels or an impaired function of platelets and in patients where hemostasis is critical.

Anesthetics also may influence blood loss by redistributing blood flow. It has been postulated that total intravenous anesthesia with propofol reduced blood loss when compared with sevoflurane-induced anesthesia. This is thought to be due to the fact that propofol selectively dilates the postcapillary, venous vascular bed, while sevoflurane causes a precapillary, arteriolar vasodilation.

Timing and amount of fluid administration

Restricted fluid administration before surgical hemostasis is achieved may contribute to the reduction of blood loss. When fluids are used cautiously until hemostasis is achieved, the intravascular pressure is not as high as it would be with liberal fluid administration, and hemostasis may be easier to achieve in the not so intensely distended veins. After the major bleeding is controlled, normovolemia must be established [2, 6, 32].

Choice of anesthetic procedure

The choice of the anesthetic given affects the perisurgical blood loss. In general, regional anesthesia seems to reduce blood loss when compared with general anesthesia [33]. Blood loss has been studied mainly for epidural and spinal anesthesia, but occasionally also in plexus anesthesia. Initially, it was thought that spinal and epidural anesthesia reduce blood loss, since they induce arterial hypotension. This may be the case. However, patients who receive epidural anesthesia, but who are kept normotensive during surgery, lose less blood than with general anesthesia. Other mechanisms may, therefore, play a role in epidural anesthesia. Peripheral venous blood pressure is also reduced, resulting in a reduced oozing from the wound. This effect is observable intra-operatively and may also extend into the postoperative period. Spontaneous ventilation, which does not increase the pressure in the vena cava (as does mechanical ventilation), has been implicated as a reason for the reduced blood loss.

The reduction of blood loss during epidural anesthesia has been demonstrated in a variety of procedures, among them gynecological, urological, and orthopedic [29] procedures. For knee replacement, hypotensive epidural anesthesia without tourniquet use reduces total blood loss even more than spinal anesthesia with a tourniquet [34]. Even in spinal surgery, epidural anesthesia in combination with general anesthesia reduces blood loss [35]. When comparing epidural with general anesthesia for elective Cesarean section for placenta previa, transfusions were reduced in the epidural group [36]. In contrast, epidural anesthesia seems not to reduce intraoperative blood loss in gastrointestinal surgery [37].

Key points

• The anesthesiologist contributes many facets to the blood management of a patient. These include preoperative measures, intra- and post-operative reductions of blood loss, and the care of the critically ill or severely injured. He/she is therefore best involved with the planning of procedures from the time the patient presents for evaluation.
• There are a variety of anesthetic methods that reduce blood losses, including:
  ◦ Positioning intra- and post-operatively
  ◦ Controlled hypotension
  ◦ Warming of the patient
  ◦ Choice of ventilation patterns
  ◦ Choice of drugs
  ◦ Timing of fluid administration
  ◦ Choice of anesthetic procedure.

• When appropriate, different methods can be combined to enhance blood sparing.

Questions for review

1. Why is it important to warm the patient before induction of anesthesia?
2. How does the choice of the anesthetic procedure affect blood loss?
3. Which two basic principles aimed at reducing blood loss underlie the positioning of patients?
4. By what mechanisms do anesthetic agents influence intraoperative blood loss?
5. What monitoring methods may be useful for patients undergoing controlled hypotension? What are you looking for during the monitoring? What would prompt you to abandon controlled hypotension?

Suggestions for further research

What drugs used for controlled hypotension are most suitable for different types of surgery, e.g., spinal surgery, Cesarean section, prostatectomy? What drugs should not be used for these types of surgery and why?

Exercises and practice cases

Obtain a description of the positions listed in Table 14.1 and practice placing a friend in these positions. Then, ask your friend to place you in these positions and note where pressure points exist and which positions are most comfortable or most uncomfortable.

What positions may be appropriate for the blood management of patients undergoing the following surgeries:
• Radical cystectomy?
• Resection of a meningioma in the posterior fossa?
• Resection of a meningioma in the spinal canal at level T10?
• Gastrectomy?
• Right total hip replacement?
• Shunt revision on the right forearm of a dialysis patient?

Homework

Check whether your hospital has positioning aids available for patients undergoing spinal surgery.

What fluid warming devices are available? What devices for warming the patient are there? When are they used?

References

1. Lee TC, Yang LC, Chen HJ. Effect of patient position and hypotensive anesthesia on inferior vena caval pressure. *Spine* 1998;**23**:941–947; discussion 947–948.
2. Schostak M, Matischak K, Müller M, *et al.* New perioperative management reduces bleeding in radical retropubic prostatectomy. *BJU Int* 2005;**96**:316–319.
3. Rohling RG, Zimmermann AP, Biro P, Haers PE, Sailer HF. Alternative methods for reduction of blood loss during elective orthognatic surgery. *Int J Adult Orthodon Orthognath Surg* 1999;**14**:77–82.
4. Orliaguet GA, Hanafi M, Meyer PG, *et al.* Is the sitting or the prone position best for surgery for posterior fossa tumours in children? *Paediatr Anaesth* 2001;**11**:541–547.
5. Moumoulidis I, Martinez Del Pero M, Brennan L, Jani P. Haemostasis in head and neck surgical procedures: Valsalva manoeuvre versus Trendelenburg tilt. *Ann R Coll Surg Engl* 2010;**92**:292–294.
6. Melendez JA, Arslan V, Fischer ME, *et al.* Perioperative outcomes of major hepatic resections under low central venous pressure anesthesia: blood loss, blood transfusion, and the risk of postoperative renal dysfunction. *J Am Coll Surg* 1998;**187**:620–625.
7. Ong SM, Taylor GJ. Can knee position save blood following total knee replacement? *Knee* 2003;**10**:81–85.
8. Phillips WA, Hensinger RN. Control of blood loss during scoliosis surgery. *Clin Orthop Relat Res* 1988;**229**:88–93.
9. Sollevi A. Hypotensive anesthesia and blood loss. *Acta Anaesthesiol Scand* 1988;**89** (Suppl):39–43.
10. Lustik SJ, Papadakos PJ, Jackman KV, Rubery PT Jr, Kaplan KL, Chhibber AK. Nicardipine versus nitroprusside for deliberate hypotension during idiopathic scoliosis repair. *J Clin Anesth* 2004;**16**:25–33.
11. Yoshida K, *et al.* Autologous blood transfusion and hypotensive anesthesia for rotational acetabular osteotomy. *Nagoya J Med Sci* 1998;**61**:131–135.
12. Degoute CS. Controlled hypotension: a guide to drug choice. *Drugs* 2007;**67**:1053–1076.
13. Purdham RS. Reduced blood loss with hemodynamic stability during controlled hypotensive anesthesia for LeFort I maxillary osteotomy using high-dose fentanyl: a retrospective study. *CRNA* 1996;**7**:33–46.
14. Testa LD, Tobias JD. Pharmacologic drugs for controlled hypotension. *J Clin Anesth* 1995;**7**:326–337.
15. Kiss H, Raffl M, Neumann D, Hutter J, Dorn U. Epinephrine-augmented hypotensive epidural anesthesia replaces tourniquet use in total knee replacement. *Clin Orthop Relat Res* 2005;**436**:184–189.
16. Choi WS, Samman N. Risks and benefits of deliberate hypotension in anaesthesia: a systematic review. *Int J Oral Maxillofac Surg* 2008;**37**:687–703.
17. Massicotte L, Lenis S, Thibeault L, Sassine MP, Seal RF, Roy A. Effect of low central venous pressure and phlebotomy on blood product transfusion requirements during liver transplantations. *Liver Transpl* 2006;**12**:117–123.
18. Dutton RP. Controlled hypotension for spinal surgery. *Eur Spine J* 2004;**13** (Suppl 1):S66–S71.
19. Qvist TF, Skovsted P, Bredgaard Sorensen M. Moderate hypotensive anaesthesia for reduction of blood loss during total hip replacement. *Acta Anaesthesiol Scand* 1982;**26**:351–353.
20. Boldt J, Weber A, Mailer K, Papsdorf M, Schuster P. Acute normovolaemic haemodilution vs controlled hypotension for reducing the use of allogeneic blood in patients undergoing radical prostatectomy. *Br J Anaesth* 1999;**82**:170–174.
21. Ahlering TE, Henderson JB, Skinner DG. Controlled hypotensive anesthesia to reduce blood loss in radical cystectomy for bladder cancer. *J Urol* 1983;**129**:953–954.
22. Lessard MR, Trépanier CA, Baribault JP, *et al.* Isoflurane-induced hypotension in orthognathic surgery. *Anesth Analg* 1989;**69**:379–383.
23. Suttner SW, Piper SN, Lang K, Hüttner I, Kumle B, Boldt J. Cerebral effects and blood sparing efficiency of sodium nitroprusside-induced hypotension alone and in combination with acute normovolaemic haemodilution. *Br J Anaesth* 2001;**87**:699–705.
24. Michelson AD, MacGregor H, Barnard MR, Kestin AS, Rohrer MJ, Valeri CR. Reversible inhibition of human platelet activation by hypothermia in vivo and in vitro. *Thromb Haemost* 1994;**71**:633–640.
25. Bock M, Müller J, Bach A, Böhrer H, Martin E, Motsch J. Effects of preinduction and intraoperative warming during major laparotomy. *Br J Anaesth* 1998;**80**:159–163.
26. Winkler M, Akça O, Birkenberg B, *et al.* Aggressive warming reduces blood loss during hip arthroplasty. *Anesth Analg* 2000;**91**:978–984.
27. Young VL, Watson ME. Prevention of perioperative hypothermia in plastic surgery. *Aesth Surg J* 2006;**26**:551–571.
28. Ruel MA, Rubens FD. Non-pharmacological strategies for blood conservation in cardiac surgery. *Can J Anaesth* 2001;**48** (4 Suppl):S13–S23.
29. Modig J, Karlstrom G. Intra- and post-operative blood loss and haemodynamics in total hip replacement when performed under lumbar epidural versus general anaesthesia. *Eur J Anaesthesiol* 1987;**4**:345–355.
30. Cullen BF, Margolis AJ, Eger EI. The effects of anesthesia and pulmonary ventilation on blood loss during elective therapeutic abortion. *Anesthesiology* 1970;**32**:108–113.
31. Kozek-Langenecker SA. The effects of drugs used in anaesthesia on platelet membrane receptors and on platelet function. *Curr Drug Targets* 2002;**3**:247–258.
32. Vretzakis G, Kleitsaki A, Stamoulis K, *et al.* Intra-operative intravenous fluid restriction reduces perioperative red

blood cell transfusion in elective cardiac surgery, especially in transfusion-prone patients: a prospective, randomized controlled trial. *J Cardiothor Surg* 2010;**5**:7

33. Guay J. The effect of neuraxial blocks on surgical blood loss and blood transfusion requirements: a meta-analysis. *J Clin Anesth* 2006;**18**:124–128

34. Juelsgaard P, Larsen UT, Sørensen JV, Madsen F, Søballe K. Hypotensive epidural anesthesia in total knee replacement without tourniquet: reduced blood loss and transfusion. *Reg Anesth Pain Med* 2001;**26**:105–110.

35. Kakiuchi M. Reduction of blood loss during spinal surgery by epidural blockade under normotensive general anesthesia. *Spine* 1997;**22**:889–894.

36. Hong JY, Jee YS, Yoon HJ, Kim SM. Comparison of general and epidural anesthesia in elective cesarean section for placenta previa totalis: maternal hemodynamics, blood loss and neonatal outcome. *Int J Obstet Anesth* 2003;**12**:12–16.

37. Fotiadis RJ, Badvie S, Weston MD, Allen-Mersh TG. Epidural analgesia in gastrointestinal surgery. *Br J Surg* 2004;**91**:828–841.

15 Use of Autologous Blood

When thinking about ways to avoid allogeneic transfusion, the first thing that comes to mind is the use of the patient's own blood. In fact, there is a wide variety of methods for autologous blood use, e.g., autologous immunotherapy, autologous stem cell use, and cord blood harvest for premature infants, just to name a few. This chapter will consider the more common forms of autologous blood use, namely preoperative autologous donation, hemodilution, and perioperative apheresis. It will describe how they impact on blood management-related patient outcome.

Objectives

1. To review how autologous blood can be used.
2. To learn how acute normovolemic hemodilution and its modifications are performed.
3. To compare the clinical importance of acute normovolemic hemodilution and preoperative autologous donation.

Definitions

Autologous blood transfusion: Blood transfusion when the donor and recipient are one and the same.

Preoperative autologous donation (PAD): Collection of the patient's own blood before an anticipated procedure. Blood is stored in a blood bank until surgery and is transfused as deemed necessary.

Hemodilution: Dilution of blood:
• *Acute hypervolemic hemodilution (AHH):* Intravascular dilution of the patient's blood components by infusion of acellular fluids to attain and maintain hypervolemia during surgery, with the intent to increase the allowable blood loss.
• *Acute normovolemic hemodilution (ANH):* A form of intraoperative autologous donation, during which the hemoglobin concentration is reduced by drawing blood and simultaneously replacing the drawn volume with acellular fluid. Blood is kept anticoagulated in blood bags at the patient's side and is retransfused as needed, ideally after surgical hemostasis is achieved.

Plasma/platelet sequestration: Selective pre- or intra-operative withdrawal of plasma or platelet-rich plasma (PRP) by apheresis. The goal is to harvest autologous blood products for intra- or post-operative use.

A brief history

To turn the patient into his/her own blood bank is not a new idea. However, preoperative autologous donation (PAD) could not be considered before storage of blood became feasible. Fantus, who founded the first blood bank in the United States, proposed preoperative autologous donation in 1937 [1]. Initially, the use of autologous blood was advocated mainly for patients with rare blood groups. Technology was not as advanced as today and liquid storage times were restricted to about 3 weeks. It was in the mid-1980s that PAD received wider

Basics of Blood Management, Second Edition. Petra Seeber and Aryeh Shander.
© 2013 John Wiley & Sons, Ltd. Published 2013 by John Wiley & Sons, Ltd.

acceptance. The acquired immune deficiency syndrome (AIDS) crisis led physicians as well as the informed public to call for safer blood. One answer was PAD. Autologous donation programs mushroomed. During the 1980s, the volume of autologous blood donations in the United States increased more than 17 times [2]. Today, the use of PAD is rather heterogeneous. Some institutions use it excessively, while others rarely recommend it to their patients.

Another way to use the patient's own blood is acute normovolemic hemodilution (ANH). The German physician Konrad Messmer first advocated intentional hemodilution. In the late 1960s [3], he reported deliberately making patients anemic and in the 1970s he reported on his clinical experiences [4]. To begin with, ANH was used for patients undergoing cardiac surgery with cardiopulmonary bypass and hypothermic arrest to reduce blood viscosity and post-bypass bleeding. It was hoped that the withdrawn autologous blood had maintained its clotting abilities so that hemostasis was improved after the reinfusion. Although hemodilution was initially described as a therapeutic measure to reduce exposure to allogeneic blood transfusion, it can be used for much more. Parallel to the development of ANH, background research on hemodilution provided a better understanding of the physiology of hemodilution, anemia tolerance, and adaptation to volume and red cell loss. All of those research areas now provide a basis for good blood management.

As time went by, PAD and ANH were modified. Plateletpheresis was introduced as a blood bank technology in 1968 [5]. In the late 1980s, this technology transferred to the operating theater, and intraoperative plateletpheresis was introduced into clinical practice [6]. The first relevant clinical trials on intraoperative plateletpheresis were published by Giordano et al. in 1988 [7]. Since then, this method has undergone further evaluation and modifications.

Preoperative autologous donation

The preoperative collection of autologous blood, and its storage and retransfusion during or after surgery with major blood loss was shown to reduce allogeneic transfusions in different procedures, such as cardiac, orthopedic, and pediatric surgeries. Therefore, it is typically used in procedures in which blood would be typed and cross-matched, i.e., procedures with an anticipated blood loss of 1000 mL or more. In some countries, physicians are even required by law to inform patients about the possibility of autologous donation before procedures with anticipated major blood loss.

Who is eligible and who is not?
The donation of blood for PAD is a relatively safe procedure. Therefore, eligibility is not greatly limited by age and weight of the patient. Children and older persons may be equally fit for donation. Even pregnancy is not a contraindication for PAD. When contemplating the eligibility of a patient for PAD, one should keep in mind that a patient who is eligible for elective surgery with anticipated major blood loss is most probably also able to donate blood.

However, preoperative donation is contraindicated in some patients. The American Association of Blood Banks (AABB) does not permit preoperative donation in cases where the hematocrit of the patient is less than 33%. Other regulatory guidelines, such on those of the Swiss Red Cross, prohibit patients with cardiovascular disease requiring heart surgery to donate blood for PAD. Other groups allow PAD in selected patients with cardiovascular risk factors [8]. No sound scientific data are available about contraindications for autologous donations and contraindications are often determined by the head of the donor center or the responsible person in the hospital. Many sick patients donate their own blood without relevant adverse effects. Sicker patients, however, have a higher incidence of adverse reactions. Generally agreed contraindications for PAD are: a recent myocardial infarction, chronic heart failure, aortic stenosis, transitory ischemic attack, arrhythmias, hypertension, and unstable angina pectoris. Also, patients with bacteremia or suspected bacteremia (diarrhea or in patients with a leukocytosis) are not fit to donate since bacteremia increases the risk for bacterial contamination of the stored blood. For practical reasons, patients with inappropriate venous access also cannot donate blood.

How it works
The theoretical basis for effective PAD is that withdrawal of blood preoperatively results in a net gain of red cell mass due to the erythropoietic response that it is hoped will be elicited by the donation. In practice, however, this approach presents a set of problems. First, effective erythropoiesis is induced only when the hematocrit falls between 30%, a level that must not be reached when donation is performed according to current guidelines. Second, many patients are iron depleted by the donation and cannot recover their red cell mass. Third, regenera-

tion of 1 unit of donated red cells takes 20–59 days and sometimes up to 6 month [8]. To get a maximum net gain in red cell mass, therefore, the ideal donation schedule starts early before elective surgery, exploiting the maximum storage time of 35–49 days (depending on the country and the blood product stored), and aimed at withdrawing the maximum amounts of blood. This may either mean donation of 2 units at a time or 1 unit every 3 days or so. Such rather tough donation schedules are rarely used. Traditional donation schedules withdraw 1 unit per week. This is a gentler approach and reduces storage time, but it produces next to no increase in red cell mass. Typically, patients are left with 1 g/dL less hemoglobin preoperatively than before commencement of donation [8]. Thus, as one author puts it, these types of donation schedule are "hardly more than the transfer of RBC from a patient into a plastic bag with little or no benefit for the patient: poorly efficacious, poorly effective, and highly inefficient" [8].

Blood can also be stored by cryopreservation, which is the storage of blood in a frozen state. This is very expensive, but may provide blood products with a much longer shelf life (up to 10 years) than products stored as a liquid. Preparation procedures are needed to prevent red cells from severe damage, and before retransfusion, deglycerolization is needed. This prolongs the time until the units are ready. The freezing process makes the red cells more prone to damage than other conservation methods. Cryopreservation is reserved for special circumstances, such as polysensitized patients with a complex antibody spectrum or patients with very rare blood groups.

Whatever donation schedule is chosen, patients need to be prepared. Informed consent must be obtained. The patient should know about the general risks of blood donation (e.g., hematoma, infection, fainting, nausea, etc.) as well as the risks unique to him/her. These may include the risks of delaying surgery in order to donate blood. Since there is the general perception among patients that autologous blood is completely safe, inherent risks need to be discussed, such as possible storage problems, technical problems with getting the donated units in time, and that autologous blood donation is no guarantee that transfusion of allogeneic blood will not be required. Where applicable, the patient needs to know that his/her blood will be tested for infections (HIV, HBV, HCV, and syphilis) and he/she will be informed of any positive result.

The patient who is anemic at the time of presentation for PAD or who develops anemia during donation may benefit from erythropoietin and iron therapy [9]. One unit of blood contains about 450 mg of iron and its donation lowers the hemoglobin level by about 1 g/dL. Therefore, iron therapy is recommended for almost all patients prior to blood donation; in rare cases it contraindicated. Giving erythropoietin and iron substantially increases a patient's ability to donate a large amount of blood, but economic considerations preclude the routine use of erythropoietin in many parts of the world. Paradoxically, it was shown in anemic and non-anemic patients performing PAD prior to major orthopedic surgery, that only the former experienced a reduction in allogeneic transfusions [10].

A word on the retransfusion of PAD blood: The common perception that autologous blood has very few side effects often leads to unnecessary transfusions. In fact, PAD increases rather than decreases overall (allogeneic + autologous) transfusions [8]. Often, the blood is transfused only because it is available or just not to disappoint the patient. Other concerns are the wastage of unused blood with blood transfused only so that it is not discarded. It is reasonable, however, to destroy units of blood if there is no good reason for transfusion, since the risk even of autologous blood does not justify transfusion just because blood is available.

Advantages and disadvantages

The use of one's own predonated blood substantially reduces the risk of contracting a transfusion-transmissible diseases, especially viral infections such as hepatitis B and C as well as human immunodeficiency virus (HIV). It also reduces immunologically-mediated hemolytic, febrile, and allergic reactions. Potentially, PAD may reduce postoperative risk of bacterial infection and cancer recurrence, since the immunomodulatory effects are fewer than with allogeneic blood transfusion. However, while PAD reduces the patient's exposure to allogeneic blood, it increases the total amount of blood transfused [11]. This may add unnecessary problems, since stored autologous blood also has hazards, including the effects of damage from storage on the immune system and oxygen delivery capacities.

The disadvantages of donating blood need to be considered as well. PAD itself is a relatively safe procedure. Nevertheless, concerns were expressed about the safety of PAD, especially in sicker or older patients. Mild side effects like diaphoresis, light-headedness, and nausea occur in about 1–3% of all donors. Studies have reported an incidence of severe reactions of 1–2% during PAD in patients at high risk, e.g., those with myocardial infarction, angina, and death [12].

It takes several weeks until autologous blood units harvested by PAD are available. During this time, the condition of the patient may worsen. Cardiac patients, cancer patients, and patients with aortic aneurysms may be eligible for PAD, but their condition may progress or they may even die if the surgical procedure is deferred. Also, the patient may be anxious about the surgical procedure and prolonging the waiting time for surgery may be a heavy burden.

PAD shares several disadvantages with allogeneic blood. One main concern is the quality of the autologous blood. Since it is stored, it undergoes the same deterioration as allogeneic blood and has the same storage damage. Improper storage as well as microbial contamination cannot be excluded. Due to mislabeling and administrative errors, incompatibility reactions are possible.

PAD is only possible for elective surgeries. The limited storage time may cause problems. Patients may deteriorate or other reasons for deferral of the surgical procedure may render the donation schedule invalid and donated units may pass their shelf life. Only a few donor centers consider frozen storage in this case. Otherwise, the blood has to be discarded.

Pregnancy is another issue to consider. The overall transfusion rate is 1–2% of all deliveries. The risk of bleeding is increased in placenta previa, Cesarean section, and a history of postpartum hemorrhage. The frequency of side effects of PAD in mothers is similar to that in other autologous donors. The fetus, however, may be more affected by anemia, hypovolemia, and hypotension. Labor may be induced by the process of donation. Prevalent anemia in pregnancy may preclude donation of considerable amounts of blood.

PAD is a very expensive method to procure autologous blood. Patients have to dedicate time and incur travel expenses. The blood bank has to engage trained personnel to perform PAD. Also, the blood requires special handling and special labeling ("autologous blood"). The blood is stored as a leukocyte-depleted unit, whole blood, or following separation into blood components. Different institutions test the blood for diseases and determine blood groups, also increasing the costs. Studies that ignored the cost reduction from the prevention of adverse effects related to allogeneic transfusions have demonstrated that PAD is more expensive than allogeneic blood. Adding to the average cost is the high discard rate (30–50%) for unused PAD blood. "Crossover," i.e., the transfusion of unused autologous blood in allogeneic recipients, was proposed to increase the cost-efficacy of PAD. It remains controversial. Many autologous donors do not meet the donor criteria set by the American FDA. Crossover is not permitted in several countries.

Hemodilution

Two distinct kinds of hemodilution—normovolemic and hypervolemic—have evolved over time. Both share a common idea behind them: Acutely diluting the patient's blood helps in that—if blood is shed during surgery—fewer blood components are lost per milliliter of blood loss.

Acute hypervolemic hemodilution

The technique of AHH is not as widespread as ANH, a technique that will be described later. Studies have suggested that AHH and ANH are equally effective in reducing a patient's exposure to donor blood and incur similar costs. Since there are, to date, not enough data about the use and safety of AHH, we will simply give the basics about AHH and will not further dwell on it.

How it works

AHH is performed by infusing considerable amounts of crystalloids or colloids [13]. It dilutes the patient's red cells within his/her body by temporarily expanding the blood volume, increasing the allowable blood loss. A target hematocrit is aimed at, e.g., 25%. During surgery, fewer blood cells are lost per milliliter of shed blood. The technique requires a patient who can tolerate hypervolemia. To prevent excessive increase in blood pressure, the vasodilating effect of anesthetic drugs is used [14].

Early literature sources recommend an infusion volume of 20 mL/kg of body weight. However, considerably higher volumes were used in other groups of patients. Kumar *et al.* [14] proposed an equation to calculate the amount of volume expansion required to achieve a particular target hematocrit:

$$\text{Volume} = \text{EBV} \times [(H_0 - H_f)/H_f] \times \text{expansion factor}$$

where EBV is the estimated blood volume of the patient; H_0 is the preoperative hematocrit; H_f is the final, postdilutional hematocrit (target); and expansion factor describes the ability of the fluid used for hemodilution to expand the plasma volume of the patient, e.g., a fluid with a volume effect of 80% would have an expansion factor of $100/80 = 1.25$.

During surgery, hypervolemia is sustained by further volume infusion as needed. To keep the patient hypervolemic during the whole surgical procedure, it is prudent to choose a fluid that has an intravascular residence time that is similar to the time of surgery.

> ## Practice tip
>
> Acute hypervolemic hemodilution is a good starter for an anesthesiologist who would like to practice blood management. Infusing 500–1000 mL of prewarmed hydroxyethyl starch in patients who will experience major blood loss is a simple, safe, and effective method to reduce blood loss.

Advantages and disadvantages

Hypervolemia causes changes in hemodynamics and provokes tissue edema. The blood pressure of the patient may increase. It was reported that such changes revert quickly due to decreased systemic vascular resistance and decreased blood viscosity. Care must be taken in patients with cardiac and autonomous nervous system disorders, where the ability to perform the compensatory adjustments for AHH may be impaired. Intact renal function is crucial to excrete the excessive volume.

Overall, AHH is simple and can be performed at low cost. It deserves, therefore, more attention. If further proof demonstrates the safety and efficacy of AHH, it is an attractive method to reduce the use of allogeneic transfusions [15].

Acute normovolemic hemodilution

ANH, endorsed by the NIH Consensus Conference on Perioperative Red Blood Cell Transfusion and the American Society of Anesthesiologists, is performed with the intent to reduce surgical blood loss.

Indications and eligibility

The classical indication for ANH is cardiac surgery to decrease blood viscosity during hypothermia. Another reason for its use is to save functional platelets and clotting factors for the time after cardiopulmonary bypass. There are many more indications for ANH. Basically, every major surgery with expected high blood loss (e.g., >1000 mL in adults) may be an indication for ANH. Besides cardiac surgery, ANH has been successfully used in orthopedic, gynecological, urological, and vascular surgery [15, 16]. All age groups have benefited from ANH—from neonates to adults and elderly persons.

A few conditions are relative contraindications for ANH. Among them are unstable angina pectoris and severe coronary artery stenosis, congestive heart failure, severe chronic obstructive pulmonary disease (if oxygenation is severely impaired), hemoglobinopathies, coagulation disorders, poor renal function, severe aortic stenosis, and major organ system failure. Anemia is only a relative contraindication. While some authors do not recommend performing ANH in patients with preoperative anemia, i.e., with a hematocrit of less than 33%, case reports show that it is possible to perform ANH also in patients with lower preoperative hematocrits [17].

How is it done?

ANH is a simple yet ingenious procedure [18, 19]. Before starting, calculation of how much blood can safely be removed from the patient is prudent. The following equation to calculate tolerable blood loss is helpful [18]:

$$ABL = EBV \times H_0 - H_T / HAV$$

where ABL is the allowable blood loss; EBV is the estimated blood volume; H_0 is the patient's initial hematocrit; H_T is the patient's target hematocrit; and HAV is the average of the initial and minimum allowable hematocrit.

Definition of a reasonable target hemoglobin requires knowledge and experience. The medical literature defines different levels of hemodilution: mild (hematocrit 25–30%), moderate (hematocrit 20–24%), and profound/severe/extreme (hematocrit <20%). Some consider a target hematocrit of less than 20%, in the absence of hypothermia and cardiopulmonary bypass, too risky, since it is considered to impair oxygen delivery. However, other authors use much lower target hematocrits without encountering unwanted side effects (e.g., in children for scoliosis surgery).

The patient receiving ANH needs at least one large-bore vascular access. Preferably, this is a central or arterial line. If this is not available, one or two peripheral venous accesses will serve as well. The vascular access is connected to a blood bag and blood drains by gravity. The blood collection bags contain an anticoagulant (citrate–phosphate–dextrose–adenosine [CPD-A]). Occasional gentle rocking of the blood bag ensures that the anticoagulant and blood mix well. It takes about 10 minutes to harvest 1 unit. To make sure the correct volume is removed, a scale may be useful to estimate the blood volume in the bag.

Blood collection is usually started after the induction of anesthesia and before surgical blood loss occurs. The blood must be labeled with the patient's name and time of withdrawal, and is stored at room temperature in the operating room. An accepted time limit for storage at room temperature is 6–8 hours. If at all possible, blood should be returned to the patient after major surgical blood loss has ceased. If required, return of the collected blood can start earlier, namely when the lowest acceptable hematocrit level is reached or when signs of hypoxia occur and none of the maneuvers described below reverses the patient's condition. Blood is returned in reverse order, namely the unit with the highest hematocrit and most clotting factors is returned last. It is recommended not to use microfilters (40 µm) for retransfusion since they may damage the platelets.

Of greatest importance in hemodilution is the maintenance of normovolemia. Withdrawn blood is substituted with acellular fluids. Usually, the first liter of withdrawn blood is replaced by a colloid, e.g., hydroxyethyl starch, in a ratio of 1:1. The remaining volume is replaced by crystalloid solutions in a ratio of 1 L of blood to 3–4 L of crystalloid. Excess administration of fluids, prior to withdrawal of blood, results in hypervolemic hemodilution and diminishes the benefits of withdrawing blood. Therefore, preoperative intravenous fluids should be limited to the necessary amount. In an adult, about half a liter of blood can be withdrawn without immediate replacement of blood volume. This provides a nearly undiluted first unit. If the patient is stable, normovolemia should be established once withdrawal of blood has commenced.

ANH is a very safe procedure, provided it is performed by experienced hands and monitored well. Routine electrocardiography (EKG) and pulse oximetry help to rule out any signs of impaired oxygen delivery. The analysis of respired gases, arterial and central venous blood pressure, arterial blood gases, and coagulation profiles may be necessary in selected cases. Regular hemoglobin checks are recommended. On-site test kits are available to obtain immediate results with minimal blood wastage.

Troubleshooting

During ANH, not only red cells, but also platelets and clotting factors are removed. There is a theoretical risk of dilutional coagulopathy. Clinically, there seems to be no increased bleeding when baseline variables are within normal range and ANH is performed according to standards. Clotting factors, although diminished, usually remain in the physiological range. Additionally, a state of hypercoagulability develops during stress, anesthesia, and surgical intervention. This hypercoagulability may be brought back toward normal by the use of ANH.

What if hypoxia occurs? ANH may have made the patient anemic and the anemia may have been increased by ongoing surgical blood loss. If there is no further surgical blood loss, blood should be returned to the patient. If surgical blood loss is ongoing, other measures should be tried first before the blood is returned prematurely. These maneuvers may be able to bridge the time until surgical hemostasis is achieved. First, check factors that may be the cause of the hypoxia. Above all, ask yourself: Is normovolemia maintained? If not, try volume substitution. Another way to increase the safety margin of your patient is oxygen therapy. The arterial oxygen content can be increased by ventilating the patient with 100% oxygen (hyperoxic ventilation). This enhances the amount of oxygen physically dissolved in the plasma. Intraoperative hemodilution may be extended beyond the transfusion trigger simply by giving 100% oxygen. Clinical trials were able to demonstrate that even signs of tissue hypoxia could be reversed simply by increasing the FiO_2. This simple maneuver helps to bridge the time until major blood loss has ceased and ANH blood can be returned [20]. Increasing the FiO_2 from 0.5 to 1.0 increases the arterial oxygen content by about 2 mL/dL. This equals a hemoglobin increase of about 1–1.5 g/dL [21].

Advantages

The beauty of ANH lies in its almost universal range of application. It can be used virtually in every type of surgery and in a wide variety of patients of different ages, weights, and comorbidities. Septicemia is also not a contraindication. Patients for elective as well as emergency surgery can benefit from the advantages of ANH. Minimal preoperative planning is needed. Patients who decline PAD often consent to ANH (Table 15.1).

ANH is a safe procedure. There is a detectable stress response in PAD, which makes this technique unsuitable for relatively sick patients. ANH is performed under general anesthesia, reducing the stress for the patient. Also, ANH is performed under the supervision of an anesthesiologist and not in a remote donor center. Close monitoring is possible under operating room conditions. ANH blood remains in the operating room near the patient. So, the risk of administrative/clerical error (wrong blood for the wrong patient) is reduced. Immediate transfusion is possible, since the blood is already in the operating room, ready for transfusion.

Storage damage to the blood is negligible. The storage time of the autologous units is so brief that deterioration of cells and clotting factors is minimal. What is transfused

Table 15.1 Comparison of preoperative autologous donation (PAD) and acute normovolemic hemodilution (ANH).

	PAD	ANH
Costs	High	Low
Applicable in emergencies	No	Yes
Storage lesions	Yes	Minimal
Risk of clerical error	Yes	No
Risk of bacterial transmission	Yes	Minimal
Risk of transfusion-transmitted diseases	No	No
Reduction of immunologically-induced complications, such as febrile and allergic reactions, ABO incompatibilities	Yes	Yes
Immunomodulation and subsequent bacterial infection and cancer recurrence	Reduced	Reduced
Eligibility of patients	Only selected patients	Almost all
Hemostatic properties of blood	Lost	Intact
Usable in patients with systemic infection	No	Yes
Inconveniences for patient	High	None
Wastage of blood	30–50%	Minimal

to the patient is fresh blood with functional platelets and clotting factors. Also, bacterial contamination of the blood is very unlikely. There is not much time for growth of the germs. Since the blood is stored at room temperature, leukocytes are fresh and active, and therefore are still bactericidal.

ANH is the most inexpensive way to harvest autologous blood. There are no costs for storage and testing. It does not require the patient's commitment to travel or to be absent from work. Also, there is no additional personnel requirement since ANH is performed by personnel in the operating room. Unlike PAD, wastage of unused blood does not usually occur, since most, if not all, blood is returned to the patient after surgery.

Several further benefits have been reported regarding ANH. Since the procedure reduces the viscosity of blood and aggregability of red cells [22], better organ perfusion and improved tissue oxygenation result. After orthopedic surgery with ANH [23], a reduced incidence of deep vein thrombosis was reported. A decreased incidence of wound infections was observed after ANH as well [5].

To date, there is no consensus about the safety of ANH. Some authors criticize ANH because of the possibility of perioperative complications (such as myocardial ischemia, elevated lactate levels, and increased blood loss). Most studies, however, have not demonstrated increased perioperative complications. A very sensitive field is heart surgery. It was claimed that hemodilution is detrimental to cardiac patients, but recent findings con-

tradict this claim. Actually, hemodilution to the extent induced by ANH may be beneficial. Patients with severe coronary artery disease or aortic stenosis have benefited from hemodilution to a target hematocrit of 28% prior to surgery. It was shown that there was not only no indication of myocardial ischemia, but also levels of cardiac enzymes indicating myocardial compromise (troponin I, creatine kinase) were no lower than in patients without hemodilution. Besides, hemodiluted patients have a better stroke volume [24–26], although this effect may be influenced by the kind of anesthetic chosen [27]. Moderate hemodilution (target hematocrit of 21–25%) may even improve renal function when compared to no hemodilution or severe hemodilution [28, 29].

To maintain normovolemia, large amounts of fluids are needed. Peripheral edema and abnormal postoperative pulmonary function and wound healing may occur. Although rare, pulmonary edema was observed following ANH. Generalized edema is more pronounced if crystalloids alone are used, and less with colloids. Peripheral edema typically resolves within 72 hours.

Advanced use

Several modifications of ANH promise better results. Among them are augmented ANH (A-ANH) and fractionation.

A patient undergoing ANH may experience anemia below their individually tolerable level as a result of surgical blood loss. In this situation, after making use of the above-mentioned maneuvers, return of the ANH blood is usually considered even before surgical blood loss ceases and perhaps even before the completion of surgery. A-ANH is a method that seeks to avoid the need for this. At the point where return of ANH blood is considered, an artificial oxygen carrier is infused. This oxygen carrier has the ability to deliver oxygen to the tissue and can bridge the time until definite surgical hemostasis is achieved. After that, the ANH blood can be given back and the extent of postoperative anemia reduced [30].

A-ANH is a safe procedure that can maintain tissue oxygenation and is efficacious in terms of avoiding allogeneic transfusion. The problem with this technique is that an artificial oxygen carrier for use in A-ANH is not available in most countries. South Africa and Russia are among the few countries that can use the benefits of artificial oxygen carriers. Classical ANH includes the withdrawal of whole blood for later retransfusion. Under certain circumstances, only a particular component of blood is required intraoperatively to provide the patient with exactly what is needed. To do this, blood harvested by ANH can be fractionated, i.e., divided into its components. Using modern cell-saving devices, whole blood can be divided into three components: red cells, platelet-poor plasma (PPP), and platelet-rich plasma (PRP). Some physicians prefer to give back part of the plasma immediately to diminish the theoretical risk of bleeding; others use the components for a targeted autologous transfusion therapy. As with other advanced methods of autologous transfusion therapy, fractionation needs further evaluation before it can be recommended for wider application [31].

Does ANH reduce postoperative anemia and does it improve the outcome?

Models of ANH show that it requires high blood loss, a high initial hematocrit, and a low target hematocrit to be effective. However, clinical studies show that ANH is able to spare patients from being given allogeneic transfusions [32–35]. A meta-analysis by Bryson et al. demonstrated clinical efficacy of ANH [36]. The blood-conserving effect was obvious in studies where at least 1000 mL of ANH blood were removed. Low-volume acute normovolemic hemodilution, during which only 5–10 mL of blood/kg are withdrawn, does not lead to significant reduction in perioperative blood loss [37].

ANH is especially useful in conjunction with a comprehensive blood management program. A multimodality approach combines the benefit of different procedures and drugs to reduce a patient's exposure to donor blood. Preoperative application of erythropoietin and iron to patients with low initial hematocrit levels has improved the effectiveness of ANH.

Platelet- and plasma-pheresis

Parallel to PAD and ANH, there are also methods to use autologous platelets and plasma selectively. Both, preoperative and intraoperative procurement methods are available, with advantages and disadvantages similar to those described for PAD and ANH.

Intraoperative autologous plateletpheresis is used mainly in cardiac surgery. Heart surgery, with its related procedures, may lead to coagulopathy. Among many other factors, a reduction in number and function of platelets due to damage caused by the extracorporeal circulation is considered an important reason for postoperative coagulopathy and subsequent increased platelet, plasma, and red cell transfusions. Perioperative plateletpheresis seeks to remove platelets from the patient's circulation before the blood is exposed to the stress of the cardiopulmonary bypass. This can be done either some days before surgery in the blood bank or directly after induction of anesthesia in the operating room.

Reasons similar to those advocating plateletpheresis also recommend plasmapheresis. Clotting factors can be kept functional when plasma is spared the effects of cardiopulmonary bypass. Plasmapheresis can be performed either preoperatively in a blood bank or directly in the operating room. As with PAD, autologous plasma can be stored for some time before surgery. When it is shock frozen, it can be kept for up to 2 years.

Platelet- or plasma-pheresis techniques used in the blood bank are similar to those used in the operating room. Apheresis techniques differ with regard to the way blood is drawn (gravity versus active), place of collection (in collection bags or directly in the centrifuge), form of the centrifuge, speed of the centrifuge (2000–6000 rotations/min), and the rate at which blood is withdrawn (60–100 mL/min).

Advantages and disadvantages

Studies have demonstrated several benefits of intraoperative allogeneic plateletpheresis, such as decreased postoperative bleeding, enhanced hemostasis due to fresh platelets and clotting factors, reduced chest tube drainage after cardiac surgery, better pulmonary function in comparison with patients undergoing no platelet sequestration [6], shorter stay in the intensive care unit, and higher postoperative fibrinogen and antithrombin III levels.

Plateletpheresis can be performed in patients in whom ANH is not possible due to anemia. As with the blood harvested by ANH, intraoperative plateletpheresis provides fresh blood products without the storage damage seen in allogeneic platelets.

Although it was shown that the quality of intraoperatively harvested platelets is superior to the quality of allogeneic platelets, concerns remain regarding the quality of the harvested units. Citrate, as part of the anticoagulant, may damage platelets. Centrifugation releases platelet granules. Red cells returned after platelet sequestration are more fragile due to processing and are prone to hemolysis during cardiopulmonary bypass. Nevertheless, the damage caused by the apheresis process is less than the combined damage of blood bank apheresis and storage. That is why freshly harvested platelets are more effective than allogeneic platelets.

The procedure of intraoperative plateletpheresis is time consuming. Depending on the device used and the hemodynamic stability of the patient, it takes 30–80 minutes to harvest therapeutic quantities of PRP. To reduce operating room time, apheresis may be performed parallel to patient preparation.

The net effect of platelet- or plasma-pheresis on blood management has yet to be fully appreciated. These are labor and equipment intensive procedures, without well-defined improvement of outcome variables. Future research will demonstrate whether such pheresis procedures should have a fixed place in blood management.

Key points

• Hemodilution is a simple, safe, convenient, and effective alternative to PAD.
• Maintaining normovolemia is imperative for successful hemodilution.
• ANH can replace PAD as an autologous blood procurement method.

Questions for review

1. What are the advantages and disadvantages of PAD?
2. What are the advantages and disadvantages of ANH?
3. Do patients with severe coronary artery stenosis have to be excluded from hemodilution? Explain your answer.
4. How is AHH performed?

Suggestions for further research

What monitoring tools may indicate tissue hypoxia under acute normovolemic hemodilution?

Homework

Find out where you can obtain blood bags for hemodilution and record the contact details and other pertinent information.

Exercises and practice cases

Calculate how much blood can be drawn for ANH in the following patients and draw conclusions about your results.
A 50-kg healthy female with a hemoglobin level of 16 g/dL
A 50-kg healthy female with a hemoglobin level of 13 g/dL
A 50-kg healthy female with a hemoglobin level of 10 g/dL
A 100-kg healthy male with a hemoglobin level of 16 g/dL
A 100-kg healthy male with a hemoglobin level of 13 g/dL
A 100-kg healthy male with a hemoglobin level of 10 g/dL

References

1. Fantus B. Blood preservation. *JAMA* 1937;**109**:128–131.
2. Popovsky M, *et al.* Preoperative autologous blood donation. In: Spiess BD, *et al.* (eds) *Perioperative Transfusion Medicine.* Baltimore, Williams and Wilkins, 1997.
3. Messmer K. Überleben von Hunden bei akuter Verminderung der O2-Transportkapazität auf 2,8g% Hämoglobin. *Pflügers Archive Physiol* 1967;**297**:R48.
4. Bauer H, Pichlmaier H, Ott E, Klövekorn WP, Sunder-Plassmann L, Messmer K. [Autotransfusion through acute, preoperative hemodilution—1st clinical experiences]. *Langenbecks Arch Chir* 1974;Suppl:185–189.
5. Spiess BD, *et al.* (eds) *Perioperative Transfusion Medicine.* Baltimore, Williams and Wilkins, 1997.
6. Christenson JT, Reuse J, Badel P, Simonet F, Schmuziger M. Plateletpheresis before redo CABG diminishes excessive blood transfusion. *Ann Thorac Surg* 1996;**62**:1373–1378; discussion 1378–1379.

7. Giordano GF, Goldman DS, Mammana RB, *et al*. Intraoperative autotransfusion in cardiac operations. Effect on intraoperative and postoperative transfusion requirements. *J Thorac Cardiovasc Surg* 1988;**96**:382–386.

8. Singbartl G. Pre-operative autologous blood donation: clinical parameters and efficacy. *Blood Transfus* 2011;**9**:10–18.

9. Tryba M. Epoetin alfa plus autologous blood donation in patients with a low hematocrit scheduled to undergo orthopedic surgery. *Semin Hematol* 1996;**33** (Suppl 2):22–24; discussion 25–26.

10. Boettner F, Altneu EI, Williams BA, Hepinstall M, Sculco TP. Nonanemic patients do not benefit from autologous blood donation before total hip replacement. *HSS J* 2009 Dec 5 [Epub ahead of print].

11. Forgie MA, Wells PS, Laupacis A, Fergusson D. Preoperative autologous donation decreases allogeneic transfusion but increases exposure to all red blood cell transfusion: results of a meta-analysis. International Study of Perioperative Transfusion (ISPOT) Investigators. *Arch Intern Med* 1998;**158**:610–616.

12. Monk TG, Goodnough LT. Blood conservation strategies to minimize allogeneic blood use in urologic surgery. *Am J Surg* 1995;**170** (6A Suppl):69S–73S.

13. Galli C, Brandes IF, Otten JE, Nagursky H, Schwarz U, Gellrich NC. [Optimized hemodilution with hydroxyethyl starch. A blood saving method in malocclusion operations]. *Mund Kiefer Gesichtschir* 2001;**5**:353–356.

14. Kumar R, Chakraborty I, Sehgal R. A prospective randomized study comparing two techniques of perioperative blood conservation: isovolemic hemodilution and hypervolemic hemodilution. *Anesth Analg* 2002;**95**:1154–1161.

15. Saricaoglu F, Akinci SB, Celiker V, Aypar U. The effect of acute normovolemic hemodilution and acute hypervolemic hemodilution on coagulation and allogeneic transfusion. *Saudi Med J* 2005;**26**:792–798.

16. Terai A, Terada N, Yoshimura K, *et al*. Use of acute normovolemic hemodilution in patients undergoing radical prostatectomy. *Urology* 2005;**65**:1152–1156.

17. Rehm M, Orth V, Kreimeier U, *et al*. Four cases of radical hysterectomy with acute normovolemic hemodilution despite low preoperative hematocrit values. *Anesth Analg* 2000;**90**:852–855.

18. Jarnagin WR, Gonen M, Maithel SK, *et al*. A prospective randomized trial of acute normovolemic hemodilution compared to standard intraoperative management in patients undergoing major hepatic resection. *Ann Surg* 2008;**248**:360–369.

19. Monk TG. Acute normovolemic hemodilution. *Anesthesiol Clin North Am* 2005;**23**:271–281, vi.

20. Habler O, Kleen M, Kemming G, Zwissler B. Hyperoxia in extreme hemodilution. *Eur Surg Res* 2002;**34**:181–187.

21. Meier J, Kemming G, Meisner F, Pape A, Habler O. Hyperoxic ventilation enables hemodilution beyond the critical myocardial hemoglobin concentration. *Eur J Med Res* 2005;**10**:462–468.

22. Gu YJ, Graaff R, de Hoog E, *et al*. Influence of hemodilution of plasma proteins on erythrocyte aggregability: an in vivo study in patients undergoing cardiopulmonary bypass. *Clin Hemorheol Microcirc* 2005;**33**:95–107.

23. Vara Thorbeck R, Rosell Pradas J, Mekinassi KL, Prados Olleta N, Guerrero Fernandez-Marcote JA. [Prevention of thromboembolic disease and post-transfusional complications using normovolemic hemodilution in arthroplasty surgery of the hip]. *Rev Chir Orthop Reparatrice Appar Mot* 1990;**76**:267–271.

24. Licker M, Ellenberger C, Sierra J, Christenson J, Diaper J, Morel D. Cardiovascular response to acute normovolemic hemodilution in patients with coronary artery diseases: Assessment with transesophageal echocardiography. *Crit Care Med* 2005;**33**:591–597.

25. Licker M, Sierra J, Kalangos A, Panos A, Diaper J, Ellenberger C. Cardioprotective effects of acute normovolemic hemodilution in patients with severe aortic stenosis undergoing valve replacement. *Transfusion* 2007;**47**: 341–350.

26. Licker M, Ellenberger C, Sierra J, Kalangos A, Diaper J, Morel D. Cardioprotective effects of acute normovolemic hemodilution in patients undergoing coronary artery bypass surgery. *Chest* 2005;**128**:838–847.

27. Lorsomradee S, Lorsomradee S. The use of a volatile anesthetic regimen protects against acute normovolemic hemodilution induced myocardial depression in patients with coronary artery disease. *Asian J Transfus Sci* 2009;**3**: 10–13.

28. Karkouti K, Beattie WS, Wijeysundera DN, *et al*. Hemodilution during cardiopulmonary bypass is an independent risk factor for acute renal failure in adult cardiac surgery. *J Thorac Cardiovasc Surg* 2005;**129**:391–400.

29. Habib RH, Zacharias A, Schwann TA, *et al*. Role of hemodilutional anemia and transfusion during cardiopulmonary bypass in renal injury after coronary revascularization: implications on operative outcome. *Crit Care Med* 2005;**33**: 1749–1756.

30. Kemming G, Habler O, Zwissler B. Augmented acute normovolemic hemodilution (A-ANH(tm)) in cardiac and non-cardiac patients. *Anasthesiol Intensivmed Notfallmed Schmerzther* 2001;**36** (Suppl 2):S107–109.

31. Potter PS. Perioperative apheresis. *Transfusion* 2004;**44** (12 Suppl):54S–57S.

32. Johnson LB, Plotkin JS, Kuo PC. Reduced transfusion requirements during major hepatic resection with use of intraoperative isovolemic hemodilution. *Am J Surg* 1998;**176**: 608–611.

33. Habler O, Schwenzer K, Zimmer K, *et al*. Effects of standardized acute normovolemic hemodilution on intraoperative allogeneic blood transfusion in patients undergoing major maxillofacial surgery. *Int J Oral Maxillofac Surg* 2004;**33**: 467–475.

34. Matot I, Scheinin O, Jurim O, Eid A. Effectiveness of acute normovolemic hemodilution to minimize allogeneic blood

transfusion in major liver resections. *Anesthesiology* 2002;**97**: 794–800.

35. Wong J, Haynes S, Dalrymple K, McCollum CN. Vascular surgical society of great britain and ireland: autologous transfusion reduces blood transfusion requirements in aortic surgery. *Br J Surg* 1999;**86**:698.

36. Bryson GL, Laupacis A, Wells GA. Does acute normovolemic hemodilution reduce perioperative allogneneic transfusion? A meta-analysis. The International Study of Perioperative Transfusion. *Anesth Analg* 1998;**86**:9–15.

37. Virmani S, Tempe DK, Pandey BC, *et al*. Acute normovolemic hemodilution is not beneficial in patients undergoing primary elective valve surgery. *Ann Card Anaesth* 2010;**13**: 34–38.

16 Cell Salvage

A traveler in a drought region needs no admonition to save water. Since his/her life depends on it, he/she will go to great length to save every drop of this precious commodity. We medical practitioners work in an environment where blood cannot just be replaced with another fluid with the same life-saving quality. Shouldn't it be as obvious to us to save every drop of the patient's life-saving blood? Cell salvage helps in this regard.

Objectives

1. To list the minimum components required for cell salvage.
2. To describe basic principles of modern cell salvage.
3. To discuss potential and controversial contraindications, and explain how to overcome them.

Definitions

Cell salvage: The process used to collect, wash, and concentrate blood shed blood during and after surgery or trauma, and return the concentrated red cells to the paient. Cell salvage can be categorized by the timing of blood collection (intra- or post-operative) and by the methods used to return the blood (direct cell salvage for unwashed blood, indirect cell salvage for washed blood).

A brief history

In 1818, Dr James Blundell was requested to visit a woman who was, as he wrote, "sinking under uterine hemorrhage." Before long and despite all efforts, she bled to death. Reflecting on the "melancholy scene" he encountered in this woman's case, Blundell considered transfusion as the possible salvation for her. To ascertain the feasibility of transferring blood, he constructed a device to be used in experiments with dogs. He bled the canines from the femoral artery, collected the blood in a funnel-shaped bowl, and retransfused the blood using a syringe connected to the bottom of the bowl. He observed that the dogs survived and he subsequently recommended this procedure to be used on patients as needed [1]. Although Blundell did not report any cases where he used autologous transfusions in humans, he is considered to be the father of autotransfusion. Of interest, the retransfusion device he constructed is thought to be one of the first autotransfusion devices.

More than 50 years later, William Highmore, also an English physician, visited a woman suffering from severe postpartum hemorrhage. On arrival in the house of the patient, Dr Highmore saw blood everywhere: on the bed, sheets, and also collected in a vessel. Furthermore, he saw his colleague struggling to stop the bleeding. Although the hemorrhage was finally stopped, the patient died 1 hour after Dr Highmore's arrival. Reflecting on this experience, Dr Highmore imagined that—since blood was available as it could be seen to have collected in the vessel—an attempt should have been made to return the blood to the patient. In 1874, he resolved: "I commend this plan [to autotransfuse] to the notice of the profession, and have resolved to use it myself in the first case of haemorrhage that may occur in my practice" [2].

Despite the fact that the feasibility of autotransfusion had been shown in animal studies and it was recommended as a potentially life-saving procedure, it took

Basics of Blood Management, Second Edition. Petra Seeber and Aryeh Shander.
© 2013 John Wiley & Sons, Ltd. Published 2013 by John Wiley & Sons, Ltd.

some time until the first report of human autotransfusion appeared in the medical literature. In 1886, John Duncan took care of a patient with a crushed leg. Since Duncan's patient had lost much blood and was moribund, Dr Duncan amputated the crushed leg and collected the blood in a bowl. Phosphate of soda was added to prevent rapid clotting, and the blood was diluted with distilled water. Afterwards, the patient's blood was returned to him. The patient survived without any reported adverse effects from the cell salvage. Dr Duncan was the first to report his experiences in returning a patient's own blood lost during surgery, "I have now performed it in a sufficient number of cases to enable me to speak with confidence as to its safety and value" [3] .

In 1914, J. Thies reported on a series of three women with ruptured ectopic pregnancies in whom he practiced cell salvage. He used a ladle to scoop blood out of the abdominal cavity. He filtered the blood through two layers of gauze, diluted it with saline, and returned it to the patient. The first patient received a transfusion of 1.5 L of blood subcutaneously; the other two patients received blood intravenously [4]. With his report, Dr Thies appears to be the first to have used cell salvage in gynecological hemorrhage, the indication for which it had been advocated decades before [2].

Cell salvage was later performed in selected cases of splenectomy, neurosurgery, and trauma. Side effects were rare even when crude methods were used. The resilience of patients is evident when we consider the case series of Griswold and Ortner [5]. One hundred patients with thorax or abdominal trauma received cell-salvaged blood. Only one of them died due to cell salvage. It was reported that this patient had multiple perforations in his small intestine and the blood used for direct autotransfusion was contaminated with fecal matter, to the extent that the infusion needle had become plugged with feces. At autopsy, the patient had multiple emboli in his lung.

The advent of a sufficient and seemingly safe blood supply influenced physicians to abandon autotransfusion for a while. Some factors rekindled the interest in autotransfusion. Physicians caring for patients who refused allogeneic blood for religious reasons looked to devise methods to use the patient's own blood. Another impetus for autotransfusion was blood shortages, e.g., during wars. The lack of blood in the Vietnam war urged Gerald Klebanoff, a surgeon of the US Air Force, to develop a simple autotransfusion device that used parts from cardiopulmonary bypass equipment [6]. His device was later marketed as the Bentley ATS 100. The system

was widely used, but some safety concerns caused its withdrawal from the market. However, the experience with this system helped to develop other systems that attempted to eliminate the problems encountered with Klebanoff's invention [7].

In the late 1960s and early 1970s, the engineer Allen "Jack" Latham developed a new form of cell salvage [8]. He introduced the Latham bowl, which had the ability to wash blood before it was retransfused. Washing the shed blood reduced much of the debris and either reduced or eliminated many of the side effects encoutered previously. Since then, the methods of washing blood have been refined and continue to be refined.

What is cell salvage?

Cell salvage is a clever means to harvest shed blood that is otherwise lost. Although losing favor in the developed world, under certain circumstances, lost blood can be harvested and returned without any additional processing. This kind of cell salvage is called direct cell salvage and it delivers unprocessed (washed) blood back to the patient. In contrast, blood collected by cell salvage equipment can be returned to the patient after being extensively processed. The processing usually consists of several steps that wash red cells. This kind of cell salvage is called indirect cell salvage.

If blood is given in the intraoperative period, it is usually harvested from the surgical field or from open body cavities during the surgical procedure. Postoperative cell salvage draws blood from drains, e.g., from the chest or other operative sites such as the spine or large joints (hip, knee).

Depending on the timing, cell salvage can be performed either solely intraoperatively or postoperatively. Sometimes, intraoperative use of a cell-saving device is continued into the postoperative period. Intra- and postoperative cell salvage can either be performed with or without blood processing.

Cell salvage equipment—from basic to sophisticated

There are a variety of methods and devices used for intra- or post-operative cell salvage—from very simple ones to complex apparatus. The choice of the method will largely depend on local circumstances, such as patient criteria, the specifics of the surgical procedure, costs, personal preference, and regulations. The following methods have been used successfully.

• **Method 1:** The simplest technique of cell salvage is that introduced by Thies [4]. To imitate his technique, it was proposed to use a sterilized soup ladle and a funnel. Blood is scooped out of the wound, filtered through several layers of gauze into a funnel and collected in a bottle. If blood bags rather than bottles are available, the funnel is connected to a rubber tubing. The tube is clamped at one end and the needle of the blood bag is inserted into this rubber tubing. The blood follows gravity into the bags (Figure 16.1) [9]. The container that collects the blood needs to contain an anticoagulant.

A very similar approach was proposed using a funnel. The funnel's smaller opening is closed with a sieve with pores of about 1 mm diameter. This funnel is sterilized and introduced into a small incision in the blood-containing abdomen, e.g., after an ectopic pregnancy. The

patient is tilted head-down, so that blood collects in the hypochondria and can flow into the funnel. It is then syringed out of the funnel into blood bags and retransfused. In this way, the blood in the funnel contains no debris larger than 1 mm [10].

• **Method 2:** If no cell-salvage equipment is available, cell salvage can be performed by assembling equipment that may be available even in areas with few resources. As an example, the following cell-salvage equipment can be assembled (which is similar to that originally proposed by Klebanoff [6]). Suction tips are connected to a roller head pump so that blood can be retrieved from the surgical field into a defoaming cardiotomy reservoir. Via an inline blood filter, blood is collected into vacuum collection bags and is returned to the patient.

Using this self-made equipment, the patient needs to be given an anticoagulant (typically heparin, 300 U/kg body weight) just prior to the expected blood loss. The device needs to be primed with an anticoagulant as well. Heparinization must be monitored closely and heparin is reversed with protamine after the procedure. It is necessary to keep in mind that the unwashed or improperly washed returned blood contains heparin and can reheparinize the patient. The protamine dose needs to be adjusted accordingly. With this method, up to 23 units of blood have been reported to be given safely [11].

• **Method 3:** If a preassembled cell-saving device is contemplated, many models are available to choose from. One low-cost model is a set that was designed for use in developing countries [12]. It consists of several components, namely:

  ○ A blood reservoir bag with a double filter system and tubing
  ○ An electrically driven blood pump with a maximum suction pressure of −40 mmHg
  ○ A 100-mL syringe and a collection bowl (for when there is electrical power failure).

    The collection bowl is fitted with a funnel, which contains a filter and a transfusion tubing set. The pump, syringe, and collection bowl are reusable after sterilization while the reservoir bag, filters, and tubing are not.

• **Method 4:** For direct postoperative cell salvage, specially designed containers are available which can be connected to the drain in the wound. The containers have a filter to remove any debris in the wound. A port in the container can be spiked and the container can be hung above the patient to allow the collected blood to return to the patient via an intravenous line using simple gravity.

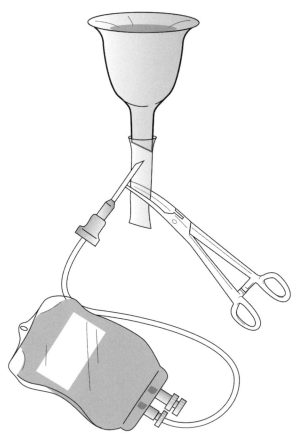

Figure 16.1 Use of blood bags for simple cell salvage.

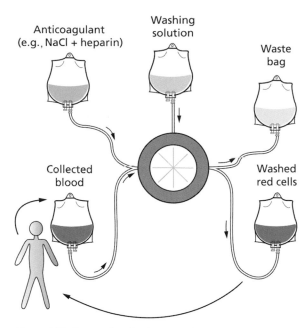

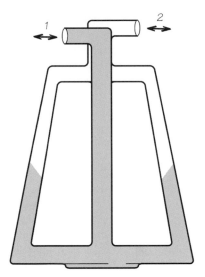

Figure 16.3 Latham bowl: 1, Port for blood (inlet and outlet); 2, port for washing solution (inlet and outlet).

Figure 16.2 Automatic cell salvage equipment.

• **Method 5:** Most developed countries with sufficient resources in their healthcare system can use computerized blood washing devices. Blood is sucked from the field and mixed with an anticoagulant. The blood runs through a filter into a reservoir or a bowl and is processed (washed). Afterwards the washed blood is automatically transferred into blood bags where it is available to be returned to the patient (Figure 16.2). The systems differ in the method used to process the blood.

How to "clean" blood

There are basically three different methods to "clean" blood—centrifugation, filtration, and sedimentation. Centrifugation is most commonly used in commercially available cell-salvage devices.

It is well known that blood constituents have different densities. Components with a high density, such as red cells, settle at the bottom of a tube, followed by components with lesser density, a process called sedimentation. If sedimentation is complete, blood will stand in different layers: blood cells at the bottom, above which is a thin layer of platelets and leukocytes (called buffy coat), followed by a wide layer of platelet-poor plasma.

It is possible to speed up the separation of blood based on density differences by means of centrifugation. In a laboratory, blood is spun to be separated for further analysis. A very similar spinning process is used to separate red cells from other blood components during cell salvage, the so-called density gradient separation. During spinning, typically at 4400 or more rotations/minute [13], red cells are packed against the outer wall of the centrifuge bowl, while other, less dense components remain, more or less, in the center of the centrifuge. Plasma, platelet remains, anticoagulant, cell debris, free hemoglobin, and other contaminants are in the plasma phase. A washing solution (sterile saline) is added. This solution dilutes the plasma supernatant, which is then removed from the centrifuge and discarded into a waste bag. After the washing process is finished, the red cell layer is pumped into blood bags and is ready for return to the patient.

Based on these simple principles, modern equipment washes blood either intermittently or continuously.

Discontinuous, intermittent blood washing

The discontinuous washing method mostly uses a Latham bowl (Figure 16.3). This looks like two bowls, with a smaller one set into a larger one. Both are turned around so that their undersides face upward. The inner bowl is stationary and holds an inlet and outlet port. The outer bowl rotates. The Baylor bowl (BRAT® bowl) is also used for discontinuous washing. In comparison with the Latham bowl, it has vertical sides [13].

A wash procedure in a Latham bowl [14] consists of three separate steps: filling or priming, washing, and emptying. Blood is collected either directly from the surgical field or from the reservoir. Blood is pumped into the rotating bowl. The centrifugal force drives the lighter supernatants medially and upward where they are removed from the outlet. The heavier red cells collect on the lateral walls of the centrifuge. When a certain red cell level is reached in the centrifuge, the filling phase ends and the washing phase begins. A washing solution, typically normal saline, enters the red cell layer on the wall of the outer bowl from below and circulates through it. The solution washes away remaining debris. Red cells from a relatively clean collection, such as from vessel injuries or from a cardiopulmonary bypass, are washed with a minimum of three times the red cell volume. A washing volume of as much as 10 times the bowl volume may be needed for contaminated blood from wounds or wound drains. At the end of the washing process, the washing solution used for the red cell layer should be clear. When the centrifuge—i.e., the outer bowl—is stopped, the red cells are pumped out of the centrifuge.

Prior to the commencement of cell washing, a set of operational settings must be selected. The first decision is the bowl size. A standard bowl holds 220–250 mL of fluid. To fill this with washable red cells, at least 500–750 mL of collected blood is needed. Bowls with a volume of 375 mL are available for cases with rapid blood loss, and bowls with a volume of about 125 mL for smaller or slower blood losses.

Another decision to be made is the pump flow rate. This can be set from 25 to more than 1000 mL/minute and is chosen according to the rate of blood loss and quality of the washed blood. The quality of the final autologous red cell concentrate prepared by the Latham bowl can partially be influenced by the operator [14]. Some parameters influencing the product quality are modifiable, while others are set by predetermined wash programs.

The elimination of waste in a Latham bowl depends on three parameters:
• **Hematocrit prior to separation:** The lower the hematocrit in the collected blood, the better the elimination of solutes. The operator can influence this hematocrit by diluting the blood in the reservoir with additional saline.
• **Hematocrit inside the bowl after the filling phase:** The higher the hematocrit, the better the elimination of solutes. A desired hematocrit level is 50–70%. The hematocrit can be increased by reducing the inflow speed of the blood that needs to be processed.

As we learned above, the fundamental principle of blood washing is sedimentation. In a centrifuge, this sedimentation can be accelerated. The longer the centrifugation, the more complete is the sedimentation. With a reduced speed of blood inflow, it takes longer to fill the bowl, prolonging centrifugation time. The increase in the length of the centrifugation period causes a higher hematocrit level in the bowl.
• **Amount of washing solution:** The more washing solution is used, the better the elimination of solutes. This, however, prolongs the washing process and reduces the amount of red cells finally recovered.

The quality of the processed blood is also influenced by parameters that are intrinsic to the system [14]. The design of the bowl determines where the washing solution enters the red cell layers. Since the washing solution is also centrifuged, it follows the centrifugal force and is driven to the center of the bowl (since the density of saline or another washing solution is lower than the density of red cells and similar to the density of plasma). In turn, red cells pushed to the wall of the bowl are not as thoroughly washed as red cells closer to the center of the bowl. Small changes to the design of the bowl can force the water to the outer parts of the bowl or force the sedimented red cells to mix. Another way to improve the washing performance is to temporarily stop or at least slow down the centrifuge. This redistributes the contents of the bowl and improves the elimination of the supernatant.

Unique to the Latham bowl is the "problem of the last bowl." If the remaining blood in the collection reservoir is not sufficient to fill the Latham bowl, the quality of this last batch of processed blood is inferior to earlier batches. The partially-filled bowl does not reach high hematocrits after separation. Attempts to solve the problem include the use of a small bowl or filling the bowl by topping it up with red cells from the already washed portion. A bowl with adjustable volume can also be used; a membrane rather than a rigid chamber wall will adjust to the amount of blood that needs to be processed.

Continuous blood washing

For a continuous blood washing setting, blood is pumped from the collection reservoir into a special centrifuge chamber. This chamber looks like a double spiral (Figure 16.4). Blood is pumped into the inner spiral of the rotating chamber. Centrifugal forces drive the red cells into the outer spiral of the chamber. On their way, they are washed by adding washing solution to the chamber. Lighter matter such as fat, washing solution containing contaminants, and plasma components drift to the middle of the chamber and are pumped out from there.

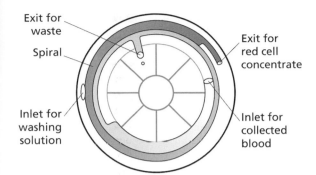

Figure 16.4 Continuous blood washing with a spiral bowl.

On its way through the spiral chamber, the red cell layer becomes ever cleaner and denser. When a certain hematocrit is reached, washed red cells are pumped into the retransfusion bag while the chamber is still rotating. The continued rotation prevents contaminants from being driven back into the red cell layer once the chamber is stopped.

In contrast to blood processing with the Latham bowl, the separation phase and washing phase in the spiral-shaped chamber work continually. The quality of the blood is constant, no matter how much blood is processed and how high the hematocrit. The bowl size does not need to be chosen according to the expected blood loss. The maximum achievable hematocrit using the continuous system is claimed to be higher than with the discontinuous system.

Filtration techniques

The second basic method of cell washing is filtration. The components of blood or a blood-containing solution have different sizes and each carries a different electrical charge. This facilitates separation by the use of appropriate filters. For cell salvage, usually ultrafiltration is used. Blood is passed over a semipermeable membrane. The hydrostatic pressure of the fluid pushes smaller molecules through the fine pores of the membrane while the larger ones are left on the original side. Depending on the membrane, either all plasma is filtered leaving mainly red cells or only water with smaller solutes is filtered, preserving plasma proteins (fibrinogen, antithrombin, etc.) and platelets.

Ultrafiltration can be used as a means of hemoconcentration. This process has been traditionally used to dialyze patients with renal failure. The method is nowadays increasingly used to concentrate the blood that remains at the end of a cardiopulmonary bypass [15]. The membrane is chosen so that most of the blood components can be given back to the patients, with only excess water and small molecular components (e.g., complement factors) filtered out. This has helped to prevent fluid overload and reduces the systemic inflammatory reaction seen after extracorporeal circulation. It also helps to reduce a patient's exposure to donor blood.

The process of ultrafiltration can also be used in a classical cell-salvage device. Salvaged blood is suspended in a solution, which typically consists of normal saline with heparin for anticoagulation. It is mixed gently and thereby washed (vortex mixing). The blood is pumped through a membrane for filtration. The membrane is chosen so that most of the plasma is filtrated and only cellular components remain [16].

Sedimentation

Non-coagulating blood that sits for some time in a container will settle into layers. The lower layer will contain red cells, with white cells and platelets in the middle layer, and plasma at the top. The rate of sedimentation depends on the quality of blood and its composition. In some disease states, the sedimentation rate is accelerated, but normally, settling occurs at only about 10 mm/hour. However, if certain colloids such as gelatin or hydroxyethyl starch (preparably high-molecular variants) are added, the sedimentation rate is up to 100 times faster than normal [17]. One part colloid is added for every two parts of blood. After 30 minutes, the red cells will have settled. The supernatant containing white cells, platelets, plasma with interleukins and free hemoglobins, etc. can be discarded, and the red cells are returned to the patient.

Blood quality after cell salvage

Unwashed blood

Unwashed blood contains whatever is in the blood leaving the wound or body cavity. Enormous differences in blood quality have been observed. Those differences depend partially on the flow (amount of blood collected over time), method of blood collection, and addition of anticoagulant. The use of substances like bone cement, glues, etc. and the area operated on (with much or little free fat) influence the quality of the final blood product.

With a high flow of blood and immediate return, intraoperatively collected blood contains most of the platelets and plasma coagulation factors. It was reported that even after a turnover as high as about five times the blood volume of the patient, coagulation was sufficient at the end of surgery [18]. With prolonged blood procurement, platelet counts vary, ranging from near normal to almost zero. Platelets are usually morphologically and functionally altered, consumed or form microaggregates.

Postoperatively collected blood has generally lost its capability to coagulate. Contact with the wound defibrinizes the blood. But it still contains activated components, such as prothrombin fragments, fibrin split products, and soluble fibrin. Fibrin split products may impair the function of fibrin and platelets [19].

Blood in the postoperative cell-salvage container has a comparatively low hematocrit. Some studies have reported hemoglobin concentrations as low as 7–12 g/dL [20]. Intact red cells for retransfusion have a near-normal survival rate. However, before red cells are ready for retransfusion, they may be damaged by processes in the wound or by the collection. This damage can lead to an increased amount of free hemoglobin in the blood.

Complement factors are activated by the process of blood collection. Leukocytes may be activated, leading to elevated cytokine levels in the blood. Especially interleukin 6, but also interleukin 1 and 8 as well as tumor necrosis factor alpha, were found to be increased in wound blood [21]. Many other immunologically active ingredients have been found in the blood, such as leukotrienes, elastase, prostaglandins, and others. When the collected blood is given back, increases in the serum levels of those substances are typically seen. These infused substances are usually cleared from the patient's blood stream within minutes to several hours and with little to no clinical consequences.

Washed blood

Washing blood reduces and sometimes entirely eliminates contaminants found in blood after collection. These contaminants include the washing solution, plasma fraction and many iatrogenically added substances (antibiotics and other medications, glues, and irrigants).

Fresh autologous red cells tolerate centrifugation well [22] so that the processed product can contain up to 80% of the lost red cells. Depending on the way the blood is processed, the hematocrit after washing lies between 52% and 80% [22]. Free hemoglobin, potassium, and protein are sufficiently reduced by the washing process. Washed blood essentially returns red cells reconstituted in saline. The product does not contain sufficient plasma coagulation factors or platelets to assure coagulation.

Washing blood eliminates approximately 80–94% of all leukocytes, although there are autotransfusion devices that eliminate only 50% of these. Leukocytes are activated

in the process of cell collecting and washing. Granulocytes, for instance, start their intrinsic functions when they are activated to a certain threshold. When this threshold is reached, changes in adhesion, migration, degranulation, and phagocytosis occur, and the respiratory burst is initiated. This may result in epithelial damage, including to the pulmonary vessels. Respiratory distress syndromes have therefore been attributed to activated leukocytes retransfused with salvaged blood. Further research has shown that other unrelated circumstances most probably trigger the pulmonary problems. Leukocytes, although slightly altered, seem not to be activated to an extent that will cause serious pulmonary problems. The current literature does not support the notion that leukocytes need to be eliminated and the use of a leukocyte-reducing filter for the sole purpose of eliminating leukocytes is not justified [23].

Besides naturally occurring substances in blood, other contaminants are also removed by the washing of blood. This also holds true for the added anticoagulant. Only a minimal heparin activity after correctly washing (0.3–0.5 U/mL) is observed. Also, hirudin derivatives used for anticoagulation during cell salvage have been shown to be reduced to an insignificant level [24]. Thus, correctly washed blood does not contain anticoagulants that would impair clotting.

Marrow fat is often present in wound blood during orthopedic surgery. It has been associated with fat embolism and related pulmonary damage due to toxic fatty acids. Damage to the pulmonary endothelium results in an increased permeability of the pulmonary vasculature. Cell-salvage equipment using a discontinuous washing process reduces the fat content in the blood, but significant amounts of fat still remain in the blood. Some physicians therefore do not return the last 50 mL of processed blood as it contains the floating fat layer. Such blood waste may be tolerable in adults, but not in the pediatric population. In this regard, continuous washing is superior to its counterparts [25].

Advantages of cell salvage

Cell salvage can be used in emergency as well as elective procedures. Several liters of blood can be salvaged intraoperatively—much more than with other methods of autologous donation. Large volumes of blood are available. Since cell salvage may be combined with other techniques of blood management, e.g., hemodilution [26], it considerably reduces the use of allogeneic transfusions. All techniques of cell salvage provide an immediately available, fresh, autologous blood product.

Since blood recovered during cell salvage is fresh and at room temperature, red cells are viable, have a near-normal osmotic membrane stability (in contrast to stored homologous blood), and a potentially normal life span. Their level of 2,3-diphosphoglycerate (2,3-DPG) is near normal [21]. This means that their oxygen-carrying capacity is no different from that of the patient's circulating blood [27]. In contrast, red cells available through donations and after cold storage are nearly devoid of 2,3-DPG and have (at least temporarily) lost their ability to release oxygen to the tissue. Cerebral and cardiac functions—dependent on available oxygen extraction—are not impaired by fresh autologous cells but are by transfused cells [27].

An important point is the outcome of patients undergoing cell salvage when compared with allogeneic transfusions. Unfortunately, there is not much data available to draw solid conclusions. However, some randomized controlled trials have demonstrated significantly lower infection rates after surgery with cell salvage when compared to using donated red cells [28]. The reason for this finding may be the absence of immunosuppression with allogeneic blood. Besides, immunosuppression associated with surgery and blood loss (reflected in a reduced frequency of natural killer cell precursors and decreased interferon gamma) can be reversed by transfusion of autologous salvaged blood, suggesting that the latter may contain immunostimulants [29]. In fact, it has been shown that the activity of neutrophils and the amount of natural killer cell precursors are enhanced [29, 30].

Some advantages of cell salvage are related to the method used. Cell salvage providing unwashed blood is a simple technique: the device is simple to use, inexpensive, easy to handle, and rapidly available in emergency situations. This makes unwashed cell salvage especially applicable where healthcare resources are limited or in mass disaster. Especially when large amounts of blood are collected in a relatively short time, e.g., during the time a surgical leak is detected until the patient is taken back to the operating room for revision, direct cell salvage is beneficial. When large amounts of blood are collectable from body cavities, e.g., from a drained hemothorax, direct retransfusion is also beneficial.

The primary advantage of cell salvage with a washing step is that activated clotting factors, free hemoglobin, and debris are removed. Computerized cell salvage markedly reduces the risk of embolism through a series of control steps, checks, valves, and sensors.

Practical considerations for cell salvage with a washing step

Before a cell salvage procedure is initiated, some basic considerations are warranted. First, the right technique and the right equipment need to be chosen. Since techniques provide different blood products with different properties, the right choice can make a difference. Factors like the procedure, comorbidities of the patient, the surgeon and the expected blood loss, cost issues, and the need for postoperative cell salvage need to be considered to make the right choice. Pediatric patients, with limited blood volume, require more thought in the choice of a cell-saving device than other patient populations. Continuous cell salvage offers distinct advantages for this population. Such devices deliver a higher hematocrit after processing. Smaller blood volumes can be processed. As mentioned above, use of the classic Latham bowl may need a refill with already washed blood. This may be difficult in small children since their small blood volume means the blood may already have been given back to the patient [31]. Therefore, continuous cell salvage is the recommended procedure in pediatric patients.

Thought should be given to the set-up of the autotransfusion device. If major blood loss is anticipated, the device should be set up prior to surgery. Patients with specific cell salvage needs will require the cell salvage to be set up accordingly, e.g., when it is necessary to prepare the equipment to ascertain that blood recovered from the surgical field is in constant contact with the circulation of the patient. To this end, the blood bag is spiked with a saline-filled infusion system and the system is connected to the patient's circulation. When the patient does not insist on constant contact of the blood with the circulation and it is questionable whether much blood can be collected, some have chosen to set up the equipment only partially (so-called "stand-by cell salvage"). Only the suction and collection reservoir are set up. If enough blood is collected, the remaining parts of the cell-salvage disposables are assembled and the blood is processed. When not much blood is collected, some disposables (e.g., the centrifuge) are not used. Another way to reduce costs with cell salvage is a modified approach. Smaller equipment is used for procedures with slow blood loss.

For an extensive procedure, physicians often use two suction tubes: one for blood leading to the collection reservoir, and the other for contaminents, e.g., irrigants, glues, and bone cement. To avoid undue blood damage, the suction tip should not suck at the blood–air interface and the suction has to be adjusted to the lowest functioning pressure.

The success of cell salvage depends on the amount of blood that can be collected and recovered for retransfusion. Typically, blood is recovered from the surgical site. Expeditious and thorough suction is needed to recover as much blood as possible. If necessary, the surgeon as well as the assistant can use a suction tip. To this end, the cell-salvage machine can be equipped with two instead of one reservoirs, with attached suction.

Practice tip Spillage from a side wound

When a wound situated on the side of a patient results in blood spillage onto the floor, sterile plastic bags can be taped immediately below the wound. Blood collects in these and can be sucked out by the suction tip of the cell-salvage equipment placed in the plastic bag.

Not all blood is collected by suction. Considerable amounts (about one-third of the total red cell recovery in one study [32]) of blood are taken up by sponges. Sponges and surgical towels soaked with blood can be rinsed in a sterile bowl containing sterile saline. After washing and wringing out of the towels, the blood is sucked into the resevior, processed, and reclaimed [27, 33].

If blood has collected in a body cavity and may be under pressure during surgical incision, it may flow out too rapidly to be collected entirely by suctioning. In such instances, a preincision drainage with a needle or similar equipment may be indicated to collect the blood. Alternatively, if a small incision only is made, the peritoneum can be "tented" to avoid spillage [10]. Afterward, the body cavity is opened in the intended manner, the remaining blood collected, and surgery continued.

Laparoscopically-guided blood salvage is also possible. It is an option when the findings in the abdomen are unclear and chances are that the bleeding problem has either already resolved itself (e.g., in a small splenic tear) or it can be solved laparoscopically [33]. Laparoscopy often provides a very good view of the bleeding source, and the hemoperitoneum can be removed. Repeated examinations are easy. When compared with methods to achieve a non-surgical management of a splenic tear, where patients wait under "transfusion protection" for the spontaneous cessation of hemorrhage, an initial laparoscopic approach may reduce the use of allogeneic blood.

Collected blood must be properly labeled. The container has to have an indication that the blood is autologous. A patient's name, date of birth, and all other identifying information, as well as the date and time of the start of blood procurement, have to be noted on the blood bags or bottles.

Autologous blood should be returned within the alloted time since it is not stored in a cold environment and not under any safety precautions prescribed for blood storage. It is recommended that the processed blood be returned within 6 hours after collection. This ensures the viability of blood cells and reduces bacterial contamination.

During the entire process of cell salvage and retransfusion, the patient must be monitored. If blood is returned postoperatively, monitoring must continue until all the blood has been returned. Monitoring includes the patient's vital signs, condition of the blood intended for return (clots?), and amount of blood coming from drains. Excessive bleeding from the drain in the presence of normal coagulation parameters is indicative of a surgical problem, not of an aquired coagulopathy [34]. Changes induced by cell salvage need to be taken into consideration when it comes to postoperative monitoring. In unwashed blood, confusion may occur in the interpretation of results of the coagulation profiles.

Anticoagulation and filters

Anticoagulant

Blood draining slowly from a wound is usually defibrinated and unable to clot. Thus, the addition of an anticoagulant is usually not necessary. Only if bleeding is brisk and the contact time of the blood with the wound is not sufficient to defibrinze all the blood will clotting not occur; otherwise an anticoagulant may be added to prevent coagulation.

Intraoperative cell salvage with or without washing requires anticoagulation as well. Either the patient is anticoagulated (as in Method 2 above) or the collected blood is anticoagulated. Typically, heparin is used as anticoagulant when a cell-salvage device calls for systemic anticoagulation. Heparin is also added to the collection reservoir. About 10 000–100 000 IU are added to 1 L of saline (typically 30 000 IU/L) and the mixture is added as blood is collected in a ratio of about 1:1.

Another anticoagulant for cell salvage is citrate in the form of citrate–phosphate–dextrose (CPD) or citrate–phosphate–dextrose–adenine (CPD-A). One part of citrate is mixed with 7–8 parts of blood. Citrate chelates calcium and thus prevents clotting. The dextrose in the citrate provides the substrate for glycolysis and preserves the metabolism in red cells. The chelating effect of citrate also protects platelets. Citrate is metabolized in the liver and should therefore be avoided in patients with significant liver damage. When calcium-containing solutions are used in the field, e.g., Ringer's solution for irrigation, CPD is also not ideal. In such patients, heparin is the anticoagulant of choice.

If a patient has a history of heparin-induced thrombocytopenia or there are other reasons not to give heparin, citrate, danaparoid or hirudin derivatives [24] are viable alternatives.

Filters

Blood filtration is recommended before the harvested blood is returned. The filter will eliminate gross debris. Typically, a standard blood filter of 170 μm is used. Since the centrifugation of blood may concentrate particular debris, a microaggregation filter (40–60-μm blood filter) is recommended. In some countries, leukocyte depletion filters are used for the return of cell-salvage blood as well, e.g., in oncology surgery or Cesarean section.

Risks and side effects of cell salvage

The risks and side effects of cell salvage are dependent on the type of procedure, the way blood is processed, and the amount of blood returned. Three groups of problems can be encountered with cell salvage: equipment malfunction, operator error, and blood-related sequelae (contamination, quality of blood). Equipment and related problems as well as operator error have been greatly reduced by microprocessor technology. Design refinements and the increased experience and credentialing of the operators make cell salvage a safe procedure.

Air embolism was reported with some cell-salvage devices. This has been attributed to infusion pumps attached directly to a reservoir and pressure applied to a retransfusion bag that contains air. To avoid this, modern cell-salvage devices do not transfuse directly from the centrifuge and have a system of air detection, which stops the system if air is detected.

If citrate is used to anticoagulate blood, hypocalcemia may occur if a large amount of citrate is returned to the patient. Checking the calcium level and administration of calcium if necessary prevent this problem.

Andecdotal case reports describe a "salvaged blood syndrome" with multiple organ failure and consumption coagulopathy following autotransfusion [28]. Although it

is known that cell salvage may cause a slight coagulopathy, especially after major blood loss and reinfusion, there is no evidence that autotransfusion itself can cause this syndrome. A large review of over 36 000 cases did not provide evidence that the "salvaged blood syndrome" is the result of autotransfusion. The incidence of coagulopathy was low (0.05%) and respiratory failure in combination with disseminated intravascular coagulation occurred in only 18 cases, all associated with major complex surgery. All patients had profound shock and received multiple transfusions. It is therefore most likely that associated problems, not the autotransfusion itself, triggered the coagulopathy [35].

There are unique risks and side effects with unwashed and washed blood.

Unwashed blood

Febrile reactions have been reported after retransfusion of collected wound blood. They are dependent on the duration of blood collection. After 6 hours of collection, febrile reactions accounted for only 2% of the total experience. If the collection period extended beyond 6 hours, more than 22% of the patients experienced febrile reactions [20]. Immunological reactions, e.g., due to cytokines in the retransfused blood, and bacterial contamination are thought to be the reason for those reactions. The great majority of febrile reactions are mild and self-limiting.

There have been a few case reports of renal dysfunction after retransfusion of unwashed blood. This event is infrequent and occurs in the presence of other risk factors. Some authors claim that free hemoglobin is the reason for the renal damage, since hemoglobin is nephrotoxic and has the ability to scavenge nitric oxide, causing microcirculatory disturbances. However, opponents of this theory claim that, once given, free hemoglobin is rapidly excreted by the kidneys. They add that normal amounts of free hemoglobin, as found in unwashed blood, are safe and excreted within 24 hours. In addition, restricting the infusion of unwashed blood to 15 mL/kg or 1 L in the adult seems to be without clinical consequences, since enough circulating haptoglobin is present to collect the free hemoglobin [21]. The impact of free hemoglobin in the blood is still controversial, although most authors agree that at least 1–2 L of unwashed blood are usually well tolerated. If renal damage does occur, markers of renal function should be assessed, autotransfusion stopped, and intravenous hydration increased.

Unwashed blood theoretically may introduce foreign materials into the circulation. Especially in orthopedic patients, bone fragments, fat, metal fragments from drills and saws, bone cement, and medications may be reinfused. Although mostly a theoretical concern, washing of blood is preferred in such procedures.

If by-products of coagulation activation are retransfused, the patient may experience a mild, subclinical coagulopathy that returns to normal within 24 hours. Activation of fibrinolysis seems to be one of the reasons for this phenomenon [36]. Although unwashed blood is given back safely in the majority of cases, there are some case reports concerning severe coagulopathies associated with increased postoperative blood loss.

The risk–benefit ratio of unwashed cell salvage may not be favorable in some situations. There may be situations when a patient loses a large volume of blood in a relatively short time after surgery. Retransfusion in this setting may be effective but may not be in the best interests of the patient, and examination of other possibilities is warranted. Is the patient coagulopathic or, more likely, does the patient need to return to the operating room? When postoperative blood loss is smaller in volume, only small amounts of wound fluid with a low hematocrit will be collected. If this is given back, the benefit to the patient regarding improvement of hemoglobin level may be small and the amount of debris given back may be relatively high. Such scenarios must be considered case by case to determine whether there is sufficient benefit to collecting unwashed blood.

Washed blood

The process of washing blood has an impact on red cell integrity and on the patient who receives the autologous blood. Normal saline is used to wash blood in the majority of cases. This has an effect on the product of cell salvage. Patients receiving the processed blood may develop a hyperchloremic metabolic acidosis, and calcium, magnesium, and proteins may decrease. This is because only sodium and chloride are present in the washing solution. Alternative washing solutions are under investigation [37]. They may prevent the drop in the pH and the electrolyte disturbances. This may be advantageous especially in surgery with major blood turnover.

Another concern with washed blood is the depletion of clotting factors and platelets. The resulting dilutional coagulopathy is infrequently observed in routine use of washed cell salvage [7].

While it is often claimed that the washing process eliminates all relevant contaminants, variations in this elimination process have been described. Free hemo-

Table 16.1 Examples of quality assurance parameters for cell-salvaged blood.

Quality marker	Cell salvage with washing step
Red cell recovery	>80%
Elimination of free hemoglobin	>90%; or <200 mg/dL
Hematocrit in autologous blood ready for retransfusion	>50%

globin may be present in much higher levels than assumed and may lead to renal dysfunction [38] (see above). It is therefore prudent to initiate routine quality assurance processes for cell salvage to insure the blood quality is as expected (Table 16.1).

Concerns and contraindications

There are concerns about the use of retrieved autologous blood in certain situations. These are when blood may be contaminated by bacteria, tumor cells, or amniotic fluid. The presence of hemoglobinopathies have been considered a relative contraindication for cell salvage. However, with some adjustments, cell salvage can be used in such situations as well.

Spread of bacterial contamination

Retransfusion of washed [39] and even unwashed blood with enteric contamination has been described [40]. Several outcome studies in trauma, colorectal, and gynecological surgery demonstrate the safety of cell washing and retransfusion where the blood is known to be contaminated with bacteria. Despite the low risk, physicians are still hesitant to use cell salvage when they consider the blood could be contaminated with bacteria.

On closer examination of this issue, one finds that a significant minority of blood used for retransfusion after (washed) cell salvage is tainted with bacteria (21–48% [41, 42]). Blood salvaged from "clean" surgical fields has been shown on occasion to grow bacteria when cultured. Regardless, upon retransfusion of this contaminated blood there seems to be no increased incidence of infection, sepsis, or other adverse effects for the patient. The bacteremia resulting from the infusion of such contaminated blood usually resolves spontaneously 24 hours after surgery. If infection occurs after surgery with autotransfusion, it is usually not related to cell salvage. The risk of complications due to infection seems to depend on other complicating factors (such as multiple injury) and not primarily on the soiling of blood. Usually, the type of bacteria cultured in the salvaged blood does not correlate with the species cultured from the site of postoperative infection [42].

Although currently a contraindication to use, bacterial contamination of blood collected for washed cell salvage carries only a theoretical risk to the patient. Published data do not support the notion of avoidance of cell salvage on the grounds of bacterial contamination.

There are some measures that can be taken to reduce either the amount of bacterial contamination in the salvaged blood or bacteria that might have been collected. When a grossly contaminated area is encountered in the surgical field, e.g., the contents of an abscess, a second suction device should be used to drain the maximally bacteria-loaded material into a separate discard container. All other blood can be collected for cell salvage. Cell washing significantly reduces, but does not completely eliminate, bacterial contamination. Leukocyte depletion filters may add to the safety of the blood collected from patients with gross bacterial contamination since they reduce the amount of bacteria infused [43]. Parenteral broad-spectrum antibiotics are recommended for patients who receive cell-salvaged blood. Timing of retransfusion is important to avoid additional bacterial growth in the collected blood. It is recommended to retransfuse blood within 6 hours after collection.

When comparing cell salvage with allogeneic transfusion, one easily comes to the conclusion that there is a proven risk of bacterial infection with allogeneic transfusion, while there is only a theoretical risk of bacterial infection with salvaged autologous blood. It may be reasonable, therefore, to favor autologous cell salvage blood over allogeneic blood, although no definitve data are available to date. Taking the above into account, one may want to join the author who wrote: "Even if sepsis is to occur, I have always maintained that it is better to have a live patient with a bacteremia than a dead patient with a sterile blood culture" [42].

Tumor cells

Extensive oncological surgery often leads to massive blood loss. Nevertheless, allogeneic transfusions should be avoided in cancer patients since they may adversely affect outcome by increasing the number of cancer relapses, reducing the time to cancer recurrence, and shortening survival time. Autotransfusion, as an alternative approach, can reduce the exposure of patients to donor blood. The question is whether autologous blood collected during oncological surgery can be retransfused safely.

Occult cancer cells are often found in the blood circulation of cancer patients prior to surgery. During surgery, pressure or manipulation of the tumor will release many more cells into the circulation. It was shown that even salvaged blood contains viable, tumorigenic cells. Due to the theoretical concern of tumor dissemination by retransfusion of cancer cells, some practitioners still refuse to use cell salvage in oncological surgery. However, this seems not to be justified as there is no convincing proof in the literature that it is detrimental for the patient. An increasing number of studies comparing recurrence and survival rates of cancer patients treated with or without cell-salvaged blood have not demonstrated any detrimental effect of autotransfusion in the oncological setting. On the contrary, there seems to be a tendency towards better outcome when compared with allogeneic transfusions [44].

To address even these theoretical concerns, methods have been tested to reduce the amount of tumor cells in the blood returned to the patient. The process of washing the blood during cell salvage eliminates or destroys a considerable amount of tumor cells. Additional reduction of the tumor cell load in the blood is achievable by the use of leukocyte depletion filters. These two methods combined greatly reduce, but do not completely eliminate, all tumor cells. However, some sources claim that the remaining tumor cells are not of any significance [45]. Some authors prefer to add cytostatics to the cell-salvage fluid to kill the tumor cells. However, since the patient is then also exposed to the cytostatics, this method has not been widely used. Although not always practical, irradiation of salvaged blood with 50 Gray can be used effectively [46]. As irradiation takes only 6–15 minutes, the blood should still be available for retransfusion within a reasonable time. The technique of blood irradiation obviously is costly and taps valuable resources. Special blood bags are needed to prevent undue hemolysis, and irradiation facilities need to be available as well as trained persons for the transfer of the blood to and from the operating room. Nevertheless, to date it seems to be the only method to completely inactivate tumor cells.

Since the postulated detrimental effects of cell salvage in oncological surgery appear not to have been substantuated [47], cell salvage currently appears to be a valuable adjunct to the treatment of life-threatening bleeding during oncological surgery. This can be understood when one follows Thomas' line of reasoning, found in a review entitled "Infected and malignant fields are an absolute contraindication to intraoperative cell salvage: fact or fiction?" It poses a series of questions to help weigh the risks and benefits of cell salvage in oncological surgery. Ask yourself: "In what percentage of cases will cells have already been disseminated? Will dormant cells be awakened simply by surgery (*or by allogeneic transfusion* [italics are ours])? What effect does the skill of the surgeon contribute? Is intravascular spread far less important than local deposits? Will reinfusing additional malignant cells negate the reduction in immunomodulation, achieved by the use of autologous blood?" [42]. After considering available facts, Thomas concluded: "However, on balance, it would appear that the use of filters, whether alone or in combination with irradiation, could produce a product that is as safe, if not safer, than allogeneic blood" [42]. In harmony with this conclusion, the latest blood conservation guidelines of The Society of Thoracic Surgeons and The Society of Cardiovascular Anesthesiologists now recommend cell salvage also for cancer patients [44].

Amniotic fluid embolism and fetal blood cells

Amniotic fluid is essentially an electrolyte solution. Toward the end of pregnancy, the fluid contains additional products, such as tissue factor, squamous cells, trophoblasts, and phospholipids (in the form of lamellar bodies resulting from fetal lung maturation), and fetal hemoglobin. Amniotic fluid can cause an amniotic embolism, which is a rare but potentially fatal complication of pregnancy. Amniotic embolus is associated with pulmonary hypertension, hypoxia, heart failure, and acute respiratory distress syndrome, as well as disseminated intravascular coagulation and uterine atonia with massive hemorrhage. The pathophysiology of amniotic fluid embolism is poorly understood. Initially, emboli of fetal debris (e.g., squamous cells, vernix, mucin) were thought to be the reason for the amniotic fluid embolism and tissue factor has been implicated as a reason for a disseminated intravascular coagulation. However, fetal squamous cells are also commonly found in the circulation of patients in labor who do not develop the syndrome. Also, during a Cesarean section, some amniotic fluid routinely enters the circulation of the mother without causing any unwanted effects. Findings suggest that amniotic fluid embolism is more akin to anaphylaxis.

The term "anaphylactoid syndrome of pregnancy" has been suggested instead.

Amniotic fluid embolism usually occurs during labor, but sometimes during abortion, abdominal trauma, and amnioinfusion. Also, in regards to cell salvage, there is a concern that amniotic embolism could be caused by the spread of amniotic contents into the circulation of the parturient. It is true that blood sucked into the cell-salvage reservoir contains many of the particles thought to be responsible for amniotic embolism. To date, there is no evidence that blood collected during Cesarean section causes amniotic embolism [48].

Washing blood reduces many of the constituents of amniotic fluid, including tissue factor. A further reduction of potentially offensive constituents is achievable with certain leukocyte-depletion filters. After cell washing and filtration, the amount of amniotic fluid constituents, such as lamellar bodies, trophoblasts, and squamous cells, are at least as low as in the mother's blood, if not lower.

Among constituents of amniotic fluid, only fetal hemoglobin increases in the mother's blood after returning the blood. Fetal hemoglobin naturally enters the mother's circulation during birth. This is without consequences unless there is an incompatibility of the blood groups, leading to complications in subsequent pregnancies. To avoid risks due to rhesus-incompatible blood, rhesus immunization of the mother is recommended. The dose of rhesus immunoglobulin should be calculated after the cell-salvaged blood is returned, since the infused fetal hemoglobin can increase the required dose of immunoglobulin.

Cell salvage and concomitant diseases

Cell salvage can be performed in patients with almost all comorbidities. While solid tumors cause some physicians to think twice before the blood is returned, malignancy of the hematopoietic system, such as leukemia and plasmacytoma, do not constitute a contraindication for cell salvage and special considerations are not needed.

Patients with hereditary anemia, e.g., spherocytosis and thalassemia [49], are also deemed safe for autologous transfusion. Sickle cell disease does not constitute a contraindication for cell salvage. Sickle cells typically develop when hemoglobin is deoxygenated and in an acidotic environment. However, in cell salvage, blood is in contact with air and is therefore oxygenated. Besides, carbon dioxide dissolves in the salvaged blood and causes a "metabolic alkalosis." Thus, in theory, sickling of red cells in the cell-salvage process is unlikely and it has been concluded that sickle cell anemia is therefore not a contraindication to cell salvage [50]. In contrast, the washing process of the autotransfusion device has been described to cause severe sickling in a blood smear obtained from the processed blood of sickle cell patients, and the author concluded that sickle cell disease may be a contraindication to cell washing [51].

Cell salvage is actually the method of choice when it comes to blood conservation of patients with certain hematological disorders. Predepositing of blood from patients with sickle cell anemia and spherocytosis is not recommended since the storage conditions (low pH, etc.) may lead to irreversible sickling in sickle cell disease and a dramatically shortened lifespan of spherocytes [50].

Indications for cell salvage

Autologous transfusions including cell salvage have been shown to reduce the use of allogeneic red cell transfusions [52, 53]. This is true for postoperative cell salvage [54] as well as for intraoperative cell salvage [55]. To make cell salvage effective, patients must be carefully selected. It has proven difficult to formulate universal criteria for patients most likely to benefit from cell salvage. In an emergency, a means of autotransfusion should be readily available whenever significant blood loss is anticipated or possible. Current guidelines suggest the following criteria for cell salvage: adults who undergo surgery with an anticipated blood loss of more than 1000 mL or more than 20% of the patient's blood; patients undergoing procedures where more than 10% are transfused allogeneically in the perioperative period; or where the mean number of transfused units is more than 1 unit. However, from the perspectives of the good quality of fresh autologous blood and cost, autotransfusion may be indicated much earlier. Interestingly, it has been calculated that setting up a modern autotransfusion device in the standby mode (using only suction and reservoir with anticoagulant) costs about the same as it does to type and cross-match 2 units of red cell concentrates [56].

Reports on successful cell salvage abound. A method of cell salvage has been used in the following procedures:
- Major vascular surgery, e.g., aortic aneurysm repair
- Thoracic and cardiac surgery or cardiac catheter interventions, e.g., coronary artery bypass surgery, valve replacement, cardiac tamponade [53, 57]
- Neurosurgery [55], e.g., for spinal fusion, basilar aneurysms, tumors

- Orthopedic surgery [26, 58], e.g., for hip and knee arthroplasty, especially bilateral or reoperations, scoliosis surgery
- Transplantation, e.g., liver transplantation
- General surgery, e.g., for exploratory laparotomy with free fluids intraperitoneally, liver surgery
- Gynecological and obstetric procedures, e.g., hysterectomy [59] and myomectomy, Cesarean section, especially in complicated placentation, ruptured ectopic pregnancy [60]
- Trauma management [18], e.g., hemothorax [61], abdominal trauma, spine surgery
- Plastic surgery [62, 63], e.g., in burn excision
- Ear–nose–throat surgery: major maxillofacial surgery
- Pediatric procedures [62, 64], e.g., craniosynostosis correction, acetabuloplasty
- Urological procedures, e. g. in prostatectomy, cystectomy.

Key points

- Cell salvage can be performed intra- or post-operatively. Blood can either be directly given back or after a washing process. The quality of blood for direct return differs greatly from the quality of washed blood. Both types of cell salvage have advantages and disadvantages.
- When life is at stake, there is no contraindication to proficient cell salvage. Relative contraindications have been cited but can be overcome by the following methods:
  ◦ **Bacterial contamination:** Cell washing, leukocyte depletion filtration, systemic broad-spectrum antibiotics
  ◦ **Contamination with tumor cells:** Cell washing, possibly no further processing required; but if desired: leukocyte depletion filtration, adding cytostatics to the blood, irradiation
  ◦ **Amniotic fluid contamination:** Cell washing and leukocyte depletion filtration.
- Cell salvage has many advantages, namely:
  ◦ Provision of the patient's own blood. This means a low risk of disease transmission, clerical error, and immunological complications
  ◦ Reducing or eliminating the use of allogeneic blood products
  ◦ Providing a blood product that contains viable, fresh red cells with a near-normal lifespan and ability to release oxygen to the tissue
  ◦ Possibly reducing costs

○ Improving outcomes of patients.
○ Making available compatible blood in elective as well as emergency surgery.

Questions for review

1. What methods are available to perform cell salvage?
2. Where does the blood that is salvaged come from?
3. What is the difference between cell salvage with washed and unwashed blood? How do these affect the quality of the blood?
4. What are the contraindications to cell salvage? Can they be overcome and if so, how?
5. Which diseases need special consideration when it comes to cell salvage?
6. Describe the different modes of anticoagulation of the salvaged blood.

Suggestions for further research

Find out if blood can be washed in your hospital and if so, whether major amounts of coagulation factors are available after this procedure.

Exercises and practice cases

> After collecting 1.5 L of blood with a hematocrit of 35%, you dilute it with 1.5 L of anticoagulant-containing solution. The cell-salvage device concentrates red cells to a hematocrit of 70% and recovers 80% of the delivered red cells.

How much blood would you get back from a typical autotransfusion device that washes the above blood?

Homework

Ask a sales representative to demonstrate a cell-salvage equipment. If possible, contact a representative for a system that uses unwashed blood and one for a system for washed blood. Record the contact details and other pertinent information.

Find out where to obtain a leukocyte-depletion filter to be used in connection with the equipment.

Check whether there are any guidelines in your hospital that guide any kind of blood salvage. If there are, obtain a copy.

References

1. Blundell J. Experiments on the transfusion of blood by the syringe. *Med Chir Trans* 1818;**9**:56ff.
2. Highmore W. Practical remarks on an overlooked source of blood-supply for transfusion in post-partum haemorrhage suggested by a recent fatal case. *Lancet* 1874:89.
3. Duncan J. On re-infusion of blood in primary and other amputations. *BMJ* 1886:192–193.
4. Thies J. Zur Behandlung der Extrauteringravidität. *Zentralblatt für Gynäkologie* 1914;**38**:1191–1193.
5. Griswold RA, Ortner AB. Use of autotransfusion in surgery of serous cavities. *Surg Gynecol Obstet* 1943;**77**:167–177.
6. Klebanoff G. Early clinical experience with a disposable unit for the intraoperative salvage and reinfusion of blood loss (intraoperative autotransfusion). *Am J Surg* 1970;**120**:718–722.
7. Laub GW, Riebman JB. Autotransfusion: methods and complications. In: Lake CL, Moore RA (eds). *Blood: Hemostasis, Transfusion, and Alternatives in the Perioperative Period*. Lippincott Williams & Wilkins, 1995, pp. 381–394.
8. Catling SJ, Williams S, Fielding AM. Cell salvage in obstetrics: an evaluation of the ability of cell salvage combined with leucocyte depletion filtration to remove amniotic fluid from operative blood loss at caesarean section. *Int J Obstet Anesth* 1999;**8**:79–84.
9. Poeschl U. Emergency autologous blood transfusion in ruptured ectopic pregnancy. *Anesthesia* 1992;**2**:Article 2.
10. Priuli G, Darate R, Perrin RX, Lankoande J, Drouet N. Multicentre experience with a simple blood salvage technique in patients with ruptured ectopic pregnancy in sub-Sahelian West Africa. *Vox Sang* 2009;**97**:317–323.
11. Heimbecker RO. History of bloodless surgery in Canada: blood recycling in the operating room. The 73rd Annual Ontario Hospital Association Convention, 1987.
12. Ovadje OO. An emergency auto-transfusion device designed for developing countries. *Intensive Care World* 1991;**8**:88–89.
13. Reeder GD. Autotransfusion theory of operation: a review of the physics and hematology. *Transfusion* 2004;**44** (12 Suppl):35S–39S.
14. Radvan J, Singbartl G, Heschel I, Rau G. [Physical principles of autotransfusion systems]. *Anasthesiol Intensivmed Notfallmed Schmerzther* 2002;**37**:689–696.
15. Eichert I, Isgro F, Kiessling AH, Saggau W. Cell saver, ultrafiltration and direct transfusion: comparative study of three blood processing techniques. *Thorac Cardiovasc Surg* 2001;**49**:149–152.
16. Shuhaiber JH, Whitehead SM. The impact of introducing an autologous intraoperative transfusion device to a community hospital. *Ann Vasc Surg* 2003;**17**:424–429.
17. Munoz M, García-Segovia S, Ariza D, Cobos A, García-Erce JA, Thomas D. Sedimentation method for preparation of postoperatively salvaged unwashed shed blood in orthopaedic surgery. *Br J Anaesth* 2010;**105**:457–465.

18. Heimbecker RO. Blood recycling eliminates need for blood. *CMAJ* 1996;**155**:275–276.

19. de Haan J, Schönberger J, Haan J, van Oeveren W, Eijgelaar A. Tissue-type plasminogen activator and fibrin monomers synergistically cause platelet dysfunction during retransfusion of shed blood after cardiopulmonary bypass. *J Thorac Cardiovasc Surg* 1993;**106**:1017–1023.

20. Waters JH, Biscotti C, Potter PS, Phillipson E. Amniotic fluid removal during cell salvage in the cesarean section patient. *Anesthesiology* 2000;**92**:1531–1536.

21. Munoz M, García-Vallejo JJ, Ruiz MD, Romero R, Olalla E, Sebastián C. Transfusion of post-operative shed blood: laboratory characteristics and clinical utility. *Eur Spine J* 2004;**13** (Suppl 1):S107–113.

22. Geiger P, Platow K, Bartl A, Völk C, Junker K, Mehrkens HH. New developments in autologous transfusion systems. *Anaesthesia* 1998;**53** (Suppl 2):32–35.

23. Innerhofer P, Wiedermann FJ. [Leucocyte activation through intra operative blood salvage]. *Anasthesiol Intensivmed Notfallmed Schmerzther* 2002;**37**:738–740.

24. Marx A, Marx A [Removal of lepirudin used as an anticoagulant in mechanical autotransfusion with Cell-Saver 5]. *Anasthesiol Intensivmed Notfallmed Schmerzther* 2001;**36**: 162–166.

25. Booke M, Fobker M, Fingerhut D, Storm M, Mortlemans Y, Van Aken H. Fat elimination during intraoperative autotransfusion: an in vitro investigation. *Anesth Analg* 1997;**85**:959–962.

26. Borghi B, Pignotti E, Montebugnoli M, *et al.* Autotransfusion in major orthopaedic surgery: experience with 1785 patients. *Br J Anaesth* 1997;**79**:662–664.

27. Ronai AK, Glass JJ, Shapiro A. Improving autologous blood harvest: recovery of red cells from sponges and suction. *Anaesth Intensive Care* 1987;**15**:421–424.

28. Vanderlinde ES, Heal JM, Blumberg N. Autologous transfusion. *BMJ* 2002;**324**:772–775.

29. Gharehbaghian A, Haque KM, Truman C, *et al.* Effect of autologous salvaged blood on postoperative natural killer cell precursor frequency. *Lancet* 2004;**363**:1025–1030.

30. Iorwerth A, Wilson C, Topley N, Pallister I. Neutrophil activity in total knee replacement: implications in preventing post-arthroplasty infection. *Knee* 2003;**10**:111–113.

31. Booke M, Hagemann O, Van Aken H, Erren M, Wüllenweber J, Bone HG. Intraoperative autotransfusion in small children: an in vitro investigation to study its feasibility. *Anesth Analg* 1999;**88**:763–765.

32. Haynes SL, Bennett JR, Torella F, McCollum CN. Does washing swabs increase the efficiency of red cell recovery by cell salvage in aortic surgery? *Vox Sang* 2005;**88**: 244–248.

33. Smith RS, Meister RK, Tsoi EK, Bohman HR. Laparoscopically guided blood salvage and autotransfusion in splenic trauma: a case report. *J Trauma* 1993;**34**:313–314.

34. Halfman-Franey M, Berg DE. Recognition and management of bleeding following cardiac surgery. *Crit Care Nurs Clin North Am* 1991;**3**:675–689.

35. Tawes RL Jr, Duvall TB. Is the "salvaged-cell syndrome" myth or reality? *Am J Surg* 1996;**172**:172–174.

36. Matsuda K, Nozawa M, Katsube S, Maezawa K, Kurosawa H. Activation of fibrinolysis by reinfusion of unwashed salvaged blood after total knee arthroplasty. *Transfus Apher Sci* 2010;**42**:33–37.

37. Sumpelmann R, Schürholz T, Marx G, Ahrenshop O, Zander R. [Massive transfusion of washed red blood cells: acid-base and electrolyth changes for different wash solutions]. *Anasthesiol Intensivmed Notfallmed Schmerzther* 2003;**38**: 587–593.

38. Gueye PM, Bertrand F, Duportail G, Lessinger JM. Extracellular haemoglobin, oxidative stress and quality of red blood cells relative to perioperative blood salvage. *Clin Chem Lab Med* 2010;**48**:677–683.

39. Brown CV, Foulkrod KH, Sadler HT, *et al.* Autologous blood transfusion during emergency trauma operations. *Arch Surg* 2010;**145**:690–694.

40. Yamada T, Ikeda A, Okamoto Y, Okamoto Y, Kanda T, Ueki M. Intraoperative blood salvage in abdominal simple total hysterectomy for uterine myoma. *Int J Gynaecol Obstet* 1997;**59**:233–236.

41. Kudo H, Fujita H, Hanada Y, Hayami H, Kondoh T, Kohmura E. Cytological and bacteriological studies of intraoperative autologous blood in neurosurgery. *Surg Neurol* 2004;**62**:195–199; discussion 199–200.

42. Thomas MJ. Infected and malignant fields are an absolute contraindication to intraoperative cell salvage: fact or fiction? *Transfus Med* 1999;**9**:269–278.

43. Waters JH, Tuohy MJ, Hobson DF, Procop G. Bacterial reduction by cell salvage washing and leukocyte depletion filtration. *Anesthesiology* 2003;**99**:652–655.

44. Society of Thoracic Surgeons Blood Conservation Guideline Task Force, Ferraris VA, Brown JR, Despotis GJ, *et al.* 2011 update to the Society of Thoracic Surgeons and the Society of Cardiovascular Anesthesiologists blood conservation clinical practice guidelines. *Ann Thorac Surg* 2011;**91**: 944–982.

45. Konsgaard UE, *et al.* The efficacy of cell saver and leucocyte depletion filter for tumour cell removal. *Anesth Analg* 1996;**82**:S244.

46. Hansen E, Bechmann V, Altmeppen J. Blood salvage in cancer surgery? *Anasthesiol Intensivmed Notfallmed Schmerzther* 2001;**36** (Suppl 2):S128–129.

47. Waters JH, Donnenberg AD. Blood salvage and cancer surgery: should we do it? *Transfusion* 2009;**49**:2016–2018.

48. Liumbruno GM, Liumbruno C, Rafanelli D. Intraoperative cell salvage in obstetrics: is it a real therapeutic option? *Transfusion* 2011;**51**:2244–2256.

49. Waters JH, Lukauskiene E, Anderson ME. Intraoperative blood salvage during cesarean delivery in a patient with beta thalassemia intermedia. *Anesth Analg* 2003;**97**: 1808–1809.

50. Dietrich GV. [Autotransfusion in special procedure and diseases]. *Anasthesiol Intensivmed Notfallmed Schmerzther* 2002;**37**:744–747.

51. Brajtbord D, Johnson D, Ramsay M, *et al*. Use of the cell saver in patients with sickle cell trait. *Anesthesiology* 1989;**70**: 878–879.

52. Carless PA, *et al*. Cell salvage for minimising perioperative allogeneic blood transfusion. *Cochrane Database Syst Rev* 2010;(4):CD001888.

53. Wang G, Bainbridge D, Martin J, Cheng D. The efficacy of an intraoperative cell saver during cardiac surgery: a meta-analysis of randomized trials. *Anesth Analg* 2009;**109**: 320–330.

54. Atay EF, Güven M, Altıntaş F, Kadıoğlu B, Ceviz E, Ipek S. Allogeneic blood transfusion decreases with postoperative autotransfusion in hip and knee arthroplasty. *Acta Orthop Traumatol Turc* 2010;**44**:306–312.

55. Bowen RE, Gardner S, Scaduto AA, Eagan M, Beckstead J. Efficacy of intraoperative cell salvage systems in pediatric idiopathic scoliosis patients undergoing posterior spinal fusion with segmental spinal instrumentation. *Spine (Phila Pa 1976)* 2010;**35**:246–251.

56. Waters JH. Indications and contraindications of cell salvage. *Transfusion* 2004;**44** (12 Suppl):40S-4S.

57. Ling-Yun G, *et al*. Autotransfusion in the management of cardiac tamponade occurring during catheter ablation of atrial fibrillation. *Chinese Med J* 2010;**123**:961–963.

58. Ashworth A, Klein AA. Cell salvage as part of a blood conservation strategy in anaesthesia. *Br J Anaesth* 2010;**105**: 401–416.

59. Wise A, Clark V. Challenges of major obstetric haemorrhage. *Best Pract Res Clin Obstet Gynaecol* 2010;**24**:353–365.

60. Yamada T, Okamoto Y, Kasamatsu H, Mori H. Intraoperative autologous blood transfusion for hemoperitoneum resulting from ectopic pregnancy or ovarian bleeding during laparoscopic surgery. *JSLS* 2003;**7**:97–100.

61. Sakamoto K, Ohmori T, Takei H, Hasuo K, Rino Y, Takanashi Y. Autologous salvaged blood transfusion in spontaneous hemopneumothorax. *Ann Thorac Surg* 2004;**78**: 705–707.

62. Fearon JA. Reducing allogenic blood transfusions during pediatric cranial vault surgical procedures: a prospective analysis of blood recycling. *Plast Reconstr Surg* 2004;**113**: 1126–1130.

63. Jeng JC, Boyd TM, Jablonski KA, Harviel JD, Jordan MH. Intraoperative blood salvage in excisional burn surgery: an analysis of yield, bacteriology, and inflammatory mediators. *J Burn Care Rehabil* 1998;**19**:305–311.

64. Ging AL, St Onge JR, Fitzgerald DC, Collazo LR, Bower LS, Shen I. Bloodless cardiac surgery and the pediatric patient: a case study. *Perfusion* 2008;**23**:131–134.

17 Blood-Derived Pharmaceuticals

Pharmaceuticals extracted from human or animal blood are increasingly used to treat coagulation problems, immunological disorders or other conditions, often in situations where formerly blood or its main components have been used. Such pharmaceuticals are or are made of what are known as blood fractions, usually proteins transported in blood, which are extracted, purified and standardized. Therapy with such pharmaceuticals, targeted to specific clinical needs, often appears to improve the outcome of patients and this can be exploited in comprehensive blood management.

Objectives

1. To list the pharmaceuticals made from blood or its fractions.
2. To describe the indications for blood-derived pharmaceuticals.
3. To learn about asanguinous therapeutic options for the indications that typically call for therapy with blood-derived pharmaceuticals.

Definitions

Plasma fraction: A more or less pure extract of human or animal blood plasma, rich in a certain plasma component. The term fractionation refers to the process of separating plasma into its components.

Orphan drug: A term coined by the legislation to describe a product that treats a rare disease.

A brief history

Whole blood was used in early transfusion therapy. Blood divided into its main components was later used as a means to expand scarce blood resources. Dividing blood into cells and plasma was rather easy, since even simple blood sedimentation could be used to produce concentrates of cellular blood components and plasma. Fractionation, a process used to further divide human plasma into its components, first started to be used in blood banking in the late 1940s with the advent of Cohn's fractionation [1]. In the first decades, albumin was the main protein produced by Cohn's fractionation. Later, by-products of plasma fractionation were increasingly used.

The therapy of hemophilia A vividly illustrates how plasma fractions have found their way into clinical practice. Once treated with whole blood and later with plasma, hemophilia A can now be treated with a plasma fraction containing mainly the missing factor VIII (FVIII). By the 1950s, a crude plasma fraction containing FVIII was used for the therapy of bleeding episodes in hemophilia A. However, the large volume needed to reach the desired FVIII level caused volume overload. Later, therefore, cryoprecipitate was used instead. During the 1970s, the process of plasma fractionation was further refined, so that fractions with improved potency of FVIII were available. Although bringing positive clinical results, pathogens were shown to be transmitted to the hemophiliacs so that virtually every hemophiliac treated with such antihemophiliac preparations was infected with various kinds of hepatitis [2]. However, in comparison to the

Basics of Blood Management, Second Edition. Petra Seeber and Aryeh Shander.
© 2013 John Wiley & Sons, Ltd. Published 2013 by John Wiley & Sons, Ltd.

effects of untreated hemophilia, hepatitis was considered a minor problem [3]. The situation changed in the early 1980s when human immunodeficiency virus (HIV) was found in antihemophiliac preparations. Half of all hemophiliacs treated with plasma-derived products contracted HIV. Therefore, methods to virus-inactivate or eliminate plasma fractions were developed. Among them was chromatography. This method enabled the blood industry to purify crude plasma fractions into more specific components. Using this method, high and ultra-high purity factor concentrates of FVIII were brought to the market. Nowadays, recombinant factor concentrates developed in parallel to the plasma-derived products are often favored over blood products [2, 3].

Apart from the fractionation of FVIII, many other fractions have been produced. In addition to the initially produced albumin, cryoprecipitate became available in the 1970s. Later, prothrombin complex concentrates were also produced. By the beginning of the 1980s, intravenous immunoglobulin was fractioned. Currently, replacement of only the missing factor, produced either in recombinant fashion or sourced from plasma, rather than administering crude products like fresh frozen plasma (FFP) or cryoprecipitate, is recommended for the majority of indications.

Constituents of plasma

About 120 different proteins have so far been detected in plasma and described. Many more have been found in proteomic and other analyses and await their identification. The major portion of plasma is made up of albumin (30–40 g), immunoglobulins (8–17 g), fibrinogen (2.5–3.5 g), transferrin (2–3 g), α1-proteinase inhibitor (1.5–2 g), and α2-macroglobulin (1.3–2 g). Most other plasma constituents, such as clotting factors, are found only in trace amounts in the plasma (see Table A.3). The constitution of plasma varies from individual to individual and over time. It may or may not contain pregnancy-related substances, certain blood group antigens, drugs, dietary components, alcohol, hormones, disease-related antibodies, cancer cells, infectious agents, cellular debris, and many, as yet unidentified, substances.

It is obvious therefore how difficult it is to fractionate a mix of thousands of compounds that are only partially identified or not known at all, and that differ with every single donor. It is (nearly) impossible to do so. Therefore, the content of most plasma fractions used for therapy is only vaguely defined. Once in a while, new constituents are found in the concentrates, with no exact knowledge as to their clinical significance [4].

Plasma fractions

Plasma fractions, the raw material of many of the blood-derived pharmaceuticals, are more or less pure extracts of human or animal blood plasma. A series of terms has been used to describe the properties of plasma fractions:
• **Activity level** is the amount of (clotting) factor in the plasma of the patient when compared with normal plasma (= specific activity, potency), measured in international units (IU). (1 IU = amount of factor present in 1 mL of normal plasma.)
• **Purity** describes how much protein is present in addition to the desired therapeutic plasma fraction. It gives the total number of units of the desired protein per milligram of total protein. Purity has nothing to do with the degree of contamination. A low purity concentrate is a crude plasma concentrate that contains the required factor or group of factors in a higher concentration than plasma. The purity is usually below 1 U/mg total protein. Intermediate purity concentrates have a purity of about 1–10 U/mg and high-purity concentrates about 50–150 U/mg. An ultra-high purity concentrate is intended to be virtually free of proteins other than the desired factor and has a purity of more than 2000 U/mg, but as such, is unstable and requires stabilizers such as albumin.
• **Intravascular or biological recovery** describes the percentage of the infused factor found intravasally immediately after infusion and is determined by the distribution space of the body. The more plasma volume per body weight, the lower the recovery of a factor. Small plasma factors distribute not only in the intravascular space, but also extravascularly, and therefore have a lower recovery than factors that remain mostly in the vessels. The presence of antibodies against the infused fraction also lowers the recovery. Table 17.1 gives the average recoveries of coagulation factor products.
• **Through (level)** is the minimum required level of factor activity. It is calculated for every single patient.

Coagulation factors

Factor mixes

Cryoprecipitate
Cryoprecipitate consists of a mix of proteins, collectively called cryoglobulins. It is a compound that precipitates

Table 17.1 Characteristics of coagulation factors needed to calculate the dose regimen.

Factor	Molecular weight (kDa)	Recovery (%)	Through level (below which abnormal surgical bleeding may occur) (%)	Half-life (h)
vWF	240–270	80–100	40	72
I (Fibrinogen)	340–320	80–100	25–30	75
II	70–72	50–60	40	60
V	330–350	80–100	15–20	12
VII	50	30–50	10	6
VIII	285–300	70–100	25–30	8–19
IX	52–55	30–50	25–30	11–27
X	55–59	30–50	15–20	50
XI	143–160	80–100	30	50–60
XIII	320	80–100	5	250

when FFP is thawed at 4 °C. FVIII, FXIII, von Willebrand factor (vWF), fibrinogen, and fibronectin are the main constituents of cryoprecipitate [5]. In the continuum from blood to blood-derived pharmaceuticals, cryoprecipitate is the plasma fraction closest to blood plasma and least pharmacologically processed. In contrast to most other factor concentrates, cryoprecipitate is not virus-attenuated.

The use of cryoprecipitate was recommended in 1996 by the Task Force of the American Society of Anesthesiologists [6] for patients with von Willebrand disease (vWD) unresponsive to desmopressin or bleeding, and for bleeding patients with fibrinogen levels below 80–100 mg/dL. Today, cryoprecipitate is used to substitute fibrinogen, either as therapy for congenital deficiency, dysfibrinogenemia, or for acquired hypofibrinogenemia, such as develops in disseminated intravascular coagulation (DIC) or thrombolysis. Cryoprecipitate is also used to treat some rare factor deficiencies, e.g., FXIII. Deficiencies of FVIII or vWF are no longer usually treated with cryoprecipitate since, although theoretically effective, better and safer alternatives exist [5]. Cryoprecipitate may no longer be available in countries where purer and safer factor concentrates for treatment of the above-mentioned factor deficiencies exist.

Prothrombin complex concentrate
There are two types of prothrombin complex concentrates (PCCs): one with "four" factors (also called PPSB) and the other with "three" factors. The "four"-factor PCC contains mainly vitamin K-dependent coagulation factors

(II, VII, IX, X, proteins S and C). FVII is missing in the "three"-factor PCC (also called a low-purity FIX concentrate). Ideally, the factors II, VII, IX, and X are evenly distributed in a ratio of 1:1:1:1, and proteins S and C are present in about 1 U/unit of FIX. Apart from the mentioned compounds, there are many other proteins (e.g., caeruloplasmin, kininogen, protein Z) in PCC, some of them as yet undefined. The coagulation factors in PCCs can also be activated; the concentrate is then called activated prothrombin complex concentrate (aPCC). A concentrate called FEIBA (factor eight inhibitor bypassing activity) also belongs to the aPCCs.

A problem of PCCs appears to be their potential thrombogenicity and ability to trigger allergic reactions. PCC therapy has occasionally been associated with myocardial infarction and DIC, but the thromboembolic risks for unactivated PCCs especially seem low enough to continue their use [7].

A "three-factor" PCC was once the favored therapy for hemophilia B. Its use has been abandoned in favor of highly purified FIX concentrates, thus avoiding potential thromboembolic complications of PCCs. "Three-factor" PCC in conjunction with recombinant human FVII (rHuFVII) may be used as a replacement for "four-factor" PCC in countries where the latter is not available.

The "four-factor" PCC is still in widespread use in countries where it is available. It is recommended for the treatment of patients with congenital or acquired deficiency of FII and FX; hemophiliacs with inhibitors (especially the activated form of PCC); bleeding during therapy with vitamin K antagonists (coumadins); or in severe liver disease-related coagulopathy. Together with fibrinogen concentrate, it is increasingly used to treat acute trauma-induced coagulopathy, thereby obviating the use of FFP. The concept of using rapidly available, blood-group independent factor concentrates instead of FFP in the early and effective correction of coagulopathy in the trauma setting is an attractive one. Preliminary results seem to indicate an improved survival when compared to FFP-based therapy [8, 9].

"Single"-factor concentrates

Technically, it is possible to fractionate most clotting factors from plasma. Additional production steps reduce the amount of other compounds found in the fraction. However, it is not possible to provide a plasma-derived product containing solely the required factor. Therefore, the term "single"-factor concentrate is somewhat misleading.

Factor VIII concentrate

The plasma coagulation FVIII is a small molecule. It consists of A-, B-, and C-domains. When activated, it loses most of the B-domain. The small FVIII:C circulates in blood bound non-covalently to the large vWF molecule. The vWF carries and protects the FVIII:C molecule and targets it to the site of injury. When the protecting influence of vWF is missing, the half-life of FVIII is reduced from 8 hours to about 8 minutes. FVIII is synthesized in the liver and endothelium, while vWF is synthesized in megakaryocytes and the endothelium. The activated FVIII activates FIX and together with FIX, activates FX.

Commercial FVIII concentrates are provided with different purity levels. Intermediate purity FVIII concentrates are prepared by precipitation. Their specific activity ranges from 2 to 5 U/mg of protein. Such concentrates contain not only FVIII but also vWF and can therefore be used as treatment for hemophilia A and vWD. Other purification steps of FVIII yield a product with a specific activity of 15–150 U/mg of protein. Such concentrates do not contain relevant amounts of vWF. High and ultra-high purity FVIII concentrates made by chromatographic methods do not contain vWF at all. Such factor concentrates contain 2000–3000 U/mg of protein. However, albumin needs to be added to these and the specific activity is reduced to 10 U/mg of protein.

FVIII concentrates can also be made from animal plasma, usually of porcine or bovine origin. However, the products may cause slight to severe thrombocytopenia and the production of such factor concentrates was discontinued in some countries [10].

von Willebrand factor concentrates

vWF is a mix of multimeric plasma glycoproteins with molecular weights ranging from 40 to 20 000 kDa. It facilitates platelet adhesion to the vessel wall by anchoring the platelet to the subendothelium. Besides, vWF is a cofactor of FVIII. When vWF is lacking or defective, patients develop vWD.

Patients with severe vWD not responding to desmopressin or other pharmacological therapies are usually treated with FVIII concentrates containing relevant amounts of vWF. In some countries, concentrates that contain mainly vWF with only small amounts of FVIII have been made available [11].

Factor IX concentrates

FIX is a naturally occurring vitamin K-dependent coagulation factor and acts as a serine protease. It can be activated either by FXI or by a complex of tissue factor and FVIIa. In the activated form, FIX activates FX.

FIX concentrates for the therapy of hemophilia B are available in different purities, ranging from low (PCC) to very high purity. Modern chromatographic purification methods have led to a product that does not have the thrombogenicity of early days. However, prolonged infusion of FIX has been associated with thromboembolic complications.

Fibrinogen

Fibrinogen is a protein that is synthesized in the liver. When thrombin proteolytically cleaves fibrinogen, fibrin develops. Fibrinogen is therefore the precursor of fibrin. When it is lacking or defective, thrombi cannot form properly and coagulation is impaired.

Human fibrinogen concentrates are available in some countries [12]. Formerly, fibrinogen therapy was administered by cryoprecipitate or FFP. These are still used in some countries. Where fibrinogen concentrates are available, they are preferred. Afibrinogenemia or dysfibrinogenemia [13], as well as other conditions leading to low fibrinogen levels, are indications for fibrinogen concentrates. Since a high fibrinogen level protects against excessive blood loss, the early substitution of lost fibrinogen during massive bleeding with fibrinogen concentrates is advocated [14]. Besides, high levels of fibrinogen may substitute for low platelet levels.

Factor XIII

FXIII is a plasma transglutaminase. In its proenzyme form, it is activated by thrombin. FXIII enhances hemostasis and wound healing, and plays an important role in pregnancy by preventing decidual bleeding.

Formerly, FXIII concentrates have been produced from human placentas. Today, commercially available concentrates are fractionated from human plasma. FXIII is used to compensate for a congenital deficiency of this factor. Furthermore, it has been used to treat badly healing wounds, problems with collagen synthesis, and vessel leakage. FXIII concentrates are also used to prevent miscarriages and perinatal bleeding in pregnant women with FXIII deficiencies, and are recommended for clot stabilization in bleeding cardiac surgery patients unresponsive to other treatment [15].

Factor XI, prothrombin, thrombin, factor X, and factor VII

FXI is a vitamin K-dependent serine protease whose activated form activates FIX (along with FVIII). A congenital deficiency has been described to have increased prevalence in Ashkenazi Jews. Even if severe, the deficiency may be clinically asymptomatic until the patient is challenged by surgical trauma. In this event, a factor concentrate may be beneficial. In some countries, virally-inactivated FXI concentrates are available for treatment [16].

Apart from thrombin which is used in surgical glues, other coagulation factors are usually not purified on an industrial scale. However, this is possible, and can be performed on the basis of the Orphan Drug Act in the United States [17]. In some European countries, coagulation factor concentrates of FX and FVII are available.

Anticoagulation factors and other therapeutically used plasma fractions

Antithrombin III

Antithrombin III is probably the most important of the four originally identified antithrombins. It is synthesized in the liver. Antithrombin III is a serine proteinase inhibitor and acts as an anticoagulant by directly binding and inactivating the serine proteases, above all thrombin, but also factors XIa, IXa, and Xa. In the absence of heparin, inactivation of serine proteinase (mostly by antithrombin III) proceeds slowly. When heparin is present, the activity of antithrombin III is increased 10–10000 times. Antithrombin III possesses not only anticoagulative but also anti-inflammatory effects.

Antithrombin III deficiency is either congenital or acquired. Patients with hereditary antithrombin III deficiency have an increased risk of thrombosis. This risk is especially high when there are other risk factors for thromboembolism, such as pregnancy and surgery. Acquired deficiency of antithrombin III develops when its production is impaired (protein catabolism is reduced, liver disease), when antithrombin III is lost (in nephrotic syndrome), or when antithrombin III is consumed (DIC, thrombosis). Septic or otherwise critically ill patients may also have low antithrombin III levels.

Antithrombin III is available as plasma-derived concentrates. These have a reported incidence of side effects of about 3%: chest tightness, dizziness, abdominal cramps, fever, and shortness of breath. All side effects are regarded as mild.

Antithrombin III concentrates are used for patients with congenital antithrombin deficiency or abnormal antithrombin. However, for these patients oral anticoagulation therapy is the first-line treatment. According to current guidelines, antithrombin concentrates are only recommended together with heparin in high-risk situations or manifest thrombosis in congenital antithrombin deficiency [18]. In acquired antithrombin III deficiency, a low antithrombin III level is associated with a worse outcome in critically ill patients. Some authorities therefore recommend high-dose antithrombin concentrates without heparin in severe sepsis complicated by DIC. Otherwise, there appear to be no indications for antithrombin concentrates, although the literature shows contradictory results [18].

Protein C

Protein C is a vitamin K-dependent factor structurally similar to other coagulation factors. It prevents the formation of blood clots by inactivating FVa and FVIIIa. Protein C needs calcium, a phospholipid surface, and protein S to cleave its target factors.

Protein C deficiency may be inherited or acquired [19]. A homozygous deficiency with factor levels below 1% is lethal unless appropriate therapy is administered. In the neonatal period, the deficiency of protein C already presents with purpura fulminans, DIC, and thrombosis [20]. As the heterozygous form of protein C deficiency often does not lead to thrombosis, its clinical relevance is a subject of debate. Apart from inherited protein C deficiency, low levels of protein C have been observed in DIC, after surgery, in tumor patients, in sepsis, and when protein C cannot be synthesized properly (vitamin K deficiency, liver disease).

Protein C is available as a plasma-derived concentrate. It has a recovery of about 44% and a half-life of 4–8 hours. Protein C is also available as a recombinant product.

For many years, protein C deficiency has been treated with FFP or prothrombin complex concentrates to replace protein C. Today, it is treated with protein C concentrates. Other possible treatment options are heparin, steroids, oral anticoagulants, or even liver transplantation [19, 21].

C1-esterase inhibitor

The C1-esterase inhibitor is the most important factor regulating the classical pathway of complementary system activation. Patients lacking C1-esterase inhibitor have an increased activation of the complementary system, leading to hereditary angioneurotic edema (Quincke's disease). Sometimes triggered by trauma or infection, the patients develop symptoms such as abdominal pain and attacks of swollen tissues, with swelling of the larynx compromising breathing. The treatment and prophylaxis options include antihistamines, androgens, tranexamic acid, and some newer agents (kallikrein inhibitor, bradykinin B2 receptor antagonist). Formerly, FFP or solvent-/detergent-treated plasma have been administered in acute attacks of angioneurotic edema. Nowadays, a recombinant product and a plasma concentrate rich in C1-esterase inhibitor are the treatment options of choice in severe angioneurotic edema.

α1-proteinase inhibitor (α1-antitrypsin)

α1-antitrypsin is a glycoprotein. It inhibits serine proteinases such as trypsin, thrombin, and renin. Its inhibition of the elastase of neutrophils is clinically important. When a congenital defect of α1-antitrypsin expression is present, tissues, especially in the lung, liver, and skin, are damaged by the uninhibited action of neutrophils and emphysema occurs. Plasma-derived α1-antitrypsin concentrates are available, but their clinical value is still debated.

Human albumin

About two-thirds of all plasma protein is albumin, making it the largest plasma protein fraction. Produced in the liver, it transports many compounds, e.g., products of hemoglobin degradation, metal ions, NO, and drugs. It renders toxins harmless while transporting them to their point of detoxification or excretion. It is a strong antioxidant and anticoagulant. Besides, albumin maintains the colloid-osmotic pressure of the plasma.

Concentrates of human albumin are available for therapy. More than 95% of the protein in the albumin concentrate is albumin. The remaining 5% consists of aggregates of prekallikrein activator, heme, aluminum, potassium, sodium, and other compounds. For therapeutic use, albumin is available in 4% or 5% solutions and in 20–25% solutions.

Clinically, albumin concentrates may support the development of edema when albumin leaves the vessels due to capillary leakage. Hypervolemia with pulmonary edema may result secondary to albumin therapy. Besides, sodium and water excretion may be reduced after albumin infusion. Other side effects of albumin infusions include viral transmission, allergic reactions, and fever. Occasionally, hypotension occurs. This has been attributed to bradykinin and other compounds present in the concentrate. Although the levels of bradykinin have been reduced in recent years, patients who are on angiotensin-converting enzyme (ACE) inhibitors and who therefore have an altered bradykinin metabolism may still react to albumin infusions with hypotension. Besides, albumin is very expensive in comparison to other volume expanders.

Albumin has been advocated as the ideal volume replacement. Formerly, human albumin was used for parenteral nutrition. This indication for albumin therapy is now obsolete, along with many other indications that have been proposed over time. Despite the existence of therapeutic alternatives, the current consensus is that albumin is indicated in massive paracentesis, therapeutic plasmapheresis, and spontaneous bacterial peritonitis in ascites [22]. Nevertheless, albumin is still widely used without sound scientific evidence. Albumin has been used as an adjunct to the therapy of fetal erythroblastosis (morbus hemolyticus neonatorum) or other causes of hyperbilirubinemia. It binds bilirubin and thus reduces the likelihood of kernicterus. Other therapies of neonatal hyperbilirubinemia are available and albumin in this setting should be obsolete.

Immunoglobulins

Immunoglobulins are a group of heterogenous molecules made up of various numbers of immunoglobulin monomers. The latter look like a Y with its arms being the Fab parts and the leg being the Fc part (Figure 17.1). In the blood, different classes of immunoglobulins are present, namely G, M, and A (IgG, IgM, IgA). IgG is the main immunoglobulin in human serum. It binds bacterial and viral antigens and antibodies, and induces their phagocytosis. IgG increases the synthesis of leukocytes and regulates mediators of inflammation. IgM increases the phagocytosis of bacteria and viruses, neutralizes toxins, inactivates autoantibodies, and regulates the complementary system. Since IgM is a pentamer or

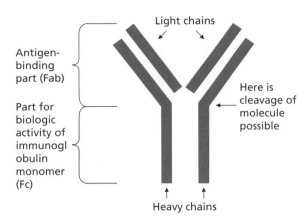

Light chains

Antigen-binding part (Fab)

Part for biologic activity of immunoglobulin monomer (Fc)

Here is cleavage of molecule possible

Heavy chains

Figure 17.1 Immunoglobulin monomer.

hexamer (consisting of 5–6 immunoglobulin monomers), it forms large agglutinates that are easily recognized by phagocytes (opsonization). IgA binds toxins, activates the complementary system, and modulates the inflammatory response as well.

In vivo, immunoglobulins have a variety of functions as part of the immune system. They are able to scavenge bacteria, viruses, and other infectious agents, as well as their toxins. They mediate cellular responses that lead to the destruction and elimination of the invaders. Besides, immunoglobulins play an important role in balancing the immune system. They can activate players in the immune system, such as macrophages and granulocytes. They can also inactivate parts of it, affecting the activation and effector functions of T and B cells, inhibit the release of proinflammatory factors, and scavenge cytokines. Autoantibodies can be regulated as well. With this knowledge, it seemed prudent to use immunoglobulins in patient's whose own immunoglobulin synthesis is insufficient (neonates, primary immune deficiency), or when a patient suffers an infection or an autoimmune diseases.

A vast variety of human plasma-derived immunoglobulin concentrates are on the market. They can be divided into two main groups: normal immunoglobulins and hyperimmunoglobulins. Normal immunoglobulins are a concentrate of one or more classes of immunoglobulins collected from a pool of the general donor population. They are made from at least 1000 donor plasmas and contain the whole spectrum of antibodies developed in this population; those against infectious agents and their toxins, as well as those directed against self (autoantibod-

ies). Hyperimmunoglobulins are made from plasmas of selected donors who have been immunized against a certain antigen. However, it is not mandatory that hyperimmunoglobulins actually have a higher than normal titer of the required antibody.

A major problem in the preparation of plasma-derived immunoglobulin concentrates is that the immunoglobulins have to remain in a form that enables them to react with their antigen. The purification process activates them, and irreversible aggregates form, which may activate the complement system, leading to unwanted effects. The standardization of immunoglobulins is difficult as well. It has been ruled that at least 95% of the protein in an immunoglobulin concentrate must be immunoglobulins (unless albumin is added). There exist major differences between the products of the different manufacturers and between batches. The actual content of the immunoglobulin concentrate, IgA content, titer of certain clinically relevant antibodies, form of fractionation and purification, and addition of stabilizers all may influence whether or not the concentrate is suitable for any specific patient.

Immunoglobulin concentrates can be administered subcutaneously, intravenously, intrathecally, or intramuscularly. Formulations for "intramuscular only" use are crude, not purified, contain many aggregates, and cannot be given intravenously, since the contaminants may elicit unwanted responses. The half-life of intravenously administered immunoglobulins is 3–5 weeks.

Immunoglobulin solutions are generally safe, but there is a residual risk of disease transmission, with newly emerging viruses contributing to this risk [23]. Nowadays, acute side effects of intravenous immunoglobulins are more common than viral transmission. About 5% of patients treated with immunoglobulins experience relevant side effects. Stabilizers, such as sucrose, have been accused of partially causing those side effects [24]. Minor side effects such as malaise, rash, fever, flu-like pains, and minor allergic reactions usually resolve after several days [25]. Major side effects, although rare, can be fatal and include anaphylactic reactions, arthritis, aseptic meningitis, irreversible renal failure, stroke, myocardial infarction and other thrombotic events [26], hemolysis, and leukopenia.

IgA deficiency is considered a contraindication to intravenous immunoglobulin. Patients lacking IgA may develop antibodies to the immunoglobulin and have an allergic reaction. If IgA deficiency is present, a concentrate with a low IgA content should be used when immunoglobulin therapy appears to be indicated.

Normal intravenous immunoglobulins of human origin
Normal intravenous immunoglobulin (IVIG) concentrates are given either to prevent or to treat a disease caused by an infectious agent or toxin, or to modify the immune system. The exact mode of action of IVIGs is not well understood and is certainly complex. The injected immunoglobulins modulate Fc receptor expression and function, the complementary system, cytokines, and the activation, differentiation and function of T and B cells. They also influence cell growth and cellular adhesion molecules [27].

IVIGs have been used in almost every condition, from diabetes to malnutrition. However, for most of the indications, proof of benefit to the patient is lacking [28]. For many of these diseases, other treatment approaches are available in addition to or instead of immunoglobulins.

Some indications currently are listed as "recommended indications," including primary and secondary immunodeficiency (including in children with AIDS), immunomodulation in immune thrombocytopenic purpura (ITP), Kawasaki disease and Guillain–Barré syndrome, and as an adjunct for bone marrow transplant [22]. Other conditions may be treated with IVIGs in situations where other therapeutic options are not feasible: rheumatological, dermatological, and neurological diseases, as well as hematological conditions such as pure red cell aplasia in parvovirus B19 infection, immune-mediated neutropenia, alloimmune neonatal thrombocytopenia, hemolytic disease of the newborn, and autoimmune hemolytic anemia [22, 29].

Hyperimmune immunoglobulins of human origin
Hyperimmune products usually have a very high titer for a specific antibody (5–8 times higher than in normal IVIG). They are routinely available, e.g., for cytomegalovirus (CMV), varicella zoster (VZV), and hepatitis B virus (HBV) infection or prevention. They can also be produced in response to a newly emerging pathogen using reconvalescent serum, as was the case with severe acute respiratory syndrome (SARS) [30].

Antisera
Fairly purified immunoglobulins given to combat or prevent a disease caused by a distinct antigen are also called antisera. Antisera are used prophylactically as passive immunization (e.g., for hepatitis A, B, tetanus, rabies) or to treat a specific disease (tetanus, botulism, etc.). The subgroup of antisera used to treat envenomation with animal venoms are also called antivenoms or antivenins.

Antisera against infectious agents or toxins are fairly purified hyperimmune sera produced from human or animal sources (e.g., horses, sheep, chicken). Animals (or sometimes humans) are vaccinated with the infectious agents or toxins and the synthesized antibodies are harvested for pharmaceutical use. Antisera are often processed to remove proteins that may cause allergies and to concentrate the desired type of antibodies. Inactive proteins may be precipitated or removed by chromatography. Immunoglobulin molecules can be cleaved further into antibody fragments [31]. Target-specific immunoglobulins (IgG) and their fragments (Fab2, Fab), as well as the choice of animal source, determine the differences in pharmacokinetic and pharmacodynamic properties of the antisera. Fab molecules have a shorter half-life than IgG molecules. However, Fab preparations seem to produce fewer allergic side effects. Lyophilized antisera consisting of Fab fragments can easily be dissolved for injection and are very stable, even when exposed to heat. This is very advantageous for use in tropical regions.

Typical side effects of antisera are allergies, the rate of which depends on the purity of the preparation and other factors. Serum sickness is a common occurrence after the administration of antisera. Its development depends on the amount of antiserum administered [32]. Serum sickness presents with fever, arthralgia, and pruritus. Although usually self-limiting, antihistamines and corticoids are used to alleviate the symptoms [32].

The dosing of antisera is important. Like other drugs, toxins, and antisera have a pharmacokinetic profile that needs to be known in order to dose the antisera correctly. A pharmacokinetic or pharmacodynamic mismatch between the antiserum and toxin may cause recurrence of the symptoms. These occur when the toxin has a longer half-life than the antiserum. To prevent late local tissue damage or coagulopathy with bleeding after snake bites, or recurrence of other phenomena, close monitoring and possibly repeated dosing of the patient in the hours and days after the envenomation or intoxication are recommended. The duration of the therapy depends on individual risk factors and on the clinical response to the therapy [33].

Anti-D-immunoglobulin
When fetal red blood cells with the Rhesus (Rh) antigen (blood group antigen D) cross the placenta, an immunological response with the production of IgM and IgG may be induced in an Rh-negative mother. The IgG molecule crosses the placenta and can act against fetal red

cells. The fetus may then suffer from hemolysis, anemia, and hydrops fetalis.

Maternal sensitization occurs when the mother is first exposed to fetal blood. In an uncomplicated pregnancy, this happens during delivery. In this case, the first child is not affected by the antibody developing after birth, but the next fetus is. When the mother is exposed to fetal blood prior to delivery, usually due to testing or obstetric complications, the current fetus is at risk for an antibody attack.

To prevent the production of antibodies, anti-D-immunoglobulin is administered to non-sensitized Rh-negative women shortly after birth or after miscarriage, threatened or induced abortion, molar pregnancy, and ectopic pregnancy, at amniocentesis and after chorionic villous sampling, and following cordocentesis. The anti-D-immunoglobulin will destroy any fetal red blood cells that have entered the maternal bloodstream, preventing the formation of maternal antibodies to the Rh factor [34].

Anti-D-immunoglobulin is also used in the therapy of other conditions, such as ITP [35].

Blood-derived pharmaceuticals in blood management

Blood banks and pharmaceutical companies all over the world offer hundreds of different blood-derived pharmaceuticals. However, since only a limited number of plasma proteins have a unique, life-conserving function, only very few diseases seem to benefit from such pharmaceuticals. Most functions in blood are performed by different proteins, so that when one is lacking, others kick in to take over the job. Others can be substituted for by non-blood therapy. Actually, for most, if not all, plasma factor deficiencies, there are non-blood alternatives.

Hemophilia A and B

While pharmaceutical [36] and physical therapies are the first-line treatment for most hemophiliacs, factor substitution plays an important additional role in the therapy of severe hemophilia. There are many products that contain FVIII and would theoretically work in the therapy of hemophilia A. Among them are FFP, cryoprecipitate, FVIII concentrates with intermediate, high or ultra-high purity, porcine FVIII concentrates, and recombinant FVIII. For the therapy of hemophilia B, FFP, prothrombin complex concentrates, activated pro-

thrombin complex concentrates, and FIX concentrates, either human plasma-derived or recombinant, are available. FFP is no real choice for these patients since, unless exchange transfusion is performed, not enough FFP can be given to raise the FIX levels sufficiently in severe hemophilia.

The choice of therapy for hemophiliac patients depends on availability, cost, and patient characteristics. For many, recombinant products are the treatment of choice. Other products such as intermediate purity concentrates have immunosuppressive effects [37]. These can be of clinical significance in already immunocompromised patients (HIV) [38]. HIV-positive patients benefit from a high purity, since this may preserve their CD4 lymphocyte count.

There exist specific recommendations for the therapy of hemophilia [39]. As a summary of some current guidelines, the following may help to direct therapy with clotting factor concentrates:

• In life-threatening bleeding, without exact knowledge of the factor lacking, recombinant FVIIa is the first-choice treatment (90–120 µg/kg). When the required factor is known, 50–70 IU/kg of a factor concentrate are infused.

• In intracerebral bleeding, a high-dose regimen of the factor needs to be started and continued until resorption of the hematoma is seen. Afterward, low-dose substitution is warranted to prevent rebleeding.

• Patients with polytrauma should have 100% factor activity until the wounds have healed.

• For surgery, the individual factor activity level should be determined before the operation and substitution is begun immediately before surgery.

• When bones are fractured or operated on, FVIII or FIX levels of 80–100% are recommended. For the time the bone is healing, a minimum factor level of 10–20% should be maintained.

• For dental work, a minimum of 30% FVII activity is recommended, together with antifibrinolytic therapy to counteract the fibrinolytic activity of the saliva.

• For gastrointestinal bleeding and bleeding into the psoas or retroperitoneum, 50% factor activity is recommended.

Recommendations like these may be not feasible in developing countries because of a limited availability of factor concentrates. In such settings, reduced infusion doses of factor concentrates have been found to be adequate [40].

Patients with hemophilia A or B and with low levels of clotting factors (<1%) are sometimes recommended to use clotting factor concentrates prophylactically. It has been claimed that this reduces severe bleeding in joints and soft tissues. However, proof that prophylactic use of clotting factor concentrates is superior to placebo in reducing bleeding is still lacking [41].

Inhibitor treatment of hemophiliac patients

The treatment of hemophilia with injection of the missing coagulation factor has one great disadvantage. The body may recognize the injected material as foreign and develop antibodies (IgG alloantibodies, inhibitors) to it. Patients who are not hemophiliacs may also develop an inhibitor. They may form alloantibodies against the endogenous FVIII idiopathically (in elderly patients), in autoimmune diseases (systemic lupus erythematosus, rheumatoid arthritis), in malignancies, as a drug reaction (penicillin, chloramphenicol, phenytoin), and during or after pregnancy.

About 10–30% of patients with severe hemophilia A and 2–5% with severe hemophilia B or mild-to-moderate hemophilia A develop inhibitors [42]. Inhibitors are detected with the Bethesda assay and the level of the inhibitor is expressed in Bethesda units (BUs). One BU is the amount of antibody that neutralizes 50% of FVIII in a 1:1 mixture of the patient's plasma and normal plasma (after 2 hours of incubation at 37°C). According to the Bethesda assay, patients can be divided into two groups: low responders with low titers of inhibitors (<10 BU), which does not increase after a challenge with FVIII; and high responders who develop a high titer of inhibitor when challenged with FVIII.

To overcome the problems in patients with inhibitors, products other than the factor concentrates can be infused. Among them are PCCs and recombinant FVIIa. Also, immunosuppressive agents to control the antibody production against clotting factors (corticosteroids, cyclophosphamide, and azathioprine) or IVIGs have been recommended for the therapy of patients with inhibitors. If these approaches fail and the patients is bleeding profusely, high-dose porcine FVIII or human FIX may be effective, providing the inhibitor is low enough (<5 BU) or lowered by plasmapheresis or protein A immunoabsorption. Another way to overcome the inhibitor is to induce immune tolerance. To this end, patients receive frequent infusions of the offending factor (e.g., daily or weekly). After months or years, the inhibitor is eliminated. However, the induction of immune tolerance fails in 20% of cases, is costly, and there are multiple adverse effects.

von Willebrand disease

Congenital vWD develops when vWF is lacking or defective. Three main types of congenital vWD are known. The most common form is Type I vWD with patients having only a moderate decrease in vWF. They typically have excessive bleeding only after a surgical challenge or trauma. Type II vWD is rare. The level of vWF is normal, but the molecule does not work properly. In the subgroup IIa vWD, vWF molecules are either not secreted or are rapidly destroyed in the circulation. In the subgroup IIb vWD, vWF molecules bind increasingly to platelets and aggregate them. Patients with Type III vWD synthesize no vWF at all. The platelet aggregation is diminished with a bleeding pattern similar to thrombocytopenia. Additionally, FVIII is impaired as well, leading to a hemophilia-like symptom pattern. There is also an acquired form of vWD which occurs when antibodies inhibit vWF or when tumors (such as lymphoid tumors) adsorb vWF onto their surface.

Desmopressin (DDAVP) is the agent of choice for the prophylaxis and therapy of most vWD patients. A test dose of DDAVP and determination of the stimulated factor levels is recommended before surgery is performed under DDAVP protection. Therapeutic options other than DDAVP include antifibrinolytics and hormones. As regards plasma fractions, vWF concentrates [43], cryoprecipitate, and FVIII concentrates containing high vWF levels [44] may be considered, sometimes in combination with IVIGs [45]. When DDAVP therapy fails, a virus-inactivated factor concentrate with sufficient levels of vWF is preferred over cryoprecipitate. Probably, the best choice is a vWF concentrate with very low levels of FVIII in order to reduce thrombotic complications [44]. Patients with a high risk of bleeding complications due to vWD may also be eligible for prophylactic measures, including infusions of factor concentrates, in order to reduce the incidence of severe bleeds [46]. In developing countries, cryoprecipitate may be the only available therapeutic blood fraction [47]. It is costly and may not be sufficiently tested for transfusion-transmissible diseases. In such settings it is especially important to explore all available non–blood-based therapeutic options before a plasma fraction is considered for therapy.

Other single (congenital) clotting factor deficiencies

Other, much less common, single-factor deficiencies can be treated with either a plasma-derived factor concentrate or another, cruder plasma fraction. Most single-factor deficiencies can be treated with recombinant FVIIa. This is probably the safest, yet most expensive, option. Table A.2 delineates the therapeutic options for the therapy of rare clotting factor deficiencies.

Therapy of vitamin K deficiency

The synthesis of many plasma factors depends on the presence of vitamin K. Mainly, these are factors II, VII, IX, and X, as well as proteins S and C. Vitamin K deficiency can be caused either by insufficient intake or by iatrogenic influences, such as therapy with vitamin K antagonists (coumadin anticoagulants) or antibiotics [48].

The treatment of vitamin K deficiency is the correction of the underlying cause and vitamin K administration. Usually, this is all it takes. Within hours, the factors are replenished. But when the therapy does not bring the desired results or the delay in response would endanger the patient, clotting factor concentrates, either recombinant or serum-derived, are prescribed.

Formerly, for emergency oral anticoagulation reversal, FFP was often prescribed. However, it was shown that FFP often does not correct the underlying deficiency. To achieve therapeutic factor levels in over-anticoagulated patients, several liters of FFP have to be infused in order to develop the desired factor levels. When FFP is used, diuretics or a partial plasma exchange have been necessary to treat the developing volume overload. To avoid this, emergency reversal is better performed using four-factor PCCs [49] or three-factor PCCs with recombinant FVIIa. They correct the factor deficiency without causing volume overload.

Bleeding in liver-related coagulopathies

All coagulation factors (apart from vWF) are synthesized in the liver. When the liver fails, the plasma coagulation is impaired as well. Besides, severe liver insufficiency is accompanied by hyperfibrinolysis, since inactivation of pro- and anti-coagulant factors in the liver is impaired. The condition is occasionally also accompanied by thrombocytopenia secondary to increased use of platelets and toxic-impaired platelet production.

Patients with liver disease-related coagulopathies can be treated without blood products, using such options as antifibrinolytics, DDAVP, vitamin K, or hormones instead. When blood products are considered, plasma fractions such as antithrombin III, PCC, and fibrinogen are recommended. However, since a liver insufficiency also affects anticoagulative factors (protein C, protein S),

the risk for thromboembolism is increased when coagulative factors are given.

Disseminated intravascular coagulation

DIC usually develops in connection with a life-threatening disorder, such as severe sepsis or polytrauma. It is initiated by a systemic activation of the coagulation process. Endotoxin- or thromboplastin-containing amniotic fluid may initiate this, resulting in increased thrombin and fibrin formation as well as activation of other plasma coagulation factors. The resulting intravascular deposits impair the microcirculation and multiorgan failure results. Fibrinolysis is increased and bleeding results. The massive use of platelets and coagulation factors depletes the blood of these, thereby accelerating bleeding. These processes continue until the offending agent is cleared from the circulation.

When DIC is diagnosed, the underlying condition has to be treated immediately to stop the continuous activation of coagulation. In parallel, hematological support needs to be initiated. However, the therapy of DIC is difficult, since bleeding and coagulation occur simultaneously. Some algorithms recommend FFP, antithrombin, heparin, activated protein C, aprotinin, platelets, fibrinogen, and PCC. However, such recommendations are not supported by hard data.

Plasma fractions used to reduce the use of other blood products

Sometimes, there are different blood-derived products available for the therapy of one condition. When this is the case, the factor with the lowest risk of adverse effects should be preferred. Since most plasma fractions are virus-inactivated, they seem to be somewhat safer than blood products that are not. By using the safer plasma fractions, use of other less safe products can be avoided. Besides, some plasma fractions may be acceptable to a patient, while cellular blood components are not. The following examples illustrate this:
• FIX concentrates containing other activated factors (such as PCCs and intermediate-purity FIX concentrates) can improve hemostasis when used in mild-to-moderate thrombocytopenia [50].
• Therapeutic apheresis procedures can be performed with a variety of agents for plasma exchange. Synthetic colloids are suitable for plasma exchange. If a patient does

not wish to resort to asanguinous therapies, albumin may be an alternative to FFP [51].
• As an alternative approach to exchange transfusion, IVIG therapy has been proposed in newborns suffering from hyperbilirubinemia secondary to hemolysis [52].
• For acute attacks of hereditary angioedema, FFP and solvent-/detergent-treated plasma may be effective treatment, but the potentially safer C1-esterase inhibitor concentrate should be used [53].

Approaches to reduce the use of blood-derived pharmaceuticals

Plasma fractions seem to be safer than untreated cellular components for transfusion. However, there is still a residual risk of transmitting diseases. Besides, plasma fractions also can impair the immune system and elicit severe side effects. They have to be prescribed with the greatest care and only in settings where the therapy promises success. If possible, plasma fractions should be avoided where possible, just as all other blood products should.

Although the reduction of the use of plasma fractions does not receive the same attention as the reduction of cellular component use, many methods have been devised to reduce the use of these blood products. The strategies described below can be remembered with the mnemonic MANAGER:
M: Monitoring and evaluation
A: Avoid blood loss
N: Need established
A: Administration
G: Generating endogenous resources
E: Existence of pharmaceutical alternatives
R: Recombinant products.

M: Monitoring

Ask yourself: Is it beneficial to obtain more information about the patient (e.g., a laboratory parameter) that could guide therapy more exactly? Would it be beneficial simply to monitor the patient rather than rushing him/her into therapy? Three examples may illustrate this.
• Pregnant women who are Rh-negative usually receive anti-D-immunoglobulin (see above). However, establishing whether the patient in question has a "weak D" (Du-positive), a complete mole, or whether the father of the child is also Rh-negative, eliminates unnecessary anti-D-immunoglobulin exposure since such patients do not need it [34].

• Patients who have been bitten by a poisonous animal can sometimes be treated with antiserum. Poison detection kits and clinical monitoring helps to see whether poison sufficient to harm the patient has been injected with the bite. If not, antiserum is not needed. When the need for antivenom is established, monitoring of the residual amount of toxin in the blood can guide the use of antivenom. This typically reduces the amount of antivenom given [54].
• Patients with clotting abnormalities may be given plasma-derived clotting factors. Using an algorithm to monitor their clotting abnormalities with tests such as thromboelastography may reduce unnecessary clotting factor therapy [55].

A: Avoid blood loss and circumstances that may lead to exposure to blood products

The use of plasma fractions can be reduced when overall blood loss is minimized. Ask yourself: Is there any way to reduce the overall blood loss of the patient? Expertise in surgical technique or the use of minimally invasive procedures can reduce blood loss and with it, the loss of plasma factors. Surgery can even be performed in patients who are coagulopathic, providing the surgical technique is meticulous. When blood loss occurs, it is sometimes possible to recover the lost blood, including plasma fractions. Concentrating and returning residual blood in a cardiopulmonary bypass by means of certain techniques allows for recovery of autologous plasma proteins, among them clotting factors, for the patient [56]. Also, ascites can be concentrated and autologous plasma proteins returned [57].

Forethought may also reduce a patient's exposure to blood products. Ask yourself: Is my patient in danger of developing a condition that may require therapy with plasma fractions? If so, can this condition be avoided? For instance, vaccination of patients at risk for a disease may make post-exposure immunoglobulin therapy unnecessary. Patients with severe hemophilia often develop hemophiliac arthropathies. They may benefit from early knee arthroplasty, since this may reduce their future use of clotting factor concentrates [58].

N: Need established (indication given?)

When a plasma fraction is considered for treatment, ask yourself: Is there a real need to expose my patient to blood products? Is there a proven benefit to the patient if I give him/her the product? Am I sure the product is not contraindicated? A thorough knowledge of the real benefits and risks of blood fractions drastically reduces their use.

A: Administration

Timing, dosing, and the route of administration have a bearing on the total amount of plasma fraction given. Therefore, ask yourself: What timing, dosing, and route of administration brings maximum benefit without exposing the patient to unnecessary plasma products? Here are some examples:

• Patients who undergo surgery with a cardiopulmonary bypass need to be anticoagulated. This is often done with heparin. When such patients require plasma factor replacement, the infusion should be withheld until after the neutralization of heparin. This reduces the amount of concentrate needed.

• The administration of coagulation factor concentrates to maintain the blood level of a patient above the through level is inversely related to the time between the boli given, which means that more frequent, smaller bolus injections reduce the total amount of coagulation factor given when compared to less frequent, but high-dose injections [59]. However, the continuous infusion of factors has totally eliminated the need for intervals between bolus injections and therefore maximally reduces the factor concentrate requirements [60].

• Dosing of snake antivenom may be varied. It has been shown that a low single-dose administration of an antivenom for neurotoxic symptoms of snake bites is as effective as a multiple high-dose regimen [61].

G: Generate endogenous resources

When plasma proteins are lacking in patients, it may still be possible to increase the production of these proteins pharmacologically. Desmopressin may raise the level of FVIII and the vWF. Vitamin K may raise the level of vitamin K-dependent plasma factors. Liver transplant patients who typically receive antiviral agents and immunoglobulins for protection against hepatitis B infection can undergo an enhanced program of vaccination; they often develop sufficient autologous hepatitis B antibodies to allow immunoglobulin therapy to be terminated [62]. Therefore, before you think about giving a plasma-derived product, check whether there is a way to activate the patient's body to help itself.

E: Existence of non-blood pharmaceutical alternatives

There are quite a few pharmaceuticals that can reduce the use of plasma fractions. Ask yourself: Is there any drug

available that may reduce the use of the plasma product? Is there anything that may replace the function of the missing protein? For example, tranexamic acid may reduce the use of cryoprecipitate in patients undergoing liver transplantation [63]. Antiviral drugs may be as effective or even superior to immunoglobulin therapy against cytomegalovirus infection in transplant recipients [64]. Immunoglobulins extracted from human milk may be a good source of immunoglobulin A for babies with immunodeficiencies or with mucosal infections [65]. This may be superior to IVIG therapy. Always make sure that you do not miss a suitable pharmacological approach.

R: Recombinant products

When a patient cannot be treated with the above measures, a recombinant product that can replenish the missing factor may be available. Therefore, ask yourself: Is there any recombinant plasma product that may meet the needs of my patient?

Key points

• Every plasma sample has a unique composition.
• Using fractionation methods, a variety of plasma fractions can be made available for therapy. Most therapy with plasma fractions is empirical. Attempts to demonstrate an improved outcome in patients receiving therapy with such products have failed for most indications.
• Optimization of the use of plasma fractions follows the same line of thought as in attempts to reduce the use of cellular blood components. MANAGER serves as a useful mnemonic to remember the approaches.

Questions for review

1. What do the following terms mean: Bethesda unit, international unit, intravascular recovery, potency, purity, specific activity, survival study, and through level.
2. What is the difference between (a) FFP and cryoprecipitate, (b) IVIGs and hyperimmune globulins, and (c) "three"-factor PCC and "four"-factor PCC?
3. What indications have been proposed for the following plasma fractions: FXIII, C1-esterase inhibitor, high-purity FVIII, albumin, fibrinogen, and IVIGs?
4. What therapeutic options exist for the following conditions, and which are based on blood and which are

not?: hemophilia A without inhibitors, patients with coumadin overdose, vWD, and hereditary angioneurotic edema.

Suggestions for further research

Find out what the term "gammaglobulins" means. What does this term stem from?

How do platelets and fibrinogen interact to form a clot? How can this knowledge be used clinically in cases of thrombopenia?

Exercises and practice cases

Refer to Table 17.1. Compare the recoveries and the molecular weight of the factors. Can you see a relationship?

Refer to Table A.2 which lists the treatment options for factor deficiencies. What non–blood-based therapeutic options are available? What factor deficiency cannot be treated adequately without resorting to donor blood products?

Use the MANAGER strategy to evaluate the therapy of the following patients. What could be done to prevent or reduce their exposure to the blood products? List all the points you find with a thorough literature search using the mnemonic MANAGER.
• Dental surgery in hemophilia B.
• A baby girl with ecchymosis and hemorrhagic bullae with a protein C activity of 3%.
• A male patient with a history of unexplained thrombocytopenia and vWD Type 2B.

Homework

List all available pharmacological and blood-based therapeutic options available in your hospital to treat patients with a deficiency of plasma proteins.

References

1. Farrugia A, Robert P. Plasma protein therapies: current and future perspectives. *Best Pract Res Clin Haematol* 2006;**19**: 243–258.
2. Kingdon HS, Lundblad RL. An adventure in biotechnology: the development of haemophilia A therapeutics—from whole-blood transfusion to recombinant DNA to gene therapy. *Biotechnol Appl Biochem* 2002;**35**:141–148.
3. Mannucci PM, Tuddenham EG. The hemophilias–from royal genes to gene therapy. *N Engl J Med* 2001;**344**: 1773–1779.
4. Romisch J, Feussner A, Vermöhlen S, Stöhr HA. A protease isolated from human plasma activating factor VII independent of tissue factor. *Blood Coagul Fibrinol* 1999;**10**:471–479.
5. Fritsma MG. Use of blood products and factor concentrates for coagulation therapy. *Clin Lab Sci* 2003;**16**:115–119.
6. Practice guidelines for blood component therapy: A report by the American Society of Anesthesiologists Task Force on Blood Component Therapy. *Anesthesiology* 1996;**84**: 732–747.
7. Franchini M, Lippi G. Prothrombin complex concentrates: an update. *Blood Transfus* 2010;**8**:149–154.
8. Schochl H, Nienaber U, Maegele M, *et al.* Transfusion in trauma: thromboelastometry-guided coagulation factor concentrate-based therapy versus standard fresh frozen plasma-based therapy. *Crit Care* 2011;**15**:R83.
9. Grottke O, Rossaint R. Prothrombin complex concentrate (PCC) for the treatment of coagulopathy associated with massive bleeding. *Wien Klin Wochenschr* 2010;**122** (Suppl 5):S23–24.
10. Hay CR. Porcine factor VIII: current status and future developments. *Haemophilia* 2002;**8** (Suppl 1):24–27; discussion 28–32.
11. Goudemand J, Negrier C, Ounnoughene N, Sultan Y. Clinical management of patients with von Willebrand's disease with a VHP vWF concentrate: the French experience. *Haemophilia* 1998;**4** (Suppl 3):48–52.
12. Kreuz W, Meili E, Peter-Salonen K, *et al.* Efficacy and tolerability of a pasteurised human fibrinogen concentrate in patients with congenital fibrinogen deficiency. *Transfus Apher Sci* 2005;**32**:247–253.
13. Parameswaran R, Dickinson JP, de Lord S, Keeling DM, Colvin BT. Spontaneous intracranial bleeding in two patients with congenital afibrinogenaemia and the role of replacement therapy. *Haemophilia* 2000;**6**:705–708.
14. Fries D, Martini WZ. Role of fibrinogen in trauma-induced coagulopathy. *Br J Anaesth* 2010;**105**:116–121.
15. Society of Thoracic Surgeons Blood Conservation Guideline Task Force, Ferraris VA, Brown JR, Despotis GJ, *et al.* 2011 update to the Society of Thoracic Surgeons and the Society of Cardiovascular Anesthesiologists blood conservation clinical practice guidelines. *Ann Thorac Surg* 2011;**91**: 944–982.
16. Liumbruno G, Bennardello F, Lattanzio A, Piccoli P, Rossetti G; Italian Society of Transfusion Medicine and Immunohaematology (SIMTI) Working Party. Recommendations for the use of antithrombin concentrates and prothrombin complex concentrates. *Blood Transfus* 2009;**7**: 325–334.

17. Josic D, Hoffer L, Buchacher A. Preparation of vitamin K-dependent proteins, such as clotting factors II, VII, IX and X and clotting inhibitor protein C. *J Chromatogr B Analyt Technol Biomed Life Sci* 2003;**790**:183–197.

18. Wiedermann CJ, Hoffmann JN, Juers M, *et al.* High-dose antithrombin III in the treatment of severe sepsis in patients with a high risk of death: efficacy and safety. *Crit Care Med* 2006;**34**:285–292.

19. Bereczky Z, Kovacs KB, Muszbek L. Protein C and protein S deficiencies: similarities and differences between two brothers playing in the same game. *Clin Chem Lab Med* 2010;**48** (Suppl 1):S53–66.

20. Radosevich M, Zhou FL, Huart JJ, Burnouf T. Chromatographic purification and properties of a therapeutic human protein C concentrate. *J Chromatogr B Analyt Technol Biomed Life Sci* 2003;**790**:199–207.

21. Bernard GR, Vincent JL, Laterre PF, *et al.* Efficacy and safety of recombinant human activated protein C for severe sepsis. *N Engl J Med* 2001;**344**:699–709.

22. Liumbruno GM, Bennardello F, Lattanzio A, Piccoli P, Rossettias G; Italian Society of Transfusion Medicine and Immunohaematology (SIMTI). Recommendations for the use of albumin and immunoglobulins. *Blood Transfus* 2009;**7**:216–234.

23. Boschetti N, Stucki M, Späth PJ, Kempf C. Virus safety of intravenous immunoglobulin: future challenges. *Clin Rev Allergy Immunol* 2005;**29**:333–344.

24. Sokos DR, Berger M, Lazarus HM. Intravenous immunoglobulin: appropriate indications and uses in hematopoietic stem cell transplantation. *Biol Blood Marrow Transplant* 2002;**8**:117–130.

25. Hamrock DJ. Adverse events associated with intravenous immunoglobulin therapy. *Int Immunopharmacol* 2006;**6**:535–542.

26. Katz U, Shoenfeld Y. Review: intravenous immunoglobulin therapy and thromboembolic complications. *Lupus* 2005;**14**:802–808.

27. Bayary J, Dasgupta S, Misra N, *et al.* Intravenous immunoglobulin in autoimmune disorders: an insight into the immunoregulatory mechanisms. *Int Immunopharmacol* 2006;**6**:528–534.

28. Aries PM, Hellmich B, Gross WL. Intravenous immunoglobulin therapy in vasculitis: speculation or evidence? *Clin Rev Allergy Immunol* 2005;**29**:237–245.

29. Arzouk N, Snanoudj R, Beauchamp-Nicoud A, *et al.* Parvovirus B19-induced anemia in renal transplantation: a role for rHuEPO in resistance to classical treatment. *Transpl Int* 2006;**19**:166–169.

30. Zhang Z, Xie YW, Hong J, *et al.* Purification of severe acute respiratory syndrome hyperimmune globulins for intravenous injection from convalescent plasma. *Transfusion* 2005;**45**:1160–1164.

31. Lovrecek D, Tomic S. A century of antivenom. *Coll Anthropol* 2011;**35**:249–258.

32. LoVecchio F, Klemens J, Roundy EB, Klemens A. Serum sickness following administration of Antivenin (Crotalidae) Polyvalent in 181 cases of presumed rattlesnake envenomation. *Wilderness Environ Med* 2003;**14**:220–221.

33. Lavonas EJ, Ruha AM, Banner W, *et al.* Unified treatment algorithm for the management of crotaline snakebite in the United States: results of an evidence-informed consensus workshop. *BMC Emerg Med* 2011;**11**:2.

34. Fung Kee Fung K. Prevention of Rh alloimmunization: are we there yet? *J Obstet Gynaecol Can* 2003;**25**:716–719.

35. Naithani R, Kumar R, Mahapatra M, Tyagi S, Mishra P. Efficacy and safety of anti-D for immune thrombocytopenic purpura in children. *Indian Pediatr* 2010;**47**:517–519.

36. Frachon X, Pommereuil M, Berthier AM, *et al.* Management options for dental extraction in hemophiliacs: a study of 55 extractions (2000–2002). *Oral Surg Oral Med Oral Pathol Oral Radiol Endod* 2005;**99**:270–275.

37. Berntrop E. Die Auswirkungen einer Substitutionstherapie auf das Immunsystem von Blutern. *Hämostaseologie* 1994:74–80.

38. Sultan Y. High purity factor VIII concentrates for the treatment of HIV-positive patients with haemophilia. *Blood Coagul Fibrinol* 1995;**6** (Suppl 2):S80–81.

39. Keeling D, Tait C, Makris M. Guideline on the selection and use of therapeutic products to treat haemophilia and other hereditary bleeding disorders. A United Kingdom Haemophilia Center Doctors' Organisation (UKHCDO) guideline approved by the British Committee for Standards in Haematology. *Haemophilia* 2008;**14**:671–684.

40. Mathews V, Viswabandya A, Baidya S, *et al.* Surgery for hemophilia in developing countries. *Semin Thromb Hemost* 2005;**31**:538–543.

41. Stobart K, Iorio A, Wu JK. Clotting factor concentrates given to prevent bleeding and bleeding-related complications in people with hemophilia A or B. *Cochrane Database Syst Rev* 2006;(2):CD003429.

42. Rodriguez-Merchan EC, Wiedel JD, Wallny T, *et al.* Elective orthopaedic surgery for inhibitor patients. *Haemophilia* 2003;**9**:625–631.

43. Goudemand J, Scharrer I, Berntorp E, *et al.* Pharmacokinetic studies on Wilfactin, a von Willebrand factor concentrate with a low factor VIII content treated with three virus-inactivation/removal methods. *J Thromb Haemost* 2005;**3**:2219–2227.

44. Federici AB. Management of von Willebrand disease with factor VIII/von Willebrand factor concentrates: results from current studies and surveys. *Blood Coagul Fibrinol* 2005;**16** (Suppl 1):S17–21.

45. Lipkind HS, Kurtis JD, Powrie R, Carpenter MW. Acquired von Willebrand disease: management of labor and delivery with intravenous dexamethasone, continuous factor concentrate, and immunoglobulin infusion. *Am J Obstet Gynecol* 2005;**192**:2067–2070.

46. Berntorp E, Petrini P. Long-term prophylaxis in von Willebrand disease. *Blood Coagul Fibrinol* 2005;**16** (Suppl 1):S23–26.

47. Mannucci PM. Management of von Willebrand disease in developing countries. *Semin Thromb Hemost* 2005;**31**: 602–609.

48. Alperin JB. Coagulopathy caused by vitamin K deficiency in critically ill, hospitalized patients. *JAMA* 1987;**258**: 1916–1919.

49. Yasaka M, Sakata T, Naritomi H, Minematsu K. Optimal dose of prothrombin complex concentrate for acute reversal of oral anticoagulation. *Thromb Res* 2005;**115**: 455–459.

50. Galan AM, Reverter JC, Pino M, *et al*. Concentrates containing factor IX could improve haemostasis under conditions of thrombocytopenia: studies in an in vitro model. *Vox Sang* 2002;**82**:113–118.

51. McLeod BC. Therapeutic apheresis: use of human serum albumin, fresh frozen plasma and cryosupernatant plasma in therapeutic plasma exchange. *Best Pract Res Clin Haematol* 2006;**19**:157–167.

52. Mundy CA. Intravenous immunoglobulin in the management of hemolytic disease of the newborn. *Neonatal Netw* 2005;**24**:17–24.

53. Longhurst HJ. Emergency treatment of acute attacks in hereditary angioedema due to C1 inhibitor deficiency: what is the evidence? *Int J Clin Pract* 2005;**59**:594–599.

54. Theakston RD. An objective approach to antivenom therapy and assessment of first-aid measures in snake bite. *Ann Trop Med Parasitol* 1997;**91**:857–865.

55. Sorensen B, Ingerslev J Tailoring haemostatic treatment to patient requirements—an update on monitoring haemostatic response using thrombelastography. *Haemophilia* 2005;**11** (Suppl 1):1–6.

56. Samolyk KA, Beckmann SR, Bissinger RC. A new practical technique to reduce allogeneic blood exposure and hospital costs while preserving clotting factors after cardiopulmonary bypass: the Hemobag. *Perfusion* 2005;**20**:343–349.

57. Borzio M, Romagnoni M, Sorgato G, *et al*. A simple method for ascites concentration and reinfusion. *Dig Dis Sci* 1995;**40**: 1054–1059.

58. Bae DK, Yoon KH, Kim HS, Song SJ. Total knee arthroplasty in hemophilic arthropathy of the knee. *J Arthroplasty* 2005;**20**:664–668.

59. Morfini M, Messori A, Longo G. Factor VIII pharmacokinetics: intermittent infusion versus continuous infusion. *Blood Coagul Fibrinol* 1996;**7** (Suppl 1):S11–14.

60. Batorova A, Martinowitz U. Continuous infusion of coagulation factors. *Haemophilia* 2002;**8**:170–177.

61. Agarwal R, Aggarwal AN, Gupta D, Behera D, Jindal SK. Low dose of snake antivenom is as effective as high dose in patients with severe neurotoxic snake envenoming. *Emerg Med J* 2005;**22**:397–399.

62. Starkel P, Stoffel M, Lerut J, Horsmans Y. Response to an experimental HBV vaccine permits withdrawal of HBIg prophylaxis in fulminant and selected chronic HBV-infected liver graft recipients. *Liver Transpl* 2005;**11**:1228–1234.

63. Boylan JF, Klinck JR, Sandler AN, *et al*. Tranexamic acid reduces blood loss, transfusion requirements, and coagulation factor use in primary orthotopic liver transplantation. *Anesthesiology* 1996;**85**:1043–1048; discussion 30A–31A.

64. Varga M, Remport A, Hídvégi M, *et al*. Comparing cytomegalovirus prophylaxis in renal transplantation: single center experience. *Transpl Infect Dis* 2005;**7**:63–67.

65. Carbonare CB, Carbonare SB, Carneiro-Sampaio MM. Secretory immunoglobulin A obtained from pooled human colostrum and milk for oral passive immunization. *Pediatr Allergy Immunol* 2005;**16**:574–581.

18 Transfusion Medicine

Medical use of blood has always been controversial. Formerly, blood letting was considered to be the cure for all ailments. Nowadays it seems that the contrary is believed, namely, that blood transfusion is a panacea. Despite rapidly increasing theoretical knowledge about human blood and its medical use, the practice of blood use seems little changed. In fact, today's medical use of blood can be compared with an "early 1900 ironclad ship operating in the rough seas of the 21st century" [1]. Comparison of the facts gleaned from the current literature on blood with current medical practice reveals a huge gap between knowledge and practice. Hopefully, this chapter will close any gap in the clinician's knowledge and practice. A further purpose of this chapter is to help clinicians see why adjustment of current practice toward a more outcome-oriented approach to the medical use of blood, i.e., blood management, is needed.

Objectives

1. To describe what is known about the benefits of allogeneic transfusions.
2. To list different methods used to define a "transfusion trigger" and to state the limitations of these.
3. To explain the risks and side effects of allogeneic transfusions.
4. To examine current guidelines for the use of red cells, platelets, white cells, and plasma, and the basis for these guidelines.
5. To define the risk–benefit ratio of blood transfusions.

Definitions

Transfusion: Infusion of blood or blood components into a living being. Blood can be derived from various sources:
• *Autologous transfusion*: Blood taken from a patient is stored and then infused into the same patient. The patient receives his/her own blood.
• *Allogeneic (= isogenic, homologous) transfusion*: Blood from another, genetically distinct individual of the same species, a blood donor, is infused.
• *Heterologous transfusion*: Blood from a different species, e.g., a cow, is infused into a human.

A brief history

Blood has always been viewed as something special. It has been credited with magic qualities and healing properties. People believed blood determined the qualities of an individual, and that such qualities could be transferred in the blood. Therefore, blood from wounded heroes was collected and drunk [2]. Blood has also been drunk in attempts to cure anemia and epilepsy. Royalty from various dynasties have bathed in blood in attempts to cure their ailments. The principle "like cures like" underlies attempts to use blood for wound care. Because blood runs out of a wound, it was thought a cure could be obtained by returning blood to the wound. Some cultures used human blood mixed with oil. In Asian cultures, kidnapped children were hung head-down over a pot

Basics of Blood Management, Second Edition. Petra Seeber and Aryeh Shander.
© 2013 John Wiley & Sons, Ltd. Published 2013 by John Wiley & Sons, Ltd.

containing hot oil and their blood was let and flowed into the oil. This "human oil" was used to cure wounds [2]. Most ancient cultures used such cruel methods to obtain and use blood for medicinal purposes. Only the ancient Hebrews were forbidden to use blood for medical purposes [3].

Aside from peroral and external use of blood, its injection has kindled the interest of poets and scientists alike. In Greek mythology there are descriptions of attempts to open a blood vessel and to instill some fluids in exchange, including, on occasions, blood. A first, yet questionable, attempt to infuse blood was made to rejuvenate Pope Innocent VIII in 1492. Nevertheless, he died, as did the boys who "donated" their blood. Later, in the 17th century, attempts were made to transfuse blood, first animal to animal, later animal to human. The indications for transfusion were psychiatric disorders. Blood of a sheep, a tame animal, was thought to calm a madman. Well, it did and he died. The first blood transfusions were unsuccessful and were therefore soon banned by authorities, among them the Pope [3].

New attempts to transfuse were made in the 19th century. At the beginning of the 1800s, James Blundell transfused a man who suffered from vomiting [4]. He died, but this did not stop Blundell from trying again. He finally succeeded in transfusing blood in 50% of his cases—a miracle indeed, considering he had no idea about blood groups. Blundell's success encouraged other physicians. In time, hundreds of patients were transfused. Problems arising during the development of blood transfusions, e.g., with blood banking, were to some extent overcome.

Apart from the challenges in the blood bank sector, other challenges had to be faced concerning the indications for transfusions. The historical work of Adams and Lundi, who claimed that oxygen transport is impaired if hemoglobin falls below 10 g/dL or if the hematocrit is below 30%, has been used in the form of the 10/30 rule as a "transfusion trigger." More recent findings have shown that Adam and Lundi's work is a valuable physiological study, but cannot be used to define a transfusion trigger. However, use of the 10/30 rule continues—no matter how deleterious the effects. John Maynard Keynes seemed to be right when he claimed: "The difficulty lies, not in the new ideas, but in escaping the old ones." History has shown that—in response to the acquired immune deficiency syndrome (AIDS) pandemic—no ill effects were observed when the transfusion trigger was lowered and substantially less blood transfused.

Guidelines were formulated to guide the decision to transfuse. Transfusion guidelines have changed considerably in developed countries within the last 25 years. Before the AIDS era, guidelines often included a special transfusion trigger in the form of a hemoglobin level warranting transfusions in all patients. With the recognition of the dangers of transfusion, the focus of guidelines has shifted more toward a patient-oriented approach to transfusion medicine that takes into account the clinical condition of the individual patient. This has been mirrored in some subsequent changes in behavior [5]. Decreased reliance on an arbitrary transfusion trigger has been observed in parallel with increased interest in autologous transfusions.

Why do physicians transfuse?

According to Spiess, "Physicians have the best of intentions in applying the therapy, but the decision to transfuse is driven by fear (i.e., of not acting, lawsuit, or adverse outcome) and emotion. The transfusion trigger, a particular hemoglobin level of discomfort in the prescribing physician, is not defined by clear physiologic parameters. To date, we do not have a real time monitor of oxygen supply and demand ... Therefore, physicians make transfusion decisions based upon their past teaching and enculturation. We are encultured to believe that giving blood saves lives, yet there is little data published to support such conclusion" [6]. Reading this, clinicians may wonder what really is behind allogeneic transfusions—science or emotion?

Current transfusion practice is extremely variable. For total knee replacement, for instance, one center may transfuse 12% of its patients, while another transfuses 87% of its patients [7]. Similar differences in transfusion practice are observed in many other procedures. The reasons for the variability are not usually due to variability in case acuity, but stem from the fact that there are no valid scientific data driving a unified transfusion practice. Therefore, surrogate decision-makers determine transfusion practice. These include industry, hierarchy, and peers, as well as the emotions and medical education history of the treating physician. A more "official" indication for transfusions is that the "transfusion trigger" has been reached. Automatically blood is ordered once a certain laboratory value appears on the patient's sheet. This seems a more scientific approach, since the physician just follows the guidelines. But is treating a laboratory value for the benefit of the patient or to reassure the physician?

In order to escape such biased decision-making, the presumed benefits of transfusion therapy should be examined in the light of medical evidence. Two basic questions require an answer: (a) Are patients for whom transfusion therapy is considered at risk for adverse outcome? and (b) Can these adverse outcomes be averted by the intended transfusion therapy? The answers to these two questions then need to be integrated into the medical decision-making for the blood management of any given patient. For ease, the decision-making process that is described below will follow the well-known mnemonic BRAND (Benefits, Risks, Alternatives, Nothing done, Decision).

What do you get when ordering a blood product?

When clinicians order a vial of penicillin, they just have to look at the vial's label to obtain a complete list of contents. Such a label is not available for most blood products, though, and no label could ever list all the constituents in the blood bag. However, better knowledge of what actually is transfused into a patient, apart from the contents on the blood bag label, should influence the clinician's therapeutic decision.

Red cell concentrates

Red cell concentrates, either sourced from whole blood donations or achieved by apheresis, vary in their properties. The apheresis product has a relatively stable red cell content (interunit variation 6%), while the product from whole blood donations varies widely in red cell content (up to two-fold variation) [8]. This leads to the delivery of red cell concentrates in varying volumes, typically between 200 and 450 mL/bag, and with varying hematocrits, typically between 50% and 70%. Less than 0.8% of the stored red cells should be hemolyzed after the median storage time. After the maximum storage time, 24-hour *in vivo* red cell survival after transfusion should be 70% (recovery rate), the remaining 30% of red cells being destroyed during the first 24 hours after transfusion.

The crudest red cell concentrates contain the cellular portion of centrifuged blood, including white cells and platelets. Other red cell concentrates from whole blood donations are buffy coat-free, i.e., with reduced

amounts of white cells and platelets. Filtration of red cell concentrates further reduces the amount of leukocytes in the unit.

Efforts are under way to standardize red cell concentrates and to reduce the variability of the contents. It was proposed that a single unit of red cells should be delivered with 50 g of hemoglobin and in additive solutions that may be able to reduce storage lesions [9]. If patients react allergically to foreign proteins or the presence of plasma proteins (antibodies) may be detrimental, red cell concentrates can also be washed with saline to remove almost all plasma (see Chapter 17).

Red cell concentrates are usually stored at low temperature, namely, normal refrigerator temperature (4 °C). This temperature reduces the metabolic rate of the red cells and possible bacterial growth. Freezing must be prevented as this would lead to hemolysis. Depending on the time and manner of storage, red cells develop various types of storage lesions [10–13]. They lose ATP and at the same time their shape. First, they develop spiculae and become echinocytes. Then, they swell and become more spherocytic. Finally, they shed their spiculae as lipid vesicles and become completely spherocytic. They lose their deformability and their osmotic resistance. Besides, they tend to aggregate and to form stacks, called "rouleau" formation [14]. The loss of ATP as well as the loss of nitric oxide during storage depresses the red blood cells' ability to vasodilate the microcirculation and nearby vessels so that they can no longer participate efficiently in the vasoregulatory process. Besides, red cell surface receptors, among others those making red cells stick to the vessel wall, are also activated during storage. Storage therefore has a proadhesive effect on red cells. During storage, red cells also lose antioxidants, resulting in oxidative damage to the red cell cytoskeleton and membrane. Hemoglobin is reduced to methemoglobin, which cannot bind oxygen. Additionally, blood stored for more than 7 days is deplete of 2,3-diphosphoglycerate (2,3-DPG), a compound needed to release oxygen to the tissues. The oxygen dissociation curve is shifted to the left and red cells cannot easily release oxygen. Besides, new antigens may be expressed on the membrane during storage [15]. So, compatibility testing performed before storage may no longer be valid after storage. Taken together, stored red blood cell concentrates are a proinflammatory, procoagulatory cocktail.

White cells, present even in leukocyte-depleted products and therefore simultaneously stored within blood packs, also impair the red cell function. They increase hemolysis and potassium level due to leakage from the red cells. Cytokines released from leukocytes accumulate in the stored blood product. Soluble lipids, being similar to platelet activating factor, accumulate. These lipids do not seem to come from white cells and therefore cannot be reduced by leukoreduction [9].

During storage, red cells as well as residual white cells and platelets undergo proteolysis, resulting in the release of their contents into the supernatant of the red blood cell concentrate. The amount of protein found in the red blood cell concentrate increases gradually over the time of storage. Theoretically, all compounds of the red cell, the proteome (see Table A.4), lipids, minerals, carbohydrates, and nucleic acids, can be found in the supernatant of red blood cell concentrates. Proteomics is shedding new light on this topic and about 200 proteins have been found in the red cell, of which about 25% are uncharacterized [16]. Table 18.1 lists some of the constituents

Table 18.1 Examples of constituents found in the supernatant of stored red cell concentrates.

Constituent	Biological activity
Adenine	Nutrient
Albumin, haptoglobin, transferrin, apolipoprotein, actin, hemoglobin (as fragments or isoforms)	Common proteins found abundantly with known functions
Alpha-1B glycoprotein	Function unknown, possibly immunoglobulin-related
Anticoagulant (e.g., citrate)	Anticoagulation
Bacteria	Sepsis
Carbonic anhydrase I	Catalyzes hydration of carbon dioxide and dehydration of bicarbonate; removal of carbon dioxide by red cells; regulation of functions in the gastrointestinal tract and kidneys (stomach acidity, acid–base and fluid balance)
cDNA clone (hypothetical protein)	Not known
Complement C4 A	Inflammation
Connective tissue-activating peptide (CTAP)	Promoter of neutrophil adhesion
Fibrinogen	Coagulation protein
Free iron	Promotes bacterial growth; modulates endogenous iron metabolism
Glucose	Added nutrient
Immunoglobulins and their fragments	Immunomodulation
Phosphate	Added nutrient
Plasticizers	Toxic (released from blood bags)
S100 calcium-binding protein	Modulates activity of leukocytes, inflammation, cell proliferation, and differentiation, including neoplastic transformation, phosphorylation; regulates enzyme activities, function of cytoskeleton and membranes, intracellular calcium homeostasis; trophicor toxic depending on concentration
Serum amyloid P (SAP)	Acute phase scavenger
Thioredoxin peroxidase B	Antioxidant, regulation of intracellular H_2O_2, may regulate gene expression
Transthyretin	Transport, binding

found in the supernatant of RBC concentrates as well as their presumed functions.

Platelet concentrates

Platelet concentrates come in two different forms: random donor platelets, which are pooled from four to eight whole blood donations, and single donor apheresis platelets.

Random donor platelet concentrates contain a minimum of 5.5×10^{10} platelets/unit in the pool and have a volume of about 150–450 mL. The random donor platelet concentrate can be made either from platelet-rich plasma (PRP platelets) or by centrifugation of the buffy coat (BC platelets). Single donor platelet units are made by apheresis. The minimum number of platelets is 3×10^{11} in a volume of 150–300 mL.

In the additive solution, platelet concentrates contain not only platelets, but also a considerable amount of plasma and red cells, as well as leukocytes, the amount depending on whether the platelets are leukocyte depleted or not.

Platelet concentrates are stored at room temperature (about 22 °C) under gentle agitation. The length of platelet storage depends on the container and the method of collection and processing. A closed system can store platelets for up to 5 days, whereas an open system (e.g., for washing and resuspension of platelets in platelet suspension medium) typically can store platelets for 24 hours only. During storage, some platelet concentrates undergo special treatment. Some units are split or hyperconcentrated for intrauterine or neonatal use; others are irradiated or leukocyte-depleted.

Platelet storage lesions lead to changes in the shape of the platelets and they lose their natural discoid form. The granule content is released and adhesive glycoproteins are expressed, severely impairing function. Stored platelets do not aggregate normally in response to aggregating agents (e.g., epinephrine). Recovery and survival are impaired, especially if the pH is below 6.0. The pH in stored platelets is lowered due to platelet metabolism. In time, stored platelets undergo proteolysis, disintegrating and shedding proteins into the platelet concentrate supernatant. Membrane proteins also change, presenting a changing pattern of antigens; therefore, antigenicity seems to increase with storage [17].

Storage also increases the incidence of transfusion reactions. The longer platelets are stored, the more side effects there are. It has been suggested that reactions to platelet transfusions result from pyrogenic and vasoactive substances accumulated during storage [18]. Since prote-

olysis is a common feature of platelet storage lesions, it would be interesting to know which proteins are released that may affect the patient. Exactly which proteins are released is difficult to say. In fact, this may change depending on the donor and storage time. Potentially, all contents of a platelet can be released once the platelet is damaged. However, as is also the case with red cells, since the proteome (all proteins in the platelet), transcriptome (all mRNA transcripts in the platelet), and all other contents of normal human platelets have not yet been described, it cannot be said with certainty what the supernatant of platelet concentrates contains. Using advanced techniques such as proteomics and transcriptomics, hundreds, if not thousands, of proteins have been found in the platelet, yet the significance of these proteins is poorly understood [19–21]. As far as is understood, platelet-derived proteins have many different functions and releasing such proteins may influence functions in the entire body. It remains to be seen whether platelet-derived clusterin influences apoptosis in transfusion recipients; whether frataxin derived from the transfusion changes iron homeostasis in the recipient; or whether the progesterone receptor-associated protein P48 found in platelets influences progesterone receptor signaling in transfused patients [20].

Granulocyte concentrates

Collection of granulocytes is difficult. The normal amount of circulating granulocytes is 30×10^7/kg. For therapy, a daily dose of more than 15×10^7/kg is recommended. Therefore, either the buffy coats of several donations are pooled or a single donor is prepared with prednisone or growth factors before donation. Blood from patients with chronic lymphatic leukemia circulate enough granulocytes to provide for the donation and these patients are sometimes asked to donate. To donate sufficient amounts, daily donations or alternate-day donations are requested. This reduces the risk of multiple donor exposure for the patient, but puts the donor at risk. Granulocyte concentrates cannot be stored and are therefore prepared for immediate transfusion.

This shows that granulocyte donations are problematic. They are rarely prescribed. When they are given, they are given ABO and RhD compatible, since they contain many red cells.

Fresh-frozen plasma

Fresh frozen plasma (FFP) is plasma that is derived from one unit of donated blood by centrifugation. It is frozen to at least −18 °C within 8 hours after donation. When thawed, it can be kept refrigerated for up to 24 hours before use. Storage in the frozen state is needed to prevent rapid loss of the coagulation factor activity, which occurs within hours after storage at room temperature. In some countries, standard FFPs are held in quarantine for 4 months, since they are allowed to be infused only after the donor presents healthy for the next donation.

Some countries also provide plasma units derived from pooled plasma. This is treated with solvent–detergent (SD-FFP) or methylene blue (MB-FFP) to reduce viral transmission. Such plasma is not kept under quarantine.

FFP contains all the components usually found in the blood; however, the number of cellular components is starkly reduced, so that only a few red cells, white cells, and platelets remain. FFP contains at least 60 g of protein/L. This proteome is a mixture of known and unknown proteins (see Table A.3) [22]. About 120 proteins have been characterized, many others have not. The main proteins in FFP are albumin, immunoglobulins, fibrinogen, and transferrin. In addition to proteins, FFP contains metabolites, cellular components, tumor markers, (pregnancy) hormones, etc. The clotting factor and other protein levels in FFP vary and are not only dependent on the donor, but also on the duration and conditions of storage. After 8 hours of storage at room temperature, 13% of factor VIII activity is lost; after 24 hours about 30% of the activity is lost. The overall loss of plasma factors participating in coagulation, anticoagulation, and clot lysis is non-proportional, with some proteins deteriorating faster than others. Finally, stored plasma is a procoagulant, because anticoagulatory proteins (protein S, protein C) deteriorate faster than procoagulatory components.

Risk factors for adverse outcome

Before a decision is made in blood management, it needs to be established whether the problem to be treated is actually outcome-relevant. Relevant outcomes are survival, development of stroke, myocardial infarction and renal failure, wound healing, ventilator-dependence, length of hospital stay, among many more.

Blood management-related risk factors for adverse outcome are anemia of any degree (long before ischemia develops) and active bleeding. Anemia is a multiplier for mortality in many different settings, such as in the perioperative period, and in patients with heart failure, chronic obstructive pulmonary disease, kidney disease,

infection, etc. [23]. Besides, anemia itself appears to endanger the patient, resulting in impaired tissue oxygenation, cardiovascular instability, heart failure with or without left ventricular hypertrophy, progressive kidney failure, respiratory failure with or without ventilator dependence, and difficulties weaning from the ventilator. It seems to be true that the more severe the anemia, the greater the risk of adverse events. Further, the sicker the patient, the less he/she can tolerate anemia.

Laboratory markers have been used as surrogate markers for the risk factors anemia and active bleeding. Curiously, arbitrary laboratory values have been adopted as "transfusion triggers." It is simply assumed that the makers reliably reflect the actual risk factors and that correction of those laboratory values improves the patient's outcome. Over time, a vast variety of such "transfusion triggers" have been tested for different blood products. The most prominent are a hemoglobin or platelet level or a certain coagulation parameter (e.g., the international normalized ratio [INR]) as a guide for the use of red cells, platelets, or plasma, respectively. Hemoglobin values are not reliable to diagnose anemia, since hypervolemia may mimic anemia. They are not even able to predict the development of ischemia in any given patient [24]. There is also no specific coagulation parameter predicting that the patient will bleed. Other transfusion triggers include surrogate markers of global hypoxia, such as an oxygen extraction ratio of less than 50% in combination with a low hemoglobin level [25], a low blood pH or a high blood lactate. Surrogate markers for a regional critical oxygen supply and impending or manifest ischemia have been tested for various organs, e.g., the brain, heart, kidney, and gut. Changes in the electroencephalogram, ST segment of the electrocardiogram, kidney function parameters, and gastrointestinal tonometry have been studied for their ability to predict development of anemic ischemia. However, many other factors can influence such values and render them invalid as surrogate markers for (clinically relevant) anemia and as transfusion triggers [26].

BRAND: Benefits of transfusions

With the diagnosis of anemia or active hemorrhage, the patient is known to be at risk for adverse outcomes. If transfusions are now considered, it has to be established whether they are able to prevent these adverse outcomes. Table 18.2 summarizes those outcome variables and whether or not they can be improved with transfusion

Table 18.2 Outcome variables and their modification by transfusion therapy.

Outcome variable	Effect of stored allogeneic red blood cell concentrates
Improved survival	No, on the contrary
Prevention of stroke in anemia	No, on the contrary
Prevention of myocardial infarction in anemia	No, on the contrary
Prevention of renal failure in anemic patients	No, on the contrary
Length of hospital stay	Prolonged
Length of ICU stay	Prolonged
Ventilator dependency	Prolonged

therapy [27–32]. Current evidence thus suggests that transfusions are associated with and the reason for [33] a worse outcome: increased rates of myocardial infarction, stroke, renal failure, infections, impaired wound healing, and consequently, decreased survival [23].

If the stringent tenets of evidence-based medicine, the precautionary principle or simply common sense was used to decide whether or not to transfuse, this intervention would be abandoned after examining the evidence for the benefit of transfusion. But physicians and other healthcare providers hold to the attitude that "blood transfusions saves lives," and continue to let "firm belief" and cultural conditioning dictate their behavior such that they "trust that blood transfusion is a 'life-giving' force" [34].

BRAND: Risks of transfusions

Effects of allogeneic transfusions in the human body

Transfusing stored blood into living human beings causes many changes in the recipient. The most striking changes appear to be induced in the microcirculation. While fresh, deformable autologous red cells squeeze through the narrow vessels of the microcirculation to deliver oxygen, stored red cells lack this ability. The hardened red cells impair the microcirculation and tissue oxygenation. Stored red cells decrease capillary perfusion, increase

sticking and transmigration of leukocytes, induce edema formation in the endothelium, and often slow the blood flow and block vessels [35]. Red cell surface receptors are also activated during storage and the cells therefore tend to adhere more to the vessel wall, contributing to a microvascular traffic jam. Besides, the stored red cells that have lost 2,3-DPG cannot unload oxygen to the tissue. Thus, transfused red cells can load oxygen, but are no longer able to unload it. Apart from the oxygen delivery of fresh red blood cells, stored red cell units obviously do not deliver sufficient oxygen but cause severe microvascular derangement. Although loss of 2,3-DPG and deformability, as well as the increased aggregatability, are partly reversible after transfusion, stored red cells do not function as expected. Oxygen uptake is not increased after transfusion, neither globally nor regionally [36]. Mixed venous oxygen saturation does not increase and lactate levels do not decrease reliably after transfusion of stored red cells [37]. What is even worse, stored red cells not only fail to function as hoped, but also impair tissue oxygenation. Indeed, after 7–14 days' storage, red cells appear to cause so many changes in the microvascular system that measurable tissue "deoxygenation" occurs after transfusion [38].

Transfusion of stored blood also changes coagulation. Stored blood contains procoagulant factors and factors promoting vasoconstriction. Exocytotic microvesicles, e.g., from red cells formed during storage, seem to be only one of the reasons why transfusions are believed to be thrombogenic [39]. In addition, different blood components are primed during storage to initiate coagulation once infused.

Allogeneic transfusions also undoubtedly exert a profound effect on the transfusion recipient's immune system [40]. Such effects have been collectively called TRIM (transfusion-related immunomodulation; see below). TRIM is a multifactoral process caused by, among many other factors, priming of neutrophils during storage, release of cytokines accumulated in the stored blood product, and the surplus of decayed blood cells flooding the reticuloendothelial system for clearance.

Outcome variables

The profoundly negative effects of allogeneic transfusions on the human microcirculation, coagulation, and immune systems result in the deterioration of many outcome variables. Allogeneic transfusions have therefore been termed a risk factor for negative clinical outcomes. On the other hand, transfusions have rarely been shown to be associated with improved outcome.

The risk of postoperative bacterial infection (wound, urinary tract, pneumonia, sepsis, abscess formation) is increased after allogeneic transfusions, a phenomenon shown for standard and leukocyte-depleted red cell concentrates, as well as for stored autologous red cells [41–45]. A meta-analysis demonstrated that transfusions increase the risk for infection after simple surgery by a factor of 3.45. Trauma surgery patients receiving transfusions are 5.3 times more likely to develop an infection than non-transfused patients [46]. Patients who are transfused are more susceptible to developing dose-dependent multiorgan failure [47], are ventilator-dependent for longer, need more vasopressors, remain longer in the intensive care unit (ICU), and have longer stays in hospital [48].

Transfusions also worsen the outcome of patients undergoing surgery for a variety of malignancies, resulting in decreased survival rates, shortened disease-free time, and increased metastasis recurrence [49, 50].

Transfusions diminish the strength of gastrointestinal anastomoses, leading to increased anastomotic leakage [51, 52]. Transfusions after gastrointestinal bleeding increase the likelihood for rebleeding and increase mortality. This is due to the transfusion reversing the hypercoagulable state that naturally develops after hemorrhage [53].

Some particular effects of allogeneic transfusions have been described in neonates. The development of chronic lung disease and retinopathy of prematurity is associated with transfusion exposure [54]. The manifold increase in levels of growth-promoting substances (insulin-like growth factor) in adult blood as compared with neonatal blood may, when transfused, accelerate angiogenesis and may damage a baby's eyes via retinal neovascularization [55]. Oxidative damage [56] by lipids in transfusions may damage the lungs of the premature. Necrotizing enterocolitis is also likely more frequent in babies who have received allogeneic transfusions [57].

A history of transfusion is a risk factor for many diseases, such as stroke and myocardial infarction [58], as well as for intracranial hemorrhage [59]. Interestingly, even infertility is associated with transfusions [60]. The reasons suggested for these associations are long-term immunomodulation and patient infection with various infectious agents causing chronic inflammation. Platelet transfusion has also been implicated as a cause of perioperative stroke [48]. Thromboembolism, deep vein thrombosis, and pulmonary embolism have been associated with many blood products [61].

Patients who suffer from ischemic heart disease are more likely to suffer deleterious effects when anemia is present [62]. This has led to the assumption that such patients benefit from generous red cell transfusion. However, quite the contrary may be the case. Evidence is accumulating demonstrating that the sicker the patient, the less allogeneic transfusions are tolerated. A liberal transfusion strategy is more often associated with reduced exercise tolerance and increased myocardial ischemia than a restrictive one [63, 64]. Patients who are transfused while suffering from an acute coronary syndrome are more likely to die than non-transfused patients with the same syndrome, even after correcting for comorbidities [65]. It has even been suggested that patients transfused to keep the hematocrit above 25% are four times more likely to die than those who are not transfused [66]. Rao et al. summarize current findings as follows: "Previous randomised studies support the conclusion that blood transfusion may, at best, be neutral with respect to survival or, at worst, be associated with either decreased survival or worsening cardiac function" [66].

Kidney function is also dependent on oxygen transport and deteriorates as patients become more anemic. However, as in the case of ischemic heart disease, transfusing anemic patients in an attempt to prevent renal damage is futile. Allogeneic transfusions even increase kidney damage. The reasons for this phenomenon are multifactorial; among those postulated are impaired oxygen unloading capacity of stored red cells, impaired microvascular perfusion with hardened red cells and other factors, leading to tissue deoxygenation rather than oxygenation [67]. Free iron from lysed transfused red cells may contribute to the kidney damage [68].

Overall, transfusions are negatively correlated with short- and long-term survival. Of course, transfused patients are usually in a more severe condition than non-transfused patients. However, when accounting for disease severity, transfusions are still associated with increased perioperative death [48]. It has been shown that patients who have undergone heart surgery and transfusion are twice as likely to die within 5 years compared to those undergoing the same procedures without receiving a transfusion. While those patients receiving transfusions were more severely ill, with correction to take account of comorbidities, transfusions still caused 70% greater mortality [69]. Transfused trauma victims are almost three times as likely to die than other non-transfused patients with the same hemoglobin level and shock severity [70].

Risks and side effects of transfusions

Risks and side effects of transfusions are a major concern and have attracted even more attention than drug-associated risks. Efforts have been made to avoid the dangers associated with them. Governments have instituted mechanisms to control transfusion-associated risks, the United Kingdom based initiative "Serious Hazards of Transfusions" (SHOT) being an example [71]. Transfusion-transmissible infections (TTIs) are considered by the public to be the greatest problem related to transfusions. This may be true in developing countries, but is not the case in developed countries. Only about 1% of events reported to the SHOT initiative were TTIs.

Other risks of transfusion are listed in Table 18.3 [72–78].

Immunomodulatory effects

An effective immune response requires the fine-tuned interaction of all parts of the immune system. Among them are CD4+ T-helper (Th) cells, which recognize antigens in combination with major histocompatibility complex (MHC) type 2 molecules, the latter being expressed only on a few cells, such as B lymphocytes and macrophages. The CD8+ cytotoxic T cells recognize antigens with MHC type 1, the latter being present on all cells with a nucleolus and on platelets. As a result of interaction, different responses occur, all with the aim of ridding the system of intruders. Depending on the mechanisms leading to activation of the immune system, different responses occur. A Th1 response results in CD4+ cell proliferation, release of interleukin (IL)-2, γ-interferon, macrophage activity, delayed-type hypersensitivity, and cytotoxicity. A Th2 response results in increased IL-4, -5, -6, and -10, B-cell activation, and antibody formation.

Immunosuppression results when the normal responses to an antigen are downregulated or modulated. Transfusions cause such changes, a condition called transfusion-related immunomodulation (TRIM). Overall, allogeneic transfusions elicit a persistent, but ineffective, immune response.

Each cellular blood component contains at least some residual platelets and leukocytes that carry MHC molecules, and so does plasma. These allow the body to identify them as foreign. Since transfusions are usually not MHC-matched, they elicit immunological reactions. These may result either in alloimmunization, tolerance, or immunosuppression.

Transfusion antigens confuse the immune system. On the one hand, transfused cells are considered self, i.e., from the same species. On the other, they are considered foreign since they have a different MHC. This kind of situation does not happen in response to other foreign material, such as bacteria. Also, since blood is given intravenously, the immune system lacks costimulation from signals originating from infected tissues and dendritic cells. This lack of costimulation results in anergy and apoptosis of T cells.

Leukocytes from the donor also influence the blood recipient. The necrotic remains of stored white cells preferentially stimulate a Th2 response. This results in increased levels of IL-4, -5, -6, and -10, B-cell activation, and antibody formation. In addition to this, the patient's Th1 response is downregulated, resulting in diminished CD4+ cell proliferation, release of IL-2, γ-interferon, macrophage activity, delayed-type hypersensitivity, and cytotoxicity.

In summary, allogeneic transfusions impair T-cell proliferation, change the CD4 +/CD8+ ratio, reduce delayed hypersensitivity reactions, and release Th2 cytokines while reducing Th1 cytokines to a lesser degree. Macrophage function, natural killer cell activity, and cellular cytolysis are also affected. The more leukocytes that are present in donated blood, the more extensive is the immunomodulation response to transfusion. Reducing the amount of donor leukocytes in blood products is therefore helpful in reducing the immunological side effects of transfusions. However, leukocyte-depleted red cells also affect the immune system, e.g., by suppression of T-cell proliferation [79].

Immune response to autologous transfusions [79, 80]

In contrast to the immune response to allogeneic transfusions, the response to an autologous transfusion is short term. Autologous red cells increase the proliferation of T cells, cytokine secretion, and B-cell activation.

Stored autologous blood seems, in part, to have the same effects on the immune system as stored allogeneic blood. Patients who receive their own preoperatively stored blood experience an impaired natural killer cell function similar in extent to that for allogeneic blood. However, when patients receive fresh autologous blood procured by intraoperative hemodilution, natural killer cell function is increased. This may explain why the postoperative infection rate is reduced in patients who only receive their own fresh blood.

Table 18.3 Risks of transfusions.

Risk	Description	Clinical consequence	Remarks
Bacterial contamination	Bacteria introduced into blood product, multiply in blood bag	Infection to severe, even lethal sepsis	Platelets especially vulnerable since they are stored at room temperature
Clerical error	Wrong blood given to the patient	Incompatibility, hemolysis, kidney failure, death	1:14 000–19 000 transfusions
Alloimmunization	Antibodies develop against blood antigens other than those of the ABO and Rhesus system	Delayed extravascular hemolysis, death	Incidence increases with increased exposure to donor blood; after 10–20 transfusions: >10%; after 100 transfusions: >30%
Febrile non-hemolytic transfusion reaction (FNHTR)	Diagnosis of exclusion; defined as an increase in body temperature of >1°C above pretransfusion value	Fever, shaking chills	Occurs especially after platelet and granulocyte transfusions; attributed to donor white cells and proinflammatory cytokines
Anaphylactic transfusion reactions	Typical anaphylactic reaction	Rapid reaction, sometimes within minutes; urticaria, bronchospasm, hypotension, anaphylactic shock, death; no fever	More allergic reactions occur during platelet transfusion than red cell or plasma transfusion
Transfusion-related acute lung injury (TRALI)	Acute lung injury within 6–24 hours after transfusion	Clinically indistinguishable from acute respiratory distress syndrome	Leukocytes infiltrate the lung, the endothelium is altered, pulmonary edema develops and hyaline membranes form, thus damaging lung tissue; severely underreported

Hemolytic transfusion reactions	Accelerated immune-mediated red cell destruction	Acute hemolysis <24 hours after transfusion: intravascular hemolysis (fever, chills, abdominal and chest pain, nausea, vomiting, hypotension, tachycardia, hemoglobinuria, flushing, renal failure, disseminated intravascular coagulation with uncontrolled bleeding) Chronic (= delayed) hemolysis: extravascular hemolysis (gradual decline in hemoglobin)	Patients with sickle cell disease are especially vulnerable to delayed hemolysis; may suppress erythropoiesis and cause hemolysis that also includes autologous red cells (bystander hemolysis)
Transfusion-associated graft-versus-host disease(TA-GvHD)	Rare, but particularly lethal complication	Symptoms develop 3–30 days after transfusion (fever, watery diarrhea, rash progressing to generalized erythroderma and desquamation). Hemorrhage, infection, and pancytopenia follow. >90% mortality within 1–3 weeks	Caused by proliferating transfused donor T lymphocytes. The donor lymphocytes recognize the recipient's cells as foreign and attack them, while the recipient's system does not identify the donor cells as foreign and as such they are tolerated
Microchimerism	"Mononuclear cell transplantation"	May predispose to autoimmune diseases, chronic graft-versus-host disease, recurrent abortion	"Transplanted" donor cells proliferate and survive in the transfusion recipient's bone marrow for months or years after transfusion
Post-transfusion purpura	Severe thrombocytopenia 1–2 weeks after transfusion	Usually self-limited, but mortality is 13%	Platelet-specific alloantibodies result in destruction of the patient's platelets
Transfusion-associated circulatory overload (TACO)	Too much or too rapid transfusion	Fluid overload (acute respiratory failure, hypertension, decreased cardiac output)	Patients at high risk: renal failure, cardiopulmonary disease, chronic anemia (already hypervolemic)
Iron overload	Transfusion-associated hemosiderosis	Oxidative tissue damage (especially the heart, pancreas)	Always occurs in long-term transfusion therapy

BRAND: "Alternatives"—other therapeutic options

There are many therapeutic and prophylactic options for anemia and active bleeding (be it due to coagulopathy or surgical reasons). Most of these options do not involve the use of allogeneic blood products. As shown in previous chapters, these options are safe and effective, and are indispensable for improving patient outcome. When compared with transfusions, they may be at least as effective in improving outcome, while having a more favorable risk–benefit ratio. Therefore, such treatments deserve their due place in the decision-making process.

BRAND: No transfusion or no therapy at all

When the use of transfusions is being contemplated, the consequences of "no transfusion" should also be considered. However, the consequences of "no transfusion" should not be confused with the consequences of "no therapy." While it may indeed be better not to transfuse the patient, appropriate blood management may still be required. Many, if not all, conditions that typically have resulted in allogeneic transfusions being given do require therapy, but not the transfusion of blood.

Anemia, for example, although only a symptom, most often needs therapy, either by remedying the underlying condition or by directly treating the anemia. If anemia is not treated, problems can ensue. Untreated anemia seems to worsen patient outcome. Depending on the severity of the anemia, the time over which it has developed, and the comorbidities of the patient, symptoms such as fatigue, palpitations and tachycardia, left ventricular hypertrophy, deterioration of kidney function, changes in mental status, dyspnea, etc. result. What is more, anemia also potentiates the ill effects of other medical conditions [81]. To date, it has not been clarified whether all kinds of anemia benefit from therapy. Since anemia may be protective to a certain degree, the value of anemia therapy in addition to therapy for the underlying disease is not fully understood. However, proof is accumulating, showing that some therapies of anemia are beneficial. The benefit depends on the kind of therapy. While patients with cardiovascular and renal dysfunction and anemia benefit from erythropoietin therapy and the resulting correction of anemia (preventing remodeling of the myocardium, improving kidney function, reducing

fatigue, etc.), patients transfused as a therapeutic strategy to correct anemia do not [81, 82].

BRAND: Decision-making

Now that several facts about allogeneic transfusions have been considered, the focus will move to structured decision-making. Decision-making is a cognitive process to select a course of action from available options. It begins with the recognition that something needs to be changed and it ends with a decision about what is to be done. Such decisions may be rational or irrational and have an influence on future success, in this case, the patient outcome. All the information available is required to make a sound decision.

Aids for decision-making, known as decision-making tools, have been devised. Using them, such as PMI or grid analysis, may help clinicians avoid overly emotional decisions. The decision should represent the most beneficial option for the patient, because it takes into account what is known to be beneficial and what is known to be detrimental. Decision-making tools also help clinicians internalize new thinking patterns and aid in transferring recent scientific evidence into routine patient care.

Transfusion guidelines

Medical practice has long been determined by guidelines. Originally, these represented a consensus of expert opinion that defined the standard of practice. More recently, a change has been made toward a more scientific, evidence-based approach to guideline formulation. This is commendable, but since hard data are missing for most of the relevant transfusion issues, the interpretation of the available evidence and therefore the resulting guidelines are still mostly based on expert opinion. This can be clearly seen when guidelines on the same topic issued by different agencies are compared.

Red cell transfusions

When current guidelines are summarized, there are basically three scenarios in which red cell transfusions are still recommended: acute major hemorrhage, severe (symptomatic) anemia, and some specific conditions (e.g., hemoglobinopathy, kernicterus). Since the benefits of red cell transfusions are questionable, guidelines state that transfusions should not be considered when a patient is able to tolerate anemia. Nevertheless, the majority of the guidelines recommend maintaining hemoglobin levels between 7 and 9 g/dL, especially in acute cases, and above 5–6 g/dL in fit, young patients with chronic anemia. Transfusions are rarely recommended if the hemoglobin level is above 10 g/dL.

None of the guidelines compares red cell transfusion with other therapeutic options. It is therefore not stated whether other approaches would lead to the same or even superior outcomes.

Guidelines also list contraindications for red cell transfusions, namely, stable acute and chronic anemia. These conditions include autoimmune anemia, megaloblastic anemia, iron deficiency, and anemia in patients with renal failure [83], all of which can be corrected by non-blood management.

Platelet transfusions

The introduction to a current platelet transfusion guideline states: "The decision to transfuse PCs [platelet concentrates] must not be based exclusively on the platelet count. The absolute indication is severe thrombocytopenia together with clinically relevant bleeding. All the other indications are more or less relative and depend on the clinical condition of the patient" [84]. An even more recent and comprehensive review of platelet transfusions came to the conclusion: "The message of all the science is to use these agents sparingly and with great thought and caution. Platelet products from the blood bank are not to be regarded to be 'normal platelets', nor should the product be regarded as 'magic'. There are suggestions that by using platelet transfusions one can make an inflammatory picture worse and potentially either increase the risk for bleeding or for thrombosis. . . . The fact that clinical behaviour is erratic and seemingly inconsistent means that as a medical industry we have failed to provide a system that supports rational and rapid decision making" [85]. It is in this context that the following platelet transfusion guidelines should be interpreted.

What do the guidelines say about platelet transfusions? It has been suggested that platelet transfusions may be considered for the following conditions:
• **Bone marrow failure** (because of disease, cytotoxic therapy, or irradiation): Without risk factors, a threshold of 5–10^9/L for platelet transfusions is considered safe [86]. Patients with chronic stable thrombocytopenia (e.g., myelodysplasia or aplastic anemia) should be transfused very restrictively, so that alloimmunization is best avoided. For this group of patients, no threshold for prophylactic platelet transfusions is indicated. When risk factors such as fever above 38 °C, fresh minor hemor-

rhage, sepsis, antibiotics, and other hemostatic impairment exist, the transfusion threshold may be lowered.
• **Thrombocytopenic patients** are believed to need a certain number of platelets to undergo procedures safely, but sound scientific evidence is lacking for the prophylactic use of platelet transfusions prior to surgical interventions [86]. In the search for guidelines, refuge was therefore taken in expert opinion. This resulted in the following recommendations: Bone marrow aspirations can be performed without platelet support given that adequate surface pressure is maintained after puncture. A platelet count between 40 and 50×10^9/L is considered desirable for lumbar puncture, epidural catheter insertion, endoscopy, intravascular catheters, liver biopsy, and laparotomy [87]. For surgery in areas where even minor bleeding could be detrimental, e.g., brain or eye surgery, guidelines recommend a platelet count of at least 100×10^9/L. The fact that some physicians perform procedures safely in patients with much lower platelet counts than those stated demonstrates there is no unequivocal agreement to these thresholds. Lumbar punctures, for example, have been performed safely with a patient platelet count of only about 20×10^9/L.

There are conditions where platelets are not recommended unless there is a life-threatening bleeding. These include platelet function disorders and autoimmune thrombocytopenias. If at all possible, other therapeutic approaches should be sought to prevent and treat bleeding and to improve platelet function and count.

There are contraindications to platelet transfusions. Platelets can cause life-threatening thrombosis in conditions where there is a risk of thrombotic consumption of platelets, e.g. thrombotic thrombocytopenic purpura, hemolytic-uremic syndrome, heparin-induced thrombocytopenia, and active disseminated intravascular coagulation.

Granulocyte transfusions

There are no evidence-based indications for granulocyte transfusions [88].

Transfusion may be considered "in prolonged 'reversible' neutropenia with an ANC (absolute neutrophil count) of less than 500/mL, which is refractory to G-CSF therapy and is associated with severe uncontrolled infection" or for congenital neutrophil dysfunction with severe uncontrolled infection [89].

Fresh frozen plasma

Apart from very rare factor deficiencies (factor V) and plasmapheresis for ADAMTS-13-related thrombotic thrombocytopenic purpura, there is no longer any indication for FFP, given the availability of products of modern medicine such as prothrombin complex concentrate (PCC), recombinant factor VIIa and fibrinogen concentrates. Therefore, some European centers have ceased to use FFP [90]. Where this is not the case, FFP is recommended only in cases of massive transfusion and in warfarin-related intracranial hemorrhage [91]. However, the basis for the latter two recommendations is scientifically weak.

Key points

- Medical decision-making is often made using the mnemonic BRAND:
  - **Benefits of transfusions:** Decades of research in the field has not shown any major benefit for patients.
  - **Risks of transfusions:** Allogeneic blood transfusions substantially alter the recipient. They also cause many diseases (TRIM, infections, etc.).
  - **Alternative therapies:** There are many therapeutic options available to treat anemia and active bleeding.
  - **No therapy:** At times, doing nothing rather than transfusing is a sound medical option. However, under certain circumstances, patients greatly benefit from therapy with drugs or methods not involving blood transfusions. "No therapy" is not an alternative to allogeneic transfusion; blood management options are.
  - **Decision:** Blood management is the path to be taken, because blood saves lives, while transfusions do not.

Questions for review

1. Why do physicians transfuse?
2. What are the benefits of allogeneic transfusions?
3. What effects do stored blood products have on the microcirculation?
4. How do allogeneic transfusions affect patient outcome?
5. What results if anemia and active bleeding are left untreated?
6. What do the following abbreviations stand for and how do the conditions present clinically? FNHTR, TACO, TRIM, TRALI, TA-GvHD, and TTI.

Suggestions for further research

Look into current guidelines for blood transfusions. Choose those that state the level of evidence on which

recommendations are based. Sort the recommendations by level and compare recommendations based on scientific evidence with those that are merely the opinion of the authors of the guidelines.

Exercises and practice cases

Mr B requests bilateral hip replacement. He agrees that you should select the most beneficial, or any combination thereof, from the following therapy options:
Use a cell saving device (intra- and post-operatively)
Operate one hip at a time, allowing for restoration of red cell mass
Preoperative autologous donation
Do nothing to prevent blood loss and transfuse allogeneically if the blood count drops
Use acute normovolemic hemodilution
You consider the following factors to be important:
Prevention of infection in the hip is of utmost importance
Hazards of allogeneic transfusions should be avoided
Patient wants to invest as little time as possible in the treatment
Overall cost of treatment, including length of stay, should be minimized

Use grid analysis to decide on the most suitable therapeutic option for this patient. What conclusion do you come to?

Homework

- Find out who is in charge of blood transfusion risk management and quality assurance at your hospital and ask for an opinion on blood management.
- Explain the risks and benefits of blood transfusion and appropriate blood management procedures to a patient.
- Find a reliable source from which to learn about the risks of infection with blood-borne diseases in your country.

References

1. Hathaway EO. Changing educational paradigms in transfusion medicine and cellular therapies: development of a profession. *Transfusion* 2005;**45** (4 Suppl):172S–188S.

2. Mahdihassan S. Blood as the earliest drug, its substitutes, preparations and latest position. *Am J Chin Med* 1986;**14**:104–109.

3. Barsoum N, Kleeman C. Now and then, the history of parenteral fluid administration. *Am J Nephrol* 2002;**22**:284–289.

4. Blundell J. Some account of a case of obstinate vomiting in which an attempt was made to prolong life, by the injection of blood into the veins. Lecturer, in conjunction with Dr. Haighton, on physiology and midwifery, at Guy's Hospital, 1818:296–301.

5. Nuttall GA, Stehling LC, Beighley CM, *et al*. Current transfusion practices of members of the american society of anesthesiologists: a survey. *Anesthesiology* 2003;**99**:1433–1443.

6. Speiss BD. Transfusion and outcome in heart surgery. *Ann Thorac Surg* 2002;**74**:986–987.

7. Gombotz H, Rehak PH, Shander A, Hofmann A. Blood use in elective surgery: the Austrian benchmark study. *Transfusion* 2007;**47**:1468–1480.

8. Hogman CF, Meryman HT. Red blood cells intended for transfusion: quality criteria revisited. *Transfusion* 2006;**46**:137–142.

9. Ho J, Sibbald WJ, Chin-Yee IH. Effects of storage on efficacy of red cell transfusion: when is it not safe? *Crit Care Med* 2003;**31** (12 Suppl):S687–697.

10. Kor DJ, Van Buskirk CM, Gajic O. Red blood cell storage lesion. *Bosn J Basic Med Sci* 2009;**9** (Suppl 1):21–27.

11. Lion N, Crettaz D, Rubin O, Tissot JD. Stored red blood cells: a changing universe waiting for its map(s). *J Proteomics* 2010;**73**:374–385.

12. Hess JR. Red cell storage. *J Proteomics* 2010;**73**:368–373.

13. Kim-Shapiro DB, Lee J, Gladwin MT. Storage lesion: role of red blood cell breakdown. *Transfusion* 2011;**51**:844–851.

14. Krugluger W, Koller M, Hopmeier P. Development of a carbohydrate antigen during storage of red cells. *Transfusion* 1994;**34**:496–500.

15. Fritsma MG. Use of blood products and factor concentrates for coagulation therapy. *Clin Lab Sci* 2003;**16**:115–119.

16. Kakhniashvili DG, Bulla LA Jr, Goodman SR. The human erythrocyte proteome: analysis by ion trap mass spectrometry. *Mol Cell Proteomics* 2004;**3**:501–509.

17. Snyder EL, Dunn BE, Giometti CS, *et al*. Protein changes occurring during storage of platelet concentrates. A two-dimensional gel electrophoretic analysis. *Transfusion* 1987;**27**:335–341.

18. Muylle L, Wouters E, De Bock R, Peetermans ME. Reactions to platelet transfusion: the effect of the storage time of the concentrate. *Transfus Med* 1992;**2**:289–293.

19. Garcia A, Prabhakar S, Brock CJ, *et al*. Extensive analysis of the human platelet proteome by two-dimensional gel electrophoresis and mass spectrometry. *Proteomics* 2004;**4**:656–668.

20. O'Neill EE, Brock CJ, von Kriegsheim AF, *et al*. Towards complete analysis of the platelet proteome. *Proteomics* 2002;**2**:288–305.

21. Gnatenko DV, Bahou WF. Recent advances in platelet transcriptomics. *Transfus Med Hemother* 2006:33.

22. Anderson NL, Polanski M, Pieper R, *et al*. The human plasma proteome: a nonredundant list developed by combination of four separate sources. *Mol Cell Proteomics* 2004;**3**:311–326.

23. Kumar A. Perioperative management of anemia: limits of blood transfusion and alternatives to it. *Cleve Clin J Med* 2009;**76** (Suppl 4):S112–118.

24. Wahr JA. Myocardial ischaemia in anaemic patients. *Br J Anaesth* 1998;**81** (Suppl 1):10–15.

25. Sehgal LR, Zebala LP, Takagi I, Curran RD, Votapka TV, Caprini JA. Evaluation of oxygen extraction ratio as a physiologic transfusion trigger in coronary artery bypass graft surgery patients. *Transfusion* 2001;**41**:591–595.

26. Engelfriet CP, Reesink HW, McCullough J, *et al*. Perioperative triggers for red cell transfusions. *Vox Sang* 2002;**82**:215–226.

27. Lelubre C, Vincent JL. Red blood cell transfusion in the critically ill patient. *Ann Intensive Care* 2011;**1**:43.

28. Wilkinson KL, Brunskill SJ, Dorée C, *et al*. The clinical effects of red blood cell transfusions: an overview of the randomized controlled trials evidence base. *Transfus Med Rev* 2011;**25**:145–155 e2.

29. Bower WF, Jin L, Underwood MJ, Lam YH, Lai PB. Peri-operative blood transfusion increases length of hospital stay and number of postoperative complications in non-cardiac surgical patients. *Hong Kong Med J* 2010;**16**:116–120.

30. Veenith T, Sharples L, Gerrard C, Valchanov K, Vuylsteke A. Survival and length of stay following blood transfusion in octogenarians following cardiac surgery. *Anaesthesia* 2010;**65**:331–336.

31. Willis P, Voeltz MD. Anemia, hemorrhage, and transfusion in percutaneous coronary intervention, acute coronary syndromes, and ST-segment elevation myocardial infarction. *Am J Cardiol* 2009;**104** (5 Suppl):34C–38C.

32. Nikolsky E, Mehran R, Sadeghi HM, *et al*. Prognostic impact of blood transfusion after primary angioplasty for acute myocardial infarction: analysis from the CADILLAC (Controlled Abciximab and Device Investigation to Lower Late Angioplasty Complications) Trial. *JACC Cardiovasc Interv* 2009;**2**:624–632.

33. Isbister JP, Shander A, Spahn DR, Erhard J, Farmer SL, Hofmann A. Adverse blood transfusion outcomes: establishing causation. *Transfus Med Rev* 2011;**25**:89–101.

34. Spiess BD. Blood transfusion: the silent epidemic. *Ann Thorac Surg* 2001;**72**:S1832–1837.

35. Arslan E, Sierko E, Waters JH, Siemionow M. Microcirculatory hemodynamics after acute blood loss followed by fresh and banked blood transfusion. *Am J Surg* 2005;**190**:456–462.

36. Fernandes CJ Jr, Akamine N, De Marco FV, De Souza JA, Lagudis S, Knobel E. Red blood cell transfusion does not increase oxygen consumption in critically ill septic patients. *Crit Care* 2001;**5**:362–367.

37. Mazza BF, Machado FR, Mazza DD, Hassmann V. Evaluation of blood transfusion effects on mixed venous oxygen saturation and lactate levels in patients with SIRS/sepsis. *Clinics (Sao Paulo)* 2005;**60**:311–316.

38. Marik PE, Sibbald WJ. Effect of stored-blood transfusion on oxygen delivery in patients with sepsis. *JAMA* 1993;**269**: 3024–3029.

39. Greenwalt TJ. The how and why of exocytic vesicles. *Transfusion* 2006;**46**:143–152.

40. Blumberg N. Deleterious clinical effects of transfusion immunomodulation: proven beyond a reasonable doubt. *Transfusion* 2005;**45** (2 Suppl):33S–39S, discussion 39S–40S.

41. Morris CD, Sepkowitz K, Fonshell C, *et al.* Prospective identification of risk factors for wound infection after lower extremity oncologic surgery. *Ann Surg Oncol* 2003;**10**: 778–782.

42. Innerhofer P, Klingler A, Klimmer C, Fries D, Nussbaumer W. Risk for postoperative infection after transfusion of white blood cell-filtered allogeneic or autologous blood components in orthopedic patients undergoing primary arthroplasty. *Transfusion* 2005;**45**:103–110.

43. Sauaia A, Alexander W, Moore EE, Stevens BR, Rosen H, Dunn TR. Autologous blood transfusion does not reduce postoperative infection rates in elective surgery. *Am J Surg* 1999;**178**:549–555.

44. Ikuta S, Miki C, Hatada T, *et al.* Allogenic blood transfusion is an independent risk factor for infective complications after less invasive gastrointestinal surgery. *Am J Surg* 2003;**185**:188–193.

45. Banbury MK, Brizzio ME, Rajeswaran J, Lytle BW, Blackstone EH. Transfusion increases the risk of postoperative infection after cardiovascular surgery. *J Am Coll Surg* 2006;**202**:131–138.

46. Hill GE, Frawley WH, Griffith KE, Forestner JE, Minei JP. Allogeneic blood transfusion increases the risk of postoperative bacterial infection: a meta-analysis. *J Trauma* 2003;**54**:908–914.

47. Moore FA, Moore EE, Sauaia A. Blood transfusion. An independent risk factor for postinjury multiple organ failure. *Arch Surg* 1997;**132**:620–624; discussion 624–625.

48. Spiess BD, Royston D, Levy JH, *et al.* Platelet transfusions during coronary artery bypass graft surgery are associated with serious adverse outcomes. *Transfusion* 2004;**44**: 1143–1148.

49. Society of Thoracic Surgeons Blood Conservation Guideline Task Force, Ferraris VA, Brown JR, Despotis GJ, *et al.* 2011 update to the Society of Thoracic Surgeons and the Society of Cardiovascular Anesthesiologists blood conservation clinical practice guidelines. *Ann Thorac Surg* 2011;**91**: 944–982.

50. Chau JK, Harris JR, Seikaly HR. Transfusion as a predictor of recurrence and survival in head and neck cancer surgery patients. *J Otolaryngol Head Neck Surg* 2010;**39**:516–522.

51. Yeh CY, Changchien CR, Wang JY, *et al.* Pelvic drainage and other risk factors for leakage after elective anterior resection in rectal cancer patients: a prospective study of 978 patients. *Ann Surg* 2005;**241**:9–13.

52. Okano T, Ohwada S, Sato Y, *et al.* Blood transfusions impair anastomotic wound healing, reduce luminol-dependent chemiluminescence, and increase interleukin-8. *Hepatogastroenterology* 2001;**48**:1669–1674.

53. Blair SD, Janvrin SB, McCollum CN, Greenhalgh RM. Effect of early blood transfusion on gastrointestinal haemorrhage. *Br J Surg* 1986;**73**:783–785.

54. Collard KJ. Is there a causal relationship between the receipt of blood transfusions and the development of chronic lung disease of prematurity? *Med Hypoth* 2006;**66**:355–364.

55. Hubler A, Knote K, Kauf E, Barz D, Schlenvoigt D, Schramm D. Does insulin-like growth factor 1 contribute in red blood cell transfusions to the pathogenesis of retinopathy of prematurity during retinal neovascularization? *Biol Neonate* 2006;**89**:92–98.

56. Collard KJ, Godeck S, Holley JE. Blood transfusion and pulmonary lipid peroxidation in ventilated premature babies. *Pediatr Pulmonol* 2005;**39**:257–261.

57. Dempsey EM, Barrington K. Short and long term outcomes following partial exchange transfusion in the polycythaemic newborn: a systematic review. *Arch Dis Child Fetal Neonatal Ed* 2006;**91**:F2–6.

58. Yamada S, Koizumi A, Iso H, *et al.* History of blood transfusion before 1990 is a risk factor for stroke and cardiovascular diseases: the Japan collaborative cohort study (JACC study). *Cerebrovasc Dis* 2005;**20**:164–171.

59. Yamada S, Koizumi A, Iso H, *et al.* Risk factors for fatal subarachnoid hemorrhage: the Japan Collaborative Cohort Study. *Stroke* 2003;**34**:2781–2787.

60. Gorgun E, Remzi FH, Goldberg JM, *et al.* Fertility is reduced after restorative proctocolectomy with ileal pouch anal anastomosis: a study of 300 patients. *Surgery* 2004;**136**: 795–803.

61. Abu-Rustum NR, Richard S, Wilton A, *et al.* Transfusion utilization during adnexal or peritoneal cancer surgery: effects on symptomatic venous thromboembolism and survival. *Gynecol Oncol* 2005;**99**:320–326.

62. Sabatine MS, Morrow DA, Giugliano RP, *et al.* Association of hemoglobin levels with clinical outcomes in acute coronary syndromes. *Circulation* 2005;**111**:2042–2049.

63. Hebert PC, Wells G, Blajchman MA, *et al.* A multicenter, randomized, controlled clinical trial of transfusion requirements in critical care. Transfusion Requirements in Critical Care Investigators, Canadian Critical Care Trials Group. *N Engl J Med* 1999;**340**:409–417.

64. Johnson RG, Thurer RL, Kruskall MS, *et al.* Comparison of two transfusion strategies after elective operations for myocardial revascularization. *J Thorac Cardiovasc Surg* 1992;**104**: 307–314.

65. Yang X, Alexander KP, Chen AY, *et al.* The implications of blood transfusions for patients with non-ST-segment eleva-

tion acute coronary syndromes: results from the CRUSADE National Quality Improvement Initiative. *J Am Coll Cardiol* 2005;**46**:1490–1495.

66. Rao SV, Jollis JG, Harrington RA, *et al.* Relationship of blood transfusion and clinical outcomes in patients with acute coronary syndromes. *JAMA* 2004;**292**:1555–1562.

67. Tsai AG, Cabrales P, Intaglietta M. Microvascular perfusion upon exchange transfusion with stored red blood cells in normovolemic anemic conditions. *Transfusion* 2004;**44**:1626–1634.

68. Habib RH, Zacharias A, Schwann TA, *et al.* Role of hemodilutional anemia and transfusion during cardiopulmonary bypass in renal injury after coronary revascularization: implications on operative outcome. *Crit Care Med* 2005;**33**:1749–1756.

69. Engoren MC, Habib RH, Zacharias A, Schwann TA, Riordan CJ, Durham SJ. Effect of blood transfusion on long-term survival after cardiac operation. *Ann Thorac Surg* 2002;**74**:1180–1186.

70. Malone DL, Dunne J, Tracy JK, Putnam AT, Scalea TM, Napolitano LM. Blood transfusion, independent of shock severity, is associated with worse outcome in trauma. *J Trauma* 2003;**54**:898–905; discussion 905–907.

71. Stainsby D, Jones H, Asher D, *et al.* Serious hazards of transfusion: a decade of hemovigilance in the UK. *Transfus Med Rev* 2006;**20**:273–282.

72. Brand A. Immunological aspects of blood transfusions. *Transpl Immunol* 2002;**10**:183–190.

73. Shaz BH, Stowell SR, Hillyer CD. Transfusion-related acute lung injury: from bedside to bench and back. *Blood* 2011;**117**:1463–1471.

74. Janatpour K, Holland PV. Noninfectious serious hazards of transfusion. *Curr Hematol Rep* 2002; **1**:149–155.

75. Nusbacher J. Blood transfusion is mononuclear cell transplantation. *Transfusion* 1994;**34**:1002–1006.

76. Vietor HE, Hallensleben E, van Bree SP, *et al.* Survival of donor cells 25 years after intrauterine transfusion. *Blood* 2000;**95**: 2709–2714.

77. Lee TH, Paglieroni T, Utter GH, *et al.* High-level long-term white blood cell microchimerism after transfusion of leuko-reduced blood components to patients resuscitated after severe traumatic injury. *Transfusion* 2005;**45**:1280–1290.

78. Langenfeld JE, Machiedo GW, Lyons M, Rush BF Jr, Dikdan G, Lysz TW. Correlation between red blood cell deformability and changes in hemodynamic function. *Surgery* 1994;**116**: 859–867.

79. Innerhofer P, Kuhbacher G. [Mechanisms of immunomodulation after transfusion of allogeneic and autologous red cell concentrate]. Anasthesiol *Intensivmed Notfallmed Schmerzther* 2002;**37**:681–684.

80. Nielsen HJ. Influence on the immune system of homologous blood transfusion and autologous blood donation: impact on the routine clinical practice/differences in oncological and non-tumour surgery? *Anasthesiol Intensivmed Notfallmed Schmerzther* 2000;**35**:642–645.

81. McCullough PA, Lepor NE. The deadly triangle of anemia, renal insufficiency, and cardiovascular disease: implications for prognosis and treatment. *Rev Cardiovasc Med* 2005;**6**:1–10.

82. Silver MR. Anemia in the long-term ventilator-dependent patient with respiratory failure. *Chest* 2005;**128** (5 Suppl 2):568S–575S.

83. KDOQI Clinical Practice Guidelines and Clinical Practice Recommendations for Anemia in Chronic Kidney Disease. *Am J Kidney Dis* 2006;**47** (5 Suppl 3):S11–145.

84. Liumbruno G, Bennardello F, Lattanzio A, *et al.* Recommendations for the transfusion of plasma and platelets. *Blood Transfus* 2009;**7**:132–150.

85. Spiess BD. Platelet transfusions: the science behind safety, risks and appropriate applications. *Best Pract Res Clin Anaesthesiol* 2010;**24**:65–83.

86. Guidelines for the use of platelet transfusions. *Br J Haematol* 2003;**122**:10–23.

87. Schiffer CA, Anderson KC, Bennett CL, *et al.* Platelet transfusion for patients with cancer: clinical practice guidelines of the American Society of Clinical Oncology. *J Clin Oncol* 2001;**19**:1519–1538.

88. Bishton M, Chopra R. The role of granulocyte transfusions in neutropenic patients. *Br J Haematol* 2004;**127**:501–508.

89. Ohsaka A, Kikuta A, Ohto H, *et al.* Guidelines for safety management of granulocyte transfusion in Japan. *Int J Hematol* 2010;**91**:201–208.

90. Kozek-Langenecker S. Do we really need FFP in Austria? *Wien Klin Wochenschr* 2010;**22** (Suppl 5):S14–15.

91. Roback JD, Caldwell S, Carson J, *et al.* Evidence-based practice guidelines for plasma transfusion. *Transfusion* 2010; **50**:1227–1239.

19 Step by Step to an Organized Blood Management Program

Blood management is a multimodal, multidisciplinary team approach that aims to optimize the patient's outcome by skillfully managing the patient's own blood. It is driven by the philosophy that the patient is at the center of attention. Blood management is best implemented within the framework of an organized and recognized program. In this chapter, help is given to assemble all the different elements of blood management into an organized program. The required background information is provided, as are the management tools. The steps in a tried-and-tested approach to establishing a program are described.

Objectives

1. To list the 10 steps that will lead to implementation of a blood management program.
2. To identify ways to educate and train different groups in blood management.
3. To acquire management skills essential for running a blood management program.

Definitions

Program: A system of services created to meet a public need, involving a series of steps that have to be carried out for goals to be achieved.

Marketing: Communicating information on an idea, product, or service in order to encourage sharing, purchase, or use of it by others. It consists of a group of activities designed to find out what customers want (market research), to increase customer awareness, and to attract customers to the object being marketed; planning and executing a concept in order to meet customers' needs.

Education: Includes all activities revolving around teaching or instructing, aimed at imparting knowledge or skills.

Why take the trouble to organize a blood management program?

Arranging for and keeping order requires energy. Since this is true also for the order needed to organize blood management, you might ask why you should invest your energy in such an endeavor. An organized blood management program is well worth the effort. Successfully implemented, a program will result in the establishment of a competence center for blood management, offering a holistic care program for patients. It will provide the ideal skill mix of well-educated and trained, up-to-date healthcare providers needed to manage patients' blood effectively. In such a center, the experience gained over time will translate into improved patient outcomes [1]. A blood management program will attract new patients for the hospital, reduce overall treatment costs, and help eliminate the adverse effects associated with transfusions. Patient and healthcare provider satisfaction will increase. Surely, these are more than enough reasons to start an organized blood management program.

Who can take the initiative to start an organized blood management program?
Once the idea has been hatched that a blood management program would be a valuable asset to a hospital, who

Basics of Blood Management, Second Edition. Petra Seeber and Aryeh Shander.
© 2013 John Wiley & Sons, Ltd. Published 2013 by John Wiley & Sons, Ltd.

should initiate the program? The best approach is to start from within the institution [2], meaning that someone already working in the hospital—usually an influential physician—should spearhead the program. It is certainly true that a successful program is driven by internal forces. However, history shows that many programs have not been started in this manner. Often, it was nurses, nursing coordinators, or individual Jehovah's Witnesses who initiated development of the program. Also, government initiatives may be the starting point for developing a blood management program. In recent times, consultants or companies in the consulting field have offered to initiate a program. These support the hospital from outside and contribute their expertise. Hospitals can hire consultants to support its own efforts to launch a program. Among the advantages of hiring a company is that external consultants can address "hot" issues with much more ease than physicians who have to be careful about internal hospital politics. This may mean that the program can progress faster than otherwise. Further, external consultants devote their whole day to program development and are not distracted by daily clinical activities. In addition, they may bring the necessary expertise to tailor the program to the needs of the hospital. They are usually acquainted with time-proven concepts, can easily implement them, and have access to forms, computer programs, agendas, statistics, and methods that may be difficult for the hospital to obtain.

Finally, *who* starts the program is not so important, as long as a program *is* started. If there are no physicians willing to adopt the program, then most probably not even the hospital administration or the head of the most influential department can bring about the required philosophical changes. However, if resourceful department heads or others are available who see the potential of the program, implementation is possible even if it is proposed by a less influential person.

Step 1: Information and education of the initiator

You as the initiator of a blood management program need to acquire the necessary knowledge and compile information about general and specific blood management-related issues. The right motivation is also required to start a blood management program because it must be sufficient to overcome the initial hurdles that have to be cleared.

Several ways of gathering the required information are feasible. If available, a dedicated program of education on blood management would be the easiest source to consult. Such a program has been developed in Canada as part of a provincial program for blood conservation (The Ontario Transfusion Coordinators) [3]. If such education is unavailable, self-education is warranted. There is more than enough educational material available. Pertinent journals and blood management-related books and brochures are good sources of information. More informal, yet very practical, education can be gained at blood management conferences, before and after dedicated lectures, and during visits to existing blood management programs. There are several Web sites that provide information about blood management-related issues and several societies that provide information and serve as a conduit for information exchange (see Appendix B for detailed information).

Another field in which you as the initiator of the program need to acquire knowledge is the specific situation of the hospital. This is best done by performing a structured initial analysis (as shown in Appendix C). In the initial analysis, hospital-specific information is gathered about the patient population, established blood management measures, current use of blood, financial implications of these issues, and personnel and their willingness and ability to adopt blood management. Information about the hospital also includes the area it serves, its market share, other blood management programs in the vicinity, and a comparison with local competitors. Information about funding opportunities is also beneficial. In addition, forces and interests outside the hospital that may help or hamper establishment of a blood management program should be known. Such an initial analysis performed in the early stages of a blood management program forms the basis for future activities. If the initial analysis identifies aspects that seem to indicate that the program cannot be implemented successfully, it may still be possible to identify another hospital that can implement the program.

After educating yourself about blood management, you are equipped to work toward instituting an organized blood management program. A continuous source of motivation is required so that you do not tire in your efforts. Early on, join others who are engaged in the same kind of project. This can be done by joining blood management forums on the Internet, any of the many societies, or by regularly communicating with colleagues who share the same commitment.

Step 1: How to proceed

- Learn as much as possible about blood management in general.
- Perform an initial analysis of the hospital you want to work with.
- Arrange for occasions that provide ongoing motivation for you.

Table 19.1 Sample outline for the first presentation.

Definition (and history) of blood management
Benefits of a blood management program (for this hospital, for the patients, physicians, etc.)
Cost issues of transfusion and blood management (general and hospital-specific)
Recommendation to go ahead with a blood management program—cite the next few steps and a time frame for them

Step 2: Your business plan

Now that the information has been gathered and sufficient motivation is available to start a blood management program, make specific plans. Put them down in a form that can be presented orally as well as in writing; the latter will be the business plan [4].

An informal business proposal

When attempting to convince others to help establish a blood management program, the informal format will most likely be chosen. Present your ideas orally and arrange your arguments well in order to win support. An oral presentation is best made to key individuals in the hospital where the program is to be initiated. The aim is to help further the program and the audience may include important administrative staff (chief executive officer [CEO], marketing director, head of the financial department, etc.). Also, key clinical staff (heads of the various medical and surgical departments, head of nursing, chief of staff, quality assurance officer, etc.) should be invited. Persons with a keen interest in blood management may also be invited. Since it may be important for the administrators to see how many key hospital staff are already willing to adopt a new approach, inviting representatives from both the administration and clinicians to a discussion may be beneficial. This may help identify the support (and resistance) the hospital administration (and you) will encounter in initiating the program. The presentation will probably have to be made several times to reach all those of importance in the hospital.

The purpose of such initial informal presentations is to establish your position as an authority in the field and to make the plan to start a blood management program known to those invited. It is also the occasion to establish some important facts, such as that blood management is better care and is beneficial to both the patients and the hospital. Current hospital data and recent key publica-

tions should be available and presented to support the argument that proceeding with blood management is the course to be taken. After Step 1, pertinent information will be available from the fundamental analysis.

Use some visual aids to support the initial presentation. An overhead projector or handouts may be used to appeal to the audience. A sample outline for this initial presentation is shown in Table 19.1.

A formal business proposal

In addition to the informal presentation, it may be useful to prepare a formal written business plan. This plan serves several purposes. Initially, the most important purpose is to provide the hospital administration with answers to key questions. This information may well be the basis for its decision to support or to reject your proposal. The business plan is also a guide for you or others who want to start the blood management program. It may stake the claims, as it were, building the framework on which the blood management program will develop. A formal business proposal usually addresses those individuals who are empowered to make decisions. After receiving the proposal, they should be able to decide whether or not to permit you to start, and they should also be able to cooperate toward the funding of the project and afford the required network access (business relations, introduction to the right people, introduction of the program to further key persons). The written proposal, therefore, mainly addresses the hospital's administration.

A formal written business proposal can be designed in various formats. If the hospital makes a form available to employees for business proposals, this form could be used. If not, select your own format. Whatever format is chosen, keep the business proposal simple and concise, and tailor its contents to the specific business context the hospital operates in.

The contents of the business proposal may vary, depending on the format. Refer to the outline of the different model structures for the written business plan in Appendix C or simply ask colleagues at conferences or via Internet discussion platforms.

No matter what format is chosen for the business proposal, some of the key features discussed below could be included.

Why do we need a blood management program?

The full scope of problems arising from untreated anemia, undetected coagulopathy or unnecessary blood loss, as well as unwarranted medical use of blood, may not be realized by all in the hospital. They may also be unaware of the specific issues of the current and emerging transfusion-related situation the hospital finds itself in. In the introduction to the business plan, briefly explain the reasons why a move toward blood management is needed. After explaining the problems (Table 19.2) [5], a statement could be made to the effect that the envisioned blood management program is the solution to the multiple problems surrounding the use and misuse of blood.

What can be anticipated if the blood management program is implemented?

General as well as hospital-specific data are required to illustrate the results expected from the program. The more hospital-specific data included, the more trustworthy the projections. General information may include statistics on patient safety, liability issues, improved outcome, and patient satisfaction. Hospital-specific projections may include an increased market share, number of patients expected to choose the hospital because of the blood management program, and benefit of improved patient outcomes, such as reduced length of stay, infection rates, and mortality.

Who will be served by the program?

It is prudent to answer the question of who initially will be served by the program directly in the formal business proposal. Although blood management is preferably mainstream medicine, for practical reasons, starting the program for a restricted population only may be better. This creates an environment in which the hospital staff can become comfortable with the new philosophies and techniques involved [6]. Later, further patient groups can be added. This makes the start easier and prevents the hospital from being overwhelmed by a flood of patients presenting for blood management. Many hospitals have chosen to start with a program for Jehovah's Witnesses and have gradually added other patient groups until universal blood management is adopted as the standard of care. To begin with, other patient populations may be those treated in a single department or even just those undergoing a specific procedure (e.g., hip replacement) or suffering from a specific disease (e.g., sickle cell patients). Refer to Step 9 below for more information on how to choose where to start.

Can the success of the program be monitored?

Progress can be monitored by setting goals for the program. This may help not only to check the program for progress and to adapt to challenges, but also to ensure the continuing support of the hospital administration. By mentioning which monitoring tools (Table 19.3) have been chosen, control of the program's success may be placed in the hands of the administration, which may encourage managers to invest in starting the program in the first place.

What is the time frame in which the proposed changes will be realized?

It may take 3–5 years until the full benefit of a program is realized. The hospital administration should be aware of this. This will prevent coordinators from being pressured unduly when the expected goals are not met within several months.

Will the program be financially taxing?

Cost projections most probably will be interest to the hospital administration. Try to answer questions such as: How much do we have to invest? Is such investment worthwhile? What is the return on investment?

Table 19.2 Why do we need the program?

Need to improve clinical outcomes
Benefits of appropriate therapy of anemia
Current and future costs rising
Patient preference
Public concern
Liability
Efficacy of allogeneic transfusions not proven

To answer the hospital administration's financial questions, prepare a rough estimate of the budgeted investment. It may be better to estimate the budget on the high side. Identify essential line-item expenses for operation of the program (Table 19.4). Typically, only costs directly related to the program are included in the budget. Other incidental costs are not included. The latter include costs for medical treatment, e.g., for blood management-related drugs and autotransfusion. Such costs will arise, but are usually offset either by savings realized by reduced

Table 19.3 Simple ways to monitor program progress.

Goal	Monitoring	Source of statistics
Reduce allogeneic transfusions	Units of blood used, procedures performed	Blood bank, transfusion meeting reports, hospital or departmental statistics of performed procedures, billing department
Increase patient share	Number of patients enrolled in program	Admission services, patient questionnaire regarding motivation to use the program
Increased patient satisfaction	Patient satisfaction score increases	Questionnaire
Reduced transfusion-associated infections	Number of infections, relation to transfusion, historical numbers of infections	Infection-tracking sheet, billing department, transfusion meeting reports
Reduced length of stay	Length of stay in comparison with historical population or with population not in the blood management program	Admission services, billing department

Table 19.4 Line-item budgeting.

Line item	Comment
Salaries of (full-time) program coordinators	When budgeting for several years, include increases in salaries
Equipment	Includes office equipment only, since the medical–surgical equipment is usually covered by the budgets of the respective departments
Staff education	Include costs for educating and training physicians, nurses, and ancillary staff; the coordinator's participation in national and international conferences, use of libraries, purchase of books and journals
Management fees	To compensate medical directors or committee members for the hours they spend on the program
Patient tracking and identification	Costs incurred depend on how patients are tracked and identified. Costs for computer specialists, printing of stickers, wristbands for patients, forms, etc.
Marketing	It will be easier to budget marketing costs if the avenues to be used to market the program have been determined; include also costs for community education, clubs, etc.
Office costs	All the miscellaneous things needed to run the program, i.e., telephone, fax, mail, pagers, stationery, postage, printing of brochures, office rent, cleaning, etc.
Miscellaneous	Depending on the scope of the program, costs for research, data analysis, grants for patients (travel costs, accommodation of families, etc.) may have to be included

allogeneic blood use or are already included in the respective departmental budgets. It is worth mentioning that implementation of the program will shift savings and expenses within hospital budgets. For instance, blood bank costs will be reduced, but pharmacy costs may increase. Such shifts need not be calculated, but the administration should be informed as necessary.

In addition to drawing up a budget, make a realistic estimate of the time frame involved and the financial goals to be reached. For instance, based on the initial analysis, it may be estimated that costs can be saved by reducing the current transfusion rate by 20% within the next 3 years. Another way to project costs and revenue is to multiply the number of new patients by the average income per patient gained by the hospital. To do so, average the income over the last 3 or 6 months and divide this figure by the average number of patients treated during this period.

The method chosen to demonstrate the financial benefits of the program depends on the type of health system in which the hospital operates. Government-run hospitals with a fixed budget and a mandate to care for the general public may not be interested in increasing patient load. Cost reductions and a reduction in the length of stay in the hospital might be more welcome. Other hospitals that are dependent on patients for income may be more concerned about increasing numbers of patients. Yet others receive income from various sources and may be interested in prestige rather than financial gain, or another motive may be of more interest. Some background information about payment modes and sources of income may help in the choice of argument to convince the hospital administration that the program is lucrative. However, no matter how revenue is estimated, budget on the low side. This will make it easier either to meet or exceed the administration's expectations.

Who will put the program into practice?

The business proposal also has to address the issue of who will share the responsibilities within the program. Outlining the structure of the program as described in Step 5 will help the reader of the business plan to understand how the program will finally operate.

Step 2: How to proceed

- Prepare an informal presentation using visual aids.
- Prepare a realistic budget and project hospital revenue.
- Write a formal business plan.

Step 3: Get help—your champions

Professionals who have been successful in implementing a blood management program emphasize the necessity of having at least one champion to implement the program [7]. Champions are those healthcare providers who work together with the initiator to achieve the goals. They are the locomotives of the venture. Champions are motivated to improve patient outcomes by managing the patient's blood or may even be eager to implement blood management as a program. Such champions are indispensable to change the behavior of healthcare providers [8, 9] and to spread the philosophy of the program [6]. Champions are opinion leaders and serve as credible messengers to establish the program. They play a vital role in setting realistic goals, participating in the development, distribution, and implementation of blood management guidelines, and in staff education.

Since champions are thus essential to the program, seek out such individuals. While working through this book and doing the homework, you have already contacted a variety of professionals who may be potential champions. Ideally, persons will be found who already practice blood management. There may be others who are convinced that changes are needed, but who are waiting for a little encouragement and support to translate their resolve for change into action by founding a blood management program. Champions are often found among anesthesiologists [3]; however, blood bank professionals, surgeons, or other professionals have given substantial support to blood management programs. Ask such professionals for help and offer to help them. They may be more than willing to provide support and do their share.

What if a suitable champion cannot be found? Then the initiator will have to create the champions. List those who may be suitable, preferably individuals in the top league, as it were—heads of departments, the CEO, or another person in a similar position. Others may also be recruited. A short guide on how to identify such individuals can be found in an article by Hiss *et al.* published in 1978 [10].

Having identified potential champions, think about what may motivate them to change their opinion and practice blood management. Usually, physicians are satisfied with the treatment they give; they claim already to have a near optimal patient outcome with no undue blood loss and no untreated anemia, and they transfuse only if it is unavoidable. This is the common belief.

Change it by benchmarking. Gather convincing data. The hardest data available are those associated with death or major morbidity. Maybe a comparison can be made between transfusion rates in the hospital and in other hospitals. If possible, begin a small-scale study. After collecting the data, come up with some simple statistics. For instance, show how many patients are anemic in a department, how many transfusions were given to patients initially presenting with anemia, or how many received transfusions mainly because of high intraoperative blood loss. Such patients are potential candidates for up-to-date blood management. Simple mathematics may convince the potential champion or at least move him/her to give the program a try.

If all else fails, be your own champion. In time, you may be successful in recruiting further champions. For the time being continue by yourself. Remember that no effort, however small, goes unnoticed; so, even if a fully-fledged program cannot be implemented, do not give up. Everything takes time, even recruiting champions. Once physicians have had the chance to come to terms with blood management, then they will volunteer to be champions.

Step 3: How to proceed

- If possible, find at least one champion, either by recruiting one or by creating one.
- If none is available initially, be your own champion.

Step 4: Get more support—convince the hospital administration

No blood management program has ever been established and continued without the ongoing support of the hospital administration. It is usually the hospital administration that initiates the profound change needed in the hospital's philosophy regarding blood use. The hospital administration must fully advocate the intended changes; otherwise required support is missing and the program will vanish. Therefore, a very important step in implementing a blood management program is to sell the program to the hospital administration [6].

In many cases, the hospital administration is represented by the CEO. The CEO is most likely confronted with new proposals every day, each of which to each presenter is very important. The CEO has now to be convinced of the importance of your program [2]. Putting yourself into the CEO's shoes for a moment will help understand what it may take to convince him/her. The CEO is responsible not only for monetary issues such as allocating limited resources, but also for patient safety, patient relations, litigation, public relations, ethical and political issues, distinguishing the hospital from competitors, etc. His/her ultimate goal is to keep the hospital running effectively. To convince the CEO, his/her concerns must be addressed in terms he/she can understand. The main aim should be to convince him/her that the program will contribute to keeping the hospital viable, now and in the future. Convey to the CEO what clear advantages result from adopting a blood management program. Be very specific using data pertinent to the hospital. For a CEO to be convinced to invest money and time in the program, he/she has to see what the return on investment will be. Show how many patients it would take to recover the invested costs. Try to model some calculations that demonstrate the extent of savings achievable. Apart from cost issues, it may also be important to reassure the CEO that the program will not interfere with hospital politics. It may be beneficial to demonstrate to the CEO that there is already interest and support in the hospital, e.g., the heads of anesthesiology, hematology, blood bank, surgery, or other surgical specialties. It is therefore prudent to come up with some champions before approaching the CEO. However, where this is not possible, suggest to the CEO that you will find out as soon as possible whether there is support among the physicians.

When you have convinced the hospital administration to implement the blood management program, ask for approval in writing. The administration may officially endorse your formal business plan or may want to create its own contract. Whatever the case, make sure that your responsibilities and authority are clearly delineated. Nothing is more frustrating than a lack of authority. If permission needs to be asked for regarding every little detail, progress will be hampered and may even make the program futile. After receiving the hospital administration's approval, it could be asked to inform others about the program's implementation and to introduce you and your plan, stating what your responsibilities are and what authority you now have (e.g., by e-mail, hospital newsletter, by inviting staff to dinner, or by walking through the hospital with you and introducing you to the heads of departments). This will pave the way for further contact with hospital staff and win their cooperation.

Step 4: How to proceed

- Identify those who represent the hospital administration.
- List points that may convince them to implement your blood management program.
- Sign a contract with the hospital for the implementation of the program.

Step 5: Structure is essential—directors, coordinators, committees

Once the hospital administration approves the business proposal, the way is paved to begin the actual work of organizing the program. The first thing to be done is to structure the program. If a thoroughly planned business proposal is already available, this will serve as a guide through the next few months' work. Both a medical and an administrative structure need to be established and effective communication facilitated.

Medical structure

As shown by experience, the greatest benefit is drawn from a formal blood management program if it is physician-driven [4]. Therefore, there should be at least one physician—still better a group of physicians—taking the lead in medical matters (the champions). If just one physician is available, he/she can be appointed medical director. If more than one physician is available, a group of medical directors, a committee, or working group could be organized. Ideally, this group represents a variety of specialties. The physicians taking the lead will develop and implement the medical part of the program and will be instrumental in providing ongoing staff education and training. They will act as role models for other healthcare providers in the program. The main task of the medical directors is clinical work, and only a small proportion of their time will be spent with administrative issues. They are the liaison between the program administration and the clinicians.

Another important task for the physicians taking the lead is to recruit a core team. All members of this core team must share a commitment to patient-centered blood management [11]. They must not only be willing but also capable of performing blood management when treating patients. The members of this core team should include the champions, the physicians taking the lead in the program, and other physicians who are already trained or are prepared to be trained in blood manage-

ment. This core team should present a suitable skill mix to offer multidisciplinary blood management. Typically, surgeons, anesthesiologists, internists, pediatricians, nursing staff, etc., are included. The names of members of the core team should be known to the administration of the blood management program so that patients wishing to use the services of the program can be referred to them. The core team members should also be well informed about the program's policies and procedures. It is advisable to have them sign a written agreement with the program, stating the rights and responsibilities of members of the core team. This may be necessary to ensure that patients wishing to benefit from a blood management service are treated according to the policies and procedures of the program. Such a written agreement serves as the durable basis for the relationship between the program and physicians, and vice versa.

Administrative structure

The administrative part of the blood management program is essential to keep the program running. Probably the most important factor is the presence of at least one dedicated coordinator [3], because experience shows no program can develop without one. The coordinator is typically not a physician, but is a member of senior nursing or technical staff or an otherwise dedicated individual with a background knowledge in blood management. He/she is essential to the daily affairs of the program [7]. His/her many responsibilities include development, organization, and supervision of program progress. The coordinator develops policies and procedures for the program, renders patient-specific decisions, gives support, assesses patients for blood management, serves as liaison between patients, physicians, the administration, and the public; organizes education and training; and collects data for quality management and research. A model job description for the coordinator can be found in Appendix C or in the literature [3]; this gives deeper insight into the many responsibilities of a blood management coordinator.

Facilitating communication

Since blood management is a team approach, communication among the members of the team is essential. Therefore, structuring a blood management program also includes paving the way for communication between all parties. These are the coordinator(s), physicians who are the program leaders, core team members, other hospital staff who only indirectly contribute to the success of the program, and also patients, their families, as well as the public. The lines of communication should always be open. To be practical, the blood management program should be located in an office within the hospital and the coordinator should be based there. The regular business hours should be known to patients and staff alike. It should be possible to contact members of the blood management program in an emergency, e.g., during the night or at weekends. All these provisions facilitate communication.

Those taking the lead in the program must communicate regularly. It is wise to schedule regular meetings. This is especially important in the initial phases of program development. During such programmed meetings, the responsibilities of each individual member of the steering group should be established. Regular meetings involving the committee of medical directors and the program's administrative personnel—the coordinator(s)—keep the lines of communication open. In addition, communication may be scheduled with other established committees, e.g., with the hospital transfusion committee, administration, public relations, nursing committees, and patient relation groups.

Step 5: How to proceed

- Recruit medical directors for the program and get them to form a committee.
- Appoint at least one dedicated blood management coordinator.
- Identify a medical–surgical and nursing core team.
- Organize an in-hospital office for the coordinator.

Step 6: Policies and procedures

Now that personnel have been recruited and the organizational background for the program has been set up, it is necessary to establish how these will work to fulfill the purposes of the program. This is determined by the policies and procedures that should now be developed. Since blood management is a multimodal approach [12] spanning the field of patient care—from first contact with the institution until completion of care—policies and procedures should mirror every modality of care [7]. The policies and procedures define acceptable and unacceptable care. They answer the question of how the program will benefit patients and how universal blood management will be established in clinical routine. Policies and procedures are designed to finally shape the behavior of all parties participating in blood management [13].

Which policies and procedures are needed depends on the scope of the blood management program. If the program serves only the patients attending one department, only a limited set of policies and procedures is needed initially. For example, if at the beginning the program only applies to orthopedics, then the use of a cardiopulmonary bypass does not need to be addressed. If the program initially serves only one specific group of patients, then policies and procedures that are unacceptable may not be required (e.g., if the program is only for Jehovah's Witnesses, policies and procedures for preoperative autologous donation for storage are not needed).

Listing surgical and medical continua helps in forming an idea as to which policies and procedures need to be developed. Continua include all methods and approaches to patient blood management offered by the program, organized according to sequence of occurrence in medical care (e.g., preoperatively, intraoperatively, postoperatively). An example of a surgical continuum is found in Appendix C. Continua can be developed for elective procedures (e.g., in gynecology, orthopedics, urology), emergencies, polytraumatized patients, intensive care of adults, radiation and chemotherapy in cancer patients, obstetrics, and the premature, neonates, and other pediatric patients. To begin with and as an aid to the development of continua, consult some review articles which list methods available for blood management [14–17].

Developing policies and procedures is no easy task; however, many sample policies and procedures are already available. Therefore, do not reinvent the wheel. First, use policies and procedures developed for your hospital. The initial analysis may show what policies and procedures are already available and need to be adapted, or are still missing and need to be developed. Appendix B contains a list of published algorithms and guidelines. Refer to them to establish your own set of policies and procedures. A list of administrative, clinical, legal, and ethical guidelines that have been established by other blood management programs can be found in Appendix C.

Typically, administrative policies and procedures are developed by the coordinator in cooperation with the medical directors and the hospital administration. Medical policies and procedures are best developed by the coordinator, group of champions, steering physicians with an interest in blood management, and pertinent nursing staff and technicians. The legal department should assist with legal policies and procedures. Staff will be more than happy to ensure that pitfalls are avoided and will probably be able to give valuable advice. They may be concerned about the impact of the program on hospital litigation. If necessary, contact experienced lawyers or hospital administrators to convince the hospital's legal department that the blood management program is no threat to the hospital.

In time, policies and procedures will change, because they need to adapt to program development and growth as well as to changing needs. During the initial development of policies and procedures, select a format that is simple to modify, allowing policies and procedures to be added or deleted as required. If the hospital has International Standards Organization (ISO) certification, contact a professional to help you to bring the program's policies and procedures in line with ISO requirements (this may be mandatory to receive funding). Lists of policies and procedures may not be all that is required; lists of those responsible and of the tools may be needed. Refer to Appendix C for a model format for a policy or procedure.

After the policies and procedures have been finalized, it is important to implement them. Initially, circulate them among those involved in the policy or procedure. Then the champions need to take the lead in putting them into practice. This requires hard work, frequent educational interventions, and encouragement.

Step 6: How to proceed

- Develop medical and surgical continua pertinent to the program.
- Identify medical, administrative, and legal/ethical issues to be regulated by policies and procedures.
- Collect available policies and procedures, tapping into either those currently applicable in the hospital or published in the literature.
- Develop a unique set of policies and procedures.

Step 7: Education—preparation for life

Healthcare practitioners' general knowledge about blood management-related issues is surprisingly scant. Medical and nursing school curricula often omit blood management. Even professionals who train in a dedicated fellowship-training program do not often learn much about the fundamentals of patient-centered blood management [18]. Further, use of autologous blood is infrequently taught, and in-depth knowledge must therefore not be assumed. Residents and young physicians in par-

ticular, those who typically carry the major clinical workload, do not know much about blood management. Therefore, when beginning a blood management program, most staff members need to enhance their knowledge and skills in blood management.

Specific educational interventions can be planned whose goal is to build a highly motivated, well-trained team of healthcare practitioners sharing a commitment to blood management. Behavioral changes are initiated through education and encouragement, and in the end all participants in the blood management program practice according to their assigned role. This ideally results in improved patient outcomes. As research has demonstrated, improvement of blood management-related behavior is achievable by education [19, 20]. There is a strong association between knowledge of transfusion indications and their use in situations where they are considered appropriate [13]. Thorough education and training can encourage multimodal use of blood management measures [21, 22]. Willingness to listen to counsel and actively seeking advice are also associated with a reduction in transfusions [13]. Therefore, educational interventions, encouragement, and fostering a spirit of mutual consultation are essential to establish and improve a blood management program.

Since education is an integral part of a blood management program, it is essential to know how to educate. Merely introducing guidelines or presenting a lecture about blood management will not change practice [23]. Forcing physicians to adhere to guidelines seldom wins their favor. How, then, can behaviors be changed? There is extensive research on this subject. Six general methods have been studied: education, feedback, participation of physicians in the effort to change, administrative interventions, financial incentives, and penalties [9]. Success in terms of changing the healthcare provider's behavior or better patient outcome varies. Mere lectures or supplies of written material do not change physicians' behavior, unless the curriculum has been specially designed to effect change. Clinical guidelines do not automatically change behaviors. The reasons may be that guidelines are impractical, physicians may not trust guidelines or they ignore them, giving in to other influences such as financial constraints, incentives, or fear of litigation. Guidelines only effect changes when they are distributed and endorsed by opinion leaders. Feedback may or may not be effective, depending on the circumstances. When physicians themselves recognize that their methods need improvement and prospective feedback is given at a time when physicians can change their behavior immediately (and not retrospectively), then feedback may be effective. In contrast, surprisingly effective in changing behavior is so-called academic detailing, an educational method involving an opinion leader talking to one person at a time. Including physicians in the change process is also very important for change. While in some instances outside pressure may change physicians' behavior (e.g., a law requiring quality assurance measures for autologous blood products), changes in practice are best started from within. Hence, educational interventions should place control in the hands of healthcare personnel. Including healthcare providers in the process of education would not undermine their authority or call their judgment into question; thus, they do not feel threatened. Administrative efforts to enforce change are effective, but most of these should be used as a last resort. Financial incentives (e.g., payment by case) or penalties (being financially personally responsible for treatment) are very effective in changing physicians' behavior. Having said all this, no single method is inherently successful in changing behavior. A combination of methods seems to be better than a single method.

Who should receive education?

Since the success of a blood management program depends on each player, all participants in the program need to be educated. First, the blood management coordinator should be well informed and keep up-to-date with current developments so as to remain an expert in blood management. The coordinator should be capable of informing physicians and other healthcare providers as well as the hospital administration.

In addition to the coordinator, all champions, directors, and members of the core team should be educated and trained in blood management in relation to their specialty. If possible, they should have a better knowledge of blood management than the average healthcare provider. Ideally, they should also know what other specialties contribute to the success of blood management. This will enable them to coordinate patient care across specialties.

Minimum levels of education and training should be defined for all other participants in the program (Table 19.5). However, these levels should not be unreasonably high so as not to deter potential participants, but rather they should be sufficiently demanding to ensure a good blood management service to patients. Education given to other persons in the program should focus on their role, specialty, and field of expertise.

Table 19.5 Whom to include in educational interventions.

Physicians
Nurses (including intensive care, anesthesia, and ward nurses)
Students (medical and nursing)
Laboratory personnel
Blood bank professionals
Visiting professionals
Administration
Ancillary staff, e.g., admission personnel
Patients and family
The public

Structured educational interventions

Maintaining the philosophy of universal blood management requires continuous education over years, and so planning is essential. Three steps are involved: (a) assessment of educational needs and wants; (b) defining the content of educational interventions; and (c) evaluation (i.e., assessment of what the blood management team has learnt and put into practice as a result).

Needs assessment

The goal of the needs assessment is to determine what the blood management team wants and needs to learn. A variety of methods can be used. The formal ones are surveys in written or oral form [24], questionnaires [25], and a literature search of pertinent information [26]. The informal ones include discussions in the hospital lounge, cafeteria, or at medical meetings, or simply, intuition. "Keeping one's ear to the ground or one's hand on the pulse of medical practice" [19] is essential. Another important way to identify educational content is by making a baseline review of current blood management practice. Using treatment policies and procedures that are to be implemented as the basis, an audit may help to identify how well current treatment conforms to such policies and procedures. For example, suppose it were planned that a cell-salvage device be used in a certain type of procedure and hemodilution in another, and that an antifibrinolytic would also be introduced. An audit may reveal that the cell-salvage device and hemodilution are already being used where possible for the majority of eligible patients, but only a few patients receive the antifibrinolytic. Education on the use of the antifibrinolytic agent should, therefore, be given the highest priority. Such an audit needs to be done regularly and continuously throughout the lifetime of the blood management program to identify current educational needs.

To change behavior, it is also wise to ask why members of the blood management team behave in a manner perceived to be unacceptable. For example, a liberal transfusion practice often results from a lack of knowledge of the pathophysiology of anemia [19]. Non-implementation of a cell-salvage device may be based on the belief that returning blood to the patient can often be detrimental. Avoidance of acute normovolemic hemodilution could be based on the understanding that it does not reduce allogeneic transfusions. Other reasons are fear of litigation or criticism for allowing a patient to continue with a low hemoglobin level. Further, some may understand that there are no risks of low-to-moderate anemia, there are benefits inherent to allogeneic transfusions experienced by all patients, and that transfusion risks are so small that they do not outweigh the benefits. Such misconceptions need to be removed.

Another obstacle to change of practice is anxiety. Seymour Handler, in his article "Does continuing medical education affect medical care: a study of improved transfusion practices" [19] summarized the situation experienced in blood management as follows: "Reduced hemoglobin values cause more symptoms in the attending physician than in the patient. The surgeon's anxiety is translated into an order for blood transfusions. Indeed, the major problem of postoperative anemia may be the surgeon's anxiety. Studying massive surgical hemorrhage without blood replacement apparently requires more courage than most surgeons can muster." Apparently, there is a strong emotional component to blood management. To implement changes in the behavior of the blood management team, consideration should be given to the anxiety and timidity exhibited when changes in policy are proposed. Knowing about such misconceptions and anxieties can help those who are responsible to design appropriate educational interventions and motivation campaigns.

Content of education

The content of the education and training offered in the blood management program depends on the result of the needs assessment and on the target students. Make a list of the envisioned educational contents, prioritize them, and add a note about the target audience to help plan such interventions. Content is also best tailored to the current situation of the program. Initially, more basic education is needed; later, updates may be sufficient. Additional *ad hoc* interventions in response to challenges

encountered or to highlight exemplary patient care may reinforce lessons learned in more formal, programmed training. Such patient-based discussions are the spice of the educational program.

In addition to medical issues, organizational issues may be the content of education, as well as team building concepts and communication.

Evaluation of education

The effects of the educational intervention should be evaluated to monitor progress, to spot weak points, and to adapt to developing needs. Several methods can be used to do so: (a) comparison of behavior before and after training, (b) comparison of performance and behavior in the hospital's program with that in other hospitals or programs, and (c) comparison of professional behavior after training with that of those in the hospital who did not receive special training. Professionals who have not changed their behavior in response to the educational intervention may thus be identified. There may be a problem that has not received due attention. When the situation is taken care of, these professionals may be more than willing to comply with the contents of the training.

"Crucial prerequisites for success in postgraduate education include the voluntary participation and active learner involvement of resident and staff physicians, as well as the education program coordinator's respect for the resident's autonomy, familiarity with their already crowded educational agenda, and accommodation of their time-consuming professional commitments" [27]. Taking these points into consideration, put the educational plan down in writing. It could be included in the schedule that every new employee receives as part of the orientation. A brief introduction to blood management and an invitation to participate could also be included. At least one annual mandatory lecture on blood management could be scheduled for nursing staff, and invitations for blood management conferences could be posted on nurses' bulletin boards. Fixed dates for scheduled education and training should be set to ensure the highest possible participation of all involved in the blood management program and that no one is overlooked.

Educational methods and tools

There is a wide variety of educational methods to choose from [28] and they can all be used to teach blood management. The best results seem to be achieved by a combination of methods, depending on local circumstances, target audience, and manpower available.

Formal one-to-one education

Formal one-to-one education is a very effective means of changing the behavior of medical professionals. It is used by pharmaceutical companies in that they regularly send representatives to physicians who are potentially in a position to effect a change in practice. This type of intervention is time consuming, although a session rarely exceeds 90 minutes. It has been shown that even short 30-minute visits to surgeons increases the likelihood of their increasing the rate of autologous donations.

Formal one-to-one education may be scheduled as a brief visit of 30–90-minutes duration [29] for which preparation is needed. Defining the goal of the visit and the take-home messages (not too many) help in arranging visits such that the goals are reached. Material needs to be gathered which supports the credibility of the source information presented. The pros and cons of the information presented need to be discussed, as do the benefits of the proposed change of behavior. Those visited should be encouraged to interact and to continue working with others in the blood management team. At the end of the session, the take-home messages should be repeated and the individual visited should be aware of the behavioral changes expected. Ideally, visual aids should be used and a short summary of the content discussed should be left with the visited person. Questions should be allowed and contact information for the visiting professional should be available after the visit.

An example of an outline for a formal one-to-one educational intervention can be found in Appendix C.

Informal one-to-one education

Situations for informal discussion of blood management-related issues arise spontaneously. They arise at the bedside, in the canteen or lounge, in the hallways, after formal meetings, etc. It is up to those concerned to take advantage of such situations. The impact of such informal one-to-one education is difficult to study, but it seems to substantially influence the person contacted. In fact, informal one-to-one education is thought to be the most effective type of educational intervention [19].

Lectures and grand rounds

Most hospitals in the world arrange regular lectures and grand rounds for professionals. Such educational interventions are either scheduled for the whole hospital or part of the in-service education of the various departments. Lectures have the advantage that many can be taught at one time, making them a relatively inexpensive type of education. However, the knowledge conveyed is limited and behavioral changes often do not occur. When lectures are used, they are best combined with other methods of education.

Conferences on blood management

Educational conferences dedicated to blood management are often of high quality. Most of the topics presented relate to blood management, making such conferences a very condensed form of education. They offer multiple opportunities to network with colleagues and discuss current topics of blood management, as well as opportunities to ask questions, formally or informally. However, such conferences are often used only by individuals who are already interested in blood management. The high cost of participation and travel may preclude most staff from attending. A solution to this problem is to send one or two members of the team who on return present selected issues to all members of the team.

Daily clinical rounds

Patients who are candidates for a certain procedure (cell salvage, minimization of iatrogenic blood loss) or who are at high risk for developing severe anemia can be visited daily by a trained member of the blood management team. Typically, a chart review is performed and the past day's therapy is discussed, as well as the next steps in blood management. When deviations from established policies and procedures are observed, personnel attending to the patient can be instructed as needed [30]. However, this approach is time consuming, especially in the initial phase of establishing a program. Yet, it is very likely to be effective, and in time, staff will be alert to the treatment needed for blood management and only a few patient cases will need to be discussed.

Retrospective peer review and audit

In transfusion medicine, peer review processes and audits have proven valuable in reducing transfusions. In some hospitals, medical records personnel check transfusion forms retrospectively for compliance with transfusion guidelines [31]. Other hospitals describe an approach where blood bank pathologists review the indications for blood transfusions and provide a written or oral review to the physician who ordered the transfusion [20]. Regular chart review can provide valuable clues about blood management practice. Using and circulating the results of such reviews, educational interventions can be tailored explicitly to address the weak points identified.

Algorithms

No matter how well designed they are, policies and procedures are of no use if they are not implemented. A great deal of time needs to be invested in implementation. Algorithms can be an aid in doing this. Implementation may involve providing technical and organizational support (e.g., immediate availability of drugs and equipment, bedside monitoring), training, and initial guidance until the algorithm has been internalized by staff.

Prospective review of blood management practice

Reviewing transfusion decisions prospectively has been shown to reduce inappropriate transfusion behavior. Blood bank personnel who are required to check the indication before blood is issued can review every transfusion order prospectively. They may be able to withhold blood products or provide instant information on a more appropriate therapy. A mandatory pathology consultation has been established before clotting factor concentrates were issued [32]. Using well-trained decision-makers for the transfusion decision has reduced the use of the blood products.

Computer systems can also be used to double-check the transfusion order [33]. They can list accepted indications and alert the physician regarding any deviations from such. The computer system can utilize laboratory results, e.g., the latest hemoglobin value or the coagulation profile, to provide further support. Similarly, computers can be used to double-check the hematological status of patients before booking the operating room for elective procedures is permitted. Similarly, a computer system can be used to double-check whether or not a patient has given informed consent for the scheduled procedure.

Self-educating documentation and order slips

Existing guidelines are often not translated into practice. Typically, published guidelines are buried in files or disappear in physicians' drawers. A convenient way to turn blood-related guidelines into practice is to design order sheets for blood management procedures, containing a short and simple form of procedure-related guidelines. Such a self-educating blood or procedure request form is a simple administrative intervention that can encourage adherence to policies and procedures [34].

Simply printing transfusion guidelines with information on acceptable and unacceptable transfusion practice on the blood request form forces the transfusing physician to read the guidelines. The front page of such a form might consist of fields to be filled in, depending on what blood product the physician plans to administer. If red cells are ordered, the fields may be the latest hemoglobin level, heart rate, blood pressure, and the presence of symptoms of anemia. The reason for the transfusion and the clinical situation (e.g., type of surgery) should be stated for all blood products. The institution's transfusion guidelines can be printed on the reverse side of the form. Mandatory completion of forms before blood is released has been instrumental in enforcing adherence to transfusion policies [20]. The beauty of this self-educating request form lies in its simplicity. No manpower is needed to instruct users, and it is well accepted, especially by junior medical staff. By reading the form, staff members instantly educate themselves. They may realize that their request does not comply with current guidelines, so they may refrain from asking for blood. Thus, they do not lose face, and therefore, this educational instrument may be well accepted.

In a similar manner to blood product request forms, request and documentation forms for blood management-related procedures may be designed to support adherence to established guidelines. Documentation forms for autologous blood use may include inclusion and exclusion criteria, a checklist of the steps involved in performing the procedure, and mandatory fields to be filled in. Other forms may include the content of the informed consent process, the algorithm used to optimize a patient's hemoglobin level prior to surgery, the procedures to draw blood samples in patients at high risk for iatrogenic blood loss, and the schedule for preoperative assessment and optimization before elective surgery is performed (e.g., booking the operating room is possible only when the patient has reached at least minimum hemoglobin level).

Combining the form with an audit process further enhances the value of the educational intervention. Requests that do not comply with guidelines may first have to be cross-checked by a blood management specialist. The compiled request and documentation forms for each month may be audited by the blood management committee.

Reading assignments and journal clubs

While reading assignments may be feasible only in the formal education setting, a journal club may make reading assignments acceptable for professionals. During a 1-hour session, one or a number of selected articles dealing with blood management can be discussed. Typically, journal club participants know in advance which articles are to be discussed and they are asked to read them before the meeting. A short presentation of the content is given to summarize the article and a discussion follows. A good communicator should be chosen to steer the discussion and to provide constructive feedback. Explicit learning objectives for each meeting together with a structured review and meeting process may contribute to the educational success of the journal club [35, 36]. When all participants are asked to contribute, they change from being passive listeners to active learners. This will help them to retain the content of the articles. Combining reading with a meal at each club meeting will make the journal club an even more pleasant experience and the opportunity to socialize may be a further incentive for participation.

Dedicated teaching programs

A very successful type of education is a specifically developed rotation, exclusively dedicated to blood management. This is a time- and resource-intensive endeavor, but seems to bring rich reward. Such a dedicated program typically includes seminars, attendance at blood management meetings, research projects, reading assignments, dedicated lectures, hands-on experience in blood management techniques (in the laboratory and in the clinical setting), and acting as consultants for physicians and patients in the blood management program, and it could conclude with formal graduation tests. Implementing such a dedicated teaching program needs much planning. The goals and objectives need to be outlined and staff need to be assigned to this program. A time period should be fixed for the participants of the program. For example, anesthesiology residents interested in transfusion issues were offered a 2-month rotation dedicated to transfusion medicine [37]. Similar programs have been designed in the field of bloodless healthcare and in blood management in general.

While such programs may, at first, seem hard to install, the benefits outweigh the disadvantages. Staff trained in such intensive programs are most likely dedicated and well trained in effective blood management. The program trainees are apt candidates for research projects. These projects can be designed to audit and substantially improve the hospital's blood management.

Use of educational tools

There are many educational tools. Per se, they do not educate but they provide help to teach. Educational tools can be distributed to persons who are motivated enough to use them themselves or the tools can be used in education and training by blood management teachers. In the latter case, they are only useful in combination with other educational interventions. Otherwise, they are ineffective in changing healthcare provider practices.

Current literature articles

Literature articles are valuable teaching tools. Therefore, the coordinator of the blood management program will want to stay up-to-date with the literature on blood management. Useful articles could be collected and distributed to others who want the information or need to have it. However, discretion is required and the choice should be selective. Flooding others with literature does not help. On the contrary, it may even make them reluctant to read articles that are especially important for them. Therefore, if the coordinator finds an interesting article about heart surgery, it should not be sent to the urologists and dermatologists in the program, but rather should be reserved for the cardiac surgeons. Interesting literature may also be sent for reading in response to a recent case. If a team is confronted with a difficult case and there is something in the literature that might help design the patient's care plan, it should be sent to all team members. The team members may be more inclined to read the article despite their tight schedule because it appears to be beneficial and relevant.

Videotapes

In situations where many persons are to be taught, videotapes may be very useful [38]. A slide show running in parallel with a recorded tape explanation could be used as an alternative.

Often videos are commercially available. Companies selling medical equipment for blood management provide videos for free. If there is no video available to fit current educational needs, a video could even be produced by program staff. In teaching environments such as universities, there are often media centers that can aid in producing the video. If a practical topic is to be taught, e.g., cell salvage or patient identification, the person performing the procedure can be followed with a video camera and comments can be added. Photographs and computerized graphics may be used to supplement the educational content. If self-production of educational videos is not possible, commercial videos may be an adequate substitute.

Videos provide a uniform method of teaching. Since the video can be used on multiple occasions, persons working in different shifts, in different departments, and even in different hospitals can be taught using the same educational content. This may compensate for the efforts required to produce a video.

Although it might seem a good idea simply to send copies of the video to healthcare providers and ask them to view it, it may be more practical to invite practitioners to prearranged video sessions. Healthcare providers may be more inclined to watch the video—discussion of the educational contents will be promoted among the audience, and the number of persons who actually watch the video can be monitored.

Samples of equipment or drugs

Samples of equipment or drugs may be useful educational tools. They may be used to provide hands-on experience or it may be possible to simply ask a sales representative to bring in some drug samples and printed information. The drugs can be issued to healthcare providers who are then asked to use them in practice. It may be of greater educational value to arrange not only for samples to be supplied but also for the assistance of a professional to demonstrate how the samples are used. For example, to introduce a tissue adhesive into practice, a sales representative might be willing to demonstrate how best to assemble the syringes, prepare the area where the adhesive is to be applied, apply the adhesive, and check its effectiveness. The representative may be able to provide some insider tips, making it easier for staff to use the product. Such an approach would help avoid suboptimal results with the adhesive; this in turn might lead to healthcare providers becoming frustrated and abandoning a method which would have been beneficial had it been used properly.

If equipment is bought, healthcare providers who are expected to use it will have to be trained in its use. If there are multiple options available and no decision has been made as to which brand is to be bought, why not borrow each model and ask those healthcare providers concerned to try them out. Sales representatives, technicians, or healthcare providers experienced in the use of the equipment should be available in the initial stages when new equipment is introduced. There are already educational guidelines available for some blood management techniques, e.g., for autotransfusion [39]. Coordinators may want to use such guidelines. These usually show concisely how to teach the essential details of the method. Often companies that produce equipment can provide educational material. Using these along with the equipment in a hospital setting may be the most effective way of training staff to use new technology.

Brochures and pictures

Brochures, pictures, charts, tables, and similar printed material may be efficient tools for educating patients, nursing staff, medical staff, and the public. They may be used to convey basic ideas and to explain various methods used in blood management. They can also be used as marketing tools. Such printed material may be made available through the marketing department of the hospital. It may be designed by the coordinator, or previously published material can be used, if permitted.

The coordinator should ensure that he/she has all the printed material available to meet the needs of the program. This would include pictures of a cell-saving device and a heart–lung machine for patient education. Charts showing how to perform acute normovolemic hemodilution may be used to educate healthcare providers. Program brochures may be available as a giveaway for patients who are treated in the blood management program and for media representatives. Written material, including current treatment algorithms, may be handed out to healthcare providers receiving their initial orientation. As the blood management program develops, printed material can be designed to be used as an effective tool in all types of educational interventions.

Role plays

Selected educational topics can best be taught in role-play settings. One example is improving the process of informed consent for blood management. Role plays may be welcome to practice this essential part of blood management. As demonstrated in a study, a 1-hour didactic lesson coupled with a 90-minute workshop with role plays tremendously improved healthcare providers' ability to inform patients about the options in blood management and to obtain a valid informed consent for the planned treatment [40].

Combinations of educational interventions

As the literature demonstrates, combinations of some of the above-mentioned educational interventions are effective in reducing allogeneic blood use [41]. For instance, the combination of audit, review of published guidelines, case presentations, and an in-service program has proven successful in substantially reducing fresh frozen plasma transfusions [42]. In another campaign to improve the awareness of physicians about transfusions guidelines, a small leaflet with the guidelines was distributed, the topic was discussed within the departments, a continuing medical education program for all staff members was set up, and questions were answered on a one-to-one basis. This combination of educational interventions reduced unjustified transfusions [43]. When planning educational interventions, a variety of methods in combination is most effective.

Step 7: How to proceed

- Identify educational needs.
- List groups of persons participating in the blood management program who should be trained.
- List educational methods within the reach of the program.
- Outline a schedule ensuring initial and continuing education of all those who should be trained.

Step 8: Marketing

Marketing, in other words "going to the market," can mean that something is obtained or something is sold. On going to the market, it is helpful to know what exactly is to be marketed. Realistic goals should also be defined before going to the market.

Posing a series of questions will help identify the product or service to be marketed—in this case, blood management. The answers to such questions as: "What service do I want to market?," "How is this product identified (name, logo)?," "What is unique and important about this service?," "Why would people be willing to use this service?," and "What is especially attractive to customers?" will clarify how the product is identified in the market. Even if the answers are obvious, it is wise to take the time to put them in writing. This is the starting point for the marketing concept.

Next, set the marketing goals. The goals may include making money, increasing the hospital's market share, retaining patients, attracting new patients, or enhancing the hospital's image. Improving patient care can also be a marketing goal. Since blood management is good clinical practice that improves patient outcome, successfully marketing blood management, in turn, also improves the outcome by convincing the patients to use this superior mode of treatment.

The next step is to define the target group. Who would look for blood management services of his/her own initiative or who can be convinced to do so? These individuals are the marketing target and include referring physicians, potential patients, the media, the public, your colleagues, or others (see Appendix C).

At this point, marketing tools need to be chosen and there are many. However, since not all marketing methods fit all target groups, a method applicable to the group has to be selected. The program's budget as well as the time and manpower available may limit the choice of marketing methods. Marketing media are chosen taking these factors into account. They might include print media, electronic media, person-to-person communication, distribution of giveaways and gimmicks, and word of mouth (see Appendix C). Presentations can be scheduled at staff orientations. The public or healthcare providers can be invited to blood management seminars. Customers of companies providing equipment for blood management can be contacted.

Another very interesting marketing tool is a club. Clubs can be founded for the chronically ill, e.g., for sickle cell disease patients. Organizing regular club meetings for the patients and their families not only attracts "customers" for the hospital, but also serves to educate those concerned about disease management and enhances adherence to a chronic drug regimen. In turn, such clubs attached to a blood management program have been shown to improve patient outcome, potentially resulting in a reduction in mortality [1].

Most probably, help will be needed to successfully market a blood management program. If available, the hospital's public relations manager can be asked for help. Also, a commercial consultant can be instrumental in designing and marketing the program. Those who are experienced in running a blood management program can share their experiences when asked for advice.

Step 8: How to proceed

- Define the marketing goals.
- List the target groups for the marketing initiative.
- Select marketing methods to address the target groups identified.
- Recruit help for marketing initiatives.

Step 9: Running the program

Once the initial hurdles have been cleared, many daily challenges encountered while running the program will have to be faced. In the following, some suggestions are given as to how such challenges can be met.

Setting priorities

At the beginning of the program there is so much to do that it cannot possibly all be done at once; therefore, it is imperative to set priorities. The burden of organization and prioritizing will fall mainly on the coordinator. Prioritizing means to limit the initial tasks to items that are really important. The contract on which the blood management program is based may already limit the field of work, thus setting the priorities. If the hospital administration has agreed to launch blood conservation in the cardiac surgery department only, then this limit should be respected, even if other departments urgently need blood conservation. If the program is limited to a special patient population, then this should be the priority. In time, the opportunity to expand the program may arise, but for practical reasons, the tasks assigned to the program must have priority.

But what if the purpose of the blood management program is described as "perioperative blood management"' or even as "hospital-wide" blood management? Then, suddenly, the program coordinator will most probably be confronted with an enormous workload. This can be compiled in a desk journal to help organize the work at hand. Whenever a new task arises, it should be noted in the journal. Once in a while, upcoming tasks need to be prioritized. If there is so much work that the coordinator is unable to do it, it needs to be limited. How can this be done?

If the first task is to demonstrate that the program can reduce transfusions, then it is best to start where most transfusions can be reduced and this place needs to be identified. Sometimes, this will be self-evident from the available hospital statistics. If, for instance, orthopedic surgeons transfuse much more than ear, nose, and throat surgeons, then the orthopedic department may deserve initial attention. If the workload needs further limiting, blood product use can be classified by disease. The hospital's information department may be able to print a list of transfusions, sorted according to diagnosis-related groups [44]. These can be ranked, starting with the diseases for which most transfusions are administered, and priorities can be listed top down. Another starting point could be where the most variations in transfusion use occur. To this end, transfusions can be classified according to surgeon. Some surgeons may transfuse more than others for the same procedure. This may be the point where transfusion use varies most and where a start can be made to lower transfusion rates. For instance, a surgeon who transfuses small amounts could be asked to describe the technique

used to help those who transfuse more to adapt their technique.

Another approach in Belgium, which began small and systemically expanded, has been described [17]. This approach divides blood management into three stages. A basic analysis of the situation in the hospital will reveal the stage at which the hospital operates. As the program progresses, the first stage will give way to the second and the third.

- **Stage 1:** Most or all patients receiving a type of surgery are transfused.
  - ○ *Strategy:* Use of systematic blood management measures that benefit all patients. A reduction of blood use is expected in all patients.
- **Stage 2:** A new class of patients who are not transfused emerges.
  - ○ *Strategy:* Try to identify prospectively which patient population is transfused and which is not. Rethink the transfusion decision and the decision on which blood management measures are used. Do they increase risks and costs for non-transfused patients? Focus blood management measures on patients who typically receive transfusions.
- **Stage 3:** Most patients receive no allogeneic transfusions. However, a small group of patients still receives major amounts of blood.
  - ○ *Strategy:* Analysis of critical incidents. Are there indicators for the critical incidents? Are there procedural changes that may reduce such critical incidents? Can blood management be improved in such situations? At what cost? Is there a safety net that can be established for the patients?

After these three stages have been completed, further progress can still be made. Every drop of blood should be considered precious. A database established in the initial phase of program development will help identify emerging problems early, as well as interteam variability and other challenges that need to be addressed. Continually adapting blood management is vital for continued progress.

Data collection propels the program

Data should be gathered from the beginning of the blood management program and stored in a database [11]. A well-designed database will provide valuable information about the progress of the program and about potential challenges. It will be a research tool, will permit comparison of the effectiveness of newly modified blood management measures, and will assist in quality control.

Table 19.6 Contents of the database.

Demographic data of patients

Patient risk factors (pre-existing diseases, drugs)

Surgery or procedures performed

Details of blood management measures (e.g., acute normovolemic hemodilution with volumes, volume replacement, etc.)

Drugs used for blood management

Outcome data (length of stay, morbidity, mortality)

Use of blood products

Designing such a database may take more time than initially anticipated, but it is well worth the effort. Permission from the hospital's ethical review board will have to be obtained initially. When this is granted, the content of the database will need to be defined. An interdisciplinary working group including the computer department may be required for this task. Listing the questions the database is to answer will help determine what data need to be collected. Working definitions for each data entry need to be defined (e.g., What is considered a deep vein thrombosis? and What is considered preoperative aspirin ingestion?). Table 19.6 lists potential contents of a blood management database.

Data to be entered into the database should be collected for every patient over the lifetime of the program. The information sets collected should be as complete as possible. In addition to the fixed content, flexible space may be left in the database. This will allow for temporary collection of additional data, e.g., for a short-term research project. Keep the database simple. Data sheets attached to patient files or hand-held computers used to enter data collected on chart review may facilitate data collection.

It should be simple to retrieve data from the database. The computer department may be able to design the database so that important data can be regularly summarized and tables, charts, and reports can be printed for the hospital administration or for research projects.

Building routine

Running a blood management program involves many routine tasks. These include patient tracking, referrals, patient transfers, patient education, obtaining informed consent, patient assessment, staff education, bookkeep-

ing, and many more. To ensure these tasks do not become a heavy burden, the coordinator needs to establish a routine and to design appropriate forms and checklists to perform tasks properly.

It is also practical to establish and publicize office hours, a phone number, e-mail address, and emergency contacts. This will give patients and healthcare providers alike the chance to contact program staff. It will also help the coordinator find time when he/she can work without disturbance.

Every morning on coming to the hospital the coordinator should know which patients are participating in the blood management program. This is where patient tracking comes in. Which patients need to be tracked daily depends on the scope of the program. Thus, selection criteria have to be established for patients who should be in the program. If the program is for orthopedic patients only, then the coordinator should be informed about all current and upcoming orthopedic patients. If the coordinator takes care of Jehovah's Witness patients, then he/she has to track them. If the coordinator wants to track all patients whose blood management needs close monitoring, he/she may want to know about all patients with low hemoglobin levels or with a coagulopathy. Whatever the case, the coordinator needs to find all the patients that fit the selection criteria. Patients may come to the blood management office to contact the program coordinator. Physicians and nurses may be instructed to inform the coordinator whenever a patient happens to fit the selection criteria. It may also be possible to retrieve the names of patients who fit the selection criteria from the hospital medical or admission computer system. The hospital's computer department may be able to connect the laboratory computer to a blood management program e-mail account to notify the coordinator about patients whose laboratory values indicate severe anemia or coagulopathy, and a visit can be scheduled. It may even be possible to adjust the admission routine to screen patients eligible for blood management. The admission clerk may ask patients if they are willing to participate in the blood management program. If they agree, the admission clerk may note this on the computer and an e-mail is automatically sent to the blood management program.

Identifying patients in the blood management program is also important. Again, which patients need to be identified depends on the scope of the program. If all eligible patients are treated according to the tenets of blood management, some hospitals differentiate between level 1 and level 2 patients, based on whether individual patients refuse transfusion under all circumstances or not. Other hospitals have decided to identify intensive

Table 19.7 Contents of an office program.

Data file with patient contact information

Data file with information about healthcare providers willing to do blood management

Forms (linked to the patient and physician database) for transfer, referrals, informed consent, information materials, marketing, etc.

Tools to schedule appointments (e.g., for preoperative recombinant human erythropoietin [rHuEPO] or iron therapy)

Filing of pertinent literature

care patients who receive special treatment to reduce iatrogenic blood loss. In other places, patients with at least a 10% risk of receiving a transfusion are identified. In practice, patient identification can involve marking the patient's chart, attaching a wristband, attaching a warning sign to the patient's bed, or entering a special note into the computer.

Some blood management programs have greatly benefited from the use of a dedicated computer program (Table 19.7) to organize the daily routine. The program supports daily tasks and contains information and tools needed daily. Tasks such as letter writing and filling in forms, keeping track of patients and physicians participating in the program, transfers, referrals, literature organization, and research can all be supported with software. It can either be designed by the hospital's computer department or by a commercial provider. Programs tested in practice are commercially available.

Forms, questionnaires, and checklists need to be designed in order to transfer established administrative policies and procedures from the paper into practice. Many of the forms used elsewhere have been published in the literature [45] or on the Internet. They can simply be adjusted to the needs of the program. As an example, Appendix C contains a transfer form with a checklist for reference.

Step 9: How to proceed

- If overwhelmed by the amount of work, set priorities and tackle one item at a time.
- Obtain a computer program that fills the program's needs.
- Design forms and checklists that facilitate routine tasks.

Step 10: Evaluation and safety

Evaluation and benchmarking

In all likelihood the goals for the blood management program were established at the business proposal stage. After some time has elapsed, it will be worthwhile to check whether these goals have been reached. Data have to be collected to do this. The database mentioned earlier can be designed to evaluate the blood management program. Which data are collected for evaluation depends on what needs to be measured. If increasing the patient load was the goal, patient numbers need to be tracked. It may also be useful to check new patients' area codes to see where they come from. Or if the goal of the program is to reduce transfusions, transfusion statistics, the procedures performed, and the patients who were treated need to be registered.

Evaluation of the program, however, does not only consist of checking to see whether the program has reached its business goals. It would be interesting to know how the program performed medically and how it is performing in comparison with other blood management programs. The purpose of this is to improve patient care and to provide information to policymakers, patients, and the public, and it may lead to available resources being used more efficiently. To benefit from such an evaluation, benchmarking is needed. Benchmarking simply means setting a point of reference or comparison to define excellent patient service. What constitutes best service currently can be determined by consulting the program's benchmarking partners. Benchmarking implies that performance is improved by adopting the best practice of benchmarking partners. Procedures that benchmarking partners use to outperform the program being evaluated are identified and adopted. In turn, benchmarking partners use features of other programs to improve where necessary.

Safety systems

Preventing hazards in the blood management program improves patient safety. Safety provisions contribute to the performance of a blood management program. By definition, blood management includes a commitment to safe patient care. Safety assurance must be a central part of the blood management program.

Organized measures to systematically prevent hazards and improve patient safety are relatively new to medicine in general and to blood management in particular. However, safety programs per se are not new. Aviation and many other businesses with the potential for causing serious accidents have systems in place to prevent serious hazards and have established a convincing safety record. What can be learned from aviation and other industrial safety systems? The overall goal is to prevent major fatal accidents. As these occur infrequently, there is no way to analyze them statistically for triggers. However, major accidents are often preceded by major and minor incidents, termed near misses. In comparison to major fatal accidents, such incidents occur much more frequently and are amenable to systematic analysis when reported. Modern safety systems analyze incidents, and a safety culture is developed. In such a safety culture the awareness of participants is raised so that notice is taken even of minor errors and near misses, and reporting encouraged. Of course, the individual reporting the incident should not have to fear any adverse consequences. An analysis is made and the reason for the near miss sought. Any intrinsic problem is identified to prevent further near misses. This is how major fatal accidents are reduced. There needs to be a clear line between acceptable and unacceptable practice, and all participants should be aware of it. Further elements of safety systems include continuing monitoring of service performance, a report system for near misses and fatalities, an initiative to analyze reported events in order to draw the necessary conclusions, and making changes to policies mirroring the commitment to avoid a recurrence of the reported event as well as adopting appropriate measures to implement these policies.

The safety concept used in aviation is also applicable in blood management. An error log can be kept to record all errors. These errors can be grouped as actual errors, potential major errors, and potential minor errors [46]. Errors can be grouped according to the processes they occur in and are typically defined as deviations from established policies. Table 19.8 provides an example of errors in a process relevant to blood management.

Once a patient hazard has been identified, policy changes need to be implemented. Three key points are essential to implement policy changes that result in increased patient safety: simplify, avoid duplication, and implement changes in a multidisciplinary fashion [26]. Keeping processes simple and guidelines concise reduces errors. Duplication of paperwork leads to errors; therefore, each set of data should be collected only once. Also, a multidisciplinary approach is essential when it comes to working on and modifying guidelines.

Table 19.8 Example of errors in the process of informed consent.

- Actual error:
  - The patient is treated contrary to his/her stated wishes
- Potential errors—major:
  - Patient did not receive information about blood management
  - Patient was not given the opportunity to fill out the informed consent form
  - Patient underwent surgery without the surgeon knowing about the patient's preferences regarding blood management
- Potential errors—minor:
  - Wrong name on patient informed consent form
  - Consent form is not filed in patient chart
  - Information is missing; not all required details of patient's wishes are recorded
  - Signature on the informed consent form is missing

Step 10: How to proceed

- Review the business goals regularly and document whether they have been met.
- Participate in benchmarking to improve the service offered by the blood management program.
- Put a safety system in place to keep a record of all errors. Correct policies and procedures after analysis of recorded safety failures.

Suggestions for further research

What are the effective methods to motivate healthcare providers? What role does motivation play in implementing a blood management program? How can others be motivated to become blood managers?

Homework

Find out what is required to obtain permission from the ethics committee to establish a blood management database.

Are there any legal restrictions on advertising by medical facilities in your country? If so, what are they?

References

1. Akinyanju OO, Otaigbe AI, Ibidapo MO. Outcome of holistic care in Nigerian patients with sickle cell anaemia. *Clin Lab Haematol* 2005;**27**:195–199.

2. Morgan TO. Blood conservation: the CEO perspective. *J Cardiothorac Vasc Anesth* 2004;**18** (4 Suppl):15S–17S.

3. Freedman J, Luke K, Monga N, *et al.* A provincial program of blood conservation: The Ontario Transfusion Coordinators (ONTraC). *Transfus Apher Sci* 2005;**33**:343–349.

4. Derderian GP. Establishing a business plan for blood conservation. *J Cardiothorac Vasc Anesth* 2004;**18** (4 Suppl): 12S–14S.

5. Spiess BD. Blood conservation: why bother? *J Cardiothorac Vasc Anesth* 2004;**18** (4 Suppl):1S–5S.

6. Morgan TO. Cost, quality, and risk: measuring and stopping the hidden costs of coronary artery bypass graft surgery. *Am J Health Syst Pharm* 2005;**62** (18 Suppl 4):S2–S5.

7. Ozawa S, Shander A, Ochani TD. A practical approach to achieving bloodless surgery. *AORN J* 2001;**74**:34–40, 42–47; quiz 48, 50–54.

8. Lomas J, Enkin M, Anderson GM, Hannah WJ, Vayda E, Singer J. Opinion leaders vs audit and feedback to implement practice guidelines. Delivery after previous cesarean section. *JAMA* 1991;**265**:2202–2207.

9. Greco PJ, Eisenberg JM. Changing physicians' practices. *N Engl J Med* 1993;**329**:1271–1273.

10. Hiss RG, *et al.* Identification of physician educational influentials in small community hospitals. *Res Med Educ* 1978;**17**:283–288.

11. Green JA. Blood conservation in cardiac surgery: the Virginia Commonwealth University (VCU) experience. *J Cardiothorac Vasc Anesth* 2004;**18** (4 Suppl):18S–23S.

12. Rosengart TK, Helm RE, DeBois WJ, Garcia N, Krieger KH, Isom OW. Open heart operations without transfusion using a multimodality blood conservation strategy in 50 Jehovah's Witness patients: implications for a "bloodless"' surgical technique. *J Am Coll Surg* 1997;**184**:618–629.

13. Salem-Schatz SR, Avorn J, Soumerai SB. Influence of knowledge and attitudes on the quality of physicians' transfusion practice. *Med Care* 1993;**31**:868–878.

14. Waters JH. Overview of blood conservation. *Transfusion* 2004;**44** (12, Suppl):1S–3S.

15. Martyn V, Farmer SL, Wren MN, *et al.* The theory and practice of bloodless surgery. *Transfus Apher Sci* 2002;**27**:29–43.

16. Shander A. Surgery without blood. *Crit Care Med* 2003;**31** (12 Suppl):S708–S714.

17. Baele P, Van der Linden P. Developing a blood conservation strategy in the surgical setting. *Acta Anaesthesiol Belg* 2002;**53**:129–136.

18. Domen RE, Rybicki LA, Popovsky MA, Milam JD. Fellowship training programs in blood banking and transfusion medicine: results of a national survey. *Am J Clin Pathol* 1996;**106**:584–587.

19. Handler S. Does continuing medical education affect medical care. A study of improved transfusion practices. *Minn Med* 1983;**66**:167–180.

20. Rehm JP, Otto PS, West WW *et al.* Hospital-wide educational program decreases red blood cell transfusions. *J Surg Res* 1998;**75**:183–186.

21. Ferraris VA, Ferraris SP. Limiting excessive postoperative blood transfusion after cardiac procedures. A review. *Tex Heart Inst J* 1995;**22**:216–230.

22. Wilson K, MacDougall L, Fergusson D, Graham I, Tinmouth A, Hébert PC. The effectiveness of interventions to reduce physician's levels of inappropriate transfusion: what can be learned from a systematic review of the literature. *Transfusion* 2002;**42**:1224–1229.

23. Salamat A, Seaton J, Watson HG. Impact of introducing guidelines on anticoagulant reversal. *Transfus Med* 2005;**15**:99–105.

24. Irving G. A survey of the use of blood and blood components among South African anaesthetists working in teaching hospitals. *S Afr Med J* 1992;**82**:324–328.

25. Rock G, Berger R, Pinkerton P, Fernandes B. A pilot study to assess physician knowledge in transfusion medicine. *Transfus Med* 2002;**12**:125–128.

26. Mancini ME. Performance improvement in transfusion medicine. What do nurses need and want? *Arch Pathol Lab Med* 1999;**123**:496–502.

27. Barnette RE, Fish DJ, Eisenstaedt RS. Modification of fresh-frozen plasma transfusion practices through educational intervention. *Transfusion* 1990;**30**:253–257.

28. Toy PT. Audit and education in transfusion medicine. *Vox Sang* 1996;**70**:1–5.

29. Soumerai SB, Salem-Schatz S, Avorn J, Casteris CS, Ross-Degnan D, Popovsky MA. A controlled trial of educational outreach to improve blood transfusion practice. *JAMA* 1993;**270**:961–966.

30. Shanberge JN. Reduction of fresh-frozen plasma use through a daily survey and education program. *Transfusion* 1987;**27**:226–227.

31. Morrison JC, Sumrall DD, Chevalier SP, Robinson SV, Morrison FS, Wiser WL. The effect of provider education on blood utilization practices. *Am J Obstet Gynecol* 1993;**169**:1240–1245.

32. Marques MB, Fritsma GA, Long JA, Adler BK Clinical pathology consultation improves coagulation factor utilization in hospitalized adults. *Am J Clin Pathol* 2003;**120**:938–943.

33. Hoeltge GA, Brown JC, Herzig RH, *et al.* Computer-assisted audits of blood component transfusion. *Cleve Clin J Med* 1989;**56**:267–272.

34. Cheng G, Wong HF, Chan A, Chui CH. The effects of a self-educating blood component request form and enforcements of transfusion guidelines on FFP and platelet usage. Queen Mary Hospital, Hong Kong. British Committee for Standards in Hematology (BCSH). *Clin Lab Haematol* 1996;**18**:83–87.

35. Lee AG, Boldt HC, Golnik KC, *et al*. Structured journal club as a tool to teach and assess resident competence in practice-based learning and improvement. *Ophthalmology* 2006;**113**: 497–500.

36. Lee AG, Boldt HC, Golnik KC, *et al*. Using the Journal Club to teach and assess competence in practice-based learning and improvement: a literature review and recommendation for implementation. *Surv Ophthalmol* 2005;**50**:542–548.

37. Growe GH, Jenkins LC, Naiman SC. Anesthesia training in transfusion medicine. *Transfus Med Rev* 1991;**5**:152–156.

38. Brooks JP, Combest TG. In-service training with videotape is useful in teaching transfusion medicine principles. *Transfusion* 1996;**36**:739–742.

39. Grainger H, Jones J, McGee D; UK Cell Salvage Action Group. Education, training and competency assessment for intraoperative cell salvage. *J Perioper Pract* 2008;**8**:536–542.

40. Goodnough LT, Hull AL, Kleinhenz ME. Informed consent for blood transfusion as a transfusion medicine educational intervention. *Transfus Med* 1994;**4**:51–55.

41. Garrioch M, Sandbach J, Pirie E, Morrison A, Todd A, Green R. Reducing red cell transfusion by audit, education and a new guideline in a large teaching hospital. *Transfus Med* 2004;**14**:25–31.

42. Ayoub MM, Clark JA. Reduction of fresh frozen plasma use with a simple education program. *Am Surg* 1989;**55**: 563–565.

43. Kakkar N, Kaur R, Dhanoa J. Improvement in fresh frozen plasma transfusion practice: results of an outcome audit. *Transfus Med* 2004;**14**:231–235.

44. Jefferies LC, Sachais BS, Young DS. Blood transfusion costs by diagnosis-related groups in 60 university hospitals in 1995. *Transfusion* 2001;**41**:522–529.

45. Gohel MS, Bulbulia RA, Slim FJ, Poskitt KR, Whyman MR. How to approach major surgery where patients refuse blood transfusion (including Jehovah's Witnesses). *Ann R Coll Surg Engl* 2005;**87**:3–14.

46. Galloway M, Woods R, Whitehead S, Gedling P. Providing feedback to users on unacceptable practice in the delivery of a hospital transfusion service—a pilot study. *Transfus Med* 2002;**12**:129–132.

20 Law, Ethics, Religion, and Blood Management

Decision-making is at times difficult, and all the more so when human lives are at stake. Having principles and laws aids in decision-making. This chapter deals with the principles and laws needed to make sound decisions in blood management. It will consider blood management from three different angles: ethical, legal, and religious. All three aspects are interwoven and must be taken into account before decisions are made.

Objectives

1. To relate the basic principles of ethics and law pertaining to blood management.
2. To list the points that need to be kept in mind when caring for a Jehovah's Witness patient.
3. To describe how a compassionate use protocol is instituted.

Definitions

Ethics: Practice of making principled choices between right and wrong, or, as Webster's dictionary put it in 1913, the "science of human duty" or "the body of rules or duty drawn from this science."

Medical ethics determines the principles of proper professional conduct concerning the rights and duties of the physicians, patients, and fellow practitioners, as well as the physicians' actions in the care of patients and interaction with their families.

Patients' rights: Fundamental claims of patients, as expressed in statutes and declarations, or generally accepted moral principles.

Compassionate use (= single patient IND, single patient access): Providing an investigational new drug (IND) to a patient on humanitarian grounds before the drug has received official approval, when the patient would otherwise not qualify for the clinical trial.

Principles as a basis for decision-making in blood management

A body of principles and regulations governs everyday decision-making in medicine, and quite a few of them relate to blood management. Picturing these as a pyramid (Figure 20.1), we see that one set of principles and regulations builds on another one. The very basis for these regulations is found in the Holy Scriptures, as I. Taylor wrote: "The completeness and consistency of its morality is the peculiar praise of the ethics which the Bible has taught." Building on the Bible's teachings and the in-built human conscience, ethics developed which—as a science—describes human duties. As a subset of such ethics, human rights were determined and eventually formulated in writing. Human rights obviously apply also to humans who are sick. Their rights, namely, patients' rights, are based on human rights and specify these to apply in the situation sick persons find themselves in. Charters and bills dealing with patients' rights go another step further and give detailed guidance. As such, they help government and non-government institutions to integrate patients' rights into their legislation or codes by adjusting them to the unique situation in the country or their field of work, respectively.

The pyramid can also be considered from top to bottom. Quite a few principles may not be adequately

Basics of Blood Management, Second Edition. Petra Seeber and Aryeh Shander.
© 2013 John Wiley & Sons, Ltd. Published 2013 by John Wiley & Sons, Ltd.

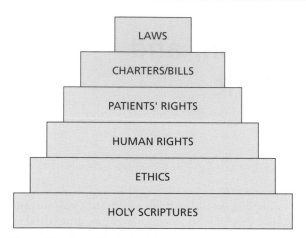

Figure 20.1 Pyramid of principles.

incorporated in the law of a country, yet deserve consideration. A look into charters or bills of patients' rights may help, and, if not available or applicable, basic human rights or principles of ethics and religion may apply.

Principles of bioethics

Many ethical principles apply to the medical field. Among them are autonomy, veracity, fidelity, right to know, beneficence, and justice. The *Belmont Report* [1], formulated in 1979, summarized these as the three "basic ethical principles," being respect for person, beneficence, and justice.

Principle of respect for persons

Respect for persons is expressed in two distinct ways: accepting the autonomy of humans and protecting those who cannot act fully autonomously.

"Autonomy, the moral right to choose and follow one's own plan of life and action, is a deeply embedded and dominant element in western culture, law, ethics, and medicine" [2]. Respecting this autonomy in medicine means that patients are allowed to voice their opinions and choices, and for these to be accepted unless they are outrightly detrimental to others. This includes that patients are given the chance to articulate their decisions intentionally, without controlling influences and informed by the required knowledge. Before a medical intervention is started, an informed consent must be obtained whenever possible. When an informed consent is not available, it must be ruled what should be done to

uphold the respect for person. There are three different ways to determine what the patient wants. The most common is to accept what the patient said before he/she became unconscious (subjective standard). If this is not known, persons who know the patient well can tell about the patient's values and what he/she had said in the past. Judgment can be rendered according to this information (substituted judgment standard). If neither of these standards is available, it is assumed what the patient would have wanted if he/she had the chance to decide.

Accepting the autonomy of a patient is based on the assumption that a patient is capable of self-determining. When this capability is wholly or in part lacking, patients are still entitled to full respect. They must be protected from harming themselves or others, but must also be allowed to follow their plan of life to the extent possible in their limited capability. Respect for persons also requires asking permission of other parties who are legitimate substitute decision-makers for the patient.

Principle of beneficence

The principle of beneficence is the obligation of a physician to benefit the patient. In addition, the Hippocratic maxim "*primum nihil nocere*" (first, do no harm; non-maleficence) is also an expression of the principle of beneficence. Non-maleficence means that no needless harm is administered intentionally.

Unless in an emergency, the physician usually has the right to decide whom he/she has a duty to and whom not; i.e., whom he/she takes as a patient and whom not. Sometimes, a physician has the legal duty to take all patients and can refuse to do so only if his/her conscience is violated. The latter may be the case when a physician has a contract with government agencies that provide healthcare for the public. No matter how the physician entered a patient–physician relationship, it is always his/her duty to adhere to the principle of beneficence.

To act in an ethical manner, procedures performed in blood management must benefit the patient and not cause any undue harm. How does this look in reality? Well, studies are urgently needed to evaluate the benefits of measures of blood management. There is a solid body of evidence that methods like cell salvage and acute normovolemic hemodilution, as well as many drugs, are able to reduce patients' exposure to donor blood, something regarded to be of benefit to the patient. When such methods and drugs are used with skill, their side effects are usually mild. The benefit of avoiding exposure to donor blood seems to exceed the harm possibly caused. Viewed from this angle, to use such methods and drugs therefore seems to be ethical. However, avoiding blood transfusions is not the main goal of blood management. As the definition of blood management states, the goal of this discipline is to improve the outcome of the patient. Currently, many blood management measures are under scrutiny regarding their ability to improve the patient's outcome and therefore benefit the patient. It is only after the availability of sound scientific data that measures of blood management can validly be considered beneficial and, with this, ethical or not.

What about the benefits of allogeneic transfusions? Despite decades of medical transfusions and the well-entrenched belief that allogeneic transfusions are beneficial, most contemporary transfusion practices are not based on solid evidence. It is known that untreated, severe anemia increases mortality. However, it is unclear whether the correction of anemia by transfusion lowers mortality rates. There is an obvious lack of evidence that allogeneic transfusions benefit the patient. In contrast, there is overwhelming evidence that such transfusions cause harm to the recipient. With currently available evidence, it is questionable whether donor blood transfusions meet the criteria for an ethical intervention.

Principle of justice

The principle of justice describes the fair allocation of scarce resources in a society. It also means that nothing good is withheld from a person who has a right to receive it or that undue burden is not imposed on a patient.

Sometimes, it has been called unjust when patients request therapy other than allogeneic transfusion. It was proposed that such patients should pay for any expenses incurred by the choice of other therapeutic options. However, this view was abandoned. Personal choices affect and sometimes increase the risks persons take. As an example, smoking increases the risk of certain diseases. Nevertheless, the expense of the treatment of smoking-related diseases is usually covered by government healthcare. Besides, nobody would ask a patient to pay for the transfusion only because it may, in the long run, be more expensive than non-blood management. The consensus is therefore as follows: Patients who refuse allogeneic transfusions for personal reasons or who want to use alternative treatment are not held liable for any costs incurred by the choice they make [3]. Blood management, whether or not it includes the use of allogeneic blood products, must be made available to all patients. It is perfectly just to offer several therapeutic options to patients and to let the patients have the final say on what they want to use.

Human rights and patients' rights

Based on basic ethical principles, human rights were formulated. In 1945, when the members of the United Nations (UN) signed the Charter of the United Nations, they declared their faith in such human rights. The official UN Declaration of Human Rights was finally signed in 1948. It includes the right to healthcare. Patients' rights as a subset of human rights were declared in parallel to the declaration of human rights.

The human rights movement gave impetus to the development of patients' rights. Another driving factor for patients' rights was the fact that medicine turned into a business, with patients as its customers. Thus, consumer rights also played a role in the definition of patients' rights. In 1962, US president Kennedy identified consumer rights when he voiced a proclamation before the US Congress and identified the rights of safety, information, choice, and voice. Over the years, consumer rights were expanded to include other rights such as patients' rights.

Derived from basic human as well as consumer rights, patients' rights were formulated by organizations such as the World Health Organization (WHO) and Consumers International. Patients' rights include the right to:
• Healthcare
• Access to information
• Choice
• Participation
• Dignity and human care
• Confidentiality
• Complaints and redress.

Such expressions of patients' rights are general and are considered basic. They are thought to be valid for all humans on earth. So, no matter where you live or under which legislation you practice medicine, you are always obliged to uphold the universal patients' rights.

Charters, bills, and laws

With an increased recognition of patients' rights, many governments and non-government organizations have included these in their body of regulations. Various international organizations have drafted bills and charters to aid in decision-making in specific countries. The European Charter of Patients' Rights (the Nice Charter of Fundamental Rights) [4], the Declaration on the Promotion of Patients' Rights in Europe (Amsterdam, 1994), the

Ljubljana Charter on Reforming Health Care (1996), and the Jakarta Declaration on Health Promotion into the 21st Century (1997) are examples. These help to develop laws that suit the countries' needs. Charters, policy-related documents recommending minimum standards for patient care, are the basis for non-governmental organizations to develop patients' rights documents. In contrast, bills are considered to be for governments and are the basis for drafting laws.

On the basis of charters and bills, governments have enacted laws focusing on patients' rights. In 1992, Finland became the first country to enact such a law. The Netherlands followed in 1995. After that, dozens of countries throughout the world have enacted patients' laws or charters [5].

Taking The Nice Charter of Fundamental Rights as an example, it can be seen that there are accepted principles that also pertain to blood management. The Charter "affirms a series of inalienable, universal rights . . . These rights transcend citizenship, attaching to a person as such. They exist even when national laws do not provide for their protection." Fourteen rights of patients were formulated. The third right (right to information) supports the ethical principle of informed consent. "Health care services, providers and professionals have to provide patient-tailored information, particularly taking into account the religious, ethnic or linguistic specificities of the patient" [4]. The fourth right (right to consent) states: "Every individual has the right of access to all information that might enable him or her to actively participate in the decisions regarding his or her health." After being informed, the patient can either consent (fourth right) or refuse (fifth right; right of free choice). Especially interesting is the 10th right (right to innovation): "Each individual has the right of access to innovative procedures, including diagnostic procedures, according to international standards." The 12th right is the right to personalized treatment: "Each individual has the right to diagnostic or therapeutic programs tailored as much as possible to his or her personal needs. The health services must guarantee, to this end, flexible programs, oriented as much as possible to the individual."

In the following, we will go into detail regarding the application of these principles in blood management.

Charters, bills, and laws concerning blood management

For a decision in blood management to be ethical, humane, and legal, certain criteria need to be met. In the following, we define and explain important legal and ethical concepts pertaining to blood management. Understanding these concepts aids in making the required principled decisions.

Informed consent

An informed consent is an expression of patient autonomy, and adhering to it is paramount for upholding this autonomy.

A valid informed consent [6] comprises four elements: (a) Consent must be given voluntarily; (b) the patient must have capacity (adults are assumed to be competent until proven otherwise); (c) consent must be specific (to the treatment and provider of the treatment); and (d) consent must be informed.

The duty of a physician is to inform his/her patient. The extent of information about a medical procedure should be proportional to its risks and its degree of invasiveness. It is commonly held that prescribing an aspirin requires an informed consent, too, but it is not as extensive as the informed consent for liver transplantation. Blood is not a drug like aspirin. The transfusion of blood is more akin to the transplantation of an organ. Furthermore, the informed public is concerned about the risks of transfusions. Informed consent for a blood transfusion is therefore required to be fairly extensive. To this end, many hospitals provide printed consent forms for blood transfusions and other invasive measures, but not for aspirin [7].

Recommendations were given about the contents of the information given to a patient prior to surgery. The information should include the following:
• A description of the recommended therapy, be it a transfusion or a feature of blood management
• Risks and benefits, especially those that lead to death or serious impairment
• Possible alternatives to the proposed procedure with their risks and benefits. In our case, this means measures to reduce the likelihood of receiving allogeneic blood and other blood management options
• What would happen if no treatment at all is administered?
• Probability of success of the intervention
• Length of recuperation
• Other important information.

Some countries have enacted laws that describe the content of the information the patients should receive before they can decide about transfusions in their healthcare plan. For instance, §13(1) of the German Transfusion Act obliges physicians to inform patients about the possibility of autologous transfusions. Similar legislation exists in other countries, such as in some states of the Unites States. With regard to an informed consent, a physician can be held liable if he/she does not inform the patient properly, if he/she does not obtain consent, or if he/she acts contrary to what the patient consented to or refused.

It was established that a patient must be informed as early as possible about the chance of receiving a transfusion. At least 24 hours must be allowed to elapse between the information about the transfusion and the actual transfusion whenever possible. The patient can then make a decision unpressured by time. In case of an emergency, the 24-hour time cannot be allotted and the patient has to decide within a shorter period.

The goal of informed consent is not just to document that a patient him/herself has made a decision about his/her medical care. It is not a "legal bulwark to be contested over and used to mark the boundaries of liability and choice" [8]. Adherence to the principle of informed consent is more than a formalistic approach to patient authority. An informed consent honors the patients' wishes. It includes the right to "say no without censure or sanction" [8]. On the part of the physician, it requires that a patient is not consciously or unconsciously manipulated and coerced to achieve a desired medical end [8]. This would betray the trust and dignity of the patient.

If an informed consent cannot be obtained, as in the case of an emergency, a physician has the privilege to treat the patient without consent. Such a situation arises when the patient's life or health is endangered and the patient has not formulated an advance directive, or the patient cannot give consent and there is no substitute decision maker (such as a person who is permitted to give legal substitute consent or to make an advance directive).

The competent adult has the right to refuse treatment. When the patient has lost consciousness or is otherwise unable to decide for him/herself, a guardian or a court order is often obtained. In a life-endangering emergency, the physician has to assume what the patient's will is. An emergency does not allow for extensive evaluation of the patient's wishes. In such situations physicians are required to do what is in the best interest of the patient. It is assumed that it is in the patient's best interest to keep him/her alive. Physicians are allowed to do the best they can to avert danger to life or health. Since transfusions are considered lifesaving, they are administered without hesitation unless there is reason to assume that the patient would decide differently (as he/she may have outlined in an advance directive).

Advance directive

An advance directive or a living will is the legal expression of a patient's wishes regarding healthcare. It is written to guarantee that the patient's wishes in regard to medical care, medication, and resuscitation are carried out when the patient is unable to communicate his/her desires. Sometimes the advance directive entails a power of attorney that gives someone decision-making powers upon the person's incompetence. Among others, decisions pertaining to blood transfusions are recorded in an advance directive. Countries differ with regard to the form of a valid advance directive. For practical reasons, the written form is preferred, sometimes signed by two witnesses or a solicitor.

Writing an advance directive is one thing, adhering to it is another. Paternalism has widely been replaced by an emphasis on patient participation, respect for autonomy, and quality of life and death [9]. However, difficulties arise when a patient is cognitively impaired. Healthcare professionals often do not consult with the advance directive or tend to engage in "soft" paternalism by making decisions that they think are in the best interest of the patient. Nevertheless, advance directives are binding, no matter whether the physician agrees with their content or not. Many legislations have laws that guide the drafting of advance directives, but few laws exist to enforce adherence to them. To avoid variations in the interpretation of advance directives caused by the ambiguity of terminology, physicians should encourage patients to clarify their wishes, whenever possible. This is especially important for planned interventions.

Pregnancy and motherhood

A patient's right to refuse treatment has sometimes been challenged when the person refusing blood is pregnant or has dependent children. The reason for the challenge is that children need care. It is assumed that the mother will die if she refuses blood transfusions and will therefore abandon her children. Forcing the mother to accept blood is justified by the will to keep the mother alive for her to take care of the children. However, if there is someone willing to take care of the children (the father or another relative, a friend), the mother may be allowed by the court to exercise her right of autonomy to decide freely [10]. In many jurisdictions, maternal–fetal duties and rights are not well defined. However, the principle of autonomy is upheld in general and applies to pregnant women as well. Physicians are not obliged to seek a court order to force a pregnant woman to take a blood transfusion. The ethical tenets of the American Medical Association and the American College of Obstetricians and Gynecologists even discourage such action [11].

Minors

Patients' rights also apply to minors. Minors, no matter how old, have the right of voice. This means that their opinion should be considered whenever reasonable possible. However, parental care and decision usually substitutes for the informed consent of the patient. Parents are responsible for their children. They are morally and legally obliged to take good care of them, providing them with the necessities of life as best as they can. To do this, they are endowed with the right to make decisions for their children. Many of the decisions parents make affect the well-being of their children. The bond between parents and children, ideally, is so tight that outsiders should refrain from intervening. In the great majority of cases, laws do not call for intervention even if the child's well-being is obviously endangered. This is the case where children have to live with smoking parents or when parents verbally abuse or divorce each other. However, when parental decisions clearly violate the well-being of their children, the principle of *parens patriae* kicks in. This means that the state has the duty to assume a parental role for the child and protect him/her from harm.

The principle of *parens patriae* also applies in situations where physicians participate in blood management [12]. It was at times claimed that parents refusing a transfusion for their child constituted an abuse of parental rights or neglect. Nonetheless, when parents demonstrate that they are willing to accept treatment for their child and look for the best possible care without blood, they are taking considerable pains to help their child in accordance with their values. "Refusal of one form of treatment in preference for a viable alternative is exercising the parental right of informed choice, not neglect" [13]. In the United States, the legal view that parents have the right to decide for their child has been upheld in many cases. For instance, the Banks case (Supreme Court, 1994) confirmed that unless there is an emergency that calls for the immediate transfusion of blood, a physician is not allowed to overrule parental refusal of a blood transfusion.

In practical terms, what should be done to avoid morally, ethically, and legally questionable treatment of minors when parents refuse transfusions? A series of steps have been proposed. In most cases, conflicts can be settled with adherence to these suggestions [13]:
• Ask yourself: "Does a truly life-threatening emergency actually exist?"

• Review non-blood medical alternatives and treat the patient without using allogeneic blood.
• If required, consult with other doctors experienced in non-blood alternative management and treat without using allogeneic blood.
• If necessary, transfer the patient to a medical team or facility experienced in blood management before his/her condition deteriorates.
• Have the outcome uncertainties, medical risks, and emotional trauma of a forced blood transfusion been fully considered? Has proper respect been shown for the parents' choice of treatment?

In case of a serious conflict, physicians and families should seek consultative assistance. Only in rare circumstances should judicial determination be sought.

Young minors are incapable of giving an informed consent. An exemption is made for minors who are mature enough to give consent. Some legislation recognizes the term mature minor or an equivalent to it. Persons may be minors under law since they have not passed the age threshold set by the government to be considered an adult. However, adolescents and even children are able to make decisions on their health. If they are mature enough to decide, their wish should be taken into consideration and respected.

The mature minor rule was created as a result of a 1967 court case in the United States, "Smith *vs* Selby." It allows healthcare providers to treat youths as adults, based upon an assessment and documentation of the young person's maturity. The mature minor rule enables the provider to ask the young person questions in order to determine whether or not the minor has the maturity to provide his/her own consent for treatment. Guidelines for an individual to be considered a mature minor include: age, living apart from parents or guardian, maturity, intelligence, economic independence, experience (general conduct of an adult?), and marital status. The age guideline does not provide a lower limit. Treating both 13- and 14-year olds as mature minors when they demonstrate key qualities of the mature minor is reasonable. Treating children aged 12 years and younger is up to the provider's best judgment.

Excursus: The physician and his/her conscience

When patients make use of their right of autonomy, they may at times make a different decision from the one the healthcare provider would. In the setting of blood management, such situations arise, for instance, when Jehovah's Witnesses opt against an allogeneic transfusion. Feelings such as guilt, frustration, and anger may arise in their healthcare providers. "A patient's refusal of care alters routine understandings of beneficence and non-maleficence and complicates caregiver roles. Suddenly, giving a blood transfusion, a routine act of beneficence, has become an act of maleficence for the patient in question" [3]. How can physicians and other healthcare providers continue with a patient's care when they feel they have difficulties accepting a patient's decision?

Here are some proposals on how to handle one's conscience when there seems to be a clash of belief systems:
• From a legal point of view, physicians are allowed to refuse to give treatment (unless in an emergency). "The frustration and guilt that caregivers experience in such situations are justified and understandable, and there is always the alternative of requesting that the patient see another caregiver who feels comfortable about providing care despite the patient's refusal of certain treatments" [3]. The early transfer of a patient to someone who can take over the case is morally and ethically justified, and often prevents further sequelae for the physician as well as for the patient (ethical transfer).
• Understand that there is something worse than death. A nurse caring for a patient refusing transfusion commented: "I felt that she and the rest of the people in the church didn't view death as the worst thing" [3].
• Try to understand why you feel the way you feel. Accepting death is often difficult. "Surgery is a warrior culture, whose practitioners are committed to battle heroically and physically against death and disease" [2]. If a physician defines his/her value by the extent he/she succeeds in "fighting" death, he/she will often be disappointed and frustrated, as one physician explains: "Even with full therapy, it wasn't very clear that this patient was going to be cured despite the best that we had to offer, but there was an opportunity for us to focus our frustration on an external factor" [3]. Make sure you do not project your own frustration about death onto your patient.
• Change your perspective: "Were (the patients) caregivers harming her by respecting her wishes? If one considers only her physical body, the answer is yes. However, if one considers the person that (the patient) saw and understood herself to be, the answer is no" [3].
• Expand the compassion for your patient as a whole person. A nurse caring for a patient who had taken a decision different from the one she would have taken

explained: "Understanding why she made her decisions and what they really meant helped us" [3].
• Learn about transfusions. Transfusions are not the panacea the media claim. A comparison of the risks and benefits of transfusions helps you to understand that you do not deprive/withhold something especially precious if you do not transfuse. On the contrary, you might even come to the conclusion that you do something good for the patient if you provide other therapeutic options.
• Learn about alternative treatments. There are many treatments you can offer your patient instead of transfusion.

Jehovah's Witnesses

Medical and ethical issues arise when patients ask for a therapy that is different from the current standard of care. In the field of blood management, Jehovah's Witnesses are a vivid example. Considering how they think, what they believe, and what special care they require will help to broaden the mind. It serves as a model of how patient care can be individualized.

Jehovah's witnesses and their attitude toward medical care

Jehovah's Witnesses love and cherish life. They consider it holy, a gift from their God, which needs to be handled with care. Unhealthy practices such as the use of tobacco, recreational drugs, and excessive alcohol are prohibited by Biblical principles. Overeating, risky hobbies, and a sedentary lifestyle are discouraged, while a healthy, balanced diet, moderate physical exercise, and personal hygiene are encouraged. When it comes to healthcare, Jehovah's Witnesses are encouraged to make a conscientious decision. Most matters of healthcare are subject to personal choice, among them organ donation, organ transplant including bone marrow transplant, and contraception.

However, where blood is concerned, Jehovah's Witnesses adhere to the Biblical command to "keep abstaining from blood." They consider blood to be as holy as life itself. For a Jehovah's Witness patient, it is more important to adhere to the Biblical command—not to take blood—than to have the chance of prolonging life. Besides, Jehovah's Witnesses consider a friendship with God a precious good and a violation of this relationship by disobedience to Biblical laws a great loss. To better understand the strong feelings involved in transfusions, one may consider the context of the Biblical command to abstain from blood. The same paragraph also likens this command to the Christian command to abstain from adultery. Forced adultery, namely rape, is a severe insult to a person and leaves scars that may last for the rest of life. The person may even not be able to continue as he/she did before. In the same manner, forced blood transfusion is a severe insult on the integrity of a Jehovah's Witness and leaves scars similar in severity to those of rape.

Jehovah's Witnesses do not take in blood, neither by mouth nor parenterally. This, however, does not mean that they refuse all medical treatment. As a group, they simply refrain from the use of blood and do not accept blood transfusions. When Jehovah's Witnesses refuse transfusions, they do not claim the "right to die," but ask to be treated with other therapeutic options.

What the physician has to do

Open-minded physicians hold that treatment is successful only if a patient is holistically treated by taking into account his/her unique physical, social, and spiritual requirements. Taking the religion of a patient into consideration is one aspect of successful treatment. Jehovah's Witnesses are entitled to have this principle applied in their healthcare. When Jehovah's Witness patients refuse conventional treatment with donor blood, physicians are called upon to tailor an individual treatment to the patient. This starts with an understanding of the patient's wishes.

Jehovah's Witnesses use a certain terminology that helps them to express their wishes regarding the use of blood in their treatment. The word "blood" in the Biblical command to "keep abstaining from blood" is interpreted as being whole blood or one of the four main components of blood, namely, plasma, red cells, white cells, and platelets. These are refused by all Jehovah's Witnesses who adhere to Bible teachings. All products made from these four main components of human blood are called fractions. Among them are proteins taken from plasma (such as coagulation factors, albumin, immunoglobulins), red cells (such as hemoglobin solutions), and platelets (such as products for wound healing). Whether or not a Jehovah's Witness considers such fractions to be blood is a matter of his/her conscience: "When it comes to fractions of any of the primary components, each Christian, after careful and prayerful meditation, must conscientiously decide for himself" [14].

Another term frequently used in connection with the care of Jehovah's Witness patients is that of a "closed circuit." According to the Biblical rule that blood that has left the body is to be discarded (Leviticus 17:13), neither donor blood nor the patient's own blood is to be transfused if it has left the body and has been stored (as in the case of preoperative autologous donation). Some patients allow physicians to use autologous blood in the course of surgery or another treatment. So, it may be possible to salvage blood from a wound, irradiate it, and give it back immediately. Often, though, patients require that blood may only be retransfused if it has not left their body entirely. It is then only possible to use the patient's blood if certain conditions are met, namely, that the patient's blood is always in contact with the body via tubing. Again, it is the patient's own conscience which decides whether or not blood has left the body once it has been taken through tubes. One Jehovah's Witness may decide it has left the body and will not allow the physician to give it back. Others have decided the blood has not left the body and consider the tubing to be an extension of the circulation. A prerequisite for the latter group of patients is that the blood is in constant contact with the body (via tubing), a set-up that is called a closed circuit (Figure 20.2). If the tubing is disconnected from the patient, the blood cannot be given back. Some details of the definition of a closed circuit are again a matter of conscience. For one Jehovah's Witness, dialysis is a closed circuit since the blood circulates continuously around a circuit and is not stored outside the body. Others accept also use of a cell saving device, although the blood is not in continuous flow. They argue that the continuous flow

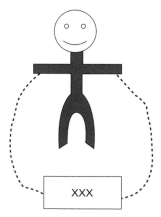

Figure 20.2 Model of a closed circuit: As an extension of the vasculature, tubing is connected to the patient. A device (the box marked "XXX") is included in the circuit. This device may be equipment for dialysis, cell salvage, oxygenation (heart–lung machine), or apheresis.

is not required since a cardiac arrest does not make blood unacceptable even though it stops blood flow temporarily. This sounds a bit confusing. However, simple communication between physicians and the patients often is enough to understand the issues that are important to a patient. The governing body of Jehovah's Witnesses summarized the issue of a patient's use of his/her own blood as follows: "A Christian must decide for himself how he will allow his own blood to be handled in the course of a surgical procedure. The same applies to medical tests and current therapies that involve extracting a small amount of one's own blood, perhaps modifying it in some way, and then reinjecting it" [15].

The above-mentioned points need to be taken into consideration when caring for a Jehovah's Witness patient (Table 20.1). To obtain an informed consent, the patient needs to be informed about the different possible uses of blood products. It is prudent to explain to the patient all fractions and all ways to use the patient's own blood. Although being extraordinarily well informed about the use of blood in medicine, most Jehovah's Witnesses are medical laymen. The physician should explain clearly what products derived from blood are available and how the patient's blood is used. It is wise to have all patients fill in a form as to what is acceptable to them and what is not. A patient presenting for the treatment of pneumonia, for instance, should be informed about such issues in the same manner as a patient who presents for a coronary artery bypass graft. Knowing the patient's opinion is extremely helpful if an emergency arises that allows no time for an in-depth evaluation of the patient's wishes.

Knowing the patient's opinion regarding the use of his/her own blood often enables a physician to adapt procedures to make them acceptable to the patient. One example is a cell-saving device. Usually, blood is sucked from the surgical field and collected in a container. If there is enough blood to be recycled, the cell saving device is set up, the blood is processed, and then given back to the patient. Some Jehovah's Witness patients may object to this procedure since it includes what they consider storage of blood outside the body. However, if the cell saving device is set up immediately before the operation starts and its tubing is connected to the patient prior to use, it may be acceptable to the patient. Similarly, other procedures can be adapted to the wishes of Jehovah's Witnesses (such as acute normovolemic hemodilution). Doing this is ethical, preserves patients' rights, and widens the array of methods that the patient allows the physician to use.

Table 20.1 Jehovah's Witnesses and their attitude toward blood.

- **Never accepted:**
  - Whole blood
  - Red cells
  - White cells
  - Platelets
  - Plasma
  - Blood that has been stored outside the body (e.g., for preoperative autologous donation)
- **Accepted by some and not by others (so-called matters of conscience):**
  - Fractions
  - Albumin (as volume substitute or as part of drugs)
  - Sera, e.g., for vaccination, Rhesus incompatibility
  - Immunoglobulins
  - Hemoglobin-based solutions
  - Coagulation factor concentrates, e.g., factor VIII, factor IX, AT III, cryoprecipitate
  - Plasma protein solutions
  - Fibrin
  - Glues containing blood derivatives
  - Bone marrow, stem cells
  - Methods with or without a closed circuit
  - Heart–lung machine
  - Extracorporeal oxygenation
  - Dialysis (e.g., continuous veno-venous hemofiltration), hemofiltration
  - Cell salvage, with or without irradiation
  - Perioperative platelet and plasma apheresis
  - Acute normovolemic hemodilution
- **Accepted:**
  - Crystalloids, colloids
  - Erythropoietin
  - Recombinant clotting factors
  - Perfluorocarbons
  - Surgical devices to achieve hemostasis
  - And many more

Patient and physician support organized by Jehovah's Witnesses

Jehovah's Witnesses are interested in the best possible medical care. Their refusal of allogeneic transfusions, however, challenges physicians to look for the best possible care without the use of donor blood. Jehovah's Witnesses support physicians in their endeavor to do that. The Watchtower Society, the legal entity of Jehovah's Witnesses, has instituted several services that are actively involved in issues pertaining to transfusions. First and foremost, it supports the patient and his/her family to receive appropriate medical care and psychological support while heeding his/her Bible-trained conscience that forbids donor blood transfusions. Second, it provides healthcare providers with valuable information regarding medical care without allogeneic transfusions and facilitates communication between the patient, physician, nurses, etc. To achieve these goals, several organizations were launched.

The Jehovah's Witness initiative in the field of blood management is spearheaded by the Hospital Information Services (HIS). Its center is in Brooklyn, New York, the world headquarters of the Watchtower Society. Many branch offices of Jehovah's Witnesses throughout the world host an HIS as well. HIS collect and provide information on transfusion-free management. They have a huge collection of articles from the medical literature and keep it updated and filed. With one mouse-click, they are able to come up with information about how to treat a specific disease or how to perform a certain procedure without donor blood. The information can be retrieved within minutes and mailed or faxed to physicians who are looking for the appropriate treatment of a Jehovah's Witness patient.

The HIS are also versed in legal and ethical issues pertaining to the refusal of transfusions. Under certain circumstances, lawyers can be asked to help if a legal dispute arises.

Besides, the HIS keep a record of physicians who are willing to treat Jehovah's Witness patients without blood transfusions. Throughout the world there exist specialists who can take care of Jehovah's Witnesses. Upon request, Jehovah's Witness patients are provided with the addresses of such cooperative physicians. This helps in preventing problems that may arise when Jehovah's Witnesses are treated by physicians who are not able or willing to treat without donor blood.

Another responsibility of the HIS is to coordinate the so-called Hospital Liaison Committees (HLC). These operate at a regional level and their members are especially trained to perform the tasks assigned to the HLC. The HLC keeps direct contact with the physicians in the region where they operate. During regular visits members search for physicians who are able and willing to treat Jehovah's Witness patients. Current information on transfusion-free management is provided. It is their aim to inform physicians and help them understand the Jehovah's Witness position. HLC are the link between

patients, physicians, and the HIS. They take good care of Jehovah's Witnesses who are sick, visit them, and support them in their path through the healthcare system.

Another group of Jehovah's Witnesses is the so-called patient-visiting group (PVG). Whether transfusions are involved or not, members of the PVG visit patients who are hospitalized in the facility the PVG is assigned to. Typically, a congregation of Jehovah's Witnesses close to the hospital provides the members of the PVG responsible for that hospital. The PVG's goals are to visit the patients, bear them company, comfort and encourage them, do pastoral work, and help them as needed, such as providing literature to read. It is its aim to make the patients comfortable and to ensure them that they are members of a loving brotherhood.

Compassionate use

As learned before, according to the Nice Charter of Fundamental Rights, patients have the right to innovation. This includes the use of new drugs if they promise to be beneficial. At times it may even seem useful to provide a patient with a drug that is not approved yet. The terms compassionate use, single-patient investigational new drug (IND), or single-patient access were coined to describe the process of getting permission to use a drug that is not approved yet. The latest official term to describe this process is "expanded access" program.

In the United States, the Food and Drug Administration (FDA) is responsible for expanded access programs. When a physician would like to use an unapproved drug for a single patient, he/she has to follow the protocol set up by the FDA. First, the physician must ask the manufacturer for permission to use the drug and to provide the product. In an emergency situation, the treating physician contacts the FDA and permission to use the drug may be given over the phone. Written documentation follows. In cases where there is no emergency, the FDA protocol as delineated in Table 20.2 should be followed.

If the request is approved, an IND number will be issued by the FDA, and the treating physician will be contacted by phone or fax, with a letter to follow. The IND is considered active upon issuance of the number. The IND sponsor, i.e., the treating physician, will then contact the drug supplier and provide the IND number. The supplier may then ship the drug directly to the treating physician.

Table 20.2 FDA protocol: Physician request for a single-patient investigational new drug (IND) for compassionate or emergency use.

Send a written request to the FDA, including:
1. A statement that an individual patient IND or an emergency IND is requested
2. Provide the diagnosis, status, and clinical history of the patient, his or her prior treatment and response to treatment, as well as the reason for requesting the proposed treatment
3. Outline a treatment plan with dosage, duration, and route of administration of the drug, etc. Provide literature that supports your intent
4. Information about the chemistry, pharmacology, toxicology, and manufacturer of the drug, or a letter of authorization issued for a previous IND request (in this case, the IND number is needed)
5. Informed consent statement (state that an informed consent and the approval of an ethics committee will be obtained before initiating the therapy)
6. Investigator qualification statement, typically the curriculum vitae of the treating physician
7. FDA Form 1571 (treating physician listed as sponsor)
8. Contact phone and fax

For further information, see the FDA home page (www.fda.gov).

Key points

• Upholding the ethical principle of autonomy by adherence to informed consent and advance directives is the *sine qua non* of medical ethics.
• To balance the ethical principles of beneficence and non-maleficence, a comprehensive evaluation of the benefits and risks of transfusions and the various features of blood management is required.
• The care of Jehovah's Witness patients poses medical and ethical challenges to the team of healthcare providers. Meeting these challenges enhances the performance of the team and spurs on the development of new methods in blood management.
• The compassionate use of a non-approved drug is ethically justified under specific circumstances. In the United States, the FDA is the board to be contacted for the initiation of a compassionate use protocol.

Questions for review

1. Which ethical principles govern medical decision-making?
2. How are patients' rights defined?
3. What is a mature minor and how can he/she contribute to decisions regarding his/her therapy?
4. What special considerations are needed when treating a Jehovah's Witness?

Suggestions for further research

Who is responsible for patients' rights? Is there a patients' right movement in your country? Does it do anything pertaining to blood management?

Homework

Learn about the legal situation of transfusions and transfusion avoidance in your country. Is there a law or a guideline on how to formulate an advance directive, a power of attorney, or a living will that is related to blood management? What is the required form of such? Are there any aids available, such as brochures or checklists? If so, obtain and file them.

Is there any legal ruling on how a patient needs to be informed about blood management options? What information needs to be included? Is a minimum time required between giving information to a patient and he/she receiving a transfusion?

Is there a law in your country that upholds patients' rights? Have there been court cases ruling on matters of blood management? If so, obtain some information on them. If there is a law, try to get the original paragraphs, read them, and file them.

Contact the nearest HLC of Jehovah's Witnesses and record its contact information. Ask it to explain its work and services. Also ask for the name, address, and contact phone of the local PVG.

Find out how to prescribe a drug that is still in experimental status/not approved. Pay particular attention to the way a compassionate use protocol is set up in your institution. Ask the following questions:
Who is entitled to institute such a compassionate use protocol? Record the address of the agency.
Who do you have to contact? (Address?)

How long does it take to get permission in an emergency?

What formalities do you have to fulfill?

References

1. National Commission for the Protection of Human Subjects of Biomedical and Behavioral Research. *The Belmont Report: Ethical Principles and Guidelines for the Protection of Human Subjects of Research.* Department of Health, Education, and Welfare, 1979.

2. McKneally MF. Witnessing death as lifesaving treatment is withheld. *Ann Thorac Surg* 2002;**74**:1430–1431; discussion 1432–1433.

3. Knuti KA, Amrein PC, Chabner BA, Lynch TJ Jr, Penson RT. Faith, identity, and leukemia: when blood products are not an option. *Oncologist* 2002;**7**:371–380.

4. Cittadinanzattiva-Active Citizenship Network Group, Cotturi G, *et al. European Charter of Patients Rights. Basis Document.* Rome, 2002.

5. Rider ME, Makela CJ. A comparative analysis of patients' rights: an international perspective. *Int J Consumer Studies* 2003;**27**:302–315.

6. Grainger B, Margolese E, Partington E. Legal and ethical considerations in blood transfusion. *Can Med Assoc J* 1997;**156** (Suppl 11):S50–S54.

7. Court EL, Robinson JA, Hocken DB. Informed consent and patient understanding of blood transfusion. *Transfus Med* 2011;**21**:183–189.

8. Guinn DE. Honor the patient's wishes. *Ann Thorac Surg* 2002;**74**:1431–1432; discussion 1432–1433.

9. Thompson T, Barbour R, Schwartz L. Adherence to advance directives in critical care decision making: vignette study. *BMJ* 2003;**327**:1011.

10. Gyamfi C, Gyamfi MM, Berkowitz RL. Ethical and medico-legal considerations in the obstetric care of a Jehovah's Witness. *Obstet Gynecol* 2003;**102**:173–180.

11. Levy JK. Jehovah's Witnesses, pregnancy, and blood transfusions: a paradigm for the autonomy rights of all pregnant women. *J Law Med Ethics* 1999;**27**:171–189.

12. Brezina PR, Moskop JC. Urgent medical decision making regarding a Jehovah's Witness minor. A case report and discussion. *NC Med J* 2007;**68**:312–316

13. Ariga T, Hayasaki S. Medical, legal and ethical considerations concerning the choice of bloodless medicine by Jehovah's Witnesses. *Leg Med (Tokyo)* 2003;**5** (Suppl 1): S72–S75.

14. Watch Tower Bible and Tract Society of New York. *The Watchtower* 2004;**125**:29–31.

15. *Keep Yourselves in God's Love.* Watch Tower Bible and Tract Society of New York, 2008, p. 218

Appendix A: Detailed Information

Table A.1 Transfusion-transmissible diseases.

Infectious agent	Causing	Likelihood
Anaplasma phagocytophilum (HGE) (rickettsia)	Ehrlichiosis	
Babesia microti (parasite)	Babesiosis, life-threatening hemolysis in immunocompromized and elderly	USA: <1:1 000 000
Chlamydia pneumoniae	Aortic aneurysm, ischemic heart disease (?)	Unclear whether TTI, but likely, since microbe in 9–46% of all healthy donors
Coxiella burnetti (Gram-negative coccobacillus)	Q fever	One case reported
CTF orbivirus (arbovirus)	Colorado tick fever (CTF)	One case reported
Cytomegalovirus (CMV) (herpes virus family)	Clinically undetectable, severe diseases with mortality in immunocompromized	Found in most donations
Epstein–Barr virus	Various diseases	Found in most donations
Filaria (nematodes, worms)	Transfused microfilaria cannot multiply since they cannot develop into adult worms, disease self-limited	
Hepatitis A virus (HAV)	Hepatitis A	USA: 1:1 000 000
Hepatitis B virus (HBV) (lipid-enveloped)	Hepatitis B	USA: 1:205 000–250 000; Canada: 1.88:100 000
Hepatitis C virus (HCV) (lipid-enveloped)	Hepatitis C	USA: 1:250 000–1,935,000; Canada: 0.35:1 000 000; UK: 1:3 000 000
Human herpes 8 virus		
Human immunodeficiency virus (HIV) (lentivirus, retrovirus)	AIDS	USA: 1:100 before testing era, currently 1:1–2 100 000 Canada: 1:10 000 000; South Africa: 2.6: 100 000

(*Continued*)

Basics of Blood Management, Second Edition. Petra Seeber and Aryeh Shander.
© 2013 John Wiley & Sons, Ltd. Published 2013 by John Wiley & Sons, Ltd.

Table A.1 *(Continued)*

Infectious agent	Causing	Likelihood
Human T-lymphotropic virus Type I and II (HTLV) (retrovirus)	Neurodegenerative disorder	USA: 1:640 000 Canada: 0.95:1 000 000
Leishmania	Leishmaniasis (visceral, cutaneous, mucosal)	Occasionally
Listeria monocytogenes		Found in platelets (case report)
New coronavirus, poss. paramyxovirus as cofactor	Severe acute respiratory syndrome (SARS)	Not known whether TTI
Parvovirus B19	Hemolytic anemia, aplastic anemia in susceptible individuals	Highly variable
Plasmodium spp.	Malaria	USA: 1–3:4 000 000; worldwide one of the more common TTIs
Protease-resistant prion protein (?)	Variant Creutzfeld–Jakob disease	
Rickettsia spp.	Rocky mountain spotted fever	One case reported
SEN virus (non-enveloped DNA virus, circovirus)	Hepatitis?	Present in blood of 1.8–24% of healthy individuals, depending on geographical region
Toxoplasma gondii	Toxoplasmosis	
Transfusion-transmitted virus (TTV)	Hepatitis?	50% of blood donated in the USA
Treponema pallidum	Syphilis	No cases in USA in last decades
Trypanosoma cruzi	Chagas disease	In endemic areas
West Nile virus	Meningoencephalitis	2.7:10,000 in endemic areas in USA

Bartonella spp. (cat scratch disease, bacillary angiomatosis), *Francisella tularensis* (Tularemia), *Borrelia burgdorferi* (Lymes disease), Japanese encephalitis virus, St Louis encephalitis virus, Western equine encephalitis virus, LaCrosse encephalitis virus, yellow fever virus, dengue virus: None of them has been reported to have caused a transfusion-transmitted disease, although theoretically possible.
TTI, transfusion-transmissible infection.

Table A.2 Treatment options for factor deficiencies.

Missing/defective factor	Incidence	Consequence of deficiency	Recommended first-line treatment	Alternatives (may not be the best therapy available)
FI (Fibrinogen)	1:1 M	Bleeding disorder	Fibrinogen concentrate	Cryoppt, FFP
FII Prothrombin	1:2 M	Bleeding disorder	PCC	FFP
FIII thromboplastin			—	
FIV Calcium	—		—	
FV	1:1 M	Bleeding disorder	rHuFVIIa	FFP
FVII	1:500 K	Bleeding disorder	rHuFVIIa	FVII (PCC with FVII works, but thrombosis risk), FFP
FVIII	1:5–10 K	Hemophilia A	Mild: DDAVP ± TA, severe: rHuFVIII; inhibitor: rHuFVIIa	FVIII; inhibitor: FEIBA, porcine FVIII, high-dose FVIII, PCC
FIX Christmas	1:30–60 K	Hemophilia B	rHuFIX; inhibitor: rHuFVIIa	High purity FIX; inhibitor: FEIBA, PCC, FFP
FX Stuart Prower	1:1 M	Bleeding disorder	PCC (with appropriate levels of FX)	FFP, low purity FIX
FXI	1:1 M	Bleeding disorder	TA, FXI concentrate	FFP
FXII Hagemann		?	Not needed for hemostasis	
FXIII	1:2 M	Bleeding disorder	FXIII concentrate	Cryoppt
von Willebrand	>1:1 K	Bleeding disorder	Mild: DDAVP ± TA, severe: vWF concentrate or FVIII with high level of vWF	FFP, cryoppt
Protein C	1:300–500	Purpura fulminans, thrombosis	Protein C concentrate	PCC, FFP
Antithrombin III		Thrombosis, heparin resistance	ATIII concentrate	rHuATIII

If not indicated otherwise, factor concentrates are plasma-derived.
K, thousand; M, million; TA, tranexamic acid; cryoppt, cryoprecipitate; FFP, fresh frozen plasma; PCC, prothrombin complex concentrate; rHuATIII, recombinant human antithrombin III; rHuFVIIa, recombinant human FVIIA; rHuFVIII, recombinant human FVIII; rHuFIX, recombinant human FIX; vWF, von Willebrand factor.

Table A.3 Plasma constituents.

Constituent	Function	Amount in plasma
Fibrinogen	Coagulation	260 mg/dL
Prothrombin	Coagulation	80–90 µg/mL
Factor V	Coagulation	0.4–1 mg/dL
Factor VII	Coagulation	0.47 µg/mL
Factor VIII	Coagulation	0.01 mg/dL
Factor IX	Coagulation	4 µg/mL
Factor X	Coagulation	6.4–10 µg/mL
Factor XI	Coagulation	0.4–0.6 mg/dL
Factor XIII	Coagulation	2.9 mg/dL
Protein C	Anticoagulation	3.9–5.9 µg/mL
Protein S	Anticoagulation	25–25 µg/mL
Vitronectin	Adhesion, complement system	0.2–0.4 mg/mL
Albumin	Transport, colloid-osmotic pressure	Main protein of serum (55–62%)
Haptoglobin	Binds free hemoglobin	27–140 mg/dL
Transferrin	Carries iron in blood	150–350 mg/dL
Ceruloplasmin	Transports Cu, phenoloxidase	20–60 mg/dL
Prealbumin	Transport	16–35 mg/dL
Antithrombin III	Anticoagulation	11–16 mg/dL
α2-Antiplasmin	Important inhibitor of plasmin and other coagulation factors	7 mg/dL
α1-Antitrypsin	Inhibits trypsin, elastase	160 mg/dL
α1-Antichymotrypsin	Inhibits chymotrypsin	45 mg/dL
C1-esterase-inhibitor	Controls activation of C1 and coagulation factors; deficiency: hereditary angioneurotic edema	24 mg/dL
α2-Macroglobulin	Inhibits thrombin, plasmin, etc., clearance of exogenous proteinases	150 mg/dL
von Willebrand factor	Coagulation	1 mg/dL
Prekallikrein	Coagulation	3.5–5 mg/dL
Plasminogen	Coagulation	7–20 mg/dL
IgG	Immunological function	1375 mg/dL
IgA 1 + 2	Immunological function	250 mg/dL
IgM	Immunological function	120 mg/dL
IgD	Immunological function	3 mg/dL
IgE	Immunological function	0.02 mg/dL
Complement 4	Immunological function	30 mg/dL
Complement 3	Immunological function	130 mg/dL

Many more plasma proteins have been characterized, among them: actin, afamin precursor, angiotensinogen precursor, apolipoprotein precursors, ATP synthase precursor, atrial natriuretic factor precursor, bullous pemphigoid antigen fragment, calgranulin A, carbonic anhydrase, cathepsin precursor, chaperonin, cholinesterase precursor, clusterin precursor, cndothelin converting enzyme, fibulin-1 precursor, ficolin 3 precursor, gamma enolase, glial fibrillary acidic protein, gravin, heparin cofactor II precursor, human psoriasin, insulin-like growth factor binding protein 3 precursor, interleukin, kininogen precursor, melanoma-associated antigen p97, mismatch repair protein, oxygen regulated protein precursor, preoxireduxin, platelet basic protein precursor, plectin, PSA precursor, putative serum amyloid A-3 precursor, selenoprotein P precursor, signal recognition particle receptor-α subunit, tetranectin precursor, vascular cell adhesion pretein 1 precursor, vinculin.

Table A.4 Identified proteins in the proteome of human red cells.

Actin	Glycophorin C
Adducin	Heat shock proteins
Aldehyde dehydrogenase	Hemoglobin
Aldolase	Hydroxyacyl gluthatione hydrolase
Aminolevulinate dehydratase	Lactate dehydrogenase
Ankyrin	Peroxireduxin 2
Aquaporin	Phosphoglucose isomerase chain A
Arginase	Phosphoribosyl pyrophosphate synthetase
ATP citrate lyase	Placental ribonuclease inhibitor
B-CAM protein	Poly (A) specific ribonuclease
Biliverdin reductase	Polyubiquitin
C1-tetrahydrofolate synthase	Presenilin-associated protein
Calcium transporting ATPase 4	Prostatic-binding protein (neuropolypeptide)
Calpain inhibitor (Calpastatin)	Purine nucleoside phosphorylase
Carbonic anhydrase	RAP2B (*Ras* oncogene)
Catalase	Rh blood D group antigen
Cofilin	Spectrin
Creatine kinase	Stomatin
D-dopachrome tautomerase	Synaptobrevin
Dematin	Thioreduxin
Duodenal cytochrome b	Transgelin
Enhancer protein	Translation initiation factor 2C
Flotilin	Tropomodulin
Glucose transporter glycoprotein	Tropomyosin
Glutaraldehyde-3-phosphate dehydrogenase	Trypsinogen
Glutathione transferase	Ubiquitin activating enzyme
Glutoredoxin	Ubiquitin isopeptidase
Glyceraldehyde-3-phosphate dehydrogenase	Zinc finger protein 180
Glycophorin	Zona pellucida binding protein

Table A.5 Definitions and equations of oxygen transport (see Chapter 2).

Definitions

Viscosity	Measure of internal friction in a laminar flow	Depends on temperature; normal for blood: 3–5 relative units (water is 1 relative unit), plasma is 1.9–2.3 relative units; can increase with slowing of blood: up to 1000 relative units because of reversible agglomeration Blood viscosity is affected by hematocrit, plasmaviscosity, cell deformability, cell aggregation
P50	Oxygen partial pressure where oxygen saturation of hemoglobin is 50%, normal value for adult hemoglobin is26.6 mmHg	A high P50 means a low affinity of hemoglobin for oxygen and vice versa

Equations

Oxygen saturation (SO_2)	(Actual O_2 content of Hb × 100)/ maximum oxygen content of Hb	
Arterial oxygen content (CaO_2)	$CaO_2 = (1.34 \times Hb \times SaO_2 + 0.003 \times PaO_2) \times 10$	
Oxygen delivery (DO_2)	$DO_2 = CO \times CaO_2$	
Oxygen consumption (VO_2)	$VO_2 = DO_2 \times O_2ER$ or $VO_2 = Q \times (CaO_2 - CvO_2)$	Normal: 110–160 mL/min x m^2
Oxygen extraction ratio (O_2 ER)	$(CaO_2 - CvO_2)/CaO_2$	Normal: 0.20–0.30

Table A.6 Definitions of basic qualities of fluids (see Chapter 6).

Quality	Description	Remarks
Osmotic pressure	Hydrostatic pressure required to oppose the movement of water through a semipermeable membrane in response to an osmotic gradient	Osmotic pressure is referred to as colloid osmotic pressure (=oncotic pressure) if it is exerted by colloids
Mole (mol)	The amount of a substance that contains 6.022×10^{23} molecules (Avogadro's number)	
Molality	Number of moles of a solute in 1 kg of a solvent	
Molarity	Number of moles of a solute in 1 L of a solvent	
Osmole (osm)	Amount of a substance that exerts an osmotic pressure of 22.4 atm in 1 L of solution	
Osmolality	Number of osmoles of a solute per kg of a solvent	Number of particles in the solution; independent of size and weight of particles, independent of any membrane; normal plasma osmolality is 287–290 mOsm/kg
Osmolarity	Number of osmoles of a solute per liter of a solvent	
Tonicity (mOsmol/kg)	Effective osmolality; the sum of the concentrations of solutes which exert an osmotic force across a membrane	Tonicity is less than osmolality; it is the property of a solution in relation to a membrane
Equivalent (Eq) = millival (mval)	One equivalent is the amount of ion required to cancel out the electrical charge of an oppositely charged monovalent ion (the valence charge of the ion is the number of equivalents there are in one mole of that ion)	For monovalent ions: 1 eq = 1 mol For divalent ions: 1 eq = 0.5 molFor trivalent ions: 1 eq = 0.333 mol
Dalton (Da)	Unit of mass used to express atomic and molecular weights that is equal to one 12th of the mass of an atom of carbon-12. It is equivalent to 1.6610^{-27} kg	

Table A.7 Facts about hemophilia A and B.

Classification:

Mild: 6–30% factor activity (muscle/joint bleeding after major trauma, usually no spontaneous bleeding)

Moderate: 1–5% factor activity (muscle/joint bleeding after minor trauma, rarely spontaneous or central nervous system bleeding)

Severe: <1% factor activity (spontaneous bleeding in muscles, joints, central nervous system) (about 70% of hemophilia A patients and 50% of hemophilia B patients have severe hemophilia)

Inhibitors:

Antibodies against the coagulation factor under consideration

Develops in about 30% of previously untreated patients now treated with rFVIII; inhibitor-development more pronounced in Hispanic and African patients

Patients on FIX concentrates develop inhibitors less frequently (1–3%)

Therapy:

Prophylactic: increasing *in vivo* clotting factor levels to more than 1% activity is sufficient to prevent most spontaneous joint bleeds

FVIII: 25–40 U/kg 3x per week

FIX: 25–40 U/kg 2x per week

Short-term prophylactic (before surgery, physical therapy or major activity): surgical procedures can safely be performed if factor concentration is perioperatively kept at a level of 50–100%

Therapeutic:

Mild hemorrhage: 20–30% factor activity required (FVIII: 10–15 U/kg; FIX: 20–30 U/kg), e.g., in severe epistaxis, persistent hematuria, dental bleeding (if unresponsive to aminocaproic acid or tranexamic acid)

Major hemorrhage: 40–50% factor activity required (FVIII: 20–25 U/kg; FIX: 40–50 U/kg), e.g., in advanced muscle/joint bleeding, hematoma of neck, tongue, pharynx, dental extraction*

Life-threatening hemorrhage: 70–100% factor activity required (FVIII: 35–50 U/kg; FIX: 70–100 U/kg; maintenance treatment with half-initial dose for 5 days to several weeks), e.g., in intracranial or gastrointestinal bleed, surgery, major traumatic bleeding

*For dental extraction, 10% activity plus oral and local antifibrinolytic agents for 7–10 days may be sufficient.
100% clotting factor activity is 1 U/mL of average normal plasma.

Appendix B: Sources of Information for Blood Management

Table B.1 Examples of current recommendations, algorithms, and guidelines pertaining to blood management.

Recommendation	Year issued
BCSH Guidelines for the use of fresh frozen plasma, cryoprecipitate, and cryosupernatant	2004, amended 2005, 2007, 2011
2011 update to the Society of Thoracic Surgeons and the Society of Cardiovascular Anesthesiologists blood conservation clinical practice guidelines.	2011
Appropriateness of allogeneic red blood cell transfusion: the international consensus conference on transfusion outcomes	2011
Detection, evaluation, and management of preoperative anaemia in the elective orthopaedic surgical patient: NATA guidelines	2011
Guideline on the management of haemophilia in the fetus and neonate	2011
Guidelines for the laboratory investigation of heritable disorders of platelet function (BCSH)	2011
NCCN Clinical Practice Guidelines in Oncology: myelodysplastic syndromes	2011
Recommendations for the transfusion management of patients in the peri-operative period. II. The intra-operative period	2011
Recommendations for the transfusion management of patients in the peri-operative period. I. The pre-operative period	2011
The American Society of Hematology 2011 evidence-based practice guideline for immune thrombocytopenia	2011
The American Society of Hematology 2011 evidence-based practice guideline for immune thrombocytopenia	2011
A United Kingdom Haemophilia Centre Doctors' Organization guideline approved by the British Committee for Standards in Haematology: guideline on the use of prophylactic factor VIII concentrate in children and adults with severe haemophilia A	2010
Active management of the third stage of labour: prevention and treatment of postpartum hemorrhage: No. 235 October 2009 (Replaces No. 88, April 2000)	2010

(Continued)

Basics of Blood Management, Second Edition. Petra Seeber and Aryeh Shander.
© 2013 John Wiley & Sons, Ltd. Published 2013 by John Wiley & Sons, Ltd.

Table B.1 (*Continued*)

Recommendation	Year issued
Acute myeloblastic leukaemias and myelodysplastic syndromes in adult patients: ESMO Clinical Practice Guidelines for diagnosis, treatment and follow-up	2010
American Society of Clinical Oncology/American Society of Hematology clinical practice guideline update on the use of epoetin and darbepoetin in adult patients with cancer	2010
Anemia and patient blood management in hip and knee surgery: a systematic review of the literature	2010
Clinical practice guidelines for the management of atypical haemolytic uraemic syndrome in the United Kingdom	2010
Clinical practice guidelines on menorrhagia: management of abnormal uterine bleeding before menopause	2010
Evidence-based practice guidelines for plasma transfusion	2010
International consensus recommendations on the management of patients with nonvariceal upper gastrointestinal bleeding	2010
Management of chronic childhood immune thrombocytopenic purpura: AIEOP consensus guidelines	2010
Prophylaxis in children and adults with haemophilia (BCSH)	2010
Significant haemoglobinopathies: guidelines for screening and diagnosis	2010
A consensus statement on the management of pregnancy and delivery in women who are carriers of or have bleeding disorders	2009
Active management of the third stage of labour: prevention and treatment of postpartum hemorrhage	2009
Anaemia management in patients with chronic kidney disease: a position statement by the Anaemia Working Group of European Renal Best Practice (ERBP)	2009
Clinical and laboratory diagnosis of von Willebrand disease: a synopsis of the 2008 NHLBI/NIH guidelines	2009
Clinical practice guideline: red blood cell transfusion in adult trauma and critical care	2009
Evidence-based recommendations on the treatment of von Willebrand disease in Italy	2009
Guideline for the Diagnosis and Management of Disseminated Intravascular Coagulation (BCSH)	2009
Guidelines for the diagnosis and management of aplastic anaemia (BCSH)	2009
International recommendations on the diagnosis and treatment of patients with acquired hemophilia A	2009
Recommendations for the use of antithrombin concentrates and prothrombin complex concentrates	2009
Antithrombotic therapy in neonates and children: American College of Chest Physicians Evidence-Based Clinical Practice Guidelines (8th Edition)	2008
Clinical practice guidelines for evaluation of anemia	2008
Erythropoietins in cancer patients: ESMO recommendations for use	2008
Guideline for the treatment of haemophilia in South Africa	2008
Guideline on the selection and use of therapeutic products to treat haemophilia and other hereditary bleeding disorders. A United Kingdom Haemophilia Center Doctors' Organisation (UKHCDO) guideline approved by the British Committee for Standards in Haematology	2008
Guidelines for the use of recombinant activated factor VII in massive obstetric haemorrhage	2008
Guidelines on the assessment of bleeding risk prior to surgery or invasive procedures (BCSH)	2008

Table B.1 (*Continued*)

Recommendation	Year issued
The CARI guidelines. Biochemical and haematological targets. Haemoglobin.	2008
von Willebrand disease (VWD): evidence-based diagnosis and management guidelines, the National Heart, Lung, and Blood Institute (NHLBI) Expert Panel report (USA)	2008
Guidelines on the use of intravenous immune globulin for hematologic conditions	2007
Use of epoetin and darbepoetin in patients with cancer: 2007 American Society of Hematology/American Society of Clinical Oncology clinical practice guideline update	2007
A practical approach to timing cord clamping in resource poor settings	2006
EORTC guidelines for the use of erythropoietic proteins in anaemic patients with cancer: 2006 update	2006
Gynaecological and obstetric management of women with inherited bleeding disorders	2005
BCSH Transfusion guidelines for neonates and older children	2004
Management of hyperbilirubinemia in the newborn infant 35 or more weeks of gestation	2004
BCSH Guidelines for the use of platelet transfusions	2003
ASCO: Platelet transfusion for patients with cancer	2001

NIH, National Institute of Health; BCSH, British Society for Haematology; ASCO, American Society of Clinical Oncology; ASA, American Society of Anesthesiologists; ACP, American College of Physicians; FFP, fresh frozen plasma; cryoppt, cryoprecipitate.

Table B.2 Books about blood management and related issues.

Title	Author	Information
Erythropoietins and Erythropoiesis	Graham Molineux, Mary A. Foote, Steven Elliott	2005
No Man's Blood	Gene Church	1986, ISBN 0-8666-155-7
The Clinical Use of Blood	World Health Organization	Information on WHO homepage
Transfusion Medicine and Alternatives to Blood Transfusion	NATA	2000 edition, information on NATA homepage
Transfusion-free Medicine and Surgery	Nicolas Jabbour	Blackwell Publishing 2005; ISBN 1405121599
A Textbook of Postpartum Hemorrhage	Christopher B-Lynch, Louis Keith, Andre Lalonde, Mahantesh Karoshi	Sapiens publishing
Your Body, Your Choice	Shannon Farmer, David Webb	Media Masters

Table B.3 Organizations and initiatives relevant for blood management.

Organization	Contact
Bloodless Healthcare International (BHI)	www.noblood.org
Bloodless Medicine Research of the University of Pisa, Italy	www.med.unipi.it/patchir/bloodl/bmr.htm
British Committee for Standardization in Hematology (BCSH)	www.bcshguidelines.com
Formerly NAAC	www.anemia.org
Medical Society for Blood Management	www.bloodmanagement.org
National Hemophilia Foundation	www.hemophilia.org
Network for the Advancement of Transfusion Alternatives (NATA)	www.nataonline.com
Ontario Nurse Transfusion Coordinators Provincial blood conservation program (ONTraC)	www.ontracprogram.com
Society for the Advancement of Blood Management (SABM)	www.sabm.org
UK blood transfusion and tissue transplantation services	www.transfusionguidelines.org
Watchtower Society	www.watchtower.org/medical_care_and_blood.htm

Appendix C: Program Tools and Forms

Basics of Blood Management, Second Edition. Petra Seeber and Aryeh Shander.
© 2013 John Wiley & Sons, Ltd. Published 2013 by John Wiley & Sons, Ltd.

Table C.1 Example of data collection in orthopedics (initial analysis).

Patient (sex/age)	Numbers of red cell units given	Procedure performed, reason for hospital stay	Length of stay	Hematocrit at first presentation	Intraoperative blood loss in mL	Pretransfusion hematocrit	Post-transfusion hematocrit	Emergency or planned admission	Units given outside accepted policies	Units given to patients who initially were anemic	Units given to patients who bled heavily intraoperatively	Comments
1												
2												
3												
4												
5												
6												

Have the blood bank provide you with the names of the patients who received red cells. Data collection is easier if every single transfusion episode is recorded rather than the summarized transfusion history of every patient.

Table C.2 Patient history: Clotting.

		Physician notes	How to proceed
Please answer the following questions		• History negative • No history taken • History positive as follows	Check kidney and liver panel, blood count, coagulation tests, drugs
Do you suffer from nose bleeds?	Yes/No	One or both sides? Drug-related? Without obvious reason (flu, dry nose, trauma)?	Labs
Do you easily get black spots?	Yes/No	Larger than 3 cm in diameter? Extremities: Medial or lateral? Trauma-related? Joint hemorrhage? Congenital or starting during lifetime?	Labs
Do you bleed for prolonged times after minor injuries, e.g., after shaving?	Yes/No	How long? Amount of bleeding? How stopped?	Labs
Are you aware of any bleeding abnormality you suffer from?	Yes/No	Diagnosis? Who diagnosed? Last consultation of physician? Therapy? Description of historical bleeding episodes	Confirm diagnosis, consult hematologist
Do any of your relatives suffer from a bleeding abnormality?	Yes/No	Diagnosis? What relative?	Confirm diagnosis, labs
Do you have or have you had prolonged menstrual bleeding (>7 days)?	Yes/No	Primary or secondary? Did Gyn provide reason?	Labs, Gyn consult
Do you suffer from kidney disease?	Yes/No	Diagnosis or symptoms	Labs, consider DDAVP
Do you suffer from a liver disease?	Yes/No	Diagnosis or symptoms	Labs, consider vitamin K, DDAVP, estrogens, antifibrinolytics
Did you ever bleed for prolonged times after surgery or having a tooth pulled?	Yes/No	Intra- or post-operative? Surgical revision needed? Rebleeding after initial hemostasis?	Confirm event
Did you ever receive a blood transfusion?	Yes/No	Reason? Blood products? Who transfused?	Confirm event
Do you take drugs ("blood thinners"), e.g., coumadin, aspirin?	Yes/No	Drug name	Stop/change
During the last 2 weeks, did you take any medication for flu, pain, psychiatric disease, epilepsy, cramps, or infection?	Yes/No	Drug name	Stop/change/treat/antagonize (?)
Do you take nutritional supplements or herbal medicines?	Yes/No	Ginkgo, ginseng, garlic, ginger, green tea, Chinese preparations, St John's wort, vitamins C or E	Reduce dose, stop 14 days prior to surgery

Table C.3 Initial analysis.

	Transfusion statistics	Organization	Established blood management	Resources
Questions	How many transfusions have been given during the last year by departments (and associated costs)? What are the top 10 procedures using blood? Which procedures are performed with >10% of patients transfused?	What are the mode of transfusion use and methods of blood management already established? How are staff educated? What area and number of patients does the hospital serve per year? Who refers patients to hospital?	Who already uses which methods of blood management?	What equipment (type, storage place, responsible person for maintenance) and personnel (number of physicians, nurses, ancillary staff, specialties, knowledge about blood management, motivation) is available? Who are the staff responsible for transfusions, blood bank, autologous blood? Who is interested in blood management? Where are there available funding opportunities?
Methods to obtain answers	Chart review, transfusion statistics, transfusion committee reports, billing department	Ask for staff education, black-board, hospital intranet, education coordinator, quality assurance files, review policies and procedures, visit blood bank, laboratory, ward, ICU	Talk to pharmacist, check policies and procedures	Survey, talk to medical technicians, surgical nurses, perfusionists, medical maintenance

What are the strengths of the hospital? For example, a very good orthopedic program? A renowned sickle cell clinic, etc.?

Table C.4 Surgical continuum.

Preoperative	Intraoperative	Postoperative
Evaluation (patient preferences, anemia, clotting, surgical)	Optimize hemostasis minimize blood loss (surgical techniques, equipment)	Minimize iatrogenic blood loss
Develop a plan of care and communicate it	Positioning	Positioning
Create lead time to optimize patients/ postponing surgeries and procedures if indicated	Embolization	Bandages, pressure applied to wounds
Optimizing hemoglobin levels (EPO, iron, vitamins, androgens)	Acute normovolemic hemodilution	Postoperative cell salvage
Treat coagulation abnormalities	Acute hypervolemic hemodilution	Optimizing anticoagulation
Optimize cardiopulmonary, renal, hepatic condition of the patient (referral to specialist)	Augmented acute normovolemic hemodilution	EPO, hematinics
Embolization	Plasmapheresis	Oxygen therapy
Informed consent	Plateletpheresis	Maintaining normothermia
Ensure availability of equipment and personnel	Synthetic and autologous tissue adhesives	Avoid hypertension
Minimize iatrogenic blood loss	Antifibrinolytics, desmopressin	Monitoring of the patient and his/her blood loss
Stop or adapt anticoagulation	Monitoring of coagulation and anticoagulation (TEG, Hepcon) Controlled hypotension Regional anesthesia Tourniquets Cell salvage Staging Packing Maintaining normothermia Induced hypothermia Ultrafiltration Retrograde priming of extracorporeal circulation circuits Oxygen therapy	Prompt intervention in case of postoperative bleeding Nutrition Judicious use of anticoagulation Antifibrinolytics

EPO, erythropoietin.

Table C.5 Job description: Coordinator of blood management program.

The coordinator plays an important role in the blood management of patients. The coordinator is responsible for establishing and running the blood management program, making (your hospital) a "Center of Excellence" in blood management

Requirements
- Thorough knowledge of the organization of a blood management program
- Basic knowledge of clinical blood management
- Understanding of patients for whom allogeneic transfusion is no option
- Computer skills, e.g., Word, Excel, e-mail, Medline
- Preferably speaking English
- Leadership and management skills
- Excellency in communication, presentation, and conflict resolution

Work environment
- Office
- Clinical area of hospital

Contacts and communication
- Within the hospital: Communicates with patients and their family/significant others; program and hospital management; medical, nursing, ancillary, and research staff
- Outside the hospital: Communicates with the media, public, national and international organizations relevant to blood management, industry, general business contacts

Accountability
- Program and hospital management

Details of responsibilities
Education and advertisement
- Together with PR department, establishes advertisement and media contact, interacts with the public to ensure progress of the blood management program
- Organizes blood management seminars for the public
- Remains up-to-date with blood management, is a source of information
- Conducts orientation sessions for new staff members regarding blood management program
- Organizes educational interventions for medical, nursing, and ancillary hospital staff
Clinical work
- Screens and interviews patients participating in the blood management program, educates patients in blood management
- Assists patients to formulate advance directives and document living wills regarding blood management
- Collects patient data, gives recommendation regarding the patient's blood management as outlined in established policies and procedures
- Liaises with patients, patient advocates, medical, nursing, and ancillary staff, and the public
- Informs patients about blood management, develops information material for patients
- Coordinates inter-hospital patient transfers and physician–patient contacts
- Coordinates and supports travel and accommodation of patients coming from far to use the service of the program
- Daily visits to patients participating in the blood management program; ensures that the patient is treated according to his/her stated will and that treatment is adequate; supports and informs the patient as needed
- Maintains 24-hour emergency contact
Data collection and research
- Assists with designing research initiatives in blood management
- Collects data for program evaluation and blood management database
- Assists with analysis and presentation of data
- Evaluates new equipment for innovative blood management

Table C.5 (*Continued*)

Management
- Coordinates and supervises service of the blood management program, develops strategies to overcome weaknesses of the program
- Corresponds in a timely fashion
- Organizes regular meetings with blood management committee, hospital administration, the public, patients, and patient advocates
- Records requests and transfers of patients in the program
- Reports about program service and other relevant data
- Works in accordance with established policies and procedures for the program
- Maintains confidentiality
- Participates regularly in training and educational interventions
- Manages finances, including preparation of realistic budgets and working within its limits

Interpersonal communication and skills
- Creates a warm, secure, harmonic, and comfortable atmosphere for patients and staff
- Is confident, competent, and professional
- Resolves conflicts
- Facilitates communication between patient and family
- Recognizes fear and anxiety, proactively provides comfort
- Is a role model for other staff members
- Addresses inappropriate behavior
- Treats patients, their family, and staff members with respect; recognizes their opinion
- Encourages staff to communicate their proposals for process and service improvement and problem solving; takes corrective measures to solve problems
- As part of a team, is observant about the work load of co-workers, supports team members to reach the goals of the blood management program using the strong points of each staff member to make the program a success

Table C.6 Model policy format.

# of policy/procedure//Name of policy/procedure *1.4.3: Transfer*. Purpose of the policy/procedure: *Describes how patients are transferred from outside hospitals to our hospital, based on their wish to participate in the blood management program.*

Step #	Step	Responsible person	Tools	Remarks
1.1	*Receive call*	*Coordinator on call*	*Mobile phone*	
1.2.	*Record essential information*	*,,*	*Flow chart "transfer" (Item No xxx)*	
1.3.	*Confirm you will call back*	*,,*		
1.4.	*Contact physician on all*	*,,*	*Physicians list (Item no xxx)*	
1.5.	*Call back*	*Physician*		
Literature:				
Date, Signatures (CEO, coordinator, medical director)				

Italics are examples.

Table C.7 Administrative policies and procedures.

Blood bank notification	What is to be done if a physician orders a transfusion that is not to be given? Convey patient-related restrictions regarding blood use to the blood bank computer to prevent unauthorized release of blood products
Budget	Document how the program receives its annual budget, how budgets can be increased, how the program is accountable for its use, and establish a book keeping mode; modes to buy
Charting and administration in the program	Develop a system to collect data, chart patient encounters, etc.; consider obtaining computerized data storage and use, develop forms and checklists for redundant procedures
Creation of lead time	Define who is doing what and how, open lines of communication
Daily work with patients on the ward	Define what the responsibilities of the coordinator are who daily visit patients on the ward. What information does he/she have to gather? Prepare a case with utensils needed during ward visits, e.g., forms, stickers, wrist bands, list of contact information, etc.
Educational interventions for hospital staff	Plan initial and continuing education; define how new staff members are reported to the program so that they can receive their orientation and can be included in educational interventions; develop information material and hand-outs for staff orientation
Informed consent	List essential components for an informed consent, develop patient education materials to explain the features of blood management so that patient is adequately informed; establish ways to document the informed consent process (advance directive, living will, consent forms, exclusion of liability) and to make the content of the patient directive known to all participants in patient care
Marketing	Define marketing strategies that support the achievement of the goals of the program and plan how to do this
Patient contacts	Establish how patients can contact the program when they want to use its service; define ways how patients enter the program when they present as emergencies as well as when they are scheduled for elective procedures; establish a "patient career'" (where the patient has to go, what he/she has to fill in, which services he/she has to receive, who has to see the patient, etc.)
Patient identification	Describe how patients in the program are identified, e.g., by wrist bands, chart stickers, note on patient identification stickers, forms in the chart, markers in the blood bank computer, identification in the admission computer, the laboratory, on the wards
Program measurement	Define goals or quality criteria (e.g., patient satisfaction, reduction of transfusions, reduction of transfusion-related morbidity and mortality, cost reduction, increase in patients) and how to measure whether these goals have been reached (e.g., patient surveys, staff surveys); establish how corrective measures are initiated when goal is not reached
Referrals	If the program is established where patients can chose a physician, there must be a procedure for how a patient is referred to a physician who is willing to take the case in accordance with the patient's preferences; keep an updated lists of physicians and their willingness to take certain patient groups, establish communication of the fact that a patient is referred to the physician, provide information about the physician to the patient (phone, office, etc.)
Screening of patients	Define which patients need to be screened regarding their eligibility to participate in the program; develop a checklist
Transferrals	There needs to be a procedure for how patients are transferred from another institution to the program or from the program to another program; describe how to transport patients, with what medical or nursing care, cost coverage, what information needs to be gained; e.g., using a check list for transferrals; define who coordinates emergency transferrals and how this person communicates
Use of donations	Establish how donations can be directed to the program; make sure this is a legally accepted way

Table C.8 Clinical guidelines.

Acute normovolemic hemodilution	Include recommendations for indications, contraindications, preparations, tools, monitoring, and documentation
Antifibrinolytics and desmopressin	For each agent, list indications, contraindications, dosing, and monitoring recommendations
Cell salvage, intra- and post-operatively	Include recommendations for indications, contraindications, preparations, tools, monitoring, and documentation. Consider patient populations requiring adaption of the method (e.g., patients with heparin sensitivity, children, Jehovah's Witnesses)
Compassionate use procedure	Outline how a compassionate use procedure is initiated, e.g., for the use of artificial oxygen carriers. Record emergency contacts and file required forms
Intraoperative platelet or plasma sequestration	Include recommendations for indications, contraindications, preparations, tools, monitoring, and documentation
Marking of autologous erythrocytes in Jehovah's Witness patients	If marking of autologous red cells is a standard diagnostic procedure in your hospital, define how this procedure is performed in patients who do not agree to take their own red cells back
Minimization of iatrogenic blood loss	Define parameters which warrant the start of efforts to minimize iatrogenic blood loss. Explain how the blood loss is reduced, e.g., using neonatal blood sample containers, etc.
Therapy of severely anemic patients who do not receive allogeneic blood	If necessary, define a minimum treatment standard for those patients
Transfusion-free care of obstetric and pediatric patients	Outline the legal and ethical implications of the transfusion-free care of the patients. Describe a decision-making process for cases with conflict potential
Use of autologous blood in patients who do not consent to allogeneic transfusions	Define how specific requests of patients are accommodated, e.g., how a closed circuit is established and maintained
Use of hematinics and erythropoietins	Include recommendations for indications, contraindications, preparations, tools, monitoring, and documentation. Standards, e.g., for a preoperative improvement of the hemoglobin level, may be helpful for the infusion center
Use of point-of-care testing	Describe the methods used and list the patients who should be assessed by the methods, and provide an algorithm which indicates appropriate therapy when the point-of-care tests are pathological
Use of recombinant clotting factors	For each agent, list indications, contraindications, dosing, and monitoring recommendations
Use of tissue adhesives	Include recommendations for indications, contraindications, preparations, tools, monitoring, and documentation, e.g., for the preparation of autologous glue, etc.

Table C.9 Legal and ethical guidelines.

Minors or parents of minors who refuse transfusions	Outline a legal way to differentiate between mature and immature minors and how to accept their wishes, and explain if and when court orders are to be obtained
Patients who refuse blood transfusion	Outline how patients who refuse transfusions are legally treated. Organize how the patient signs a release of liability, an advance directive, and/or a sheet to document detailed wishes pertinent to the planned care. Adapt the consent forms used
Physician participation	Define how to ensure that physicians keep their promise to take care of patients according to present patient values and in accordance with program policy and procedures, e.g., as a contract between the hospital and the physician. If necessary, set a minimum education level in blood management required for physicians
Pregnant women who refuse transfusions	Define the status of pregnant women who refuse transfusions. Consider also what will happen to the newborn when the mother refuses transfusions for the newborn. Think about bioethical consultations and ways to resolve conflicts with or without using the service of a court of justice

Table C.10 Media for marketing.

Print media:
- Newspapers: Which one serves the area I want to advertise in? What is their readership? Do they publish my advertisements?
- Brochures: Is there one to which I should add my service? Do I need a brochure for my program?
- Posters: Am I allowed to place posters in strategically important spots, e.g., in nursing homes, on the roadside, etc.?
- Newsletters: Do I have or can I create a mailing list? What will be the content? Is it interesting? Who will contribute to the content?
- Direct mail: With what purpose?

Electronic media:
- Website: Do I have my own or participate in an existing one?
- E-mail: Do I have a mailing list (current and potential patients). Do I need permission to contact them by e-mail? What will I say?
- Radio: Is there a radio station? Reasonable rate? Help produce content for them. Send your ads.
- TV: Is there a TV station? Costs? Content?

Person to person:
- Seminars: Content? How to promote them? Who will be the speakers? Costs? Handouts?
- Giveaways, gimmicks: The key-ring theory—useful? Will it last? Is it supposed to last?
- Word of mouth: Ambassadors, physicians, staff, religious and community groups

Table C.11 Target groups for marketing.

Referring physicians
- Information letters about the initiation of the program sent to physicians in the vicinity and in the area the hospital serves or the area the program will serve (may be greater than the usual area the hospital serves)
- Occasional information letters, e.g., once a year, about the ongoing development of the program and news regarding the program
- Information and recommendation letters to physicians who have referred patient previously, thanking for the good cooperation
- Seminars, information sessions
- Homepage, patient-oriented

Potential patients who already wish to avoid transfusions
- Regularly send information about blood management
- Sell key chains for emergencies, etc.
- Information sessions regarding blood management, seminars, use questionnaires and follow-up
- Homepage, patient-oriented
- Register program in program lists, hit lists, etc.
- Gadgets as presents, e.g., pens
- Clubs for patient groups that continually require blood management (e.g., sickle cell patients)

Media, the public
- Report about the program and spectacular cases in the media
- Invite media to report
- Provide press releases, compile information material designed for media representatives
- Homepage

Colleagues
- Participation in meetings
- Publications
- Invite speakers
- Organize sessions for mutual exchange of experiences

Table C.12 Structures for business plans [1, 2].

Proposal 1

Introduction

History of blood management, no proven efficacy of transfusions, current trends and data

Business purpose

Feasibility and desirability of the program, benefits for patient care and revenue; continued reinforcement, that administrative support is essential

Operations plan

Structure of the program, roles of the key players—physician director and coordinator; short- and long-term goals

Financial analysis

Cite historical trends in blood use of the hospital, relate them to costs, project into the future, integrate the costs of the program, calculate return on investment

Market assessment

Two basic markets for blood management: bloodless medicine for Jehovah's Witnesses and blood safety for the general public; mention existence or non-existence of competing programs in the area

Risk–benefit analysis

Very few risks associated (non-performance of program staff, failure to reach goals), many benefits

Recommendations

Establish follow-up contact and time frame; recommend a contract for at least 3 years

Proposal 2

Background

Description of the current situation of blood management in general and in the hospital, reasons to change current situation

Purpose and objectives

State that the implementation of a formal blood management program is planned, cite its objectives

Strategies

Describe in general what will be done to fulfill the purpose of the program (e.g., optimize blood use, introduce methods that reduce use of allogeneic blood transfusions, participate in research)

Benefits

For the patient, for the hospital, for the staff, for the society

Structure

Briefly explain the implementation of a physician director, a coordinator and possible, committees

Financial

Project savings, calculate costs of the program, approximate the expected return on investment

Next steps and time frame

Immediate next steps, short-, median-, and long-term goals

Appendix

Job description of the coordinator; sources and references; tables and model calculations of key numbers using hospital data

Proposal 3: The four "P's" of program development

Purpose: A general statement of the program

Philosophy: Assumptions and beliefs about the blood management program. Who is served? How? With what intention?

Policy: Precise statements of the do's and don't's. Responsibilities are briefly stated

Procedures: Precise definitions of the policies

Followed by goals and objectives:

- Goals are overall statements that direct the program in a certain direction. Goals may be classified as immediate, intermediate, and long-term
- Objectives are the specific statements that touch on the patient care and the part played by all participants in the program. They are designed based on the above-formulated objectives. They define the behavioral changes that are intended to be achieved

1. Gagliardi K. Inservice education: a commitment to excellence. *Can J Med Technol* 1991;**53**:18–23.
2. Derderian GP. Establishing a business plan for blood conservation. *J Cardiothorac Vasc Anesth* 2004;**18** (4 Suppl):12S–14S.

Table C.13 Example outline of a formal one-to-one educational intervention.

Goals of the visit:
- Introduce yourself as the blood management coordinator
- Inform the visited individual about the goals, objectives, and structure of the planned blood management program
- Identify the benefits the program brings for the hospital in general and the visited individual in particular
- Define the role of the visited individual in the blood management program
- Encourage the visited individual to assume an active role in the program
- Provide information about the next steps that are planned to bring the program into existence
- Provide contact information

Materials/visual aids to be used/left:
- Summary of the accepted business proposal for the blood management program
- Chart of the structure of the blood management program
- Information sheet for visited individual with take-home messages
- Business card of the coordinator
- Outline of the presentation
- Allow for questions
- Leave information sheet

Table C.14 Form for transfer of patients from outside hospitals into the program.

Transfer
Date: .... Time: .... Coordinator: ....
Name of patient: .... Date of birth: ....
Reason for transfer: ....
Baseline disease: ....
Medical history: ....
....

Clinical data:
Last Hb/Hct: g/dL/mmol/dL/% of coags? ... .
Active bleeding: Yes/no? where? how much? therapy initiated? ....
....
Current medication

Drug/mode of application	Dose	Remarks

Transport
Continuous intravenous therapy? Yes/ no
Monitoring? EKG, intravenous line? Arterial line? Central line? PAC? Others? Yes/no, which......................
Is patient stable for transport? Yes/no

(Continued)

Table C.14 *(Continued)*

Transferring hospital

Name of hospital .... Ward .... Cooperative Yes/no?

Treating physician: ....Phone: ....

Insurance? ....

Name of person who wishes transfer: .... Phone: ....

Checklist: Transfer

☐ Contact in-hospital physician. Contacted physician ... .Time ....

☐ Inform about patient. Transfer possible? Yes/no

☐ Check status of patient transfer. ☐ Stabile (no monitoring); ☐ not critical (constant monitoring); ☐ critical

If transfer, ask local physician to (a) contact transferring physician in 15 minutes time; (b) book a bed for patient

Contact person, who asked for transfer

☐ Call person who asked for transfer (time)

Ask to:

• Inform treating physician about transfer
• Tell treating physician that your in-hospital physician will contact him/her shortly
• Issue transport papers
• Organize transfer
• Ask nursing staff to make a copy of the patient file
• Provide information about trip to your hospital
• Ask for return-call

Caveat: When transport not cooperative, then transfer still possible (against will of treating physician)

Caveat: Inform and document information about: Transport costs? No insurance during transport? No liability?

Notes:

☐ Patient travels by him/herself, takes care of his/her own travel arrangements (give advice regarding travel)

☐ Patient cannot travel alone

Stable, without monitoring	Not critical, need for monitoring	Critically ill
Organize patient transport	Organize ambulance, possibly with emergency physician	Organize ambulance with intensivist, mobile intensive care unit, helicopter

☐ Help required. Do you have transport certificate/payment certificate?

☐ Call emergency transport coordination center (Phone: XXXXX)

☐ Call person who asked for transfer and inform about organized transfer

☐ Call treating physician

☐ Inform in-hospital physician about transfer time

Patient arrived: Date .... Time ....

Remarks ....

Appendix D: Teaching Aids: Research and Projects

This appendix provides a number of model projects and a teaching story. These are meant to help with teaching blood management.

Student projects

Project 1

Aim: Familiarize students with methods to reduce blood loss and manage anemia and bleeding without the use of donor blood. Provide an overview of the possibilities available at the student's hospital.

Task: List all specialties and subspecialties offered in the hospital. Then approach each of them and ask for methods of how to manage patients without donor blood or how to reduce the probability of allogeneic blood transfusion exposure. List all drugs and methods available, and describe the rationale for their use. Note whether the methods are used routinely, occasionally, or never.

Project 2

Aim: Encourage students to reflect on current patient's rights and ethics.

Task:

1. Find out about the right patients have to determine whether they want to have a transfusion or not. Please, give the paragraphs of your current law, not your personal opinion.
   - Can patients express their wishes concerning blood products?
   - Are patients allowed to have a valid advance directive?
   - Are you as physician bound to accept the refusal of a treatment, even if it seems to be contrary to what you think is good for a patient?
   - Can minors express their wishes and do you have to accept them?
   - Can parents say what they want for their baby and can you overrule them in an ethical manner?
   - Do you have to call for a court order in case of a mature person/a minor?
   - What happens if you do and if you do not accept the wish of a patient?
2. Give your personal response to the questions above.

Survey your fellow workers about their opinion about the following questions. Analyze their answers in the light of what you learned during your study of current law and ethics.
   - Would you accept blood transfusion if you were patient?
   - At which hemoglobin level would you like to be transfused?
   - Would you transfuse a mature patient if he or she refuses transfusion?
   - Would you use therapies that can reduce the likelihood of transfusions even if they were more expensive than blood transfusions?
   - What do you think is the most important reason for reducing patient exposure to donor blood?

Project 3

Aim: Students get to know available blood products.

Task: List all the ways blood is used for therapy in the hospital. (Do not include diagnostic procedures.) List all means of donor-blood use and all possible ways to use a patient's own blood. Describe each product, its production, indications, contraindications, risks, costs for one unit/one vial, and how often it is used in the hospital (e.g., 10 000 units of erythrocyte concentrates/year) and how has to be discarded.

Basics of Blood Management, Second Edition. Petra Seeber and Aryeh Shander.
© 2013 John Wiley & Sons, Ltd. Published 2013 by John Wiley & Sons, Ltd.

Project 4

Aim: Broaden the horizon of your students.

Task: Research traditional medicine in your country. Find out which methods are used in traditional medicine to treat anemia, coagulation disorders, reduce blood loss, etc. List as many possibilities as you can find (herbs, venoms, acupuncture, diet, etc.), describe them, and relate how they are proposed to work. Note whether the method is accepted in hospital treatment or only used by traditional healers.

Project 5

Aim: Practice integrating newly acquired knowledge into a plan of care.

Task: Develop a care plan for a severely anemic patient who is bleeding heavily from the upper gastrointestinal tract and for whom no donor blood is available. Follow the algorithms you have learned and develop a systematic plan. Explain every step of your plan and discuss therapeutic options, if available. Write the management plan for each day of 1 week. Provide the rationale for every step.

The following questions are meant to be a guide only:
• What information would you obtain by history taking and physical examination?

• What diagnostic procedures do you order?
• What laboratory diagnostics do you order?
• What therapeutic measures do you take? (immediately, tomorrow, and next week)
• Which treatments are urgent and which ones can wait?
• Prescribe with timing and dose regimen.
• What do you do if the patient is allergic to the prescribed drugs? (give a hint for every prescribed drug)
• Whom do you involve in the care of the patient?

Teaching with stories

While reading the following hospital fairy tale, think about your own hospital and its potentials to use existing features for a blood management program. Analyze the story and answer the questions below. Think about how you would answer the same questions from the perspective of the hospital you work in.
• How is the patient identified?
• What is done to comply with legal requirements?
• What steps are taken to ensure the patient's wishes are heeded?
• What direct support does the patient receive?

A hospital fairy tale

Once upon a time, in a distant land, there was a smart medical student named Tony. One day, he got a bad cough, so he went to see a doctor. Happily, it was not pneumonia. But there was something about his heartbeat that made his family doctor listen a little longer than normal. After he had completed his examination, the doctor explained that there was a heart murmur that needed further evaluation and Tony was sent to a heart specialist. The specialist concluded that Tony's heart needed surgery. This was unexpected news. He had never been seriously sick and now, suddenly, he had to undergo surgery. A million things went through his mind. What now?

Tony was a smart student and he thought about what could happen to him during surgery. He was not so bothered about the actual surgery. He would be fast asleep. But what about afterwards? During his studies he had joined physicians when they explained heart surgery to other patients. No problem! Everything was routine. But now he was the patient, and he had a strange feeling in his belly. No, of course he wasn't afraid. But time and again he thought about the blood he would receive. Would it be safe enough? Deep inside he had some doubts.

Tony had heard about many successful heart surgeries performed without the use of donor blood. After a night of discussing the pros and cons with his parents, he decided to give it a try. There was a blood management program in a nearby town. Without further delay, he called to make an appointment. A friendly voice on the telephone invited him to visit the next day and asked him to bring along a copy of his medical records.

The next morning, Tony got up early to be at the hospital on time. He had never been there before. While on the bus Tony tried to imagine the type of hospital it would be. Most probably it would be one of the huge glass buildings he had seen on TV. High-tech equipment was what he expected and much more. Then again, maybe not. He just knew this hospital must be something very special.

To his surprise, he found that the hospital was not the shining glass building he had expected. Rather, he found himself standing in front of one of those hospitals built years ago. The building was made of red bricks. Flowers were planted along the pavement toward the main hospital entrance.

Hesitantly, Tony followed the path to the hospital reception. A poster in the hallway caught his attention. Big letters said: "No Blood? No Problem." Never before had Tony seen anything like this. It was so different from the posters he was used to seeing: "Give blood, save lives." Tony looked around. Nothing was as he had imagined. The atmosphere in the hospital was rather familiar, almost cosy. Tony relaxed. The smile of the old lady at the reception was contagious. He smiled back and followed the signs to the blood management coordinator's office.

Another smiling face welcomed Tony. A young lady offered him a seat. Mr Dam, the lady said, was still with another patient but he would be with him soon. The lady brought him a cup of jasmine tea and chocolate chip cookies and left him alone in Mr Dam's office. Tony let his eyes wander. His attention was caught by a huge pin board full of cards and photos. Obviously, many patients had expressed their thanks by dropping a line.

It was not before long that the door opened and a man entered the room. The coordinator introduced himself, "Laban Dam," and he gave Tony's hand a good shake. Taking some papers from a shelf, Mr Dam took a seat.

Tony told him about his heart murmur and his concerns about receiving someone else's blood. The coordinator listened carefully, nodding occasionally. When Tony had finished, Mr Dam said: "No problem! I will refer you to a heart surgeon who is experienced in doing the procedure without the use of donor blood. Let's discuss some details. Here I have a form for an advance directive. We will go over every point and I will explain all you need to know." The coordinator took the patient education material and went over it with Tony. Tony had so many questions. Using the pictures and charts in the education material, Mr Dam patiently explained everything. By the end, Tony knew all about the use of his own blood in a cell saving device, about hemodilution, the heart–lung machine, plasma expanders, human and recombinant clotting factors, and even about artificial oxygen carriers. Tony was relieved. He could easily fill in his advance directive and the consent form, allowing the physician to use the methods he chose. He felt that he was in competent hands.

What followed seemed to be mere routine for the coordinator. He had a look on his computer and gave Tony the name and the telephone number of his surgeon, Dr Lucas. A short message informed Dr Lucas about Tony's upcoming visit, and an e-mail to the blood bank ensured that it was informed about Tony's decision regarding the use of his own donor blood. Mr Dam asked to see the copies of Tony's medical records. A short glimpse at Tony's blood count told him that everything was all right. Otherwise, the coordinator would have alerted Dr Lucas right from the start. Tony was amazed. So much professionalism!

A few days later, Tony met with Dr Lucas. He was a tall man in his fifties. His calm personality was really reassuring. After reading through Tony's documents, taking his history and a physical examination, the surgeon explained the procedure. Tony's curiosity was satisfied by Dr Lucas' friendly explanations. Dr Lucas had especially emphasized what measures he would take to reduce any unnecessary blood loss. As a future physician, Tony was fascinated and for a while he nearly forgot that he was the patient and not the physician. Since Tony's condition and especially his blood count were excellent, there was no reason to wait for the surgery. Had that not been the case, his surgery would have been postponed until erythropoietin and hematinics had done their part. Tony was scheduled for next Monday at 2 p.m.

On Monday morning, Tony traveled alone to the hospital. His parents couldn't make it, since both had caught a cold. Admittedly, Tony was nervous. But as soon as he entered the corridor and saw the smiling lady at the reception, again he felt an inner calm. He was convinced Dr Lucas and his team would know what to do.

Tony went to the admissions office. The clerk entered Tony's personal data into the computer. She asked if he was a participant in the blood management program and entered Tony's positive response into the computer. Now, every print-out on any form would not only state Tony's name and date of birth but also his status in the blood management program. When all required papers were printed, Tony was handed a folder containing his new medical documents. The clerk took him to the office of the coordinator. When he entered he felt quite at home. The same friendly face welcomed him. Mr Dam checked Tony's folder. Everything was all right. A sticker was attached to his folder indicating his participation in the program. Copies of his advance directive and his signed consent form were also put into the folder. Now every physician—no matter what specialty— would be informed about his decision regarding the use of blood. After a little small-talk, Mr Dam took Tony to the ward and introduced him to Ms Florence Shiphrah, one of the nurses in the pre-op holding area.

Right away, Florence started with her work. She attached a wrist band to Tony's arm. The bracelet had a distinct color that indicated his blood management status. Florence was well informed. She didn't take as much blood as Tony was used to from his home hospital. Also, the nurses seemed to participate in saving every drop of blood. It was real team work!

As Tony was wheeled to the operating room he had the impression that everything was ready for him. He saw the cell saving device already set up. While he wondered why a weighing scale was needed in an operating room, he drifted off to sleep.

(Continued)

Tony tried to remember what had happened. His mind was so cloudy that it took quite a while until he realized that he was in a bed. The surroundings didn't look familiar at all. He felt drowsy. Hadn't he just had surgery? Yes, he remembered remotely. His eyes scanned his surroundings. Suddenly he shuddered. Blood! Three bags were hanging on a pole over his head. Tony felt a flush of adrenaline working through his body. It nearly made him sit up! But then he felt a warm hand resting reassuringly on his shoulder. Tony turned his head and saw the brown eyes of Florence. She seemed to have noticed his startled glance at the blood above his head and said: "It is your own." Phew! Tony relaxed. Mr Dam had told him before that there might be blood remaining from cell salvage and hemodilution. This would be given back to him after surgery. Tony again felt drowsy. Calmly he gave in to his medication.

Tony didn't know how long he had been asleep. He heard a noise as if someone was turning pages and opened his eyes. This time, his mind was much clearer. Mr Dam was about to check his chart. Tony's hoarse "hello" made Mr Dam turn his attention towards him. "Everything went well. There was some blood loss during surgery but not too much. And the blood coming from your drains is only minimal. You can rest assured. It's all right." Tony nodded and leaned back on his pillow. Florence approached Mr Dam and reported her findings about Tony. There was no reason to assume complications would develop. Even if they did—there would be several pairs of eyes ready to register any change in his condition. Help would be available immediately to prevent further blood loss. Before Mr Dam left the room he offered to keep Tony's parents informed about the progress he was making.

Three days had passed since Tony's surgery. He had recovered well and was ready to go home. Florence came into the room to give him last instructions. He was told what to do to speed up his recovery, which food to eat, how to take his iron tablets, and when to come back. Tony's parents had sent friends to give him a ride home. Before he finally went home, he stopped by Mr Dam's office to thank him for his extraordinary service. Tony's eyes again rested on the pin board with the many cards and pictures. Tony was sure the card he would send would soon join the collection on the board.

Index

Basics of Blood Management, Second Edition. Petra Seeber and Aryeh Shander.
© 2013 John Wiley & Sons, Ltd. Published 2013 by John Wiley & Sons, Ltd.

Index compiled by Terry Halliday